The Human Genome in Health and Disease

The Human Genome in Health and Disease

Editor: Victor Fargo

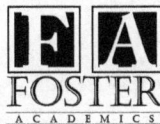

FA
FOSTER
ACADEMICS

www.fosteracademics.com

www.fosteracademics.com

FA FOSTER
ACADEMICS

Cataloging-in-Publication Data

The human genome in health and disease / edited by Victor Fargo.
    p. cm.
Includes bibliographical references and index.
ISBN 978-1-63242-696-3
1. Human genome. 2. Health--Genetic aspects. 3. Medical genetics. 4. Diseases.
I. Fargo, Victor.
RB155 .H86 2019
616.042--dc23

© Foster Academics, 2019

Foster Academics,
118-35 Queens Blvd., Suite 400,
Forest Hills, NY 11375, USA

ISBN 978-1-63242-696-3 (Hardback)

Contents

Preface

Over the recent decade, advancements and applications have progressed exponentially. This has led to the increased interest in this field and projects are being conducted to enhance knowledge. The main objective of this book is to present some of the critical challenges and provide insights into possible solutions. This book will answer the varied questions that arise in the field and also provide an increased scope for furthering studies.

The human genome refers to the complete set of nucleic acid sequences in humans. It is encoded as DNA in the 23 chromosome pairs. The human genome is over 3 billion base pairs long. Any abnormality in the structure or function of these genes or chromosomes can result in a genetic disorder. Knockouts and mutations in specific genes can have severe consequences in terms of gene function and gene expression. Genetic diseases may occur due to a single gene or due to multiple genes. Over 6000 diseases in humans can be attributed to single-gene defects. When multiple genes contribute to a genetic disorder, such as in the case of diabetes, heart disease, obesity, asthma or autoimmune diseases, it is difficult to study and treat them. A number of diseases are also related to large-scale genomic abnormalities. Nondisjunction of entire chromosomes can lead to disorders such as Turner Syndrome and Down syndrome. This book contains some path-breaking studies on the human genome and its relevance to health care. The topics included in this book on the human genome are of utmost significance and bound to provide incredible insights to readers. It is a vital tool for all researching and studying this field.

I hope that this book, with its visionary approach, will be a valuable addition and will promote interest among readers. Each of the authors has provided their extraordinary competence in their specific fields by providing different perspectives as they come from diverse nations and regions. I thank them for their contributions.

Editor

Hypomethylation coordinates antagonistically with hypermethylation in cancer development

Garima Kushwaha[1,2], Mikhail Dozmorov[3], Jonathan D. Wren[4], Jing Qiu[5], Huidong Shi[6,7]* and Dong Xu[1,2,8]*

Abstract

Background: Methylation changes are frequent in cancers, but understanding how hyper- and hypomethylated region changes coordinate, associate with genomic features, and affect gene expression is needed to better understand their biological significance. The functional significance of hypermethylation is well studied, but that of hypomethylation remains limited. Here, with paired expression and methylation samples gathered from a patient/control cohort, we attempt to better characterize the gene expression and methylation changes that take place in cancer from B cell chronic lymphocyte leukemia (B-CLL) samples.

Results: Across the dataset, we found that consistent differentially hypomethylated regions (C-DMRs) across samples were relatively few compared to the many poorly consistent hypo- and highly conserved hyper-DMRs. However, genes in the hypo-C-DMRs tended to be associated with functions antagonistic to those in the hyper-C-DMRs, like differentiation, cell-cycle regulation and proliferation, suggesting coordinated regulation of methylation changes. Hypo-C-DMRs in B-CLL were found enriched in key signaling pathways like B cell receptor and p53 pathways and genes/motifs essential for B lymphopoiesis. Hypo-C-DMRs tended to be proximal to genes with elevated expression in contrast to the transcription silencing-mechanism imposed by hypermethylation. Hypo-C-DMRs tended to be enriched in the regions of activating H4K4me1/2/3, H3K79me2, and H3K27ac histone modifications. In comparison, the polycomb repressive complex 2 (PRC2) signature, marked by *EZH2*, *SUZ12*, *CTCF* binding-sites, repressive H3K27me3 marks, and "repressed/poised promoter" states were associated with hyper-C-DMRs. Most hypo-C-DMRs were found in introns (36 %), 3′ untranslated regions (29 %), and intergenic regions (24 %). Many of these genic regions also overlapped with enhancers. The methylation of CpGs from 3′UTR exons was found to have weak but positive correlation with gene expression. In contrast, methylation in the 5′UTR was negatively correlated with expression. To better characterize the overlap between methylation and expression changes, we identified correlation modules that associate with "apoptosis" and "leukocyte activation".

Conclusions: Despite clinical heterogeneity in disease presentation, a number of methylation changes, both hypo and hyper, appear to be common in B-CLL. Hypomethylation appears to play an active, targeted, and complementary role in cancer progression, and it interplays with hypermethylation in a coordinated fashion in the cancer process.

Keywords: Epigenetic regulation, DNA methylation, Hypomethylation, CLL, Cancer, Signaling pathway, 3′UTR, Enhancer

* Correspondence: hshi@gru.edu; xudong@missouri.edu
[6]GRU Cancer Center, Georgia Regents University, Augusta, GA 30912, USA
[1]Christopher S. Bond Life Sciences Center, University of Missouri, Columbia, MO 65211, USA
Full list of author information is available at the end of the article

Background

Loss of DNA methylation, also known as hypomethylation, in cancer cells relative to normal cells was one of the first-described epigenetic changes in human cancers. Hypomethylation has been detected at both a global level and on a local scale [1] in cancer genomes. Many cancer types have been reported to have global loss of methylation like glioblastoma [2], ovarian epithelial carcinoma [3], prostate metastatic tumors [4], B cell chronic lymphocytic leukemia [5, 6], hepatocellular carcinoma [7], cervical cancer [8], colon adenocarcinoma [9], and Wilms' tumor [10]. However, the biological significance of DNA hypomethylation remains understudied owning to its unclear role in carcinogenesis, in contrast to hypermethylation, which is commonly viewed as a transcription silencing mechanism [11, 12]. Yet, hypomethylation of DNA, despite its unclear role, has been linked to tumor progression [8, 13] in different tumor types and in individual specimens [3, 14]. Also, some experiments have indicated the importance of induced DNA hypomethylation in oncogenesis by using DNA methylation inhibitors in vivo and in vitro [15, 16]. However, the role of hypomethylation is not clearly understood. Hence, it is critical to analyze hypomethylation data in depth to achieve a better understanding of its biological roles in carcinogenesis.

DNA hypomethylation in cancer is often seen in satellite DNAs, Arthrobacter luteus (ALU) repeats, and long interspersed nuclear elements (LINEs) [17, 18], etc. These DNA repeats comprise approximately half of the genome. Hence, DNA hypomethylation is generally considered a global phenomenon not suitable for use as a biomarker. One advantage of the global hypomethylation phenomenon (as it pertains to its genome composition) is that it is often considered a technique to balance focal and conserved hypermethylation in the promoter regions of key genes. Also, it is believed that these hypomethylated genomic regions are randomly spread over the genome, mostly in repetitive regions whose functions, if any, are unclear. Again, this reported disadvantage might actually be an advantage due to recent findings indicating that ALU elements can act as enhancers [19], which further emphasizes the need for defining the role of hypomethylation in cancers.

As part of our study of hypomethylation patterns, we used B cell chronic lymphocytic leukemia (B-CLL) as an example case. This B-CLL cancer type has a predominant global hypomethylation as its characteristic feature [5, 6], and it is the most common form of blood cancer. It is a clinically heterogeneous disease, with some patients experiencing rapid disease progression and others living for decades without requiring treatment [20]. Although a number of cellular and molecular prognostic markers, i.e., surface markers *ZAP70* and *CD38*, cytogenetic abnormalities, and IGHV mutational status [21–23], have been identified to help classify CLL into molecular and clinical subgroups and to predict their course of progression, they do not provide clear insight into the underlying biology necessary to develop better targeted and more effective treatments.

In addition to various molecular and genetic changes, several genome-wide DNA methylation studies have identified many aberrantly methylated genes in CLL samples [24]. Initially, DNA hypermethylation in CLL patients was found to affect 4.8 % of CpG islands on average [25]. Furthermore, hypermethylation in the promoters of tumor suppressor genes such as *DAPK1* [26], *SFRP1* [27], and *ID4* [28] genes involved in apoptosis, cell cycle regulators *p16* and *p15* [29], and prognostic markers *ZAP70* [21] and *TWIST2* [30] were identified. DNA methylation changes were also found to be associated with disease progression in the E_μ-TCL1 transgenic mouse model of CLL [28]. In addition to hypermethylation, hypomethylation of proto-oncogenes has also been observed particularly in liver tumors and leukemia such as the *c-fos, c-myc, ras, Erb-A1* [31], and the *bcl-2* gene [32]. Along with this, many studies have indicated widespread hypomethylation compared to instances of hypermethylation, particularly in the CLL cancer type. However, a detailed account on the genome-wide hypomethylation pattern and its contributing role towards cancer development has not been conducted for CLL. Hence, it is clear that an in-depth methylation analysis focusing more on hypomethylation can be very helpful to unveil the underlying mechanism regulating the disease.

Here, we studied the genome-wide DNA methylation pattern in CLL and investigated whether hypomethylation is also consistent at some locations like hypermethylation across multiple CLL patients. We also investigated the biological role of consistent hypomethylation towards tumor initiation and progression; and finally, we compared instances of consistent hypomethylation to that of consistent hypermethylation. We characterized the epigenetic context of hyper- and hypomethylated regions in CLL and further investigated association of hypomethylation with change in expression of the neighborhood genes along with their potential mechanism of influence.

Results

Methylation data analysis

In order to study genome-wide methylation changes in the CLL genome, we computed differentially methylated regions (DMRs) from genome-wide methylation data of 30 samples from publically available CLL samples in GEO (http://www.ncbi.nlm.nih.gov/geo/). DMRs of size 1000 bp were obtained by comparing each patient sample against each control normal sample individually using Fisher's exact test. False discovery rate (FDR) was used to correct for multiple testing errors with a q value threshold of 0.01. Hence, three sets of DMRs were obtained by comparing all 30 CLL samples against each of the three control samples.

Entropy and permutation analysis

Having obtained a list of all hypo- and hyper-DMRs for each CLL against each control sample, we first plotted the distribution of the number of samples in which each DMR (hypo and hyper) existed. Figure 1a shows that the majority of hypo-DMRs are present in less than 50 % of samples. Out of the DMRs present in 20 or more samples, hyper-DMRs outnumbered hypo-DMRs. This showed that overall hypomethylated regions are less conserved than hypermethylated regions across samples.

Next, in order to check randomness in contrast to conservation of methylation change in each 1000 bp region across all CLL samples, methylation entropies were calculated using a probability distribution of methylation changes for each region. Figure 1b shows this opposite pattern of entropy and average methylation change. This plot shows that a high percentage methylation of specific regions is more consistent across all patients; however, as the average methylation goes down, their conservation tends to fluctuate, thereby leading to an increase in entropy (Fig. 1b). After comparing these methylation entropies for each region against the average methylation change across 30 CLL samples, we observed a negative correlation (Pearson correlation = −0.22, p value <0.05) in each of the 3-control sample tests.

Identification of consistent differentially methylated regions (C-DMRs)

In order to obtain consistent DMRs, a binomial test was used to check the significance of each DMR with the probability of being hypo/hypermethylated in 25 or more CLL samples (q value <0.01). Hence, three lists of significant DMRs were obtained for each control sample. Next, 658 hypo- and 982 hypermethylated regions that were found common in all three lists and referred to as C-DMRs (see Tables S1–S4 in Additional file 1 and Additional file 2 for lists and details).

To further check the statistical significance of our lists of hypo- and hyper-C-DMRs, we performed two permutation tests, one by permuting samples and the other by permuting methylation values for 1000 bp regions (see Methods in Additional file 1 for more details). The sample permutation test helped in detecting whether we observed hyper/hypo-C-DMR patterns by chance if there was no difference among cancer vs. normal samples. On the other hand, the methylated region permutation test detected whether hyper/hypo-C-DMR pattern can occur by chance if there is no difference between regions. In both permutation tests, all of our obtained C-DMRs had q values <0.05, showing the statistical significance of hyper- and hypo-C-DMRs in cancer samples against normal and non-DMRs.

Differences in positional genomic location analysis of hyper- and hypo-C-DMRs

By checking the genomic-location distribution of C-DMRs, we found that a higher number of hyper-C-DMRs mapped to promoters (64 %) and 5′UTRs (43 %) as compared to hypo-C-DMRs (14 % for promoters and 12 % for 5′UTR) and genomic background regions (30 % for promoters and 29 % for 5′UTRs). A higher percentage of promoter and 5′UTR hypermethylation confirmed their role in interfering with transcription factor binding (Fig. 2a, b). However, hypo-C-DMRs outnumbered both hyper-C-DMRs and background genomic regions for 3′UTRs (29 % in hypo-C-DMRs, 8 % in hyper-C-DMRs, and 7 % in background) and introns (36 % in hypo-C-DMRs, 4 % in hyper-C-DMRs, and 15 % in background). There were also more hypo-C-DMRs (24 %) in the intergenic regions than hyper-C-DMRs (18 %), but comparable with genomic background regions (26 %). CpG sites from hypo- and hyper-C-DMRs were also checked against "weak/strong enhancer regions" chromatin states as defined by chromHMM [33] and were found coming mostly from intronic and intergenic regions on a genome. (Figure S6 in Additional file 1). Strong enhancers were overlapped more by hypo-C-DMRs in comparison to hyper-C-DMRs. Genes overlapping with hypomethylated strong enhancers were *ELN, GTF2I, KLC1, MIF4GD, MIR6821, MOB2, PTBP1, RGS3, SH3BGRL3, TBC1D14, TCIRG1,* and *VASH2.*

Across each sample data, we found 25–30 % of all DMRs as hypomethylated, and only 10–15 % hypermethylated, as shown in Figure S1 in Additional file 1. However, they were not targeted for any specific chromosomal region (Figure S2 in Additional file 1). Also, only 100 hypo-C-DMRs (15.2 %) co-localized with CpG islands, while 955 out of 982 hyper-C-DMRs (97.2 %) co-localized with CpG islands. Hypo-C-DMRs were mostly present in regions outside CpG islands and shores (Fig. 2c). Next, Fig. 2d shows that almost half of hypo-C-DMRs (46 %) were present on non-repeat regions along with ones mapped on the repeat regions. Overall, hypo-C-DMRs were found more in 3′UTR, intronic, and intergenic regions, mostly outside CpG islands and overlapping both repeat and non-repeat regions over enhancers. Additional file 3 lists the genes with genic-regions overlapped by these C-DMRs.

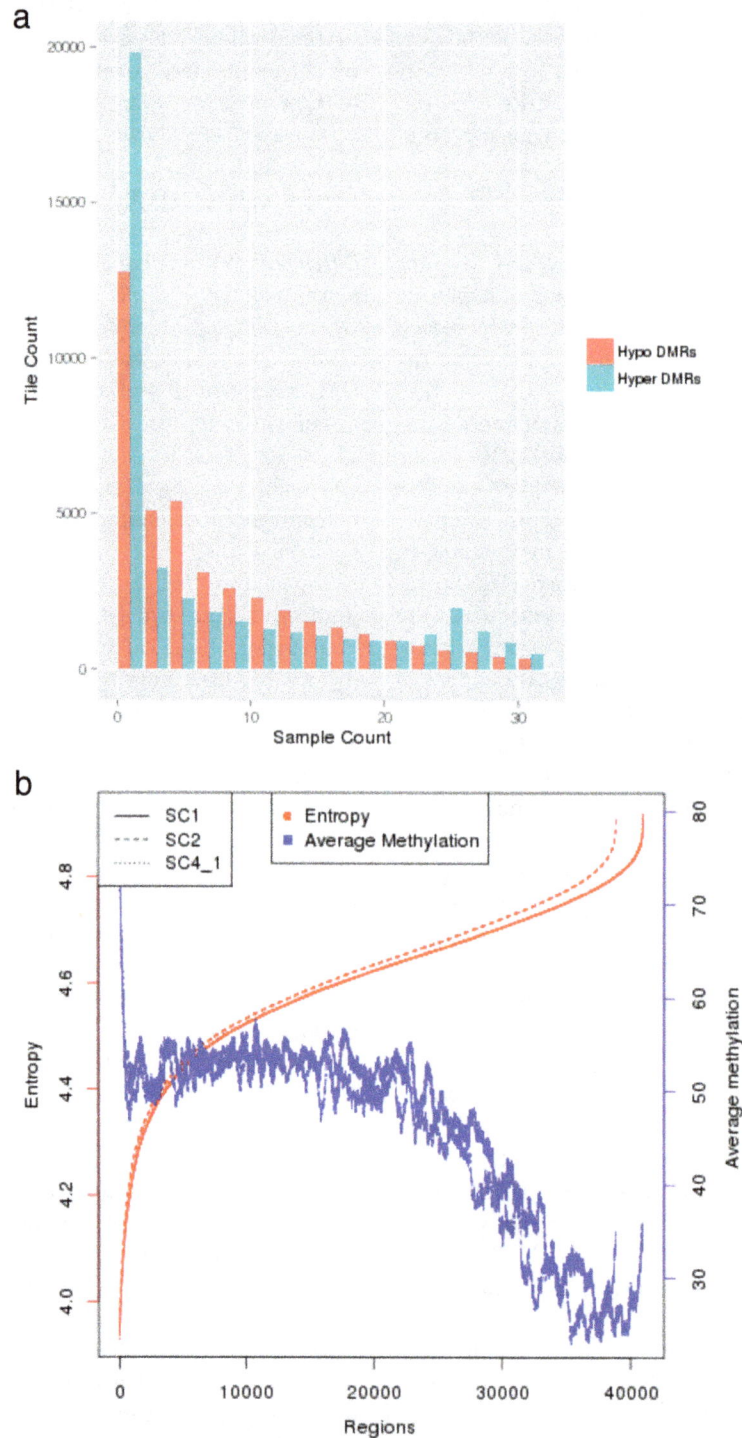

Fig. 1 Overall representation of methylation. **a** Distribution of hyper/hypo-DMRs (tiles) over number of samples. This illustration shows that a higher proportion of hypo-DMRs (compared to hyper-DMRs) are consistent in small subsets of samples. It also shows the presence of few hypo-DMRs present in all 30 samples. **b** Relationship between average methylation difference across all CLL patients against control samples (SC1, SC2, and SC4_1) and methylation entropy per 1000 bp region

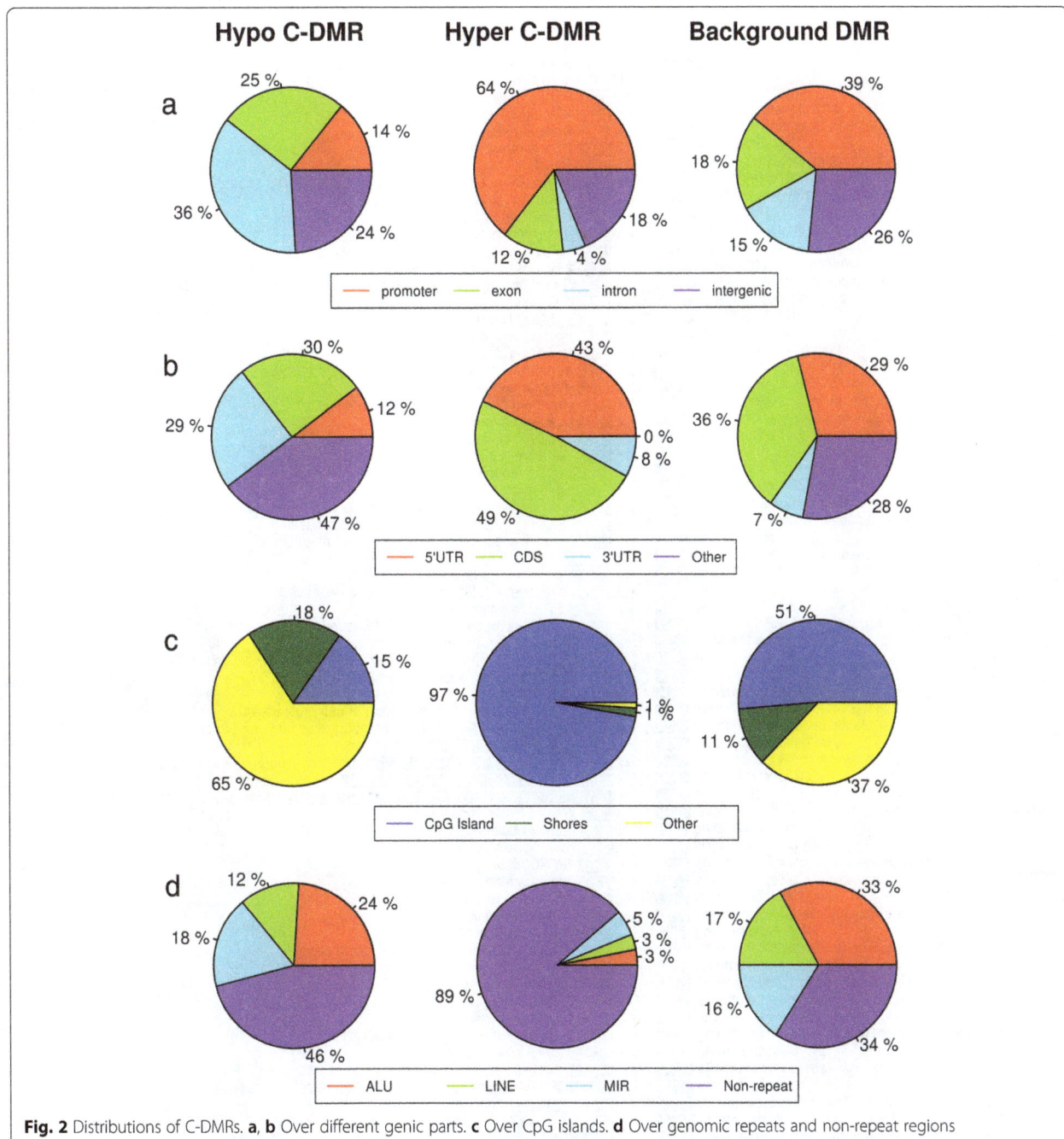

Fig. 2 Distributions of C-DMRs. **a, b** Over different genic parts. **c** Over CpG islands. **d** Over genomic repeats and non-repeat regions

Enrichment of KEGG pathways, GO annotations and phenotypes

For our obtained lists of hypo- and hyper-C-DMRs, we performed enrichment analysis of genes overlapped by C-DMRs (Additional file 3) for gene ontology (GO) [34] categories and KEGG [35] pathways. The most significantly enriched KEGG pathways in hypo-C-DMRs were "B cell receptor (BCR) signaling pathway" (adjusted p value (p.adj) = 2.21E-02), "$p53$ signaling pathway" (p.adj = 3.69E-02), and "pathways in cancer" (p.adj = 3.69E-02), along with a few other signaling pathways

and pathways involved in cancer. In contrast, hyper-C-DMRs were not enriched for any leukemia-related pathway such as *BCR* signaling. Hyper-C-DMRs were enriched for "neuroactive ligand-receptor interaction" (p.adj = 7.29E-05) and for the "calcium-signaling pathway" (p.adj = 9.86E-03) (Fig. 3). See Additional file 4 for complete enrichment results.

Among the GO annotations, the most important and significantly enriched biological processes for hypo-C-DMRs were "negative regulation of transcription" (p.adj = 4.28E-02), "chromatin modification" (p.adj = 3.92E-02),

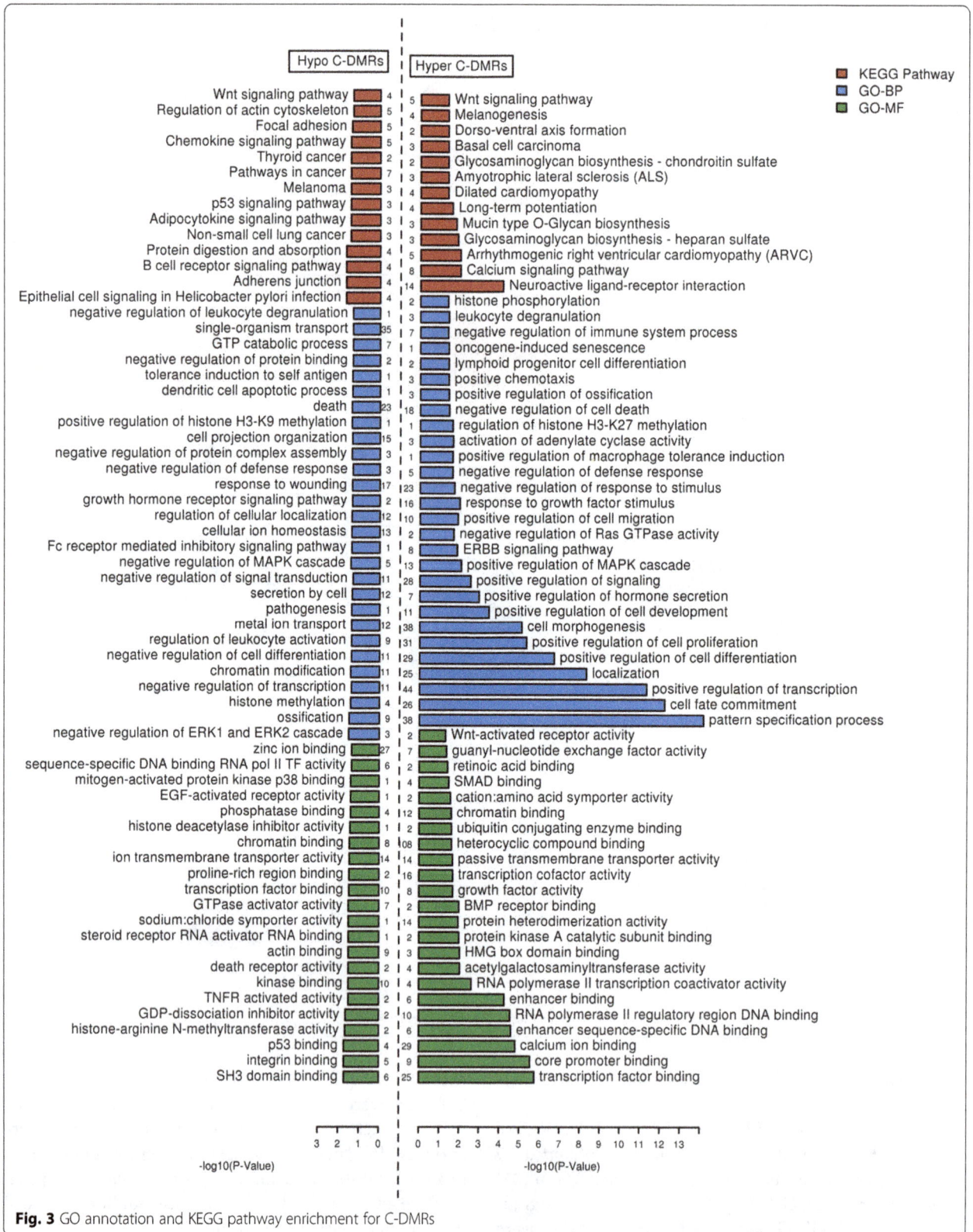

Fig. 3 GO annotation and KEGG pathway enrichment for C-DMRs

"regulation of signaling" (p.adj = 3.92E-02), "histone methylation" (p.adj = 3.92E-02); "positive regulation of histone H3-K9 methylation" (p.adj = 4.29E-02), "protein alkylation" (p.adj = 4.28E-02), "programmed cell death" (p.adj = 4.30E-02), "negative regulation of cell proliferation" (p.adj = 4.40E-02), and "negative regulation of leukocyte differentiation" (p.adj = 3.04E-02), "leukocyte activation" (p.adj = 4.28E-02), and "cell morphogenesis involved in differentiation" (p.adj = 4.29E-02). On the other hand, hyper-C-DMRs were enriched for processes which are antagonistic to the processes enriched in hypo-C-DMRs. Hyper-C-DMRs were enriched for processes like "positive regulation of transcription" (p.adj = 4.81E-12) and "positive regulation of cell differentiation" (p.adj = 1.99E-07), "positive regulation cell proliferation" (p.adj = 4.75E-06), "regulation of signaling" (p.adj = 3.53E-05) with more processes related to "cell-fate commitment" (p.adj = 6.09E-13), "cell morphogenesis involved in differentiation" (p.adj = 7.69E-08), and similar processes like "protein and cell localization" (p.adj = 4.77E-06). Also, hypo-C-DMRs were enriched for "H3K9 methylation" but hyper for "H3-K27 methylation."

Molecular functions (Fig. 3) showed a strong enrichment for binding functions like "protein binding" (like integrin, p.adj = 1.92E-02), "SH3 domain binding" (p.adj = 1.92E-02), "p53 binding" (p.adj = 1.92E-02), "histone-arginine N-methyltransferase activity" (p.adj = 2.20E-02), "tumor necrosis factor-activated receptor activity" (p.adj = 3.20E-02), GTPase regulator activity (p.adj = 3.20E-02), and "transcription factor binding" (p.adj = 3.40E-02) in hypo-C-DMRs. In comparison, hyper-C-DMRs were specifically highly enriched for "sequence-specific DNA binding" (p.adj = 5.49E-32), transcription factor (or regulator, p.adj = 3.86E-25), and trans-membrane transporter activity (p.adj = 6.58E-03), along with also metal/ion (calcium, p.adj = 6.72E-07) and "enhancer binding" (p.adj = 5.47E-05). In summary, both C-DMR types (hypo and hyper) affected similar processes but in different directions, with hypomethylation focusing on transcription and leukocyte activation and hypermethylation focusing on transcription suppression through transcription factors and cell-fate commitment.

We did not observe any differences in enriched phenotypes between hypo- and hyper-C-DMRs. Specific associations with the hematopoietic system, homeostasis/metabolism, mortality/aging, immune system, and growth/size phenotype were enriched in both types of C-DMRs, except embryogenesis (or related terms like differentiation), which was specific to hypermethylation. Genes falling under each enriched top attribute are listed in Additional file 5. These results suggest the importance of both hypo-and hyper-C-DMRs in CLL, and emphasize the functional significance of hypo-C-DMRs.

Enrichment of TFBS, histone modifications, and chromatin states

Next, in order to identify epigenomic signatures associated with both C-DMRs, we systematically tested for enrichment in transcription factor binding sites (TFBSs), histone modification marks, and chromatin states provided by ENCODE project [36].

TFBS enrichment analysis identified EZH2 as strongly associated with hyper-C-DMRs (p.adj = 1.70E-23), in contrast to hypo-C-DMRs (p.adj = 4.27E-05, Fig. 4a). On the contrary, *EBF1*, *POL2*, *CHD2*, *WHIP*, and *TBLR1* were strongly associated with hypo-C-DMRs (p.adj = 2.53E-37, 1.06E-30, 2.17E-22, 6.024E-22, and 5.78E-19, respectively), in contrast to hyper-C-DMRs (p.adj = 1.65E-09 and 3.50E-07) (Fig. 4). Other than these, the HAIB dataset in ENCODE showed additional B lymphopoiesis-related enriched TFBS like *RUNX3* (p.adj = 3.58E-31), *TCF3* (p.adj = 4.04E-14), *PU.1* (p.adj = 7.42E-11), and *PAX5* (p.adj = 7.43E-11). Both hyper- and hypo-C-DMRs were enriched in *ZNF143*, *CTCF*, *MAZ*, and *MXI1* TFBSs (Fig. 4a). These findings were confirmed by using TFBS data from all cell lines provided by the ENCODE project (Figure S3 (a), S4 in Additional file 1 and Additional file 6).

Among histone modification marks, we found H3K27me3 to be highly enriched in hyper-C-DMRs (Fig. 4b, p.adj = 2.31E-40). On the contrary, hypo-C-DMRs were strongly enriched in H3K4me1 (p.adj = 1.11E-54), H3K27ac (p.adj = 1.22E-38), and H3K79me2 (p.adj = 1.44E-34) histone modification marks (Fig. 4b). Both C-DMRs were enriched in H3K4me2, H3K4me3, and H2AZ histone modification marks (Fig. 4a). The specificity of the H3K27me3 mark for hyper-C-DMRs was confirmed by using histone modification data from all cell lines provided by the ENCODE project (Figure S3 (b) in Additional file 1 and Additional file 6).

Furthermore, hyper-C-DMRs were significantly enriched for homeobox, *E2F* and TATAbox/promoter motifs, and hypo-C-DMRS for *ETS*, *IRF4*, *EGR*, *ZFX*, *RUNX1*, *PU.1*, *Pax5*, *BATF*, *Erra*, and *bZIP* motifs (Table S5 in Additional file 1). All motifs enriched for hypo-C-DMR have been shown to contribute to cell proliferation, B cell development and pathogenesis of lymphomas [37–39].

Using chromatin state annotations from multiple cell lines (Figure S3 (c) in Additional file 1 and Additional file 6), we found hyper-C-DMRs to be enriched in "repressed" (p.adj = 5.63E-182) and "poised promoters" (p.adj = 1.24E-69) chromatin states (Fig. 4c). In contrast, hypo-C-DMRs were consistently enriched in both "strong/weak enhancers" (p.adj = 6.73E-36 for both) and "weak transcription" (p.adj = 2.73E-24). Both C-DMRs were similarly enriched in "weak promoters" (p.adj = 1.70E-19 and 2.93E-15 for hyper- and hypo-C-DMRs, respectively). These results suggest that distant enhancer regions tend to be hypomethylated in cancer whereas regions associated with repressed or poised transcription are hypermethylated.

Also, 17,811 hyper- and 15,599 hypo-differentially methylated regions (DMRs) were obtained from pooled CLL and control sample comparison (Table S2 in Additional file 1). Each of these region lists exhaustively included all hyper- and hypo-C-DMRs, respectively. KEGG and GO annotation enrichment analysis of

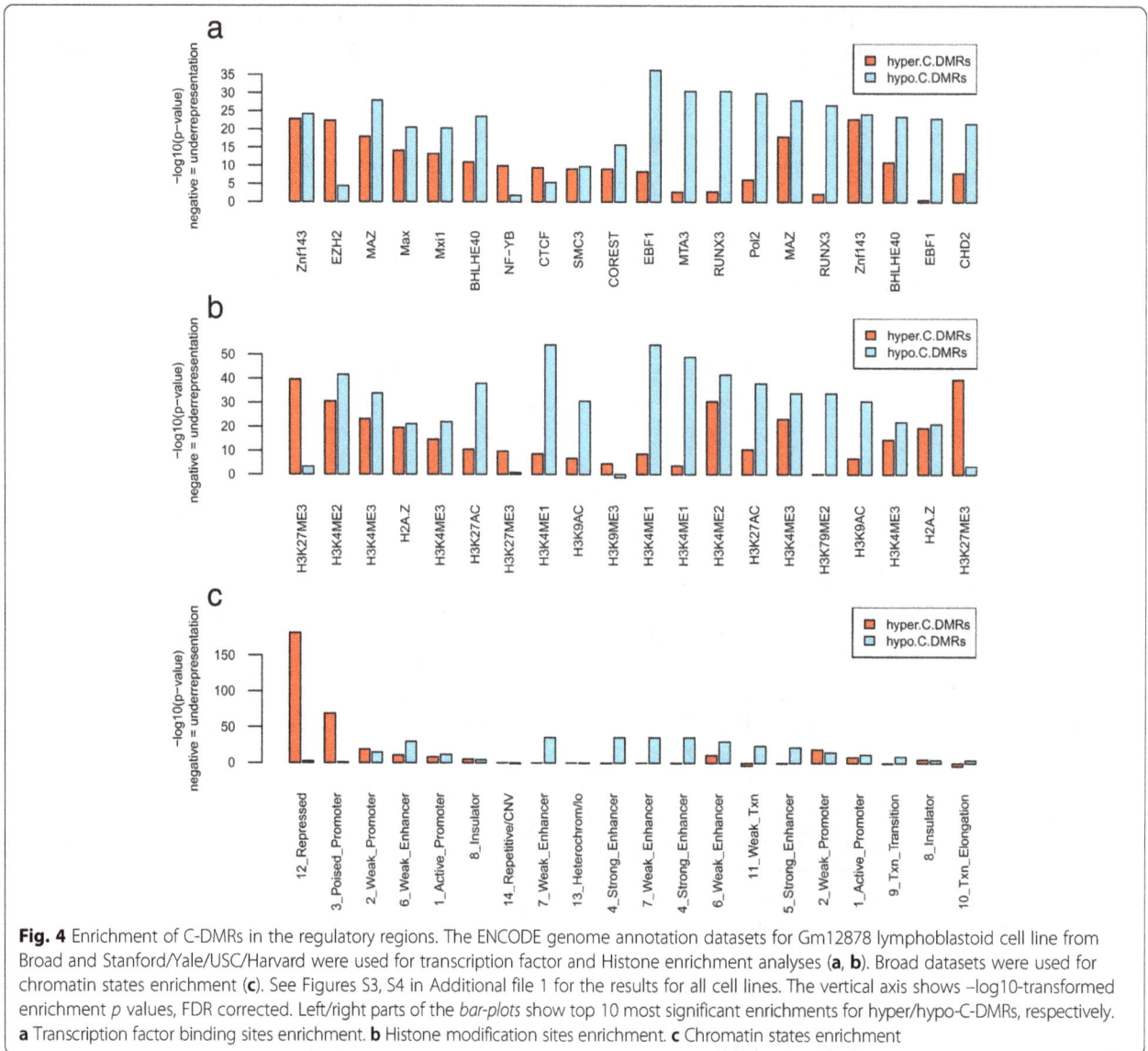

Fig. 4 Enrichment of C-DMRs in the regulatory regions. The ENCODE genome annotation datasets for Gm12878 lymphoblastoid cell line from Broad and Stanford/Yale/USC/Harvard were used for transcription factor and Histone enrichment analyses (**a**, **b**). Broad datasets were used for chromatin states enrichment (**c**). See Figures S3, S4 in Additional file 1 for the results for all cell lines. The vertical axis shows –log10-transformed enrichment *p* values, FDR corrected. Left/right parts of the *bar-plots* show top 10 most significant enrichments for hyper/hypo-C-DMRs, respectively. **a** Transcription factor binding sites enrichment. **b** Histone modification sites enrichment. **c** Chromatin states enrichment

pooled sample DMRs also showed a strong enrichment of similar terms (Additional files 1 and 4). Results from pooled sample analysis show that C-DMRs are more specific and significant subset of DMRs that are consistently present in all samples.

Expression data analysis

Expression profiles in relation with methylation

Next, we looked at the association between gene expression changes and methylation differences. For this, expression values of all transcripts from 19 matching CLL samples were divided into four expression quartiles and referred to as lowest to highest expression groups. Methylation profiles for genes in each of these quartiles were then extracted for comparison. Figure 5a shows a significant reduction of methylation at gene boundaries for all expression quartile groups. At the peripheral region, methylation in the highest

expression genes is reduced the most. Towards the center, methylation of CpGs and expression has an inverse relationship, with the lowest expression genes having the lowest percent methylation. Overall, average methylation for whole gene regions for all genes had a negative correlation (Pearson correlation = –0.07; *p* value = 3.1E-09) with expression.

Next, we looked for expression (transcript FPKM values) and methylation (for overlapped CpG sites) relationship in exons and introns individually (Fig. 5d, e). We observed that among exons (Fig. 5d), transcripts in the lowest expression quartile had the highest and most distinct methylation pattern. Overall, all exons combined from transcripts in all expression quartiles had a negative correlation (corr = –0.13; *p* value <2.2E-16). For introns (Fig. 5e), this relationship appeared to be opposite with the highest expression quartile transcripts showing the highest methylation but almost no correlation

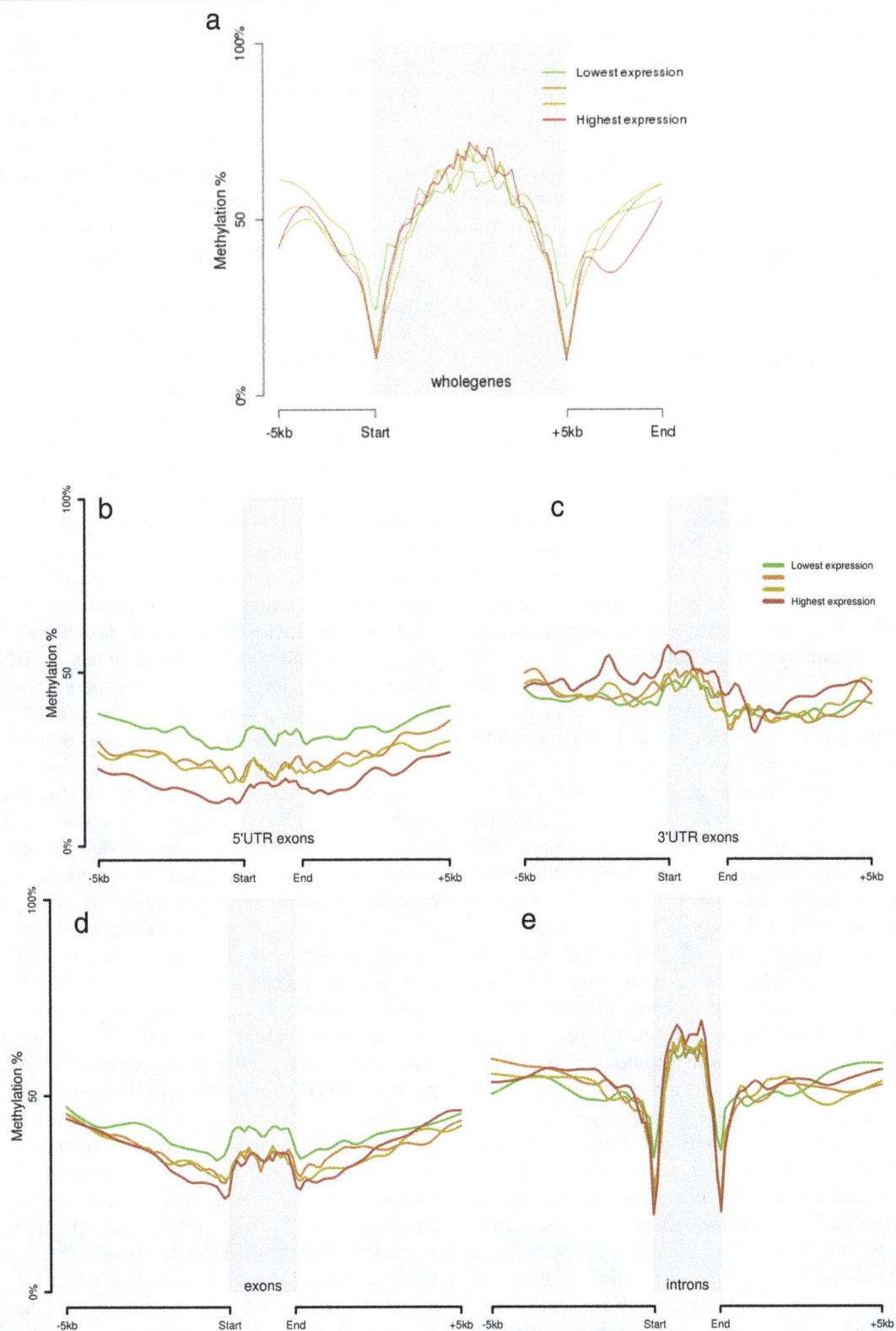

Fig. 5 Association between DNA methylation and expression in CLL samples. **a** Local regression showing methylation levels of whole genes stratified by expression quartiles in CLL samples. **b** Local regression showing methylation levels within 5′ and 3′UTRs for different transcripts stratified by expression quartiles. **c** Methylation levels within exons and introns for transcripts in different expression quartiles. **d** Methylation levels at exon boundary in different expression quartiles. **e** Methylation levels at intron boundary in different expression quartiles

(corr = −0.02; *p* value = 6.2E-2). Also, we identified a very clear distinction in methylation patterns from different expression quartiles in exons specifically from 5'UTRs (Fig. 5b). Overall, 5'UTRs had a negative correlation between methylation and expression (corr = −0.2; *p* value <2.2E-16). Conversely, exons from 3'UTRs had the opposite methylation pattern (Fig. 5c). 3'UTR exons from the highest expression quartile genes had the highest methylation (Fig. 5d, Figure S8 in Additional file 1) and overall, they had weak but positive correlation (corr = 0.1; *p* value = 2.4E-3). In summary, we observed different methylation effects on expression for different genic regions, particularly within exons from 5'UTR and 3'UTR that related to methylation changes at widespread genomic locations in CLL.

Correlation module analysis

In order to further investigate the role of 3'UTR methylation change on expression, we used both expression and methylation data to construct co-expression and co-differential methylation network modules, respectively. These modules were generated using the weighted gene correlation network analysis (WGCNA) framework [40]. For this, we selected 1780 transcripts from 19 matching CLL samples, from which both expression and average 3'UTR methylation data were available.

WGCNA identified 21 co-expression modules with sizes ranging from 41 to 181 transcripts from the expression data and 17 co-differential methylation modules with sizes ranging from 37 to 284 transcripts from the methylation data (average of all CpGs within 3'UTRs). Methylation values of transcripts in each CLL sample were compared against methylation of transcripts from one common control sample, individually. Differential methylation values for all transcripts in all CLL samples were thus obtained. Correlation network modules in each dataset were obtained using hierarchical clustering of pairwise gene correlation structures using WGCNA. WGCNA does not use gene ontology information but clusters the interconnected genes defined as branches of a hierarchical cluster tree. Hence, modules are initially labeled by arbitrary integers and then coded by colors for each dataset. Since clustering for module generation has no gene annotation or functional information, functional interpretation for each module in each dataset was further obtained by conducting a GO enrichment analysis. GO enrichment analyses revealed unique and significant enrichment of various GO terms, providing evidence of a functional role for each module as a whole (Additional file 7; Tables S2, S3, S8, and S9 in Additional file 1). Overall, different biological processes for different modules implied biological significance of clustering transcripts in separate modules in both expression and methylation data.

Next, to investigate the relationship between expression and methylation modules, these modules were matched by pairwise comparison of each methylation module to each expression module using two methods. First, they were compared to measure a statistically significant overlap of genes in each pair. Second, we used network-based statistics to assess whether the density and connectivity patterns of genes were also preserved in a two-paired set of modules with significant gene overlaps. The second method generated a composite statistic value, i.e., $Z_{summary}$, using a permutation test to measure the strength of methylation module and expression module preservation. Also, knowing the $Z_{summary}$ statistic bias towards a module with a large size, a rank-based statistic *medianRank* was used in the second method to measure their relative preservation irrespective of module size. The medianRank is the statistic calculated from observed preservation values and does not conduct any permutation test against background gene modules.

From network preservation tests, we found that expression and differential methylation modules in general exhibited relatively few overlapping genes (Additional file 7) although some of the overlaps were statistically significant. The most significant overlaps (p.adj < 0.05) were observed between large co-expression modules and co-differential methylation modules, enriched for same GO terms (Table 1 and Additional file 7; Table S4 in Additional file 1). Figure 6a reports the number of common genes resulting from pairwise module overlap analysis. The statistical significance of each pair as shown by a color scale was computed to see if the numbers of common genes were obtained according to an iterative pattern and not by chance. WGCNA arbitrarily color-code modules for visual identification, so all color-module associations described here do not have any additional meaning outside of this specific analysis. The most significant overlap as shown in Fig. 6a was for "turquoise" color-coded expression module with "magenta," "yellow", and "midnight blue" methylation module. The turquoise expression module also had the highest $Z_{summary}$ ($Z_{summary}$ = 28) and median rank from network-based statistic method (Fig. 6b). GO enrichment analysis of the turquoise expression module showed enrichment of "*TNFR*," "cell adhesion," "leukocyte proliferation," and "apoptosis/cell death." All the overlapping methylation modules which were color-coded in magenta (enriched for "*EGF*" p.adj = 1.60E-02), yellow (enriched for "focal adhesion and kinases"), midnight blue (enriched for "cofactor and ion binding") were enriched for growth factor and regulation of "Ras protein signal transduction," "kinase activity," and "ion binding." Hence, we see that the most significantly overlapping and preserved modules in CLL samples were the ones involved in cancer development. This also indicates the regulatory role of 3′UTR methylation on expression change in cancer.

Also, "green," "pink," "blue," "black," and "grey60" color-coded expression modules were the other top

Table 1 Significant overlap and preserved modules in WGCNA of 3′UTR methylation and expression

Methylation module (size)	Expression module (size)	Overlap count (p value)	$Z_{summary}$	Median rank	Functional annotation	Gene symbols
Magenta (79)	Turquoise (181)	20 (6.17E-05)	28	6	Regulation of Ras protein signal transduction	ABCC3,ALS2CL,ATG16L2,COG8,DNASE1, DOCK9,ESPL1,PDE4D,TMEM63C,TNFAIP2, TNFRSF4,TTLL1,UQCC1,ZNF385A
Red (101)	Grey60 (52)	9 (2.04E-03)	13	19	Cell division and chromosome partitioning/cytoskeleton	CHID1,FDXR,HERC2,HERC6,MYO9B, SEPT5,UBXN7
Yellow (165)	Turquoise (181)	28 (3.18E-03)	28	6	Kinases	ATG16L2,BMP1,C1orf159,CLUH,COL6A2, CRTC1,DAGLA,DNAH3,ENTHD2,EPHA10, FAM101B,FAM53A,GPR56,IGF1R,LAMC3, NLRP2,NR3C2,OPLAH,PITPNM2,PPP2R2B, PRKCA,PTPRK,RASGRF1,STK32C,THNSL2
Turquoise (284)	Blue (176)	41 (4.83E-03)	13	18	Signaling and apoptosis, cell cycle checkpoint	ACOXL,ANKH,ARHGEF18,B3GAT3,CCAR1, CCDC137,CKB,CREM,DDX39A,DFFB,DNAJB12, FAIM3,HUS1,ITPK1,KIAA0930,LRPAP1,MGRN1, MRPS24,NADK,NRARP,NUBPL,NUP155, OSBPL7,PHF14,PIP5K1A,PPFIA3,PSTPIP1, PTMA,RALBP1,RIN3,RPS6KB2,SH3BP2,SH3TC1, TP53I3,TRAF4,TRIB2,TSSC1,USP42
Brown (197)	Light green (49)	12 (5.48E-03)	9.8	9	Apoptosis/cell death	UEVLD,UNC13B,DTNB,BANP,IRF7,CCNL2, INTS9,FNTA,RBM19,DNASE1,GRB7
Midnightblue (45)	Turquoise (181)	10 (1.24E-02)	28	6	Ion binding	ABLIM2,ACE,COMMD1,ELFN2,GLT1D1, HAUS7,TOM1
Turquoise (284)	Midnight blue (55)	15 (2.11E-02)	12	2	Nucleotide binding	ADCY9,AGTRAP,BSDC1,INO80E,MCHR1, MTHFSD,NADK,P4HB,PDE8A,POR,RAB3A, RPS19BP1,SMUG1,SOX12,STX8

modules showing a strong preservation ($Z_{summary}$ >10) and low median rank (Fig. 6b). All these four modules were again enriched for "zinc ion binding," "regulation of transcription," and "apoptosis". They overlapped with "light cyan," "midnight blue," "black," and "turquoise" methylation modules. Biological processes like "cell division," "chromosome partitioning/cytoskeleton," and "GTPase regulator activity" were enriched in both "grey60" (second least rank = 5, $Z_{summary}$ = 13) expression module along with its overlapping red methylation module (Additional file 7). An additional network analysis was carried out using expression and average methylation of whole genes (not just 3′UTRs) that are non-coding (i.e., transcripts that do not encode a protein product) along with 3′UTR methylation. Results from this analysis can be accessed in Additional file 7. This non-coding RNA analysis also gave results similar to the 3′UTRs, including overlap of modules enriched for similar cancer-related terms. Hence, we see that significantly preserved expression and methylation modules were enriched for similar cancer-related biological processes like leukocyte proliferation, apoptosis, signal transduction, and cell-cycle regulation. Our observation from network preservation of expression and 3′UTR methylation change provides clues for a better understanding of the contribution made by the regulatory role imposed by 3′UTR methylation overexpression.

Next, a correlation analysis between methylation and expression modules was conducted using module *eigengene* (aka *eigennode*) that is intuitively understood as a weighted average of the variable profiles in a module. Although the composition of co-expression and co-differential methylation modules can vary, we observed multiple strong Pearson correlations between many expression and methylation module eigengenes as shown in Fig. 7, and Tables S6 and S12 in Additional file 7. For example, in our non-coding gene analysis, eigengenes of "red" methylation module was highly negatively correlated (corr = −0.97, p value = 5.75E-12) to a "brown" expression module. The red methylation module was enriched for "regulation of cell cycle" and "intracellular signal cascade" and "brown" expression module for apoptosis and leukocyte proliferation as per GO analysis, showcasing complimentary functional annotations involved in cancer regulation (Tables S8 and S9 in Additional file 7). Similarly, eigengenes of the blue methylation module were significantly and positively correlated (corr = 0.95, p value = 1.22E-09) to the "dark red" expression module, both of which were enriched for "protein localization" or "intracellular transport" (Figure S6 in Additional file 7). Also, we saw both significantly positive and negative correlations in 3′UTR methylation to expression modules and occasionally for the same module. For example, red expression module (enriched for "kinases and nucleotide binding") was negatively correlated with "green" (enriched for "nucleotide binding" and "positive regulation of apoptosis") and positively correlated with "midnight blue" and "tan" (both enriched for "nucleotide binding")

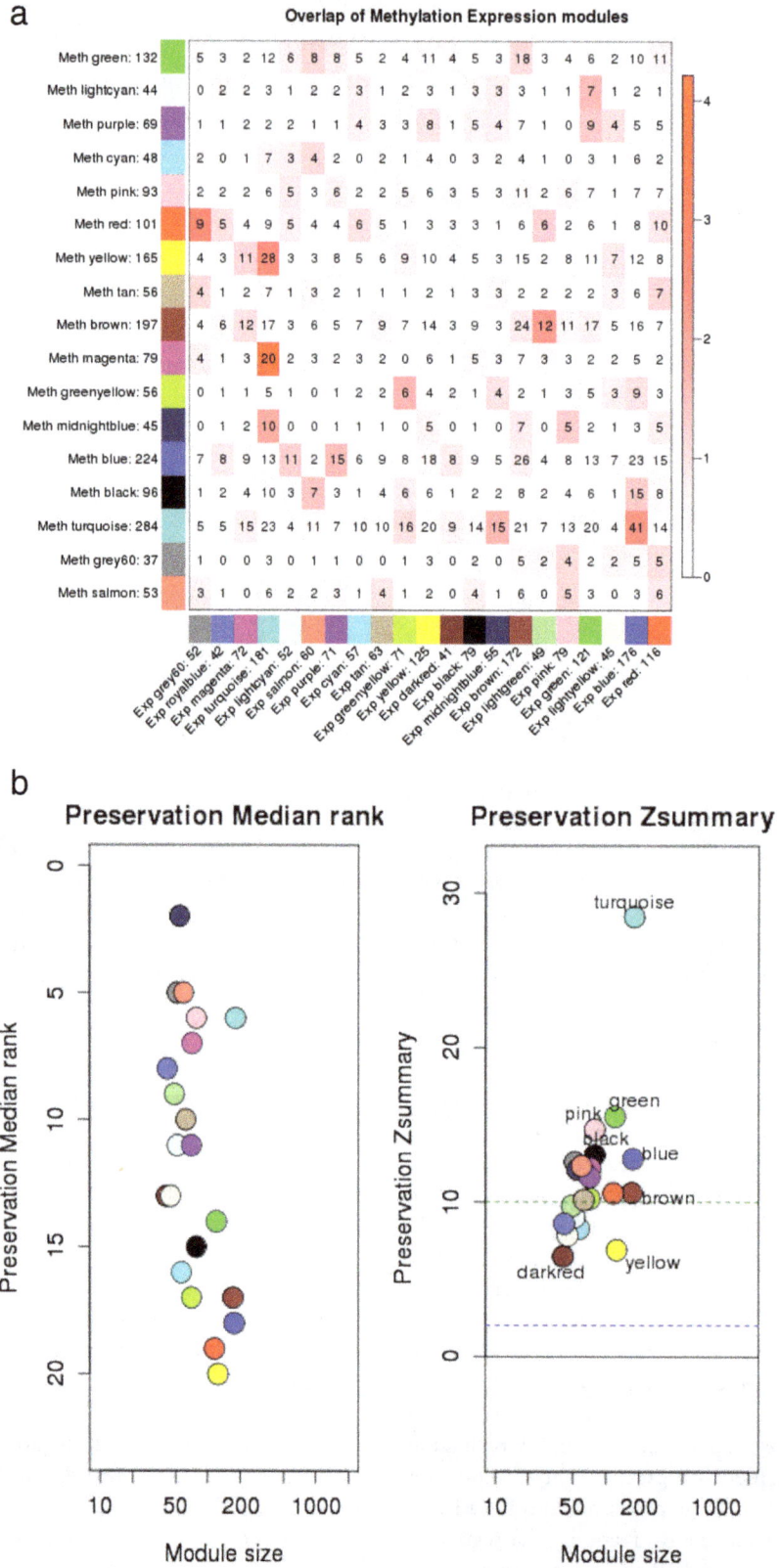

Fig. 6 (See legend on next page.)

Fig. 6 Module preservation. **a** Table showing gene overlap between each pair of methylation and expression modules. Each *row* of the table corresponds to one methylation module (labeled by color as well as text), and each *column* corresponds to one expression module. *Numbers* in the table indicate gene counts in the intersection of the corresponding modules. *Coloring* of the table encodes – log(p), with p being the Fisher's exact test *p* value for the overlap of the two modules. The stronger the *red color*, the more significant the overlap is between a methylation module for 3′UTR and an expression module. **b** Plot showing statistical analysis results for module preservation test to check preservation of 3′ UTR methylation modules against expression modules based on the density and connectivity patterns of genes in each module. The *left panel* shows the medianRank of the observed preservation statics and the *right panel* shows the distribution of $Z_{summary}$ statistics obtained from a permutation analysis for each methylation module. A module with a lower median rank tends to exhibit stronger observed preservation statistics than a module with a higher median rank. The $Z_{summary}$ statistic of a given module summarizes the evidence that the network connections of the module are more significantly preserved than those of random set of genes of equal size. The significance thresholds for $Z_{summary}$ are $Z_{summary} < 2$ implies no evidence that the module is preserved, $2 < Z_{summary} < 10$ implies weak to moderate evidence, and $Z_{summary} > 10$ implies strong evidence for module preservation between co-expression module and 3′UTR methylation module

3′UTR methylation modules. All together within the 3′UTR methylation correlations, we observed a majority of positive correlated modules of lower significance compared to negative correlated modules of high significance. Correlation in different directions can be assumed to be due to location of methylation differences within exons or introns, as we saw in our previous analysis and the direction of methylation change. Overall, we observed significant correlations in modules enriched for cancer-related terms, giving evidence of the role of methylation change in 3′UTRs towards tumorigenesis.

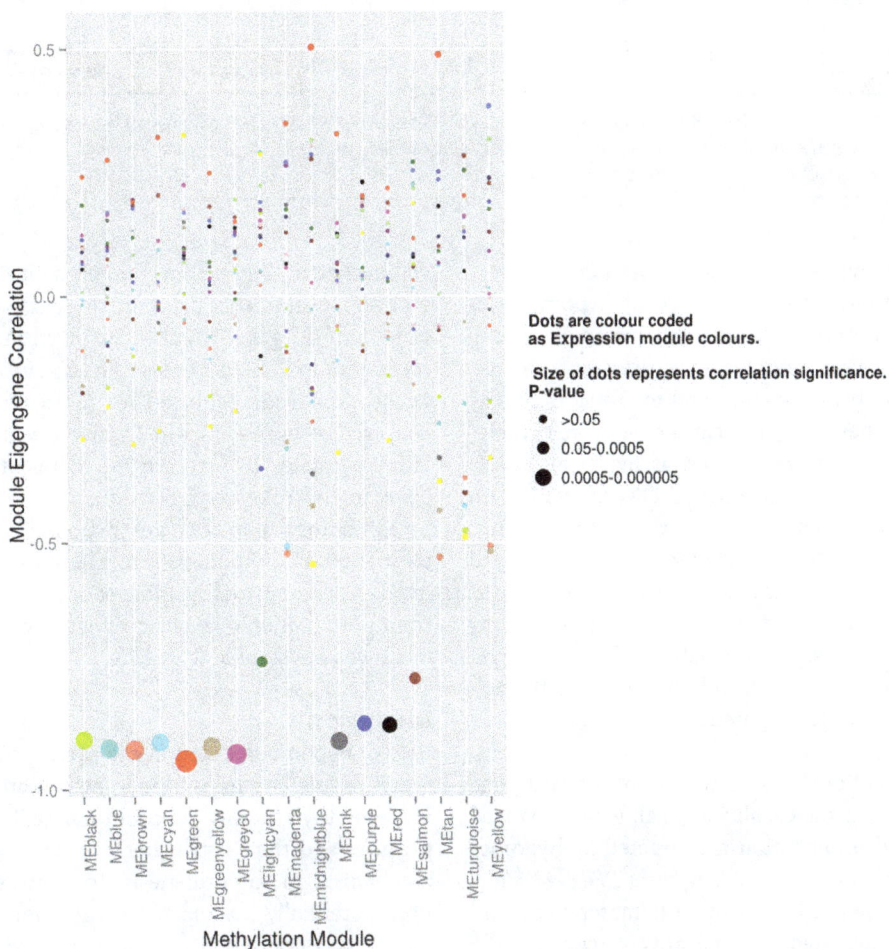

Fig. 7 Pairwise correlation between each methylation module to each expression module. Plot showing correlation between eigengenes of each 3′ UTR methylation and expression modules. X-axis shows all 17 differential methylation modules, and Y-axis shows the module eigengene correlation value for each of the 21 different color-coded dots representing 21 expression modules. Statistical significance of each correlation was calculated and represented by dot size for each corresponding methylation module

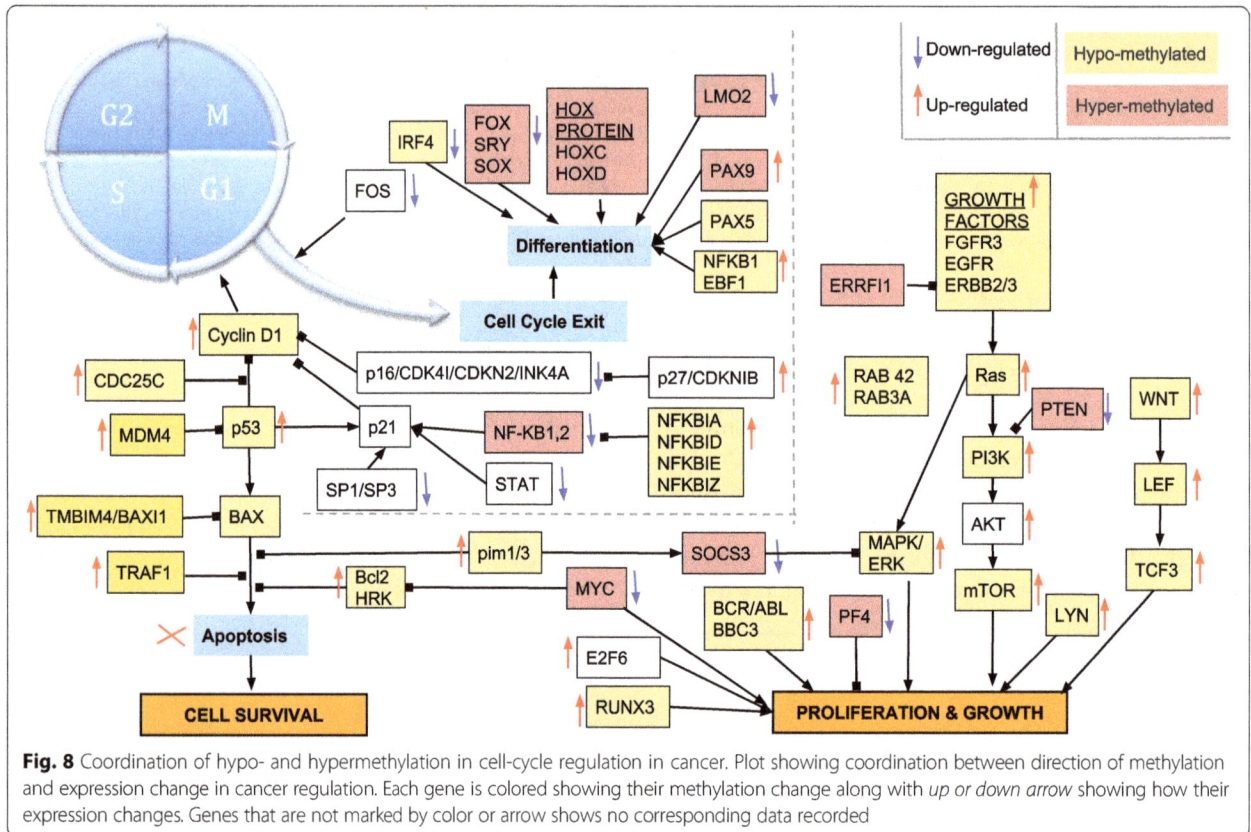

Fig. 8 Coordination of hypo- and hypermethylation in cell-cycle regulation in cancer. Plot showing coordination between direction of methylation and expression change in cancer regulation. Each gene is colored showing their methylation change along with *up or down arrow* showing how their expression changes. Genes that are not marked by color or arrow shows no corresponding data recorded

Interplay between hypo- and hypermethylation
Also, while describing the importance of hypomethylation in CLL, we described the overall interplay among hyper/hypomethylation and gene expression change. Figure 8 shows both methylation and expression change information together for key cancer and cell cycle-regulating genes. Genes are marked as hypo- or hypermethylated if any of the respective C-DMRs overlap on them. As observed from all our enrichment analyses, Fig. 8 shows that growth and proliferation is dominated by hypomethylation whereas hypermethylation blocks cell-cycle exiting and differentiation. We can see many instances where opposite methylation changes target genes in the same process but still coordinate with each other towards cancer development. Both hyper- and hypomethylation changes were found within the same network based on functional role or direction of target gene in the network. For instance, although, all genes involved in cell growth and proliferation are targeted by hypomethylation and have activated transcription, *PF4*—which is known to be involved in inhibition of hematopoiesis and *PTEN*, is hypermethylated. *PF4* negatively regulates the *PI3K-AKT/PKB* signaling pathway and acts as a tumor-suppressor and hence, hypermethylated and repressed. Similarly, in order to drive the cell cycle forward to progress through subsequent phases of cell cycle and escape

cell-cycle exit, Fig. 8 shows much complementary coordination of opposite methylation changes. We can see how the *FOS* gene, which is involved in cell-cycle exit is repressed in CLL samples but *CyclinD1* and its other genes, which are required for G1-S phase transition in cell-cycle progression are hypomethylated. Hypomethylation of genes involved in G1-S transition, thereby enables uncontrolled cell division. Also, all genes involved in inhibiting apoptosis are hypomethylated leading to their transcription activation. These examples show how hypo- and hypermethylation coordinate with each other to impose a double negative effect towards the same goal of cancer development in CLL.

Discussion
Role of hypomethylation in cell-cycle regulation, histone modification, and transcription activation in CLL
Hypermethylation at the promoter region of tumor suppressors and their subsequent silencing is a well-studied mechanism of tumorigenesis. In contrast, hypomethylation, potentially leading to upregulation of oncogenes, is not fully understood. Also, genic hypomethylation is often considered as a random and non-consistent process due to a particularly predominant demethylation process in mature B cells in CLL samples. In this study, we showed that consistent hypomethylated

regions (referred to here as hypo-C-DMRs) account for a significant pattern of methylation changes in CLL with a distinctive pattern of gene expression and regulatory associations.

In particular, we observed that both hypo- and hyper-C-DMRs were enriched for similar biological processes but in an opposite direction. For example, hyper-C-DMRs were enriched for "positive regulation of cell differentiation", but hypo-C-DMRs were enriched for "negative regulation of cell differentiation." We also observed a significant enrichment of BCR signaling associated with hypo-C-DMRs. This further strengthens the importance of hypomethylation in CLL since BCR is a central pathogenic mechanism in B cell malignancies, including CLL [41]. In addition, GO annotations relate to transcription regulation, chromatin modification, apoptosis, cell proliferation, leukocyte differentiation, and signal transduction were enriched for hypo-C-DMR, which also defines their functional role in cancer development.

Also, the most significantly enriched TFBS for hypo-C-DMRs was EBF1, which is a transcription factor that is critical for both B lymphopoiesis and B cell function [42]. EBF1, in collaboration with a hierarchy of partner proteins, including E2A, Runx1, and Pax5 (also enriched in motif analysis) activates the B cell transcriptome and represses programs of alternate hematopoietic lineages. DNA binding by EBF1 has also been linked to changes in epigenetic marks on their target genes. Binding of EBF1 and other factors including E2A have also been correlated with H3K4me1 at target genes, which is also the most enriched histone modification mark in our analysis. H3K4me1 is in fact known to facilitate additional epigenetic modifications necessary for transcription [43]. RUNX3, TCF3, PU.1, and PAX5 are also key transcription factors in B lymphopoiesis and cell proliferation. Other TFBS enriched for hypo-C-DMRs were POL2, CHD2, WHIP, and TBLR1. CHD2 is a DNA-binding helicase that specifically binds to the promoter of target genes, leading to chromatin remodeling and promoting their expression [44]. WHIP is a protein that binds to DNA polymerase delta and increases the initiation frequency of DNA polymerase delta-mediated DNA synthesis [45]. TBLR1 is a key regulator of different properties of the BCL-3 [46] that acts as an oncogenic protein through multiple mechanisms that include the induction of cyclin D1 expression and also inhibits cell apoptosis through induction of the E3 ligase of p53, MDM2 [47, 48]. Among other enriched histone modifications, H3K79 di-methylation is known for regulating the initiation of DNA replication [49], and H3K36me3 is found in actively transcribed gene bodies of genes involved in G1/S transition in a cell cycle [50]. Presence of hypo-C-DMR overlapping enhancers and weak promoters further emphasize their role in activation of

transcription. Overall, both enriched TFBS and histone modifications are known to relate to B lymphopoiesis, transcription activation, and cancer development.

In contrast to hypo-C-DMRs, hyper-C-DMRs, which are known to regulate the expression silencing mechanism, were implicated by the enrichment of EZH2. EZH2 contains a histone methyltransferase SET domain that methylates histone tails on gene promoters to repress their transcription initiation, and this domain is an important component of the polycomb repressive complex 2 (PRC2). The PRC2 protein EZH2 is also known to preferentially methylate Lysine 27 on histone 3 (H3K27) [51] and also H3K9 under certain conditions. H3K27me3 and H3K9me3 were both enriched for hyper-LSDMRs in our analysis as well. H3K4me3, H3K9me3, and H3K27me3 co-localizes with most polycomb target proteins like SUZ12, CTBP2, and EZH2-binding sites enriched in hyper-C-DMRs (Additional file 1; Figure S5). Several other studies [51, 52] have reported DNA methylation and tumor suppressors in cancers marked with polycomb proteins enriched with EZH2 and H3K27me3. This study also elucidates the known mechanism of hyper-C-DMR in gene silencing and promoting cancer development. Further, enrichment of repressor chromatin region for hyper-C-DMRs confirms their role in silencing the expression of target genes.

Our motif enrichment analysis showed hypermethylation enriched for motifs like homeobox and TATAbox, which are usually present in promoter regions and thus silence many key genes. In contrast, hypomethylation was enriched in motifs of transcription activator binding genes, such as ETS [38], ZFX [37], cMYC [39] (Table 1), which are again involved in cell growth, apoptosis, and metabolism, processes necessary for tumor progression. Enriched transcription factor motifs like Ikaros (IKZF) and PU.1 govern B cell lineage priming, which involves changes in histone modifications and chromatin structure of genes encoding molecules important for the establishment of a B cell program [53]. Other significant classes of motifs enriched in hypo-C-DMRs were motifs containing ETS domain in genes like Elk1 and Fli and RHD domain in genes like NFAT and NFkB-p65. These genes are downstream nuclear targets of Ras-MAP kinase signaling and are also known as oncogenic transcription activators, specific to [54] cell survival and proliferation.

Methylation pattern in exons, introns, and 3'UTRs

In addition to evidence of transcription activation, we observed that hypomethylation in CLL mostly targets intronic, intergenic, and 3'UTR regions. Regarding the relationship between methylation and expression change with respect to genic locations, we found negative correlation for methylation in exons and whole transcript expression within 30 CLL samples. But, this correlation within exons was inconsistent in UTRs. Exons in 5′UTRs seem to act more like promoters, but exons in 3′UTRs had the opposite effect on expression. Hence, these findings suggest that in contrast to a gene expression-inhibiting role of increasing methylation associated with 5′UTR exons, methylation in 3′UTR exons is in fact required in the normal transcription process.

Regulation of expression by 3′UTR methylation pattern

Our co-expression and co-methylation network analysis revealed that both transcriptome and methylome can be organized into modules. Genes in co-methylation and co-expression modules were found highly enriched for specific gene ontology categories, underscoring their functional importance. Many 3′UTR modules associated with methylation changes were found to have moderate to strong preservation with expression modules. Also, the most preserved module had functional annotations related to signaling and growth and proliferation. Hence, preserved 3′UTR methylation and expression modules revealed the ability of 3′UTR methylation to dictate their expression. The regulatory behavior of methylation change could, therefore, be detected—not only in 5′UTR, promoters, and gene bodies—but also in 3′UTRs in CLL. Also, significantly correlated 3′UTR methylation and expression modules were enriched for biologically important pathways involved in signaling cascade, apoptosis, and cell proliferation. These results provide a fine-grained look at the interaction among 3′UTR co-methylation and co-expression modules altered in CLL.

In summary, we report that hypomethylation of DNA appears to facilitate the aberrant expression of proto-oncogenes/oncogenes, potentially stimulating cell proliferation in CLL. We observed that apart from global hypomethylation of repeat sequences, there also exists site-specific hypomethylation of certain genes and genic regions, especially in genes linked with signaling pathways (e.g., *BCR, LYN RAB8A, NFKBIB*), chromatin modifications (e.g., *CHD2, CHD3, SMARCB1*), cell growth and development (e.g., *EBF1, EGR1, EGFR, ERBB2, MYC*), apoptosis inhibition (e.g., *BCL2, TRAF1*), and promoting cell proliferation (e.g., *CCND1, LYN, BCL3*). We observed 3′UTRs to possess a high percentage of hypo-DMRs consistent in the majority of our test samples. We report genes with 3′UTR consistent hypomethylation in CLL like *LIF* and *PIM3*. Along with that, we also report genes with consistent hypermethylation in CLL in 3′UTRs like *HMX2* and other genic regions. We also

observed that methylation changes at 3′UTR had significant correlation with expression along with overlapping network modules in both datasets. Our findings, thus, suggest that hypomethylation in different genic regions might exhibit a significant deleterious effect on gene expression that results in malignant transformation and/or tumor progression.

Conclusions

We observed that hypomethylated regions were less consistent over the genome among different samples, in contrast to hypermethylation loci. However, some hypomethylated regions were highly consistent in most of the samples, and their functional analysis revealed their potential biological significance in CLL.

We observed hypomethylation at many genes containing key TFBS involved in cell growth and development, histone remodeling, apoptosis, and cellular proliferation. We found hypomethylation in many key signaling regulators consistent in majority of samples, which do not appear to be random events or a non-specific part of global hypomethylation. In addition, this study contributes to our understanding about the relationship between methylation and expression levels in CLL samples. Results from positional analyses for genic location indicate that the conventional model of methylation regulating expression in an antagonistic manner is most common. However, we also uncovered an interesting and conflicting relationship between methylation and expression for methylation occurring in exons of 3′UTRs. Specifically, we found evidence of a loss of DNA methylation that not only causes genomic instability but also potentially activates many genes mainly in signaling pathways like *BCR* in CLL. Finally, we showed that 3′UTR methylome and transcriptome are organized into biologically meaningful modules with significant correlations and strong-to-moderate preservation of their density and connections between two datasets. The preserved modules were also found as functionally related indicating the role of 3′UTR methylation in expression regulation.

Methods
Data sources

Publicly available reduced representation bisulfite sequencing (RRBS) methylation for 30 CLL and three control samples were obtained from the GEO website (http://www.ncbi.nlm.nih.gov/geo/query/acc.cgi?acc=GSE66121). Control samples were CD19+ B cells isolated from peripheral blood of normal controls. Human genome annotation data from the UCSC genome browser (hg19 genome assembly), such as Refseq and

UCSC genes, CpG islands, Vista Enhancers, ENCODE Transcription Factor ChIP-Seq, and RepeatMasker Tracks, were used to annotate differentially methylated regions of interest. For genes with multiple isoforms, the longest one was used as the reference. Promoter regions were selected from −2 kb upstream to the transcription start site of each gene.

Read mapping and % methylation

The bisulfite-treated sequencing reads in DNA methylation data for CD19+ B cells were mapped to bisulfite-converted human genome using Bismark [55] (using Bowtie). Bismark was used also to obtain the genome-wide cytosine methylation calls at a base resolution in the CpG context. Additional file 8 provides read mapping count tables for each sample.

Sequencing reads from RNA-seq experiments were mapped using Bowtie with known ENSEMBL transcripts as gene models. After mapping, FPKM values for each gene/transcript were calculated by Cufflinks [56] and differentially expressed (DE) genes were defined by abs(ln(fold-change)) > 1.5. FDR-corrected $p <$ 0.05 for all DE genes were calculated by Cuffdiff [57]. Next, the over enriched GO categories were obtained based on a .05 FDR cutoff using the GO-seq R package.

DMR calculation

Considering the high correlation between methylation of adjacent CpGs, the methylation information obtained from RRBS data was summarized on 1000 bp tiling windows (step-size 1000 bp) with minimum 3 CpGs and minimum 10 reads mapped on each CpG using the R package, *methylKit* [58]. For DMR calculation, pairwise comparison of 1000 bp tiles in each of the 30 tumor samples against each control normal sample was performed using Fisher's exact test. From each such test, differential methylation values were obtained only for the regions that were common between CLL and control sample. Thirty such tests were conducted for each control sample. Next, in order to ensure comparable statistics, only those regions that had differential values from each of the 30 tests were used. This gave us 41,421 common regions obtained from the first control sample comparison tests. Similarly, 39,327 and 41,359 regions were obtained from each of the other two control samples.

Entropy calculation

Also, the methylation entropy across all CLL samples was calculated in order to see probability distribution of methylation changes for each 1000 bp region across all samples. Entropy for each sample was computed as follows:

The methylation vector m_r of region r across N samples was defined as,

$$m_{r=}m_{r,1}, m_{r,2}, ..., m_{r,5}, ..., m_{r,N}$$

where $m_{r,s}$ represents the methylation level in sample s. The sum of methylation levels of region r in samples ($\Sigma_{S=1}^{N} m_{r,s}$) was treated as a total methylation value. The ratio of methylation level of region in sample relative to the total value was defined as the relative methylation probability, $p_{s/r} = m_{r,s}/\Sigma_{S=1}^{N} m_{r,s}$. The original Shannon entropy of the region can be calculated as $H_o = -\sum_{S=1}^{N} p_r^{\underline{k}} \log_2 \left(p_{s/r} \right)$.

Enrichment analysis

Enrichment analysis of genes overlapped by C-DMRs for GO categories and KEGG pathways was performed using GOStats R package [59]. Gene set enrichment for gene symbols overlapping hypo-C-DMRs was also performed using GeneDecks [60] to highlight shared descriptors between pairs of genes based on annotations within the GeneCards compendium of human genes.

The epigenomic enrichment analysis of C-DMRs was performed using Genome Runner [61]. Briefly, genomic coordinates of hyper- and hypo-C-DMRs were collected and tested for co-localization with three groups of genome annotation datasets: (1) chromatin state segmentation by HMM from ENCODE/Broad, (2) histone modifications by ChIP-seq from ENCODE/Broad Institute and ENCODE/Stanford/Yale/USC/Harvard, and (3) experimentally validated transcription factor binding sites from ENCODE/Broad Institute and ENCODE/Stanford/Yale/USC/Harvard. Genomic regions annotated by the ENCODE with any functional/regulatory information (~80 % of the whole genome) were used as a "background" to estimate co-localizations that can occur by chance. p values were calculated using Chi-square test and corrected for multiple testing using FDR.

Motif analysis was also carried out using Homer [62] software after retrieving sequences around each DMR CpG along with those around non-DMR CpGs randomly chosen as a background.

Expression in relation to methylation analysis

To associate gene expression changes with methylation differences, all CpG average methylation values were paired with the average expression of transcripts they overlap in all CLL samples. Estimated expression profiles of all transcripts were divided into four expression quartiles and referred to as lowest to highest expression groups within all transcripts. The positional enrichment analysis for each gene region was performed using Homer, and R scripts were used to calculate and plot smoothened density estimates. Locfit library was used for fitting local regression, likelihood models, and related smoothing procedures.

Correlation of whole transcript expression to methylation of CpGs within each specific gene region was calculated by using the Pearson correlation coefficient. For correlation calculation average methylation of CpGs (across all CLL samples) in a specific gene region and average expression of the whole transcript corresponding to these CpGs were used.

Correlation module analysis

From 19 matching CLL samples from both methylation and expression data, we obtained differential methylation and differential expression (FPKM) for 3′UTRs of 1780 transcripts. For this, whole transcript expression and average methylation for all CpGs in each of its 3′ UTRs were used. Differential expression and 3′UTR methylation for each transcript was then computed by comparing each CLL sample individually against one common control sample.

We then used differential expression and methylation value matrices to identify co-expression and co-differential methylation network modules through the WGCNA R package (see Additional file 7 for more details), individually on each dataset. WGCNA computes networks by calculating each gene-to-gene pairwise correlation and interconnection strength by checking number of shared neighbors. It then finally generates modules using hierarchical clustering. Tables S1 and S2 in Additional file 7 provide a list of 10 top hub genes (genes with most significant module membership) in each module, and Additional file 9 consists of module membership values for all genes in each expression and methylation module.

After constructing modules in each dataset, we checked to see if any of the modules in one dataset were preserved in any of the modules from the other data set using two approaches: cross tabulation and network-based statistics. In cross tabulation, overlaps of the constituent genes in each pair of modules from the two data sets were calculated and Fisher's exact test was used to assign a p value to each overlap. In the second method, we used network module preservation statistics (NP) described in and implemented in [63] the WGCNA R package. The NP method not only assesses the significant overlap of genes, but also whether the density and connectivity patterns of modules defined in a reference data set are preserved in a test data set. We considered expression data as reference data and methylation data as test data. This NP statistic test calculates statistic values based on density and connectivity preservation within reference and test modules. From calculated statistic values, the NP test in the WGCNA package module was used to obtain two values, (1) the median rank,

which is the rank for the average of the observed preservation static values and (2) a composite module preservation statistic referred to as $Z_{summary}$ using a permutation test. Thus, we reported a $Z_{summary}$ for each expression module in the methylation modules.

Also, since WGCNA groups together highly correlated variables to generate modules, we summarized the variable profiles in each module to a single representative, i.e., the module eigengene. The module eigengene, which is defined as the first principal component of the standardized matrix containing variables in the module was used to calculate the correlation between expression and methylation within non-coding genes and 3′UTRs.

Also, since non-coding genes do not translate and do not undergo post-transcription changes (i.e., stripping 3′ UTRs) with no defined UTR or a gene body region (or in other words—whole portion can be identified as UTR), we also conducted the same network analysis by including non-coding genes.

Additional files

Additional file 1: Additional Figures, Tables and Methods. This is a "docx" file, which includes various additional figures, tables and methods that are referred in the main text supporting this research.

Additional file 2: List of C-DMRs. This is an "xls" file providing coordinates for hyper- and hypo-C-DMRs common across all control tests in separate

Additional file 3: Gene lists for C-DMRs. This is an "xls" file providing a list of genes overlapped by common hyper and hypo-C-DMRs in separate excel sheets, respectively. It also consists of excel sheets for genes overlapping different gene regions for hypo- and hyper-C-

Additional file 4: KEGG and GO enrichment analysis results. This is an "xls" format file that provides enrichment test results from GOStats package for KEGG pathways and GO biological processes for both hyper- and hypo-C-DMRs and DMRs from pooled sample analysis in separate

Additional file 5: Phenotype enrichment analysis results. This is an "xls" format file that provides enrichment results for phenotype with different phenotype descriptors, their enrichment p values along with their count and names of their corresponding genes sharing that descriptor for both

Additional file 6: ENCODE enrichment results. This is an "xls" file that provides the ENCODE epi-genomic mark enrichment analysis results from Gm12878 cell line with the name and the description of the datasets, enrichment p values that are adjusted for multiple testing using FDR, for hypo/hyper-C-DMRs in separate excel sheets, respectively, along with the name of the regulatory mark. It also consists of enrichment analysis results from all ENCODE cell lines for each regulatory mark in hypo- and

Additional file 7: WGCNA. This is a "docx" file that describes correlation modules in details, together with the step-by-step description of WGCNA analysis. WGCNA description includes data cleaning and preprocessing, adjacency topological overlap matrix construction, module detection, calculation of various module measures, and description of preservation statistics methods used. It includes tables and figures for both 3′UTR methylation and non-coding gene data, and their relation with

Additional file 8: Read mapping details. This file provides the mapping statistics for all the samples in both RRBS and RNA-seq datasets. Table S1 lists the number of RRBS reads obtained, their % that is uniquely mapped on human genome (hg19) along with total number of CpGs analyzed from each sample. Table S2 lists the number of RNA-seq reads obtained and their % that is uniquely mapped on human genome (hg19) for each

Additional file 9: Gene module membership. This is an "xls" file that provides the matrix for transcript's module membership or eigengene-based connectivity measure of each transcript for each methylation and expression module for 3'UTRs in separate excel sheet, respectively.

Competing interests

The authors declare that they have no competing interests.

Authors' contributions

GK developed the hypothesis and performed all the analyses and drafted the manuscript. MD and JDW performed epigenomic enrichment analysis, and contributed to figure preparation and writing of the manuscript. JQ contributed and verified the statistical testing used in the project. HS contributed datasets and conceptualization of the project. DX and HS contributed to the development of the method, data analysis, and manuscript writing along with jointly directing the project. All authors read and approved the final manuscript.

Acknowledgements

We thank Drs. Andrew Smith, Kristen Taylor, Jeffrey Bryan, Michael Wang, and Joseph L. Wiemels for their helpful discussions.

Declarations

This article has been published as part of *Human Genomics* Volume 10 Supplement 2, 2016: From genes to systems genomics: human genomics. The full contents of the supplement are available online at http://humgenomics.biomedcentral.com/articles/supple ments/volume-10-supplement-2.

Funding

This work was supported in part by the National Institute of Health (Grants CA134304 and DA025779).

Author details

[1]Christopher S. Bond Life Sciences Center, University of Missouri, Columbia, MO 65211, USA. [2]Informatics Institute, University of Missouri, Columbia, MO 65211, USA. [3]Department of Biostatistics, Virginia Commonwealth University, Richmond, VA 23225, USA. [4]Arthritis and Clinical Immunology Program, Oklahoma Medical Research Foundation, Oklahoma City, OK 73104, USA. [5]Department of Applied Economics & Statistics, University of Delaware, Newark, DE 19716, USA. [6]GRU Cancer Center, Georgia Regents University, Augusta, GA 30912, USA. [7]Department of Biochemistry and Molecular Biology, Georgia Regents University, Augusta, GA 30912, USA. [8]Department of Computer Science, University of Missouri, Columbia, MO 65211, USA.

References

1. Feinberg AP, Vogelstein B. Hypomethylation distinguishes genes of some human cancers from their normal counterparts. Nature. 1983;301(5895):89–92.
2. Cadieux B, Ching TT, VandenBerg SR, Costello JF. Genome-wide hypomethylation in human glioblastomas associated with specific copy number alteration, methylenetetrahydrofolate reductase allele status, and increased proliferation. Cancer Res. 2006;66(17):8469–76. doi:10.1158/0008-5472.CAN-06-1547.
3. Widschwendter M, Jiang G, Woods C, Muller HM, Fiegl H, Goebel G, et al. DNA hypomethylation and ovarian cancer biology. Cancer Res. 2004;64 (13):4472–80. doi:10.1158/0008-5472.CAN-04-0238.
4. Brothman AR, Swanson G, Maxwell TM, Cui J, Murphy KJ, Herrick J, et al. Global hypomethylation is common in prostate cancer cells: a quantitative predictor for clinical outcome? Cancer Genet Cytogenet. 2005;156(1):31–6. doi:10.1016/j.cancergencyto.2004.04.004.
5. Wahlfors J, Hiltunen H, Heinonen K, Hamalainen E, Alhonen L, Janne J. Genomic hypomethylation in human chronic lymphocytic leukemia. Blood. 1992;80(8):2074–80.
6. Kulis M, Heath S, Bibikova M, Queiros AC, Navarro A, Clot G, et al. Epigenomic analysis detects widespread gene-body DNA hypomethylation in chronic lymphocytic leukemia. Nat Genet. 2012;44(11):1236–42. doi:10.1038/ng.2443.
7. Lin CH, Hsieh SY, Sheen IS, Lee WC, Chen TC, Shyu WC, et al. Genome-wide hypomethylation in hepatocellular carcinogenesis. Cancer Res. 2001;61(10):4238–43.
8. Kim YI, Giuliano A, Hatch KD, Schneider A, Nour MA, Dallal GE, et al. Global DNA hypomethylation increases progressively in cervical dysplasia and carcinoma. Cancer. 1994;74(3):893–9.
9. Feinberg AP, Gehrke CW, Kuo KC, Ehrlich M. Reduced genomic 5-methylcytosine content in human colonic neoplasia. Cancer Res. 1988;48 (5):1159–61.
10. Ehrlich M, Jiang G, Fiala E, Dome JS, Yu MC, Long TI, et al. Hypomethylation and hypermethylation of DNA in Wilms tumors. Oncogene. 2002;21(43):6694–702. doi:10.1038/sj.onc.1205890.
11. De Smet C, Lurquin C, Lethe B, Martelange V, Boon T. DNA methylation is the primary silencing mechanism for a set of germ line- and tumor-specific genes with a CpG-rich promoter. Mol Cell Biol. 1999;19(11):7327–35.
12. Li M, Balch C, Montgomery JS, Jeong M, Chung JH, Yan P, et al. Integrated analysis of DNA methylation and gene expression reveals specific signaling pathways associated with platinum resistance in ovarian cancer. BMC Med Genet. 2009;2:34. doi:10.1186/1755-8794-2-34.
13. Pulukuri SM, Estes N, Patel J, Rao JS. Demethylation-linked activation of urokinase plasminogen activator is involved in progression of prostate cancer. Cancer Res. 2007;67(3):930–9. doi:10.1158/0008-5472.can-06-2892.
14. Jackson K, Yu MC, Arakawa K, Fiala E, Youn B, Fiegl H, et al. DNA hypomethylation is prevalent even in low-grade breast cancers. Cancer Biol Ther. 2004;3(12):1225–31.
15. Ateeq B, Unterberger A, Szyf M, Rabbani SA. Pharmacological inhibition of DNA methylation induces proinvasive and prometastatic genes in vitro and in vivo. Neoplasia (New York, NY). 2008;10(3):266–78.
16. Denda A, Rao PM, Rajalakshmi S, Sarma DS. 5-azacytidine potentiates initiation induced by carcinogens in rat liver. Carcinogenesis. 1985;6(1):145–6.
17. Qu G, Dubeau L, Narayan A, Yu MC, Ehrlich M. Satellite DNA hypomethylation vs. overall genomic hypomethylation in ovarian epithelial tumors of different malignant potential. Mutat Res. 1999;423(1-2):91–101.
18. Rodriguez J, Vives L, Jorda M, Morales C, Munoz M, Vendrell E, et al. Genome-wide tracking of unmethylated DNA Alu repeats in normal and cancer cells. Nucleic Acids Res. 2008;36(3):770–84. doi:10.1093/nar/gkm1105.
19. Su M, Han D, Boyd-Kirkup J, Yu X, Han JD. Evolution of Alu elements toward enhancers. Cell Rep. 2014;7(2):376–85. doi:10.1016/j.celrep.2014.03.011.
20. Gribben JG. How I treat CLL up front. Blood. 2010;115(2):187–97. doi:10.1182/blood-2009-08-207126.
21. Crespo M, Bosch F, Villamor N, Bellosillo B, Colomer D, Rozman M, et al. ZAP-70 expression as a surrogate for immunoglobulin-variable-region mutations in chronic lymphocytic leukemia. N Engl J Med. 2003;348(18):1764–75. doi:10.1056/NEJMoa023143.
22. Damle RN, Wasil T, Fais F, Ghiotto F, Valetto A, Allen SL, et al. Ig V gene mutation status and CD38 expression as novel prognostic indicators in chronic lymphocytic leukemia. Blood. 1999;94(6):1840–7.
23. Hamblin TJ, Davis Z, Gardiner A, Oscier DG, Stevenson FK. Unmutated Ig V(H) genes are associated with a more aggressive form of chronic lymphocytic leukemia. Blood. 1999;94(6):1848–54.
24. Kanduri M, Cahill N, Goransson H, Enstrom C, Ryan F, Isaksson A, et al. Differential genome-wide array-based methylation profiles in prognostic subsets of chronic lymphocytic leukemia. Blood. 2010;115(2):296–305. doi:10.1182/blood-2009-07-232868.
25. Rush LJ, Raval A, Funchain P, Johnson AJ, Smith L, Lucas DM, et al. Epigenetic profiling in chronic lymphocytic leukemia reveals novel methylation targets. Cancer Res. 2004;64(7):2424–33.
26. Raval A, Tanner SM, Byrd JC, Angerman EB, Perko JD, Chen SS, et al. Downregulation of death-associated protein kinase 1 (DAPK1) in chronic lymphocytic leukemia. Cell. 2007;129(5):879–90. doi:10.1016/j.cell.2007.03.043.
27. Liu TH, Raval A, Chen SS, Matkovic JJ, Byrd JC, Plass C. CpG island methylation and expression of the secreted frizzled-related protein gene family in chronic lymphocytic leukemia. Cancer Res. 2006;66(2):653–8. doi:10.1158/0008-5472.can-05-3712.

28. Chen SS, Claus R, Lucas DM, Yu L, Qian J, Ruppert AS, et al. Silencing of the inhibitor of DNA binding protein 4 (ID4) contributes to the pathogenesis of mouse and human CLL. Blood. 2011;117(3):862–71. doi:10.1182/blood-2010-05-284638.

29. Seeliger B, Wilop S, Osieka R, Galm O, Jost E. CpG island methylation patterns in chronic lymphocytic leukemia. Leuk Lymphoma. 2009;50(3):419–26. doi:10.1080/10428190902756594.

30. Raval A, Lucas DM, Matkovic JJ, Bennett KL, Liyanarachchi S, Young DC, et al. TWIST2 demonstrates differential methylation in immunoglobulin variable heavy chain mutated and unmutated chronic lymphocytic leukemia. J Clin Oncol Off J Am Soc Clin Oncol. 2005;23(17):3877–85. doi:10.1200/jco.2005.02.196.

31. Lipsanen V, Leinonen P, Alhonen L, Janne J. Hypomethylation of ornithine decarboxylase gene and erb-A1 oncogene in human chronic lymphatic leukemia. Blood. 1988;72(6):2042–4.

32. Hanada M, Delia D, Aiello A, Stadtmauer E, Reed JC. bcl-2 gene hypomethylation and high-level expression in B-cell chronic lymphocytic leukemia. Blood. 1993;82(6):1820–8.

33. Ernst J, Kheradpour P, Mikkelsen TS, Shoresh N, Ward LD, Epstein CB, et al. Mapping and analysis of chromatin state dynamics in nine human cell types. Nature. 2011;473(7345):43–9. doi:10.1038/nature09906.

34. Ashburner M, Ball CA, Blake JA, Botstein D, Butler H, Cherry JM, et al. Gene ontology: tool for the unification of biology. The Gene Ontology Consortium. Nat Genet. 2000;25(1):25–9. doi:10.1038/75556.

35. Kanehisa M, Goto S, Furumichi M, Tanabe M, Hirakawa M. KEGG for representation and analysis of molecular networks involving diseases and drugs. Nucleic Acids Res. 2010;38(Database issue):D355–60. doi:10.1093/nar/gkp896.

36. Birney E, Stamatoyannopoulos JA, Dutta A, Guigo R, Gingeras TR, Margulies EH, et al. Identification and analysis of functional elements in 1 % of the human genome by the ENCODE pilot project. Nature. 2007;447(7146):799–816. doi:10.1038/nature05874.

37. Filion GJ, Zhenilo S, Salozhin S, Yamada D, Prokhortchouk E, Defossez PA. A family of human zinc finger proteins that bind methylated DNA and repress transcription. Mol Cell Biol. 2006;26(1):169–81. doi:10.1128/mcb.26.1.169-181.2006.

38. Hogart A, Lichtenberg J, Ajay SS, Anderson S, Margulies EH, Bodine DM. Genome-wide DNA methylation profiles in hematopoietic stem and progenitor cells reveal overrepresentation of ETS transcription factor binding sites. Genome Res. 2012;22(8):1407–18. doi:10.1101/gr.132878.111.

39. Miller DM, Thomas SD, Islam A, Muench D, Sedoris K. c-Myc and cancer metabolism. Clin Cancer Res. 2012;18(20):5546–53. doi:10.1158/1078-0432.ccr-12-0977.

40. Langfelder P, Horvath S. WGCNA: an R package for weighted correlation network analysis. BMC Bioinf. 2008;9:559. doi:10.1186/1471-2105-9-559.

41. Chiorazzi N, Ferrarini M. B cell chronic lymphocytic leukemia: lessons learned from studies of the B cell antigen receptor. Annu Rev Immunol. 2003;21:841–94. doi:10.1146/annurev.immunol.21.120601.141018.

42. Hagman J, Ramirez J, Lukin K. B lymphocyte lineage specification, commitment and epigenetic control of transcription by early B cell factor 1. Curr Top Microbiol Immunol. 2012;356:17–38. doi:10.1007/82_2011_139.

43. Robertson AG, Bilenky M, Tam A, Zhao Y, Zeng T, Thiessen N, et al. Genome-wide relationship between histone H3 lysine 4 mono- and tri-methylation and transcription factor binding. Genome Res. 2008;18(12):1906–17. doi:10.1101/gr.078519.108.

44. Hazan RB, Qiao R, Keren R, Badano I, Suyama K. Cadherin switch in tumor progression. Ann N Y Acad Sci. 2004;1014:155–63.

45. Tsurimoto T, Shinozaki A, Yano M, Seki M, Enomoto T. Human Werner helicase interacting protein 1 (WRNIP1) functions as a novel modulator for DNA polymerase delta. Genes to cells : devoted to molecular & cellular mechanisms. 2005;10(1):13–22. doi:10.1111/j.1365-2443.2004.00812.x.

46. Yoon HG, Chan DW, Huang ZQ, Li J, Fondell JD, Qin J, et al. Purification and functional characterization of the human N-CoR complex: the roles of HDAC3, TBL1 and TBLR1. The EMBO journal. 2003;22(6):1336–46. doi:10.1093/emboj/cdg120.

47. Kashatus D, Cogswell P, Baldwin AS. Expression of the Bcl-3 proto-oncogene suppresses p53 activation. Genes Dev. 2006;20(2):225–35. doi:10.1101/gad.1352206.

48. Massoumi R, Chmielarska K, Hennecke K, Pfeifer A, Fassler R. Cyld inhibits tumor cell proliferation by blocking Bcl-3-dependent NF-kappaB signaling. Cell. 2006;125(4):665–77. doi:10.1016/j.cell.2006.03.041.

49. Fu H, Maunakea AK, Martin MM, Huang L, Zhang Y, Ryan M, et al. Methylation of histone H3 on lysine 79 associates with a group of

replication origins and helps limit DNA replication once per cell cycle. PLoS Genet. 2013;9(6), e1003542. doi:10.1371/journal.pgen.1003542.

50. Sims 3rd RJ, Reinberg D. Processing the H3K36me3 signature. Nat Genet. 2009;41(3):270–1. doi:10.1038/ng0309-270.

51. Cao R, Wang L, Wang H, Xia L, Erdjument-Bromage H, Tempst P, et al. Role of histone H3 lysine 27 methylation in Polycomb-group silencing. Science. 2002;298(5595):1039–43. doi:10.1126/science.1076997.

52. Reddington JP, Perricone SM, Nestor CE, Reichmann J, Youngson NA, Suzuki M, et al. Redistribution of H3K27me3 upon DNA hypomethylation results in de-repression of Polycomb target genes. Genome Biol. 2013;14(3):R25. doi:10.1186/gb-2013-14-3-r25.

53. Ng SY, Yoshida T, Zhang J, Georgopoulos K. Genome-wide lineage-specific transcriptional networks underscore Ikaros-dependent lymphoid priming in hematopoietic stem cells. Immunity. 2009;30(4):493–507. doi:10.1016/j.immuni.2009.01.014.

54. Fujita T, Nolan GP, Liou HC, Scott ML, Baltimore D. The candidate proto-oncogene bcl-3 encodes a transcriptional coactivator that activates through NF-kappa B p50 homodimers. Genes Dev. 1993;7(7B):1354–63.

55. Krueger F, Andrews SR. Bismark: a flexible aligner and methylation caller for Bisulfite-Seq applications. Bioinformatics (Oxford, England). 2011;27(11):1571–2. doi:10.1093/bioinformatics/btr167.

56. Trapnell C, Williams BA, Pertea G, Mortazavi A, Kwan G, van Baren MJ, et al. Transcript assembly and quantification by RNA-Seq reveals unannotated transcripts and isoform switching during cell differentiation. Nat Biotechnol. 2010;28(5):511–5. doi:10.1038/nbt.1621.

57. Trapnell C, Hendrickson DG, Sauvageau M, Goff L, Rinn JL, Pachter L. Differential analysis of gene regulation at transcript resolution with RNA-seq. Nat Biotechnol. 2013;31(1):46–53. doi:10.1038/nbt.2450.

58. Akalin A, Kormaksson M, Li S, Garrett-Bakelman FE, Figueroa ME, Melnick A, et al. methylKit: a comprehensive R package for the analysis of genome-wide DNA methylation profiles. Genome Biol. 2012;13(10):R87. doi:10.1186/gb-2012-13-10-r87.

59. Falcon S, Gentleman R. Using GOstats to test gene lists for GO term association. Bioinformatics (Oxford, England). 2007;23(2):257–8. doi:10.1093/bioinformatics/btl567.

60. Stelzer G, Inger A, Olender T, Iny-Stein T, Dalah I, Harel A, et al. GeneDecks: paralog hunting and gene-set distillation with GeneCards annotation. OMICS. 2009;13(6):477–87. doi:10.1089/omi.2009.0069.

61. Dozmorov MG, Cara LR, Giles CB, Wren JD. GenomeRunner: automating genome exploration. Bioinformatics (Oxford, England). 2012;28(3):419–20. doi:10.1093/bioinformatics/btr666.

62. Heinz S, Benner C, Spann N, Bertolino E, Lin YC, Laslo P, et al. Simple combinations of lineage-determining transcription factors prime cis-regulatory elements required for macrophage and B cell identities. Mol Cell. 2010;38(4):576–89. doi:10.1016/j.molcel.2010.05.004.

63. Langfelder P, Luo R, Oldham MC, Horvath S. Is my network module preserved and reproducible? PLoS Comput Biol. 2011;7(1), e1001057. doi:10.1371/journal.pcbi.1001057.

2-deoxy-2-[18]fluoro-D-glucose PET/CT (18FDG PET/CT) may not be a viable biomarker in Pompe disease

U. Plöckinger[1]* , V. Prasad[2,3], A. Ziagaki[1], N. Tiling[1] and A. Poellinger[4]

Abstract

Background: Pompe disease (PD) is an autosomal recessive, lysosomal storage disease due to a mutation of the acid α-glucosidase (*GAA*) gene. In adult patients, PD is characterized by slowly progressive limb-girdle and trunk myopathy and restrictive respiratory insufficiency. Enzyme replacement therapy (ERT) is available, improving or stabilizing muscle-function in some and slowing deterioration in other patients. Unfortunately, there is no biomarker available to indicate therapeutic efficacy and/or disease activity. Whole body MRI depicts all skeletal muscles demonstrating foci of atrophic muscles, i.e., late and irreversible pathological changes. Any method indicating the localizations of increased muscle glycogen storage, muscle inflammation and/or degradation could possibly help identifying newly afflicted tissue and may be of prognostic value. We therefore investigated 2-deoxy-2-[18]fluoro-D-glucose (FDG) PET, a biomarker for glucose-metabolism, as a tool to evaluate disease activity and prognosis in PD.

Methods: In a pilot study, we investigated four patients by FDG dynamic PET/CT while on ERT. One patient had FDG-PET/CT twice, before and after 12 months on ERT. Dynamic FDG-PET/CT quantifies the metabolic rate of glucose utilisation in mg/ml/min. MRI was performed in parallel with pelvic and thigh muscles semi-quantitatively scored for atrophy and disease-activity.

Results: None of the muscles analysed showed a focally increased FDG-uptake. Thus, quantification of muscle glucose metabolism could not be calculated. However, increased FDG-uptake, i.e., increased glucose utilisation, was observed in the respiratory muscles of one patient with severe, restrictive respiratory failure. In contrast, specific MRI sequences showed oedematous as well as atrophic muscle areas in PD.

Conclusions: Our pilot study demonstrates that FDG-uptake does not correlate with glycogen storage in vivo. In contrast, MRI is an excellent tool to demonstrate the extent of muscle involvement. Specific MRI sequences may even demonstrate early changes possibly allowing prognostic predictions or localization of early stages of PD.

Keywords: Pompe disease, 2-deoxy-2-[18]fluoro-D-glucose PET/CT, Biomarker, MRI

Background

Pompe disease (OMIM 232300) or glycogenosis type 2 is a lysosomal storage disease characterized by a mutation of the acid α-glucosidase (*GAA*) gene. Pompe disease (PD) is inherited in an autosomal recessive mode. Manifestations of PD in adult patients are a myopathy of limb-girdle and trunk muscles, with restrictive respiratory insufficiency as a possible complication. The disease is chronic and slowly progressive with some patients becoming wheel-chair-bound and respirator-dependent. The available enzyme replacement therapy effectively improves or stabilizes muscle function in some and slows deterioration of the disease in other patients [1, 2].

The phenotype/genotype correlation is poor and many patients harbour private mutations. Thus, genotyping is unable to predict the clinical course of an individual patient [3]. Clinical monitoring, i.e., follow-up of the individual patient, relies mainly either on semi-quantitative analysis of muscle function, like 6-min walk test, quick

* Correspondence: Ursula.Ploeckinger@charite.de
[1]Kompetenzzentrum Seltene Stoffwechselkrankheiten, Interdisziplinäres Stoffwechsel-Centrum: Endokrinologie, Diabetes und Stoffwechsel, Charité Universitätsmedizin Berlin, Augustenburger Platz 1, Campus Virchow-Klinikum, 13352 Berlin, Germany
Full list of author information is available at the end of the article

motor function test [4] or magnetic resonance tomographic imaging (MRI) of limb-girdle, paravertebral and thighs musculature and sometimes proximal arm musculature, or in rare cases, repeated muscle biopsies. Respiratory function is evaluated by lung function testing [forced expiratory vital capacity (FVC) and vital capacity (VC)], both while seated and supine. However, these clinical evaluations are flawed by a high intra- and inter-observer variation, as is the case for functional testing [6-min walk test [5, 6] and quick motor function test [4]. In addition, the test-results vary depending on the patient's sex, age and day-to-day state of health. A reliable positive predictive result is therefore difficult to achieve and intra-individual variability is high. Due to the lack of more sensitive and accurate measurements, the 6-min walk test is defined as the gold-standard and has been used in clinical studies for the evaluation of motor function in adult patients with PD [3, 7].

Biochemical parameters, i.e., muscle enzymes like aspartate aminotransferase/glutamat-pyruvat-transaminase (AST/GOT), alanine aminotransferase/glutamat-oxalacetat-transaminase (ALT/GPT), creatinine-kinase (CK) or lactate dehydrogenase (LDH) are non-specifically increased in PD and fail to correlate with disease severity or activity. The glucose tetra-saccharide, Glcalpha1-6Glcalpha1-4glcalpha1-4Glc (Glc(4)), is a glycogen-derived limit dextrin that correlates with the extent of glycogen accumulation in skeletal muscle. A retrospective analysis of clinical records of 208 patients evaluated for PD by this approach showed Glc(4) having 94% sensitivity and 84% specificity for the diagnosis of PD. However, while indicating the overall disease burden, Glc(4) provided no information on the location and distribution of excess glycogen accumulation [8]. In addition Glc(4) excretion in adult-onset PD is low and ERT-induced declines may be very small [8].

MRI imaging demonstrates the distribution pattern of muscular atrophy, compensatory muscular hypertrophy and vacuolised muscle fibres. A study with 34 adult-onset PD patients compared whole body muscle MRI using T1w and 3-point Dixon imaging of thighs and the lower trunk region to a wide range of functional scales. This comparison demonstrated a strong correlation between muscle strength, muscle functional scales and the degree of muscle fatty replacement in muscle MRI. In addition, muscle MRI detected mild degree of fatty replacement in para-spinal muscles in pre-symptomatic patients [9]. Others used either quantitative proton-density fat-fraction (PDFF) whole-body MRI or quantitative MRI in late-onset PD and compared the results with manual muscle testing. According to their results, MRI was more sensitive than physical examination for detection of abnormalities in multiple muscle groups [10, 11]. Yet, the rather slow disease progression in PD is one difficulty for MRI monitoring of muscles changes. A retrospective study by Carlier et al. using quantitative MRI demonstrated muscle fatty infiltration increase on average by 0.9%/year, with the hamstring and adductor muscles showing the fastest degradation. Muscle water T2 mapping revealed that 32% of all muscles had abnormally high T2 in at least one of two successive examinations. When muscle water T2 was abnormal, fatty degenerative changes increased by 0.61%/year. Enzyme replacement therapy resulted in 0.68%/year slow-down of the muscle fatty infiltration, in both muscles with normal and high T2s [12]. Unfortunately, most MRI findings all indicate a rather late event in the course of the disease, i.e., muscle atrophy. Furthermore, an overall slow-down of muscle fatty infiltration of 0.68%/year may not allow an individual prognosis, neither on the natural course of the disease nor on the effectiveness of enzyme replacement therapy. In addition, MRI imaging poses a burden on patients with claustrophobia, is difficult to perform in patients with respiratory insufficiency in the supine position and can be painful due to the long duration of laying still on a hard bench.

Muscle biopsies using ultrastructural examination of the tissue demonstrated reduced lysosomal glycogen after 6 months of ERT, consistent with stabilization of the disease that was not represented in the MRI images acquired parallel to the biopsies [13]. However, muscle biopsies are fraught due to (i) changing tissue localization at repeated biopsies and (ii) the invasiveness of the procedure.

Thus, to date, none of the aforementioned methods allow for a simple, reproducible measurement of disease activity, localization of active disease and monitoring of therapeutic efficacy.

Glucose and/or FDG uptake by the cell is a receptor-mediated process. Glucose binds to the membrane bound glucose-transporter (GLUT), as does FDG. The receptor-ligand complex is taken up into the cell by endocytosis. There the receptor separates from its substrate in early endosomes and is passed on to recycling endosomes and, subsequently, stored in the GLUT-containing vesicular compartment. Once inside the cell, FDG is phosphorylated to FDG-6P, which cannot enter the glycolytic pathways and is therefore trapped within the cell (Fig. 1).

The mutation of acid α-glucosidase (GAA) gene leads to reduced concentration/activity of the enzyme. This results in a defective metabolism of lysosomal glycogen with tissue-specific glycogen accumulation. We hypothesized that the uptake of 2-deoxy-2-[18]fluoro-D-glucose should lead to an accumulation of the labelled glucose molecule in cells with pathological glycogen storage. The extent of accumulation would indicate the extent of glycogen storage, correlating with disease activity and possible therapeutic efficacy. The method would therefore allow for early detection of active foci of glycogen deposits, well before fat accumulation or muscle atrophy occurs.

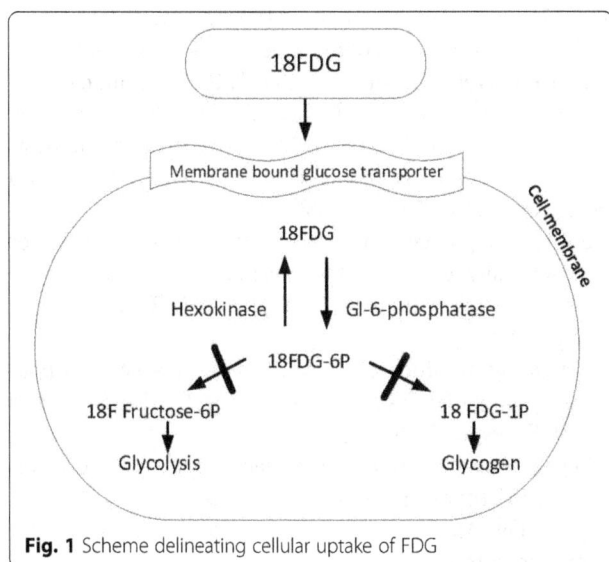

Fig. 1 Scheme delineating cellular uptake of FDG

We therefore undertook an explorative study investigating the usefulness of dynamic FDG-PET as an indicator of disease activity in late-onset PD and compared these results to routinely performed quantitative whole-body muscle MRI.

Methods

We performed five FDG dynamic PET/CTs in four patients with late onset PD. In one patient, FDG-PET/CT was performed twice, before and 1 year after the initiation of ERT, while in all other patients FDG-PET/CT took place during ongoing ERT. Patient characteristics are given in Table 1.

FDG-PET Acquisition Dynamic FDG-PET allows to quantify the metabolic rate of utilisation of glucose in mg/ml/min. Patients were kept fasting for more than 6 h, and serum glucose was measured prior to the injection of FDG. Patients were given 350 MBq of FDG as slow bolus over 20 s, and scanning was performed with the patients supine. Dynamic images were acquired over 60 min in list-mode immediately after the injection of

the tracer. Images were reconstructed as follows: 3×20 s, 8×30 s, 5×1 min, 5×2 min, 4×5 min and 2×10 min. After the dynamic images, whole body images were acquired from base of skull to mid-thigh with 1.5 min/bed position. Lean body mass maximum standardized uptake value (SUVmax) was calculated for involved muscles; region of interest was drawn on the muscles showing hyperintensity on MRI. In addition, background activity was measured on the subcutaneous fat at the level of gluteus muscle as well as over the left ventricular cavity. For correction of the PET images, we used a CT attenuation correction map.

MRI: standard T1w spin echo (SE) of the pelvis and thigh muscles was performed (TR = 472 ms, TE = 18 ms) and muscle fatty degenerative changes were scored according to a 5-grade modified Mercuri score (grade 0: normal, grade1: < 25%; grade 2: > 25% and < 50%; grade 3: > 50% and < 75%; grade 4: > 75%). Short TI inversion recovery (STIR) sequences of the same body regions were acquired with TR = 3240 ms, TE = 42 ms. Finally, after administration of 0.1 mmol/kg of a gadolinium-based contrast agent (Gadovist; Bayer Healthcare), a T1w fat-sat sequence was acquired (TR = 709 ms, TE = 18 ms). All MR scans were acquired axially. For STIR and T1w fat-sat contrast-enhanced (CE) images hyperintensities were again scored according to a 5-grade modified Mercuri score (grade 0: no hyperintensities, grade 1: mild; grade 2: moderate; grade 3: intermediate; grade 4: severe amount of hyperintensities). All MRIs were performed within 6 months of the FDG-PET. An experienced radiologist (AP) analysed the MRI scans. Fatty infiltration as a marker for muscular atrophy was scored based on T1w scans. Hyperintensities in T1w FS CE and STIR scans show hypervascularisation or leakage of contrast material and oedema, respectively. The following pelvic and thigh muscles were scored: autochthonous back muscle, iliopsoas, gluteus maximus, medius and minimus (lateral, mid, medial) quadriceps femoris, sartorius, obturator and pectineus. Activity and atrophy on MRI were scored as follows: from 0 to 4 (0 = no atrophy; 1 = minimal, 2 = moderate, 4 =

Table 1 Patients characteristics

Patient number	1	2	3	4
Age (years)	51	59	27	45
Years of ERT	1.5	6.5	7	0
Sex	M	M	M	M
Age at diagnosis (years)	50	45	20	44
Mutation	c.(336-13 T > G); (1927G > A)	IVC-45 T > G; 536bpDel (IVS16 + 102_IVS17 + 31)	c.32-13 T > G; c.1128_1129delinsC	c-32-13 T > G; c.2214G > A
6-min walk test (m)	484	204	201	510
Wheelchair bound	No	No	No	No
Respiratory failure	Yes	Yes	Yes	No

[a]*SD* standard deviation

severe). The FDG-uptake in the abovementioned muscles was visually analysed. An example for the analysis of MRI images is given in Fig. 2.

Statistics

Statistical analysis was performed using STATISTICA 6.0 and IBM SPSS Statistics (IBM, Armonk, NY), Version 21. Data were calculated as median and interquartile range, for correlation Spearman's coefficient of correlation was used. A p value < 0.05 was considered significant.

Results

Four male patients (median age 48, interquartile range 36–55 years) participated in this explorative study. All patients were on ERT. One patient was investigated twice, before and after 1 year on ERT. All the patients demonstrated clinical improvement compared to before ERT and had either a stable (patients AB, FR) or slowly progressive (patients GH, SK) course of their disease. Details of the mutation and further clinical characteristics are indicated in Table 1. Classification [14] of disease severity of was moderate (one patient) and severe (three patients).

MRI fatty infiltration in T1w images as a sign for muscular atrophy was found in all patients to varying degrees and localizations (Table 2) and correlated well with the clinical status of the patients. For all four patients, the most atrophic muscles were the intrinsic back muscles (autochthonous back muscles) and the gluteus muscles, especially the gluteus minimus. Muscles with a high degree of atrophy (score = 4) showed only low signal-intensity in STIR and T1w FS CE images (score = 0–1; score = 2 only in one case and muscle). When there was no evidence of muscular atrophy (T1w score = 0), the STIR and T1w FS CE images mostly also scored 0 in these locations. However, in two patients there were muscles without atrophic changes but with elevated STIR and T1w FS CE values. Highest score for both STIR and T1w FS CE were observed when muscular atrophy scores were between 1 and 3 (Fig. 3). Atrophy scores 0–2 positively correlated with T1w and STIR (Spearman's R: 0.693, $p < 0.05$)

and T1w and T1w FS CE values (Spearman's R: 0.644, $p <$ 0.05). In contrast, atrophy scores 2-4 demonstrated a negative correlation for T1w and STIR (Spearman's R: – 0.426, $p < 0.05$) and for T1w and T1w FS CE, respectively (Spearman's R: – 0.334, $p < 0.05$). There was a strong positive correlation between STIR and T1w FS CE values (Spearman's R: 0.854, $p < 0.05$).

For all sequences, measured alterations were rather symmetrically distributed (Spearman's R for atrophy = 0.875, $p < 0.05$; activity = 0.829 $p < 0.05$; T1w FS CE = 0.92 $p < 0.05$).

Assuming an alpha error of 0.05, we receive an a posteriori power of 1.000, 0.987 and 0.958 for T1, STIR and T1FSCE, respectively.

Repeated MRI in one patient demonstrated a reduction of the MRI scores at the tensor fasciae latae muscle after 1 year (Fig. 4). No other muscle group showed similar improvements.

FDG-PET/CT. None of the muscles and/or regions of muscles demonstrating hyperintensity on MRI showed a quantifiable focally increased FDG metabolism. Nor did we detect increased FDG-metabolism in trunk or thigh muscles. Thus, dynamic PET quantification of glucose metabolism in muscles could not be calculated. Figure 5 gives an example of the results of FDG-PET.

FDG-PET was positive in one patient with respiratory failure. We observed a high uptake of FDG in the respiratory muscles. This clearly demonstrates the increased glucose metabolism due to the high muscle workload in a patient with restrictive respiratory insufficiency (Fig. 5).

Discussion

Our pilot study confirms the usefulness of MRI to delineate affected muscles in PD [9, 12, 14–16]. The pattern of involvement was similar in patients with and without ERT [14] and disease severity and duration were correlated to quantitative MRI findings.

We analysed 26 different muscle regions of the pelvis and thighs in four different patients with late onset PD. Within individual patients, there were considerable differences in

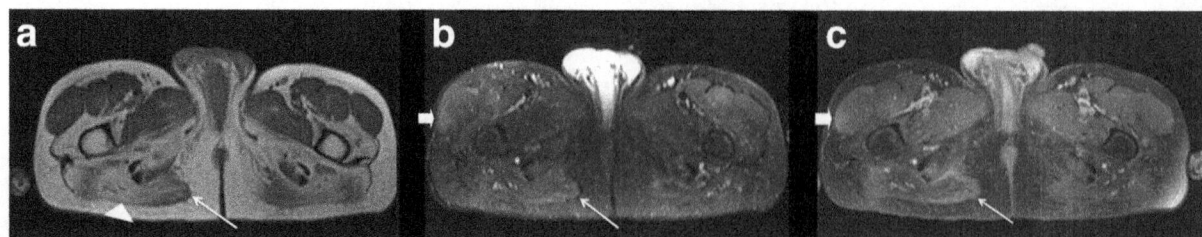

Fig. 2 MR scans of a Pompe patient at the level just below the pelvic floor. There are different stages of muscular inflammation, or atrophy respectively, visible: T1w images show fatty atrophy in various muscles, pronounced in the middle part of the gluteus maximus (**a**, arrow head). The medial part of the gluteus maximus shows only beginning atrophy at T1w (**a**, arrow) together with high signal in the STIR images (**b**). T1w FS scans also display high signal after gadolinium administration (**c**). While the tensor fasciae latae muscle (wide arrow) seems to be unaffected in the T1w images, there is high signal on STIR and T1w FS scans suggesting early changes

Table 2 Semi-quantitative results of MRI evaluation for each muscle group in Pompe disease

Muscle	T1w (Median)	T1w (IQR[a])	STIR (Median)	STIR (IQR[a])	T1 FS CE (Median)	T1 FS CE (IQR[a])
Intrinsic back muscles (lower back)	3.0	3.0–3.0	0.0	0.0–3.0	0.0	0.0–3.0
Iliopsoas	2.0	0.5–3.5	1.0	0.0–2.5	1.5	0.0–2.5
Gluteus maximus (lateral)	2.0	0.5–4.0	1.0	0.0–2.0	1.5	0.5–2.0
Gluteus maximus (center)	0.0	0.0–1.5	0.0	0.0–1.5	0.0	0.0–1.5
Gluteus maximus (medial)	1.5	0.0–3.0	1.0	0.0–2.0	1.0	0.0–2.5
Gluteus medius (ventral)	2.0	1.0–3.5	1.5	1.0–2.0	2.0	1.0–3.5
Gluteus medius (dorsal)	3.5	1.5–4.0	1.0	0.0–1.5	0.5	0.0–1.5
Gluteus minimus (ventral)	4.0	3.5–4.0	0.5	0.0–1.5	0.5	0.0–1.5
Gluteus minimus (dorsal)	4.0	3.5–4.0	0.5	0.0–1.5	0.5	0.0–1.5
Rectus femoris	0.0	0.0–0.0	0.0	0.0–0.0	0.0	0.0–0.0
Sartorius	0.0	0.0–0.0	0.0	0.0–0.0	0.0	0.0–0.0
Obturator ext.	1.0	0.5–2.0	0.0	0.0–0.5	0.0	0.0–0.5
Pectineus	0.0	0.0–2.5	0.0	0.0–0.0	0.0	0.0–0.0

[a]Interquartile range

T1 images were scored according to a 5-grade score (grade 0: normal, grade 1: < 25%; grade 2: > 25% and < 50%; grade 3: > 50% and < 75%; grade 4: > 75%). STIR and T1w fat-sat contrast-enhanced (CE) images were scored according to a 5-grade score (grade 0: no hyperintensities, grade1: mild; grade 2: moderate; grade 3: intermediate; grade 4: severe amount of hyperintensities)

muscular atrophy of different muscles ranging from no visible atrophy (score = 0) to severe atrophy (score = 4) with the intrinsic back muscles and the gluteus minimus muscle displaying the highest scores of atrophy. We found no observable atrophy in the quadriceps femoris (rectus femoris) and sartorius muscle. Why these muscles display minor damage while others are heavily involved is a matter of debate and was also observed in earlier studies [13, 15]. Van

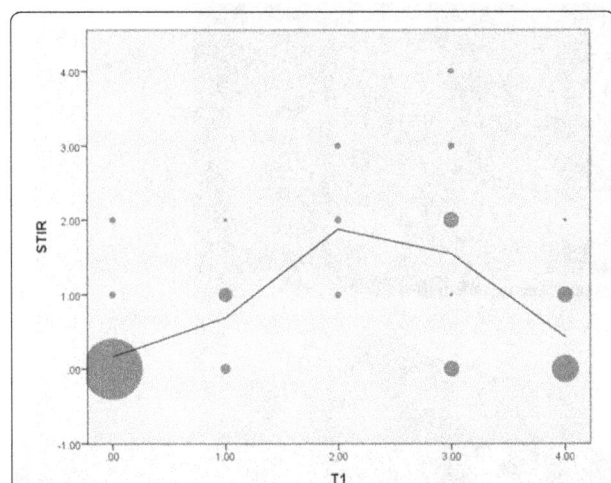

Fig. 3 Scatterplot between the semi-quantitative assessment of T1 (atrophy) and STIR (muscle oedema): the size of the circle displays the number of muscle regions. Most muscle regions showed no atrophy (T1 = 0) and no oedema (STIR = 0). As atrophy increases so does muscular oedema, but only up to a score of T1 = 2. From there, further atrophy is associated with less oedema. Of note, some muscles showing no atrophy (T1 = 0) already exhibited oedema, possibly an early sign of affected muscle

der Ploeg et al. [13] suggests that muscle groups, like the gluteus muscles and intrinsic back muscles, performing continuous or repetitive contraction are more prone to earlier damage than muscles that are subject to relatively intermittent contraction.

STIR images revealing muscular oedema were only partly in line with the results of the T1w images showing atrophy: when muscular atrophy was not visible (score = 0) in most of the muscles analysed there was also no oedema. Oedematous changes increased with increasing atrophy, but only up to an atrophy score of 2–3 (correlation of Spearman's R: 0.693). When atrophy was more prevalent (score 4) oedematous changes decreased (Spearman's R: − 0.426). None of the T1w changes with a score of 4 showed an oedema score higher than 2. As a rule, similar changes as for the STIR images were noted for the T1w FS CE images in most of the muscles analysed.

The varying degree of atrophy and oedema/inflammation in different muscles in a given individual with PD—besides the already mentioned predilection of certain muscles—indicates a temporal heterogeneity of muscular changes. We hypothesize that disease manifestation in a muscle initially demonstrates only little atrophy but an increasing amount of oedema and inflammatory changes as reflected by increased STIR and T1w FS CE values. Of note, in some muscles, oedematous and inflammatory changes were visible in muscles showing no atrophy at all, consistent with results by van der Ploeg et al. [13].

After this initial stage, atrophic, oedematous and inflammatory changes seem to develop rather synchronously up to the point when inflammation and oedema are less visible, but atrophy further increases. Finally, at

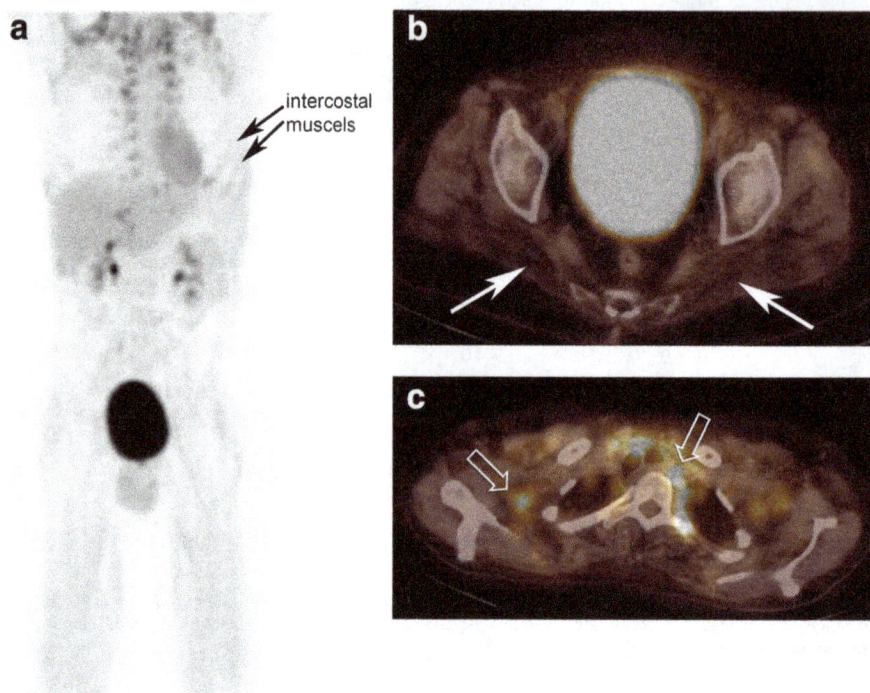

Fig. 4 a Maximum intensity projection image showing the paravertebral brown fat as well as intercostal muscle. **b** Upper panel showing fused FDG PET/CT image with gluteus muscle atrophy and almost no FDG-uptake (white arrows). **c** Lower panel showing paravertebral and axillary brown fat (open arrows)

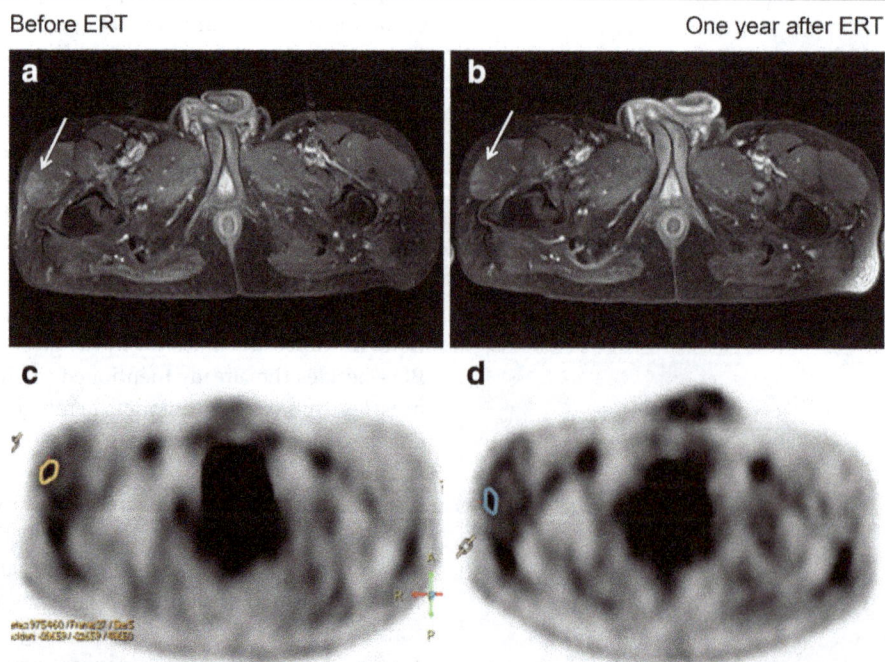

Fig. 5 MRI (**a**, **b**) and FDG PET (**c**, **d**) before and after 1 year of ERT. MRI shows slight improvement, i.e., less hyperintensity of the tensor fasciae latae muscle (arrow) in the T1w sequence after gadolinium administration 1 year after ERT. FDG-PET show no significantly different tracer uptake in the region of interest (orange and blue lines) pre- and post-therapy

the end-stage of this process affected muscles display fatty infiltration as a result of atrophy but no more inflammation or oedema.

This study is the first study that used gadolinium-enhanced MR imaging for the evaluation of non-cardiac muscle involvement in late-onset PD patients. Gadolinium-based studies have shown benefits in other forms of myositis for differentiation and staging [17]. In the present study, we found a strong positive correlation between STIR and T1 FS CE images ($R = 0.854$). However, there was one significant difference between the STIR and T1 FS CE images, with the gadolinium-based T1 images showing higher values on the modified Mercuri scale. This may indicate that T1 FS CE might be more sensitive to early muscle changes in late-onset PD patients. If gadolinium studies are really necessary for early detection needs to be evaluated in further studies, especially in light of the problem of gadolinium deposition that was first described in 2014 [18].

Due to MRI limitations (claustrophobia, non-MRI compatible devices, severe respiratory disease) [10], alternative approaches like bio-impedance measurement to assess the relative proportions of fatty and muscle tissue may give a correlation between the degree of replacement of the muscle tissue with fatty tissue and the severity of the disease evaluated clinically [19], diagnosing the late phase of the disease.

In conclusion, MRI is an excellent tool to demonstrate the extent of muscle involvement in late-onset PD. MRI may even pick up early, i.e., oedematous stages of the disease. Focusing on these early signs may allow more specific training early on to set against subsequent muscular atrophy. Whether these early changes may allow prognostic predictions has yet to be demonstrated.

In well-prepared (after 6-h fast, serum glucose < 150 mg/dl and adequate rest prior to image acquisition) non-PD patients no or only faint muscular FDG uptake can be observed. We hypothesized that in PD FDG-PET/CT would delineate increased accumulation of glucose into glycogen-enriched depots and thus diagnose the early phases of the disease. In α-glucosidase-deficient muscles lysosomal glycogen breakdown and thus glucose and energy production are reduced. To compensate for reduced glucose production, increased glucose and in analogy FDG uptake may be an option in these cells. In α-glucosidase-deficient muscles intra-cytoplasmatic GLUT4 expression is increased in damaged and normal in unafflicted muscle fibres [20]. We hypothesized that this increased GLUT4 expression may correlate with an increased glucose and thus an increased FDG uptake as well.

This information may then translate in improved local physiotherapy and/or anti-inflammatory treatment. Unfortunately, no focally increased FDG accumulation in relation or unrelated to MRI-signal changes could be demonstrated. Thus, dynamic PET quantification of glycogen deposition in muscles could not be calculated. There might be multiple explanations for this result. Nutritional status, i.e., fasting or post-prandial application of the tracer may be an issue. We injected FDG in fasting patients and thus glycolysis may have prevailed glycogenesis. This is in line with our observation of an increased uptake in the respiratory muscles in the patient with severe restrictive respiratory failure. Due to the high workload of respiratory muscles glucose metabolism was increased as it was visualized in the FDG PET/CT. Again, this would indicate a rather late state of the disease, as the increased metabolic needs are correlated with a significantly increased workload on the few remaining/surviving muscles. On the other hand, with the patient supine, the energy requirement of all other muscles was low and therefore no increased glucose metabolism could be observed.

In addition, glucose uptake via GLUT4 occurs either post-prandially insulin-stimulated or during exercise [21]. However, all patients were investigated after an overnight resting phase without increased muscular energy needs. Whether post-exercise FDG may have given different results, remains to be investigated.

Alternatively, deposition of the tracer into glycogen may not have taken place at all. Glycogen is synthesized from the activated glucose-donor, uridine diphosphate glucose (UDP-glucose), catalysed by glycogen synthase, the key regulatory enzyme in glycogenesis. To be incorporated into glycogen, FDG has to be modified by glucose-6-phosphate isomerase which catalyses the second step during glycolysis. It has been suggested that the substitution of the C-2 hydroxyl moiety by ^{18}F prevents this process [22]. Subsequently, FDG could possibly not be integrated into glycogen. A new tracer, 18F-N-(methyl-(2-fluoroethyl)-1H-[1,2,3]triazole-4-yl) glucosamine (^{18}F-NFTG), recently developed, may be a more effective biomarker in PD. So far, 18F-NFTG PET has been used in animal tumour models to visualize tumours of the upper thorax where the rate of glycogen synthesis is cell-cycle regulated and enhanced during the non-proliferating stage of cancer cells [22]. Whether the myopathy of PD is a feasible target for integrating this new tracer for demonstrating early glycogen accumulation remains to be demonstrated.

Conclusions

In conclusion, MRI delineated the localisation and extent of muscle atrophy in all patients. Changes in the STIR and gadolinium-based T1w sequences probably show the activity of the disease and can serve as earlier markers in the disease process than late changes revealed by fatty infiltration of atrophic muscles as measured by T1-weighted sequences.

FDG PET/CT did not demonstrate increased uptake in glycogen, neither in the early nor late phase of the tracer accumulation. A positive signal was detected by FDG PET/CT in the patient with respiratory failure. Due to the increased respiratory muscle workload, glucose utilisation and thus FDG-uptake was increased as well.

Abbreviations

^{18}F: ^{18}Fluoro; ^{18}F-NFTG: 18F-N-(methyl-(2-fluoroethyl)-1H-[1,2,3]triazole-4-yl) glucosamine; CE: Contrast enhanced; CK: Creatinine kinase; CT: Computer tomography; ERT: Enzyme replacement therapy; FDG: 2-deoxy-2-[18]fluoro-D-glucose; FVC: Forced expiratory vital capacity; *GAA*: Acid α-glucosidase gene; Glc(4): Glcalpha1-6Glcalpha1-4glcalpha1-4Glc; GOT: Glutamat-Oxalacetet-Transaminase; GPT: Glutamat-Pyruvat-Transaminase; GS: Glycogen synthase; LDH: Lactate dehydrogenase; MBq: Megabecquerel; MRI: Magnetic resonance imaging; OMIM: Online Mendelian Inheritance in Man; PD: Pompe disease; PDFF: Proton-density fat-fraction; PET: Positron emission tomography; SD: Standard deviation; SE: Spin echo; STIR: Short TI inversion recovery; T1: T1-weighted image; TE: Echo time; TI: Inversion time; TR: Repetition time; VC: Vital capacity; Years: Years

Acknowledgements
Not applicable.

Funding
The investigation was funded by an unrestricted grant from Sanofi Genzyme to Ursula Plöckinger. Sanofi Genzyme was not involved in the design of the study, collection, analysis and interpretation of data or in writing the manuscript.

Authors' contributions
UP conceived the study in cooperation with VP and AP. UP cared for the patients and drafted the manuscript with the technical details concerning FDG-PET/CT and MRI written by VP and AP, respectively. VP was responsible for the implementation and interpretation of the FDG-PET/CT, AP was responsible for the implementation and interpretation of the MRIs. NT collected the clinical details from the patients' files. AZ was responsible for the legal aspects of the study, critically read the manuscript and helped with the revised version. All authors read and approved the final manuscript.

Competing interests
Ursula Plöckinger was the recipient of an unrestricted grant by Genzyme, Germany, received speaker honorarium from Sanofi Genzyme, Germany; BioMarin Germany, and a research grant from Pfizer, Germany. Nikolaus Tiling has received a speaker honorarium from Shire, Germany and Sanofi Genzyme, Germany. V. Prasad, A. Poellinger and A. Ziagaki have nothing to declare.

Author details
[1]Kompetenzzentrum Seltene Stoffwechselkrankheiten, Interdisziplinäres Stoffwechsel-Centrum: Endokrinologie, Diabetes und Stoffwechsel, Charité Universitätsmedizin Berlin, Augustenburger Platz 1, Campus Virchow-Klinikum, 13352 Berlin, Germany. [2]Department of Nuclear Medicine, Charité Universitätsmedizin Berlin, Berlin, Germany. [3]Department of Nuclear Medicine Universitätsklinik Ulm, Ulm, Germany. [4]Department of Diagnostic, Interventional and Pediatric Radiology, Inselspital Bern University Hospital, University of Bern, Bern, Switzerland.

References

1. Schuller A, Kornblum C, Deschauer M, Vorgerd M, Schrank B, Mengel E, et al. Diagnosis and therapy of late onset Pompe disease. Nervenarzt. 2013;84: 1467–72.
2. Teener JW. Late-onset Pompe's disease. Semin Neurol. 2012;32:506–11.
3. Regnery C, Kornblum C, Hanisch F, Vielhaber S, Strigl-Pill N, Grunert B, et al. 36 months observational clinical study of 38 adult Pompe disease patients under alglucosidase alfa enzyme replacement therapy. J Inherit Metab Dis. 2012;35:837–45.
4. van Capelle CI, van der Beek NA, de Vries JM, van Doorn PA, Duivenvoorden HJ, Leshner RT, et al. The quick motor function test: a new tool to rate clinical severity and motor function in Pompe patients. J Inherit Metab Dis. 2012;35:317–23.
5. Casanova C, Celli BR, Barria P, Casas A, Cote C, de Torres JP, et al. The 6-min walk distance in healthy subjects: reference standards from seven countries. Eur Respir J. 2011;37:150–6.
6. Laboratories ATSCoPSfCPF. ATS statement: guidelines for the six-minute walk test. Am J Respir Crit Care Med. 2002;166:111–7.
7. Andreassen CS, Schlutter JM, Vissing J, Andersen H. Effect of enzyme replacement therapy on isokinetic strength for all major muscle groups in four patients with Pompe disease-a long-term follow-up. Mol Genet Metab. 2014;112:40–3.
8. Young SP, Piraud M, Goldstein JL, Zhang H, Rehder C, Laforet P, et al. Assessing disease severity in Pompe disease: the roles of a urinary glucose tetrasaccharide biomarker and imaging techniques. Am J Med Genet Part C Sem Med Genet. 2012;160c:50–8.
9. Figueroa-Bonaparte S, Segovia S, Llauger J, Belmonte I, Pedrosa I, Alejaldre A, et al. Muscle MRI findings in childhood/adult onset Pompe disease correlate with muscle function. PLoS One. 2016;11:e0163493. https://doi.org/10.1371/journal.pone.0163493.
10. Horvath JJ, Austin SL, Case LE, Greene KB, Jones HN, Soher BJ, et al. Correlation between quantitative whole-body muscle magnetic resonance imaging and clinical muscle weakness in Pompe disease. Muscle Nerve. 2015;51:722–30.
11. Pichiecchio A, Berardinelli A, Moggio M, Rossi M, Balottin U, Comi GP, et al. Asymptomatic Pompe disease: can muscle magnetic resonance imaging facilitate diagnosis? Muscle Nerve. 2016;53:326–7.
12. Carlier PG, Azzabou N, de Sousa PL, Hicks A, Boisserie JM, Amadon A, et al. Skeletal muscle quantitative nuclear magnetic resonance imaging follow-up of adult Pompe patients. J Inherit Metab Dis. 2015;38:565–72.
13. van der Ploeg A, Carlier PG, Carlier RY, Kissel JT, Schoser B, Wenninger S, et al. Prospective exploratory muscle biopsy, imaging, and functional assessment in patients with late-onset Pompe disease treated with alglucosidase alfa: the EMBASSY study. Mol Genet Metab. 2016;119:115–23.
14. Alejaldre A, Diaz-Manera J, Ravaglia S, Tibaldi EC, D'Amore F, Moris G, et al. Trunk muscle involvement in late-onset Pompe disease: study of thirty patients. Neuromuscul Disord. 2012;22(Suppl 2):S148–54.
15. Carlier RY, Laforet P, Wary C, Mompoint D, Laloui K, Pellegrini N, et al. Whole-body muscle MRI in 20 patients suffering from late onset Pompe disease: involvement patterns. Neuromuscul Disord. 2011;21:791–9.
16. Gruhn KM, Heyer CM, Guttsches AK, Rehmann R, Nicolas V, Schmidt-Wilcke T, et al. Muscle imaging data in late-onset Pompe disease reveal a correlation between the pre-existing degree of lipomatous muscle alterations and the efficacy of long-term enzyme replacement therapy. MGM Rep. 2015;3:58–64.
17. Schulze M, Kotter I, Ernemann U, Fenchel M, Tzaribatchev N, Claussen CD, et al. MRI findings in inflammatory muscle diseases and their noninflammatory mimics. AJR. 2009;192:1708–16.
18. Kanda T, Ishii K, Kawaguchi H, Kitajima K, Takenaka D. High signal intensity in the dentate nucleus and globus pallidus on unenhanced T1-weighted MR images: relationship with increasing cumulative dose of a gadolinium-based contrast material. Radiology. 2014;270:834–41.
19. Rozdzynska-Swiatkowska A, Jurkiewicz E, Tylki-Szymanska A. Bioimpedance analysis as a method to evaluate the proportion of fatty and muscle tissues in progressive myopathy in Pompe disease. JIMD Rep. 2016;26:45–51.
20. Orth M, Mundegar RR. Effect of acid maltase deficiency on the endosomal/lysosomal system and glucose transporter 4. NMD. 2003;13:49–54.
21. Lauritzen HP, Schertzer JD. Measuring GLUT4 translocation in mature muscle fibers. Am J Physiol Endocrinol Metab. 2010;299:E169–79.

3

Genome-wide DNA methylation analysis reveals hypomethylation in the low-CpG promoter regions in lymphoblastoid cell lines

Itsuki Taniguchi[1], Chihiro Iwaya[1], Keizo Ohnaka[2], Hiroki Shibata[1] and Ken Yamamoto[3]*

Abstract

Background: Epidemiological studies of DNA methylation profiles may uncover the molecular mechanisms through which genetic and environmental factors contribute to the risk of multifactorial diseases. There are two types of commonly used DNA bioresources, peripheral blood cells (PBCs) and EBV-transformed lymphoblastoid cell lines (LCLs), which are available for genetic epidemiological studies. Therefore, to extend our knowledge of the difference in DNA methylation status between LCLs and PBCs is important in human population studies that use these DNA sources to elucidate the epigenetic risks for multifactorial diseases. We analyzed the methylation status of the autosomes for 192 and 92 DNA samples that were obtained from PBCs and LCLs, respectively, using a human methylation 450 K array. After excluding SNP-associated methylation sites and low-call sites, 400,240 sites were subjected to analysis using a generalized linear model with cell type, sex, and age as the independent variables.

Results: We found that the large proportion of sites showed lower methylation levels in LCLs compared with PBCs, which is consistent with previous reports. We also found that significantly different methylation sites tend to be located on the outside of the CpG island and in a region relatively far from the transcription start site. Additionally, we observed that the methylation change of the sites in the low-CpG promoter region was remarkable. Finally, it was shown that the correlation between the chronological age and ageing-associated methylation sites in *ELOVL2* and *FHL2* in the LCLs was weaker than that in the PBCs.

Conclusions: The methylation levels of highly methylated sites of the low-CpG-density promoters in PBCs decreased in the LCLs, suggesting that the methylation sites located in low-CpG-density promoters could be sensitive to demethylation in LCLs. Despite being generated from a single cell type, LCLs may not always be a proxy for DNA from PBCs in studies of epigenome-wide analysis attempting to elucidate the role of epigenetic change in disease risks.

Keywords: DNA methylation, Lymphoblastoid cell lines, Epigenome-wide analysis, Epigenetic epidemiology, Human methylation array

Background

The DNA obtained from EBV-transformed immortalized lymphoblastoid cell lines (LCLs) and peripheral blood cells (PBCs) are commonly used in medical genetic studies. LCLs can be generated from both healthy individuals and patients and supply an unlimited source of genomic DNA. Additionally, LCLs and PBCs have been successfully used for gene expression analyses [1].

DNA methylation is one of the important epigenetic mechanisms regulating gene expression. In addition to sequence variants, it is increasingly accepted that this DNA modification may be implicated in the susceptibility of various multifactorial diseases [2–4]. Recent developments in technology for human genome analysis have enabled us to identify disease-related DNA methylation changes at the genome-wide level. Because it is essential

* Correspondence: yamamoto_ken@med.kurume-u.ac.jp
[3]Department of Medical Biochemistry, Kurume University School of Medicine, 67 Asahi-machi, Kurume, Fukuoka 830-0011, Japan
Full list of author information is available at the end of the article

to use relatively large samples in searching for genes that are susceptible to multifactorial diseases, the DNA sources are limited to LCLs, PBCs, and saliva. However, it is known that DNA methylation status varies between cell types [5]. Therefore, to extend our knowledge of the difference in DNA methylation status between LCLs and PBCs is important in human population studies that use these DNA sources to elucidate the epigenetic risks for multifactorial diseases.

To this end, we designed experiments to compare the DNA methylation status between LCLs and PBCs at an epigenome-wide level using approximately 400,000 methylation data sites from 92 LCL and 192 PBC samples obtained using the Human Methylation 450 K array. We analyzed global differences in methylation profiles and the degree of difference in methylation level of each site in terms of location (inside or outside the CpG island, the distance from transcription start site and promoter type) between LCLs and PBCs. Additionally, the association strength of methylation levels at the ageing-related methylation sites in *FHL2* and *ELOVL2* with chronological age was compared between LCLs and PBCs.

Methods
Subjects
EBV-transformed LCLs derived from 92 healthy Japanese subjects were provided by the Riken Bioresource Center Cell Bank [6]. PBCs were obtained from 192 participants of a baseline survey of the general population from a Fukuoka-based cohort study [7, 8]. This study was performed in accordance with the principles of the Declaration of Helsinki and was approved by the Institutional Review Board at Kyushu University.

DNA methylation chip assay
Genomic DNA was bisulfite-treated using the EZ-96 DNA Methylation Kit (Zymo Research Corporation, Orange, CA), which combines bisulfite conversion and DNA cleanup in a 96-well plate. Genome-wide DNA methylation profiles were obtained using the Illumina HumanMethylation450 BeadChip (Illumina, San Diego, CA) according to the manufacturer's instructions. The GenomeStudio V2011.1 (Methylation Module version 1.9.0) was employed to determine the beta values that reflected the estimated methylation level for each CpG site. The beta value was calculated as: Max(-signal for methylation, 0)/[Max(signal for methylation, 0) + Max(signal for unmethylation, 0) + 100]. Using this metric, the DNA methylation level was represented by a number between 0 (no methylation) and 1 (complete methylation). The signal intensities were

normalized to the internal controls and background prior to beta value calculation.

Selection and classification of DNA methylation sites
Among 473,864 methylation sites on the autosomes, 1305 sites showing low calls (<0.95) were removed for further analyses. To eliminate SNP-associated methylation sites, we screened the nearest SNP for each methylation site using the dbSNP135 database (SNPs categorized in weight = 1 group, http://www.ncbi.nlm.nih.gov/SNP/). We found 72,318 sites in which SNPs were located on the C or G site. Additionally, one methylation site demonstrated an outlier value. After removing these sites; 400,240 methylation sites on the array were available for further analyses. Based on the CpG Islands (CGI) track of the UCSC table browser of the UCSC Genome Bioinformatics database (http://genome.ucsc.edu/index.html), the 400,240 sites on autosomes were classified into two groups, CGI-sites (135,674 sites, inside of CGI) or non-CGI-sites (264,566 sites, outside the CGI). Among the non-CGI sites, 95,625 sites were located near CGI (±2,000 bases) that were classified in a shore group. The distance between the methylation site and the nearest transcription start site (TSS) was calculated using the NCBI RefSeq database. The physical positions on the human genome were based on the Genome Reference Consortium Human Build 37 (GRCh37, http://www.ncbi.nlm.nih.gov/assembly/). Of 400,240 probes, 159,688 demonstrated a TSS between −500 bases and +2,000 bases; among these, 85,700 sites could be classified into high-CpG-density promoters (HCP), intermediate-CpG-density promoters (ICP) and low-CpG-density promoters (LCP), as reported by Mikkelsen et al. [9] (69,836, 10,719, and 5145 in HCP, ICP, and LCP, respectively).

Statistical analysis
To evaluate the difference in methylation level of each site, the data were analyzed using modeling individual Illumina beta values using a generalized linear model (glm) with cell type (LCLs or PBCs), age and sex as the independent variables. P values and the difference in methylation level for each cell type were obtained. The statistical power to detect methylation differences of 0.25 and 0.5 between 192 PBCs and 92 LCLs was estimated to be 50.2 and 97.5%, respectively at a significance level of $P = 0.05$ using G*Power 3.1 software [10]. A principal component analysis (PCA) was performed using the beta values for the 400,240 sites, and the first and second principal component scores for each sample were plotted. The regression analysis was performed using the chronological age of the subjects and the beta values of cg06639320 and cg16867657 for *FHL2* and *ELOVL2*, respectively, with adjustments for sex. These analyses were performed using R (release 2.15.2).

Results

Comparison of global DNA methylation profiles between LCLs and PBCs

To assess the global difference of DNA methylation levels between LCLs and PBCs, we performed a PCA using the methylation data of 400,240 sites on autosomes obtained using the 450 K methylation array. As shown in Fig. 1a, the LCL and PBC groups were clearly distinguished by their first principal component score. Additionally, the PBC samples were distributed within a narrow range, whereas the LCL samples showed a relatively wide range in the second principal component score. These results suggest that there is a global difference in DNA methylation levels between these cell types and that the levels are more diverse in LCLs than in PBCs.

We then examined the difference in methylation level for each site using a glm adjusted for age and sex. As shown in the volcano plot in Fig. 1b, the sites showing lower levels in LCL than in PBC were predominant (low-met-LCL group). The 138,871 sites (34.7% of the total) showed $-\log_{10}(P$ value$) > 10$; among these sites, 85.1% were in the low-met-LCL group. This inclination was observed in each autosome (Additional file 1: Figure S1). Therefore, it was suggested that the main difference in DNA methylation between LCLs and PBCs was hypomethylation in the LCLs and that the change in methylation levels occurred globally in the autosomes.

Hypomethylation observed in the LCLs occurs at sites outside the GpG island

We next assessed the distribution of the difference in methylation levels between LCLs and PBLs in terms of the location of the site (inside or outside the CpG island) (named CGI-site or non-CGI-site). As shown in Fig. 2a,

the distribution of difference was dissimilar between them; the proportion of the sites showing a low P value was larger in the non-CGI-site group (black solid line) than in the CGI-site group (black dashed line). This trend was apparent in the low-met-LCL group (compare the red solid and dashed lines), whereas a dissimilarity of distribution was not observed in the high-met-LCL group (compare the blue solid and dashed lines). These results prompted us to further classify the non-CGI-sites into shore or non-shore groups because the CGI shores were suggested to contribute to tissue-specific DNA methylation [11, 12]. However, we did not find significant differences in the distribution between the shore and non-shore group of the low-met-LCL (Fig. 2b). Taken together, these results suggested that the majority of hypomethylation observed in the LCLs occurred at sites outside the CGIs regardless of shores.

Comparison of the difference in DNA methylation levels observed among LCLs and PBCs in terms of distance from the transcription start site

We further examined the relationship between the distance from the TSS and the difference in DNA methylation levels observed among LCLs and PBCs. We plotted $-\log_{10}(P$ value$)$ for each site against the distance from the nearest TSS (shown in gray dots in Fig. 3a) and indicated a proportion of the site showing $-\log_{10}(P$ value$) > 10$, 25, and 50 in blue, green, and pink dots, respectively (Fig. 3a). The proportion was calculated by dividing the number of the sites meeting the P value criteria by the total number of sites within ±50 bases of window size. We found that the proportion of significantly different sites was lower near the TSS. For instance, approximately 25% of the sites near the TSS

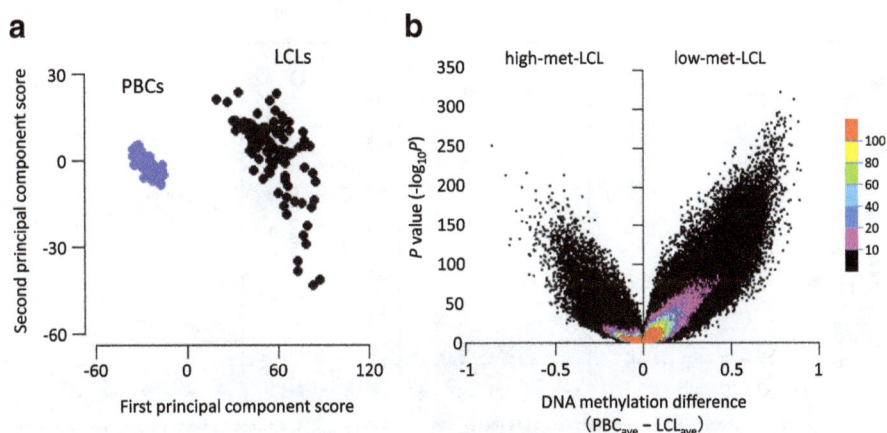

Fig. 1 Global difference in the DNA methylation level between the LCLs and PBCs. **a** Principal component analysis (PCA) plot. PCA was performed using the methylation level of the 400,240 sites on autosomes. The LCL and PBC samples are shown in *black* and *blue dots*, respectively. **b** Volcano plot with the difference of the average of DNA methylation level on the *x*-axis and the *P* value ($-\log_{10}P$) obtained via glm analysis on the *y*-axis. Each *color* shows the dot density ($100 < n$, $80 < n \leq 100$, $60 < n \leq 80$, $40 < n \leq 60$, $20 < n \leq 40$, $10 < n \leq 20$ and $n \leq 10$ per unit area (0.002×1 for *x* and *y*-axis, respectively) in *red, yellow, green, sky blue, blue, pink,* and *black*, respectively)

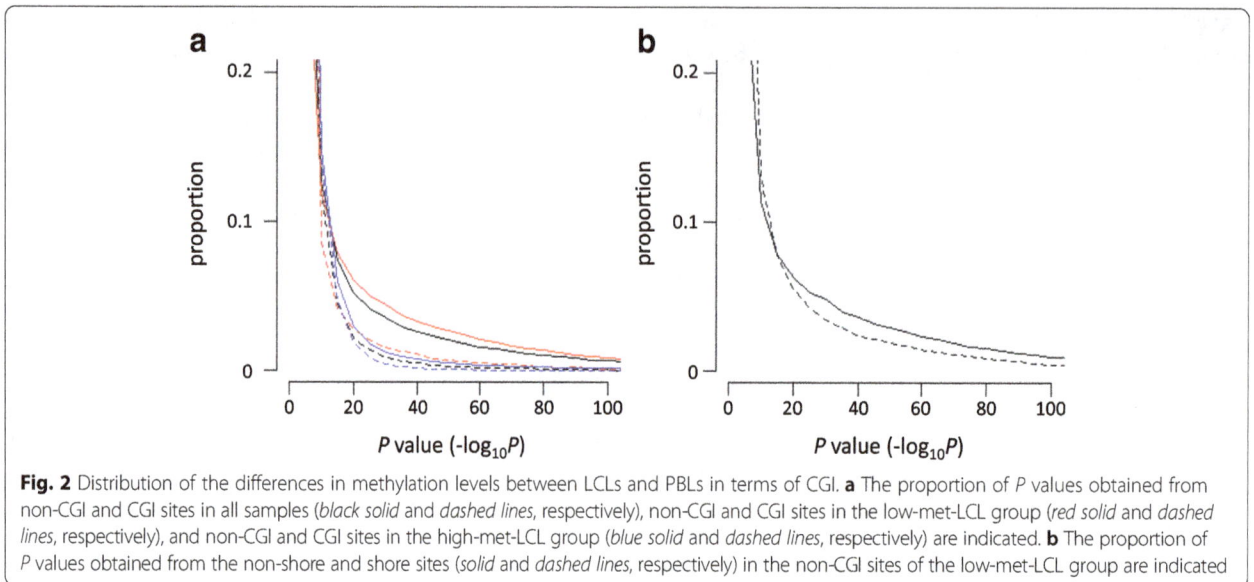

Fig. 2 Distribution of the differences in methylation levels between LCLs and PBLs in terms of CGI. **a** The proportion of P values obtained from non-CGI and CGI sites in all samples (*black solid* and *dashed lines*, respectively), non-CGI and CGI sites in the low-met-LCL group (*red solid* and *dashed lines*, respectively), and non-CGI and CGI sites in the high-met-LCL group (*blue solid* and *dashed lines*, respectively) are indicated. **b** The proportion of P values obtained from the non-shore and shore sites (*solid* and *dashed lines*, respectively) in the non-CGI sites of the low-met-LCL group are indicated

showed – $\log_{10}(P$ value$) > 10$, whereas this proportion increased to approximately 45% for the sites located approximately ±1000 bases from the TSS in the low-met-LCL group (blue dots, left panel of Fig. 3a). This trend was also observed even in the lower P value threshold group (green and pink dots) and in the high-met-LCL group (right panel of Fig. 3a). We then analyzed the sites showing – $\log_{10}(P$-value$) > 10$ separately for CGI- and non-CGI-site groups. As shown in Fig. 3b, the proportion of non-CGI-sites near the TSS was high in both the low- and high-met-LCL groups (red and blue dots, respectively, Fig. 3b). However, the lowest proportion was observed near the TSS in the case of CGI-sites (pink and sky blue dots for low- and high-met-LCL groups, respectively, Fig. 3b). These results

suggested that the low CpG promoter would show a more significant difference in DNA methylation levels than the high CpG promoter.

The methylation sites located in low CpG promoters could be sensitive to demethylation in LCLs

To assess whether the promoter type affects the difference in DNA methylation levels between LCLs and PBCs, the methylation sites located in HCP, LCP and ICP were extracted based on the data set of Mikkelsen et al. [9] (69,836, 10,719, and 5,145, in HCP, ICP, and LCP, respectively), and analyzed the distribution of – $\log_{10}(P$ value$)$ in all, low- and high-met-LCL groups (Fig. 4). It was shown that the proportion of differentially methylated sites was higher in the LCPs than the HCPs.

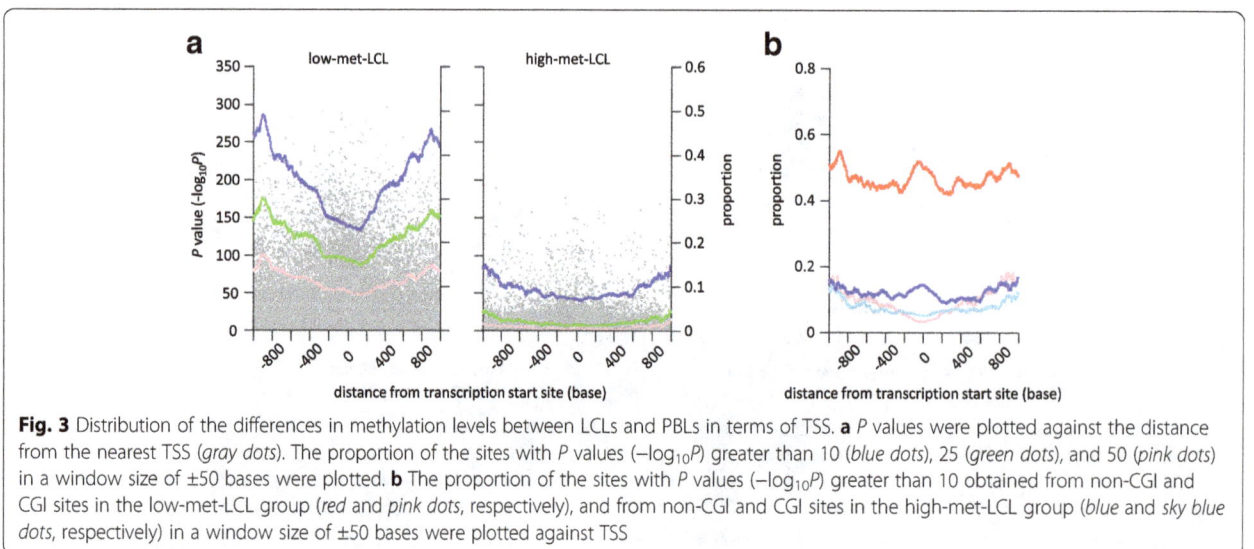

Fig. 3 Distribution of the differences in methylation levels between LCLs and PBLs in terms of TSS. **a** P values were plotted against the distance from the nearest TSS (*gray dots*). The proportion of the sites with P values (−$\log_{10}P$) greater than 10 (*blue dots*), 25 (*green dots*), and 50 (*pink dots*) in a window size of ±50 bases were plotted. **b** The proportion of the sites with P values (−$\log_{10}P$) greater than 10 obtained from non-CGI and CGI sites in the low-met-LCL group (*red and pink dots*, respectively), and from non-CGI and CGI sites in the high-met-LCL group (*blue and sky blue dots*, respectively) in a window size of ±50 bases were plotted against TSS

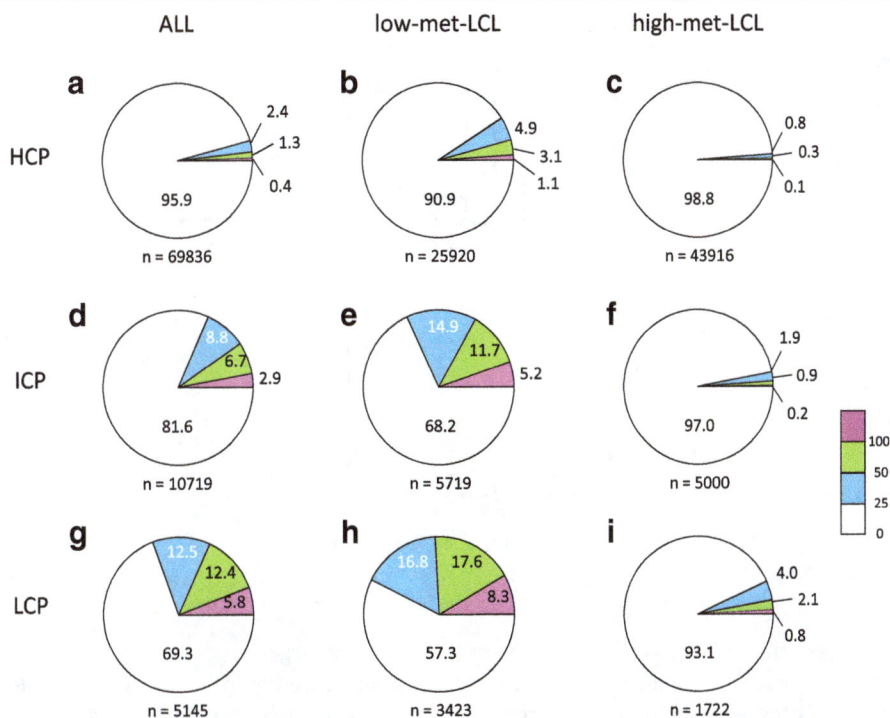

Fig. 4 Difference in methylation levels between LCLs and PBLs in terms of promoter type. The proportion of the sites with P values ($-\log_{10}P$) ≤ 25, 25 ~ 50, 50 ~ 100, and ≥ 100 are indicated in *white*, *blue*, *green*, and *red*, respectively. The results obtained from the HCP, ICP, and LCP sites in all samples (**a**, **d**, and **g**, respectively) in the low-met-LCL group (**b**, **e**, and **h**, respectively) and in the high-met-LCL (**c**, **f**, and **i**, respectively) are shown

In the LCPs, the proportion of the sites showing $-\log_{10}(P$ value) > 25 was 30.7%, whereas that in HCPs was 4.1% in all sites (compare Fig. 4a, g). This was more pronounced in the low-met-LCL group (compare Fig. 4b, c, h, i). The sites located in ICPs showed intermediate values between HCPs and LCPs (Fig. 4d–f). These results suggested that the methylation sites located in low CpG promoters could be sensitive to demethylation in LCLs.

To further assess promoter type differences, we compared the HCPs and LCPs methylation level profiles. As shown in Fig. 5, nearly half of the sites in LCPs showed more than 0.6 methylation levels, whereas almost all sites in HCPs were hypomethylated in PBCs. Additionally, it was observed that the methylation levels of highly methylated sites of the LCPs decreased in the LCLs. Therefore, we concluded that highly methylated sites of LCPs caused the difference in DNA methylation levels observed between HCPs and LCPs, especially in the low-met-LCL group.

Comparison between LCLs and PBCs regarding the association between ageing-related CpG sites and chronological age

Using DNA obtained from PBCs, it has been reported that the methylation levels of several CpG sites are associated with chronological age. However, it remains unclear whether LCLs should be utilized for studies on epigenetic ageing biomarkers. To address this issue, we performed a regression analysis for chronological age and known ageing-related CpG sites located in *FHL2* and *ELOVL2* [13, 14]. *FHL2* encodes a member of the four-and-a-half-LIM-only protein family which is suggested to have a role in the assembly of extracellular membranes and in transformation of normal myoblasts to rhabdomyosarcoma cells (OMIN 602633). *ELOVL2* encodes an enzyme which catalyzes the first and rate-limiting reaction of the long-chain fatty acids elongation cycle (OMIM 611814). As shown in Fig. 6a, the methylation level of the PBCs was highly correlated with chronological age (blue dots, $P = 1.7E\text{-}18$ and $r^2 = 0.33$ for *FHL2*, $P = 3.1E\text{-}25$ and $r^2 = 0.44$ for *ELOVL2*). In contrast, the methylation level of the LCLs was varied and the association was weak (black dots, $P = 0.04$ and $r^2 = 0.05$ for *FHL2*, $P = 1.9E\text{-}5$ and $r^2 = 0.18$ for *ELOVL2*). Therefore, these results suggest that DNA obtained from LCLs may not always be an alternative to DNA from PBCs.

Discussion

In this study, we used a 450 K methylation array to investigate the methylation differences between LCLs and PBCs, which are commonly used in genetic epidemiological

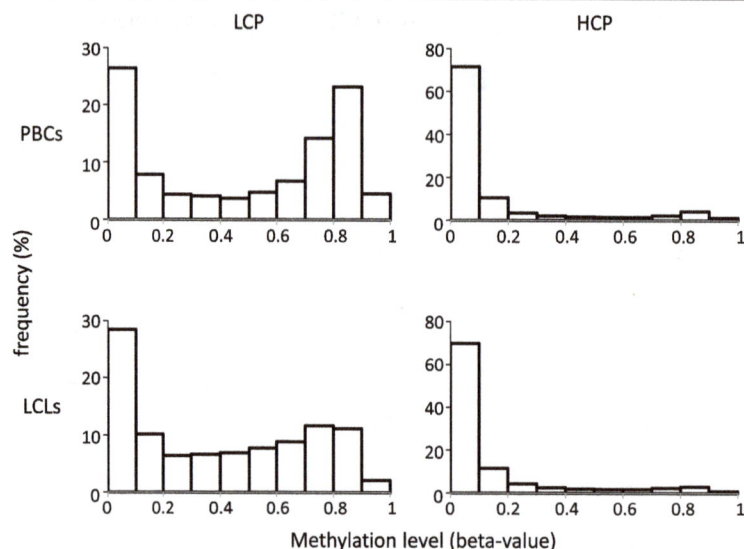

Fig. 5 Distribution of the methylation levels of the sites in the LCPs and HCPs. The frequency in the LCLs and PBCs are shown separately

studies. In all genomes, the majority of the sites in the LCLs showed lower methylation levels than those of the PBCs, and these sites were primarily located in non-CGI regions. Additionally, we found that differentially methylated sites were predominantly located in the LCP region.

Although a relatively small sample number and number of methylation sites were analyzed, previous studies showed that methylation status in LCLs is different from that of PBCs and that the methylation level in LCLs is lower than that of PBCs in the majority of sites [15–20].

Because a large number of samples and more sites were examined, we could investigate the differences in methylation levels between LCLs and PBCs in terms of CGI location, distance from TSS and promoter type as characterized by CG density. We found that a fraction showing a significant difference in methylation level between the LCLs and PBCs was observed near the TSS in the non-CGI sites but not in the CGI sites. This result suggests that the difference in the methylation level of these cell types would be high in the genes in which the promoter shows a low GC content.

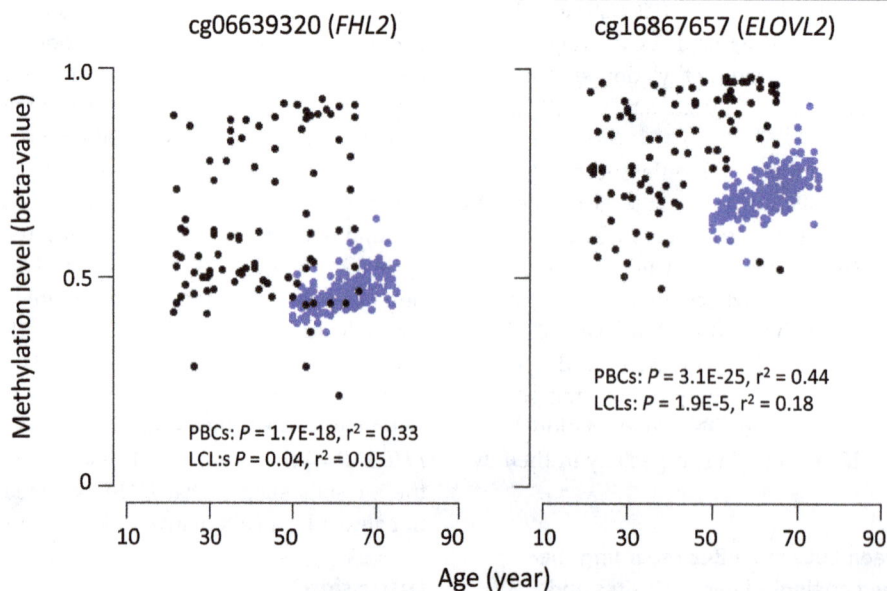

Fig. 6 Regression analyses of the methylation levels and chronological age at the *FHL2* and *ELOVL2* loci. The methylation levels in the LCLs (*black dots*) and PBCs (*blue dots*) were plotted against the age of the donors at the time of providing the specimens. The P values and r^2 were obtained by correcting for sex

We found that significantly different methylation sites were predominant in LCPs but not in HCPs. It has been demonstrated that LCPs are generally associated with tissue-specific genes, whereas HCPs are associated with two classes of genes, including ubiquitous "housekeeping" genes and highly regulated "key developmental" genes [9, 21, 22]. Therefore, our results suggest that the methylation sites located in promoters classified as LCP could have a functional role in distinguishing between LCLs and PBCs by regulating the corresponding gene expression.

The epigenome-wide association studies using human population samples to identify the disease risk loci and epigenomes that are affected by intrinsic or extrinsic factors, such as ageing and smoking, have been progressing [13, 14, 23, 24]. We evaluated the differences in association strength between well-known ageing methylation sites and the chronological age of the samples between LCLs and PBCs and found that the correlation was more significant in PBCs than LCLs. This was due to a larger variance of methylation levels in LCLs than in PBCs. In addition to the differences in cell type, artificial experimental processes, including in vitro culture, culture period and culture freezing, and thawing could cause the large variances in data observed in the LCLs. Therefore, we concluded that DNA obtained from LCLs may not always be a proxy for DNA from PBCs in studies of epigenome-wide analysis attempting to elucidate the role of epigenetic change in disease risks.

Conclusion

There is a global difference in DNA methylation levels between LCLs and PBCs, and the main difference was hypomethylation in the LCLs. The methylation levels of highly methylated sites of the low-CpG-density promoters in PBCs decreased in the LCLs, suggesting that the methylation sites located in low-CpG-density promoters could be sensitive to demethylation in LCLs. The correlation between well-known ageing methylation sites and the chronological age of the samples was more significant in PBCs than LCLs, indicating that despite being generated from a single cell type, LCLs may not always be a proxy for DNA from PBCs in studies of epigenome-wide analysis attempting to elucidate the role of epigenetic change in disease risks.

Abbreviations

CGI: CpG Island; ELOVL2: Elongation of very long chain fatty acids protein 2; FHL2: Four and a half LIM domains 2; Glm: Generalized linear model; HCP: High-CpG-density promoter; ICP: Intermediate-CpG-density promoter; LCL: Lymphoblastoid cell line; LCP: Low-CpG-density promoter; PBC: Peripheral blood cell; PCA: Principal component analysis; TSS: Transcription start site

Acknowledgements

We thank all of the people who have continuously supported the population-based cohort study, the Kyushu University Fukuoka Cohort Study. We also thank Ms. Miki Sonoda for her technical assistance.

Funding

This work was supported by KAKENHI Grant Number 15 K08290 from the Japan Society for the Promotion of Science.

Authors' contributions

KO performed the sample collection KO. KY performed the DNA methylation chip experiments. IT, CI, and KY performed the statistical and bioinformatics analyses. HS supervised the research. All authors wrote and approved the manuscript.

Competing interests

The authors declare that they have no competing interests.

Author details

[1]Division of Genomics, Medical Institute of Bioregulation, Kyushu University, 3-1-1 Maidashi, Higashi-ku, Fukuoka 812-8582, Japan. [2]Department of Geriatric Medicine, Graduate School of Medical Sciences, Kyushu University, 3-1-1 Maidashi, Higashi-ku, Fukuoka 812-8582, Japan. [3]Department of Medical Biochemistry, Kurume University School of Medicine, 67 Asahi-machi, Kurume, Fukuoka 830-0011, Japan.

References

1. Powell JE, Henders AK, McRae AF, Wright MJ, Martin NG, Dermitzakis ET, Montgomery GW, Visscher PM. Genetic control of gene expression in whole blood and lymphoblastoid cell lines is largely independent. Genome Res. 2012;22:456–66.
2. Ordovás JM, Smith CE. Epigenetics and cardiovascular disease. Nat Rev Cardiol. 2010;7:510–19.
3. Costenbader KH, Gay S, Alarcón-Riquelme ME, Iaccarino L, Doria A. Genes, epigenetic regulation and environmental factors: which is the most relevant in developing autoimmune diseases? Autoimmun Rev. 2012;11:604–9.
4. Keating ST, El-Osta A. Epigenetic changes in diabetes. Clin Genet. 2013;84:1–10.
5. Ziller MJ, Gu H, Müller F, Donaghey J, Tsai LT, Kohlbacher O, De Jager PL, Rosen ED, Bennett DA, Bernstein BE, et al. Charting a dynamic DNA methylation landscape of the human genome. Nature. 2013;500:477–81.
6. Iwakawa M, Goto M, Noda S, Sagara M, Yamada S, Yamamoto N, Kawakami Y, Matsui Y, Miyazawa Y, Yamazaki H, et al. DNA repair capacity measured by high throughput alkaline comet assays in EBV-transformed cell lines and peripheral blood cells from cancer patients and healthy volunteers. Mutat Res. 2005;588:1–6.
7. Nanri A, Yoshida D, Yamaji T, Mizoue T, Takayanagi R, Kono S. Dietary patterns and C-reactive protein in Japanese men and women. Am J Clin Nutr. 2008;87:1488–96.
8. Yoshida D, Toyomura K, Fukumoto J, Ueda N, Ohnaka K, Adachi M, Takayanagi R, Kono S. Waist circumference and cardiovascular risk factors in Japanese men and women. J Atheroscler Thromb. 2009;16:431–41.
9. Mikkelsen TS, Ku M, Jaffe DB, Issac B, Lieberman E, Giannoukos G, Alvarez P, Brockman W, Kim TK, Koche RP, et al. Genome-wide maps of chromatin state in pluripotent and lineage-committed cells. Nature. 2007;448:553–60.
10. Faul F, Erdfelder E, Lang AG, Buchner A. G*Power 3: a flexible statistical power analysis program for the social, behavioral, and biomedical sciences. Behav Res Methods. 2007;39:175–91.
11. Irizarry RA, Ladd-Acosta C, Wen B, Wu Z, Montano C, Onyango P, Cui H, Gabo K, Rongione M, Webster M, et al. The human colon cancer methylome shows similar hypo- and hypermethylation at conserved tissue-specific CpG island shores. Nat Genet. 2009;41:178–86.

12. Doi A, Park IH, Wen B, Murakami P, Aryee MJ, Irizarry R, Herb B, Ladd-Acosta C, Rho J, Loewer S, et al. Differential methylation of tissue- and cancer-specific CpG island shores distinguishes human induced pluripotent stem cells, embryonic stem cells and fibroblasts. Nat Genet. 2009;41:1350–53.

13. Garagnani P, Bacalini MG, Pirazzini C, Gori D, Giuliani C, Mari D, Di Blasio AM, Gentilini D, Vitale G, Collino S, et al. Methylation of ELOVL2 gene as a new epigenetic marker of age. Aging Cell. 2012;11:1132–4.

14. Hannum G, Guinney J, Zhao L, Zhang L, Hughes G, Sadda S, Klotzle B, Bibikova M, Fan JB, Gao Y, et al. Genome-wide methylation profiles reveal quantitative views of human aging rates. Mol Cell. 2013;49:359–67.

15. Brennan EP, Ehrich M, Brazil DP, Crean JK, Murphy M, Sadlier DM, Martin F, Godson C, McKnight AJ, van den Boom D, et al. Comparative analysis of DNA methylation profiles in peripheral blood leukocytes versus lymphoblastoid cell lines. Epigenetics. 2009;4:159–64.

16. Sun YV, Turner ST, Smith JA, Hammond PI, Lazarus A, Van De Rostyne JL, Cunningham JM, Kardia SL. Comparison of the DNA methylation profiles of human peripheral blood cells and transformed B-lymphocytes. Hum Genet. 2010;127:651–8.

17. Grafodatskaya D, Choufani S, Ferreira JC, Butcher DT, Lou Y, Zhao C, Scherer SW, Weksberg R. EBV transformation and cell culturing destabilizes DNA methylation in human lymphoblastoid cell lines. Genomics. 2010;95:73–83.

18. Sugawara H, Iwamoto K, Bundo M, Ueda J, Ishigooka J, Kato T. Comprehensive DNA methylation analysis of human peripheral blood leukocytes and lymphoblastoid cell lines. Epigenetics. 2011;6:508–15.

19. Åberg K, Khachane AN, Rudolf G, Nerella S, Fugman DA, Tischfield JA, van den Oord EJ. Methylome-wide comparison of human genomic DNA extracted from whole blood and from EBV-transformed lymphocyte cell lines. Eur J Hum Genet. 2012;20:953–5.

20. Thompson TM, Sharfi D, Lee M, Yrigollen CM, Naumova OY, Grigorenko EL. Comparison of whole-genome DNA methylation patterns in whole blood, saliva, and lymphoblastoid cell lines. Behav Genet. 2013;43:168–76.

21. Weber M, Hellmann I, Stadler MB, Ramos L, Pääbo S, Rebhan M, Schübeler D. Distribution, silencing potential and evolutionary impact of promoter DNA methylation in the human genome. Nat Genet. 2007;39:457–66.

22. Koga Y, Pelizzola M, Cheng E, Krauthammer M, Sznol M, Ariyan S, Narayan D, Molinaro AM, Halaban R, Weissman SM. Genome-wide screen of promoter methylation identifies novel markers in melanoma. Genome Res. 2009;19:1462–70.

23. Breitling LP, Yang R, Korn B, Burwinkel B, Brenner H. Tobacco-smoking-related differential DNA methylation: 27 K discovery and replication. Am J Hum Genet. 2011;88:450–7.

24. Wan ES, Qiu W, Baccarelli A, Carey VJ, Bacherman H, Rennard SI, Agusti A, Anderson W, Lomas DA, Demeo DL. Cigarette smoking behaviors and time since quitting are associated with differential DNA methylation across the human genome. Hum Mol Genet. 2012;21:3073–82.

4

Evaluating somatic tumor mutation detection without matched normal samples

Jamie K. Teer[1][*], Yonghong Zhang[1], Lu Chen[2], Eric A. Welsh[1], W. Douglas Cress[2], Steven A. Eschrich[1] and Anders E. Berglund[1]

Abstract

Background: Observations of recurrent somatic mutations in tumors have led to identification and definition of signaling and other pathways that are important for cancer progression and therapeutic targeting. As tumor cells contain both an individual's inherited genetic variants and somatic mutations, challenges arise in distinguishing these events in massively parallel sequencing datasets. Typically, both a tumor sample and a "normal" sample from the same individual are sequenced and compared; variants observed only in the tumor are considered to be somatic mutations. However, this approach requires two samples for each individual.

Results: We evaluate a method of detecting somatic mutations in tumor samples for which only a subset of normal samples are available. We describe tuning of the method for detection of mutations in tumors, filtering to remove inherited variants, and comparison of detected mutations to several matched tumor/normal analysis methods. Filtering steps include the use of population variation datasets to remove inherited variants as well a subset of normal samples to remove technical artifacts. We then directly compare mutation detection with tumor-only and tumor-normal approaches using the same sets of samples. Comparisons are performed using an internal targeted gene sequencing dataset ($n = 3380$) as well as whole exome sequencing data from The Cancer Genome Atlas project ($n = 250$). Tumor-only mutation detection shows similar recall (43–60%) but lesser precision (20–21%) to current matched tumor/normal approaches (recall 43–73%, precision 30–82%) when compared to a "gold-standard" tumor/normal approach. The inclusion of a small pool of normal samples improves precision, although many variants are still uniquely detected in the tumor-only analysis.

Conclusions: A detailed method for somatic mutation detection without matched normal samples enables study of larger numbers of tumor samples, as well as tumor samples for which a matched normal is not available. As sensitivity/recall is similar to tumor/normal mutation detection but precision is lower, tumor-only detection is more appropriate for classification of samples based on known mutations. Although matched tumor-normal analysis is preferred due to higher precision, we demonstrate that mutation detection without matched normal samples is possible for certain applications.

Keywords: Somatic mutation, Cancer genomics, Next-generation sequencing, Precision medicine

Background

Methods for massively parallel sequencing analysis have matured, even as sequencing technologies have undergone continued, rapid improvement. Detection of somatic mutations in cancer samples has proven to be challenging due to the presence of inherited germline variants, sample heterogeneity, and genomic instability. Somatic mutations can be identified from massively parallel sequencing data by directly comparing the DNA sequence from tumor samples with their matched normal samples. This allows subtraction of the germline variants shared by all cells in an individual, leaving only acquired somatic mutations. Somatic mutations include the important driver mutations that give a cell the growth advantage leading to tumorigenesis [1]. The paired tumor/normal approach to precisely identify somatic mutations has been used in landscape studies that have identified commonly mutated positions and genes in a wide variety of cancers, including recent publications by The Cancer Genome Atlas consortium (for review, see Watson et al. [2]). There are several

* Correspondence: Jamie.Teer@moffitt.org
[1]Department of Biostatistics and Bioinformatics, H. Lee Moffitt Cancer Center and Research Institute, Tampa, FL 33612, USA
Full list of author information is available at the end of the article

implementations, including VarScan [3, 4], Shimmer [5], SomaticSniper [6], Strelka [7], and MuTect [8]. However, this approach effectively doubles the number of samples that must be sequenced and analyzed and limits investigation to those tumor samples for which a matched normal tissue sample is available. This approach is theoretically sound and widely used, and many methods have been compared and evaluated, including in the crowdsourced DREAM challenge [9] and others [10]. However, the efficacy of somatic mutation detection without matched normal samples has not been widely studied. Recently, Jones et al. reported that tumor-only mutation detection resulted in large numbers of false positive detections and concluded that tumor-only detection should be used with caution, even though the approach is common in clinical testing [11].

As part of the Total Cancer Care® (TCC) project [12], we have developed a large tumor bank consisting of 26,473 frozen tumor samples. Through collaboration with a pharmaceutical partner, Merck & Co., 3917 samples from 3380 unique individuals were subjected to targeted gene sequencing (TGS) covering 1321 genes of interest. Here, we describe and evaluate a detailed approach for somatic mutation detection without matched normal samples based on a Genome Analysis ToolKit (GATK) [13, 14] pipeline. Although GATK is built on a model assuming a diploid genome that is often not applicable in tumor samples, the tool is widely used for somatic mutation detection. We therefore deliberately choose to evaluate this approach because of the disconnect between theoretical concerns and widespread use. We describe the effect of various filters on mutation detection rates and compare tumor-only mutation detection to paired tumor-normal comparison approaches using TGS data and whole exome sequencing (WES) data from the TCGA project (250 samples from 5 diseases). This study expands on the findings of Jones et al. to allow for a better understanding of the limitations and potential utility of tumor-only mutation detection. We finally describe the detailed pipeline built for this evaluation from publically available analysis tools, allowing researchers to evaluate and utilize tumor-only mutation detection themselves.

Methods

Experimental design
The objectives of this study were to define a specific methodology to detect somatic mutations without matched normal samples and to evaluate its performance. As a subset of tumor samples did have a matched normal sample, mutations were also directly compared between tumor-only and tumor-normal mutation detection strategies to calculate precision and recall.

Study cohorts
A cohort of samples from 3380 unique individuals (2575 primary solid tumors, 675 metastatic solid tumor, and 130 hematologic malignancies) from the TCC project was utilized in this study (Fig. 1a). Samples were classified according to site of tumor origin (Additional file 1: Table S1). The sites with the highest number of samples include the lung, large bowel, breast, kidney, ovary, and skin. These samples were subjected to TGS across the protein coding exons of 1321 genes covering 3.8 megabases (Additional file 2: Table S2). The median number of reads aligning per sample was 15,283,830. The read depth was consistent across tissue sites of origin with a median depth coverage of 141× (Additional file 3: Figure S1d). The median percentage of targeted bases which covered ≥ 10× across samples was 93.7%. Altogether, 53.4 million reads were generated, for a total of 4.8 trillion bases.

To identify potential batch effects or other confounding factors, a principal component analysis (PCA) was performed on various sequence metrics, including missing values, mutation counts, read counts, and transition/

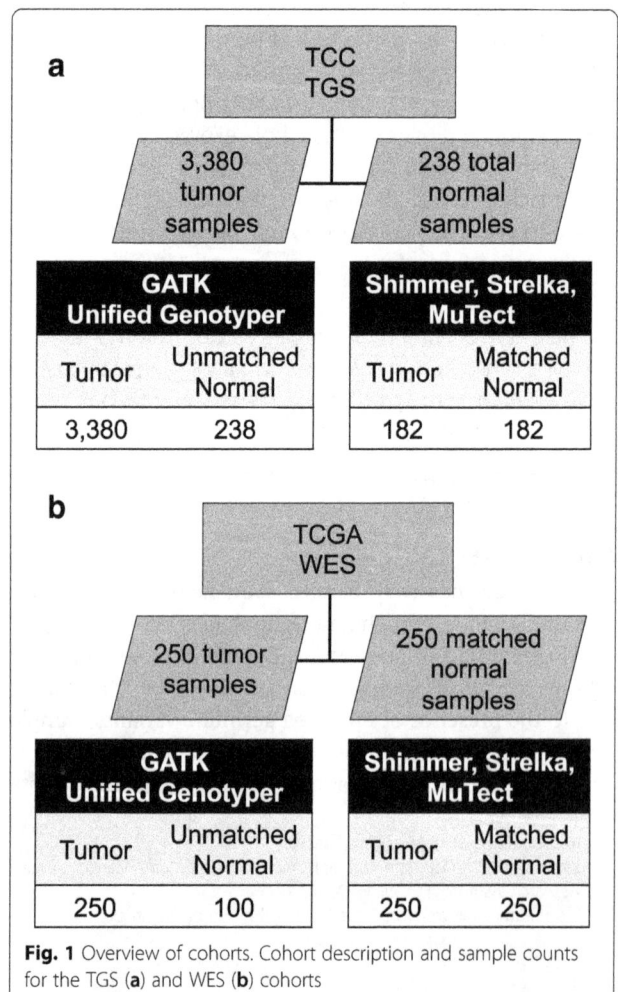

Fig. 1 Overview of cohorts. Cohort description and sample counts for the TGS (**a**) and WES (**b**) cohorts

transversion ratios. The majority of samples were grouped together, with two smaller subgroups showing some deviation (Additional file 3: Figure S1a). PCA loadings showed that the 1st component subgroup (tailing out to the right) was affected by missing values and the 2nd component subgroup (tailing to the bottom left) was affected by mutation counts (presumed to be samples with a hyper-mutator phenotype) (Additional file 3: Figure S1b) It was noted that the sites of origin did not cluster together, suggesting that the batch effects were not responsible for similarities between samples within a site of origin.

To assess the extent of potential sample issues using sequencing data and clinical metadata alone, the balance of sequence reads aligning to the X and Y chromosomes was examined to infer gender, which was then matched to clinical data for each patient. The ratio of sequence reads on chromosome X compared to chromosome Y varied over 7 logs, but formed a very distinct bi-modal pattern (Additional file 3: Figure S1c). The high ratio peak was inferred to be female, and empirical cutoffs were set to determine gender across the cohort (male ≤ 4, female ≥ 5.75). Of all samples with determined gender, 0.7% showed a discrepant gender call and were excluded from further analysis.

As a part of the TCC cohort, 238 adjacent normal tissue samples were available from individuals with cancer, which were used to create a normal pool for filtering purposes. Of these, 182 normal samples were paired with a primary tumor sample: matched tumor/normal mutation detection software was applied to these pairs for comparison to tumor-only mutation detection.

WES was also included from a cohort of 250 samples assembled from five different cancers characterized as part of The Cancer Genome Atlas (TCGA) project (Fig. 1b). Fifty tumors each were selected from acute myeloid leukemia (LAML), glioblastoma multiforme (GBM), lung adenocarcinoma (LUAD), ovarian serous cystadenocarcinoma (OV), and skin cutaneous melanoma (SKCM) (Additional file 4: Table S3). These samples each had a matched normal sample, which was used for the matched tumor/normal mutation identification methods. One hundred of these normal samples were selected for a normal pool, which was used for tumor-only mutation detection.

Tissue samples and consent
Tissue samples were collected according to the TCC methods and consent protocols detailed by Fenstermacher et al. [12].

TGS sequencing
DNA was subjected to solution-hybridization-selection using SureSelect technology (Agilent Technologies, Santa Clara, CA) targeting 1321 genes. Samples were then sequenced on GAIIx sequencers using a 90 bp, paired-end configuration (Illumina, Inc., San Diego, CA).

Analysis—alignment
Sequence reads were aligned to the human reference genome (hs37d5) using the Burrows-Wheeler Aligner (BWA) version 0.5.9-r16 [15]. Duplicate reads were marked with Picard-Tools 1.56 (http://broadinstitute.github.io/picard/). Indel realignment and base quality score recalibration were performed with GATK [13, 14]. GenomeAnalysisTKLite-2.2 was used as it was one of the last freely available versions and therefore usable by a wider audience. Samtools v0.1.16 was used for BAM file handling.

Analysis—tumor-only genotype determination
Multi-sample genotype determination was performed with GATK UnifiedGenotyper. Variant confidence/quality by depth (QD) metric was excluded from Variant Quality Score Recalibration (VQSR), as we have previously found this to penalize variants deviating from the expected 50% alternate allele frequencies. Further modifications to the pipeline are described in Additional file 5. Sequence variants were annotated with ANNOVAR [16], and additional information was included from 1000 Genomes [17] (20110521 release), ESP (http://evs.gs.washington.edu/EVS/, version ESP6500SI-V2), and COSMIC [18] version 61.

Analysis—matched tumor/normal mutation detection
Tumor-normal mutation detection of SNVs and indels was performed with Shimmer [5] (−minqual 20 −mapqual 16), Strelka [7] (v1.0.13, default settings), and MuTect [8] (v1.1.4, −max_alt_alleles_in_normal_count 3 −max_alt_allele_in_normal_fraction 0.05). In the MuTect analysis, indels were called using GATK SomaticIndelDetector.

Analysis—secondary
BEDTools [19] was used for overlap calculations. The analysis pipeline, VCF filtering scripts, and other analysis scripts were written in Perl, bash, and R. Principal component analysis was performed using Evince (v2.5.5 (Prediktera AB, Umeå, Sweden)) (http://www.prediktera.se/).

Precision (positive predictive value) was calculated as follows: mutations observed in both test method (GATK tumor-only) and standard method (MuTect) (true positives) divided by total mutations called in test method.

$$Precision = \frac{tp}{tp + fp}$$
$$= \frac{\text{mutations observed in test AND standard methods}}{\text{total mutations observed in test method}}$$

Recall (sensitivity) was calculated as follows: mutations observed in both test method and standard method (true positives) divided by total mutations called in standard method.

$$\text{Recall} = \frac{tp}{tp + fn}$$

$$= \frac{\text{mutations observed in test AND standard methods}}{\text{total mutations observed in standard method}}$$

Results

Genotype calling and VQSR tuning

Somatic mutations were identified from tumor samples using BWA [15] alignments and GATK [14] quality improvement and genotype determination. GATK's Unified-Genotyper module has the ability to determine the exact genotype of each sample at every variant position when using the multi-sample detection mode. This returns not only a list of variants seen in each sample but also whether non-variant samples have the reference genotype or are "missing" at a position due to insufficient data. This approach is critical to ensure precise classification of samples as mutated or reference for downstream phenotype association analyses. We initially followed the best practices guidelines with several adjustments (see Additional file 5).

BWA-GATK mutation detection was applied to the TGS dataset, and VQSR FILTER status was examined. A high rate of PASS putative mutations was observed, with about 5% of variants being assigned the least specific "SNPto100" tranche. However, with near-default discovery and VQSR settings, only 3.8% of the COSMIC v61 [18] mutations seen more than five times had a value of PASS (Additional file 3: Figure S2b), while 60% were in the least specific tranche (SNPto100). Neither VQSR tuning (removing Haplotype-Score and percentBadVariants) nor adding a cancer mutation training set (COSMIC v61 mutations seen more than once) greatly increased PASS count. The variant list was then filtered on the target regions plus 25 flanking base pairs (total size = 4.9 megabases) before VQSR, resulting in a large increase in the number of final passing COSMIC variants, 86.4%. This also resulted in a greater proportion of all variants passing filter (Additional file 3: Figure S2a). Finally, the target-region pre-filtering was combined with cancer-specific VQSR settings and training, and a COSMIC pass rate of 98.0% was observed. The overall pass rate also increased to 95.5%, suggesting these settings may have reduced specificity (as fewer positions are filtered) but have allowed very high sensitivity for known cancer mutations.

WES samples were less impacted by GATK settings (Additional file 3: Figure S2c, d). The overall PASS rates were slightly higher than in the TGS data, and COSMIC mutations had a much higher PASS rate with default settings (66.3% in WES vs. 3.8% in TGS). No COSMIC mutations were observed in the SNPto100 tranche with any applied settings. Tuned settings applied to the TGS cohort above were also applied to the WES dataset and also increased the proportion of both COSMIC and all PASS mutations. As was observed in the TGS cohort, the highest PASS rate in the WES cohort occurred when the mutations were first target-filtered, and then, VQSR was run using COSMIC training. While less critical, tumor-specific settings benefit whole exome sequencing as well by ensuring known somatic mutations are not falsely removed.

Efficacy of various filtering strategies

Several strategies were applied to enrich for somatic mutations. A median of 3328 potential mutations per sample was detected with the tuned BWA-GATK pipeline (Fig. 2a, "All"). The 1000 Genomes project [17, 20] has cataloged common inherited genetic variation across many different populations around the globe. Variants seen in this dataset were excluded as a first-pass filter for inherited variation, which decreased the putative mutation rate to a median of 608 per sample (Fig. 2a, "minus 1000 Genomes"). The NHLBI Exome Sequencing Project (ESP) dataset, which includes 6503 individuals, was used for further filtering. Although we expected that the large increase in "control" sample numbers would result in the exclusion of many more rare inherited variants, the median mutation count dropped only to 526 (Fig. 2a, "minus ESP"). Several larger population databases have recently become available. We examined the efficacy of filtering with ExAC [21] and KAVIAR [22]. ExAC includes data from > 60,000 whole exomes, although we used the non-TCGA download to avoid filtering known somatic mutations. KAVIAR includes > 13,000 whole genomes and > 64,000 whole exomes (including the ExAC database) and excludes cancer genomes. Although cancer samples should be absent from these databases, we observed common somatic mutations in both, necessitating the use of an allele frequency cutoff. We found that removing variants present in these databases at ≥ 1% allele frequency further decreases the number of detected mutations (Additional file 3: Figure S3a).

Many putative variants are likely artifacts arising from improper sequence alignment [23, 24], and these artifacts tend to be common across samples. We reasoned that variants observed commonly in tumor samples and also in a pool of normal samples are not likely to be cancer driver mutations and are more likely artifacts, especially when common population variants have already been removed. Potential artifacts were identified in a pool of 238 normal samples using the tuned BWA-GATK pipeline. Although these were matched samples, they were treated as unmatched: any mutation observed in this normal pool dataset at greater than or equal to 5% population allele frequency was removed. This dramatically reduced the number of putative tumor mutations to a median of 109 per sample (Fig. 2a, "minus Normal ≥ 5%"). A stricter filter

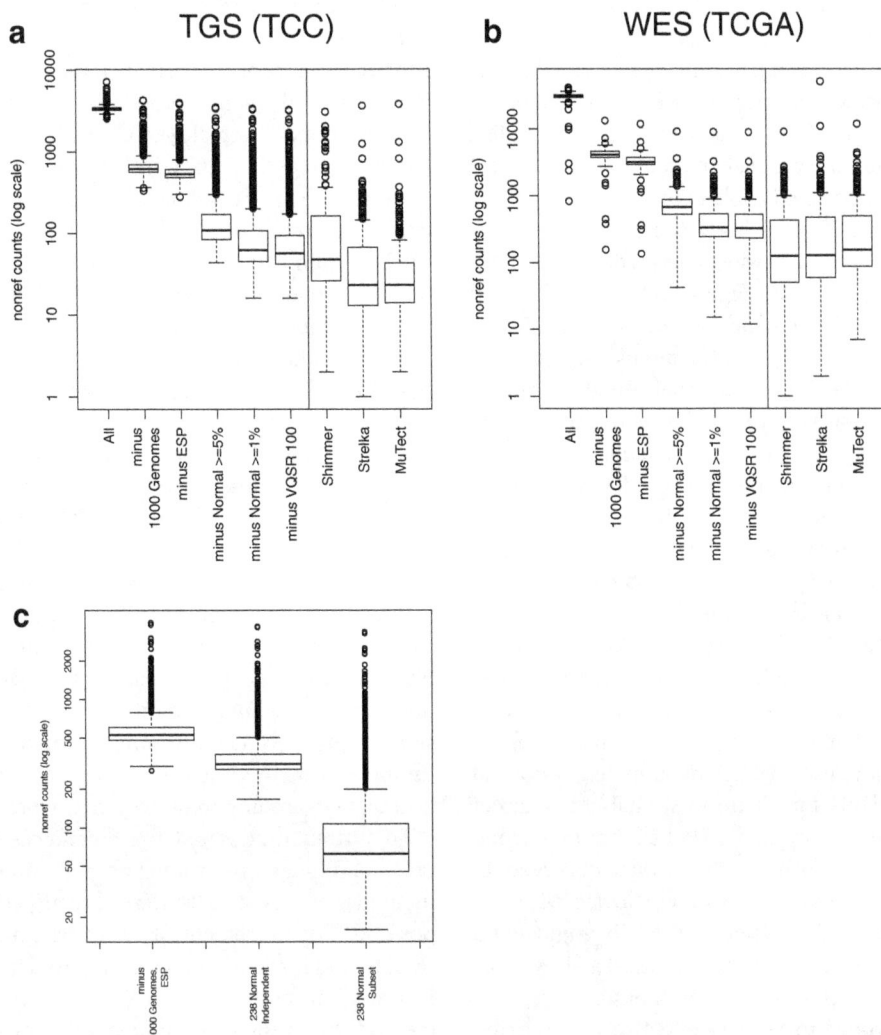

Fig. 2 Tumor-only mutation counts with filtering. **a** Boxplot showing numbers of mutations detected in the TGS cohort using tumor-only methods after each filtering step (left) and using matched tumor-normal methods on 182 sample pairs (right). **b** Boxplot showing numbers of mutations detected in the WES cohort using tumor-only methods after each filtering step (left) and using matched tumor-normal methods (right). **c** Boxplot demonstrating that in the TGS cohort, analyzing the normal samples independent of the tumor samples results in reduced ability to remove potential artifacts. GATK variant detection on all tumor and normal samples together, followed by isolation of the normal subset to annotate the tumor samples, results in the removal of more potential artifacts. Median counts are indicated by the dark line in the middle of the box. The bottom and top of the box are the first and third quartiles, respectively. The whiskers represent the most extreme points within 1.5 times the interquartile range. The y-axes are in a log scale

of no more than 1% normal allele frequency further reduced the median putative mutation count to 62 (Fig. 2a, Additional file 3: Figure S3a, "minusNormal ≥ 1%"). Finally, excluding the VQSR Tranche100 variants resulted in a final median mutation count of 57 ("minus VQSR 100"). This resulted in a final median mutation rate of 11.6/megabase investigated.

A subset of the TGS cohort also had matched adjacent normal samples, allowing for a direct comparison of matched tumor/normal mutation methods to our tumor-only pipeline. We applied three different commonly used algorithms for detection of mutations using matched tumor/normal pairs: Shimmer, Strelka, and MuTect. These

methods have performed reasonably well in comparisons [9, 10] and are all capable of detecting single nucleotide and deletion/insertion mutations. Somatic mutations were identified in 182 matched primary tumor/normal pairs using Shimmer, Strelka, and MuTect, resulting in a median mutation count of 48.0 per sample (9.83/megabase), 23.0 per sample (4.71/megabase), and 23.0 per sample (4.71/megabase), respectively (Fig. 2a, right-hand side).

The same filtering strategy was applied to the WES cohort tumor-only analysis. As different TCGA Genome Sequencing Centers used different targeted capture designs, the refSeq coding exons (plus 25 flanking base pairs) were used as target regions. Although all 250 tumors had a matched normal sample in the TCGA dataset, a subset of 100 was selected for the normal pool and analyzed together with the tumor samples using the GATK tumor-only mutation detection strategy. Putative mutation counts were determined after each sequentially applied filter. Mutation counts were higher than the TGS cohort due to the larger target size (whole exome vs. 1321 genes). As observed for the TGS cohort, the median putative mutation count decreased with each additional filter (Fig. 2b, Additional file 3: Figure S3b): all detected (31,335), minus 1000 genomes (4099.5), minus ESP (3180.5), minus normal $\geq 5\%$ (680), minus normal $\geq 1\%$ (335), minus Tranche100 (327). A final mutation rate of 7.6/megabase was observed within the refSeq coding target (43.0 megabases, including 25 bp flanking regions). The difference between mutation rates of TGS and WES is most likely due to the differences in cohort makeup (the TGS cohort has more samples from the more highly mutated tumor types). Importantly, the pattern of putative mutation count decrease was similar in the TGS and WES cohorts: large initial decreases when removing 1000 genome variants; modest decreases after further excluding ESP, KAVIAR, and ExAC; and then large decreases after further filtering with a normal pool.

As the WES cohort used TCGA data, matched normal samples were available for all tumors, enabling a direct comparison of tumor-only and matched tumor/normal mutation detection. Similar to the results observed in the TGS cohort, mutation counts were lower with the matched tumor/normal methods (Fig. 2b, right-hand side): Shimmer 125 (2.9/megabase), Strelka 128 (3.0/megabase), and MuTect 154.5 (3.6/megabase).

Normal pools proved to be very effective in removing putative variants in both TGS and WES cohorts. Titration experiments were performed to determine filtering effectiveness using fewer normal samples. The resulting mutation counts were compared after filtering with decreasing numbers of normal samples: from 238 down to 12 (TGS cohort) and from 100 down to 20 (WES cohort). Surprisingly, the amount of putative mutations remaining after removing variants with normal sample allele frequency $\geq 1\%$ was stable down to 25 samples (TGS) and 20 samples (WES) (Additional file 3: Figure S4a, b). Furthermore, the exact method of mutation detection in the normal pool affected the results. When the TGS normal samples were analyzed in a separate, independent GATK run, the number of putative artifacts removed was less then when the normal samples were analyzed together with the tumor samples (Fig. 3c). This is likely due to increased prior probability of detection when variants are observed in other samples using GATK multi-sample genotype detection. This suggests it is beneficial to analyze all samples together and then extract the normal samples for frequency calculations.

Precision, recall, and sensitivity for known tumor mutations

Mutation detection performance was examined by comparing results of each method at each mutated position. MuTect tumor/normal was used as a truth set due to its common usage in TCGA analyses, as well as its reasonable performance in evaluations of tumor/normal methods. Precision and recall were calculated for each sample against MuTect tumor/normal using GATK tumor-only, Strelka tumor/normal, and Shimmer tumor/normal (Fig. 3a, b). GATK tumor-only recall at all positions was similar to Shimmer and slightly decreased compared to Strelka in both TGS and WES datasets. However, the GATK tumor-only precision was much lower than the Strelka in TGS, and much lower than both Strelka and Shimmer in WES data. We also noted precision and recall heterogeneity across samples for each method. Precision and recall were calculated at subsequent filter levels, which demonstrated increasing precision and slightly decreasing recall with each additional filter (Additional file 3: Figures S5 and S6). Although many inherited variants are removed by population filters, precision only moderately increases due to the large number of remaining variants. This suggests it is not possible to precisely identify somatic mutations with current tumor-only methods and that both population filters and a normal pool are important to increase precision.

To further understand the differences between tumor-only and matched tumor-normal mutation detection methods, genotype calls were directly compared at each position. The agreement of calls was counted within each sample, and median values are displayed in Additional file 3: Figure S7. In both TGS and WES cohorts, the tumor-only method shows the most unique mutations. This was more pronounced in the WES dataset, which agrees with the earlier observation of a larger difference in mutation counts between tumor-only and tumor-normal methods (Fig. 2). Interestingly, Shimmer called many more unique mutations than other tumor-normal methods in the TGS dataset, but MuTect called many more unique mutations in the WES cohort. Positions at which all methods made the same mutation call were the more common ($\sim$ 5-fold) than any other combination of two or more methods. Despite this agreement, we noticed that many positions were called by some tumor/normal methods and not others (Additional file 3: Figure S8). Strelka had the highest degree of overlap with the other two methods in both cohorts.

Sensitivity for known cancer mutations was assessed by determining the fraction of COSMIC mutations observed in each dataset. 43.5% of those positions observed commonly in COSMIC (more than 20 times) were also observed in the tumor-only TGS analysis (Fig. 3c, right). This fraction decreased as the less common mutations were considered, likely due to the increased numbers of

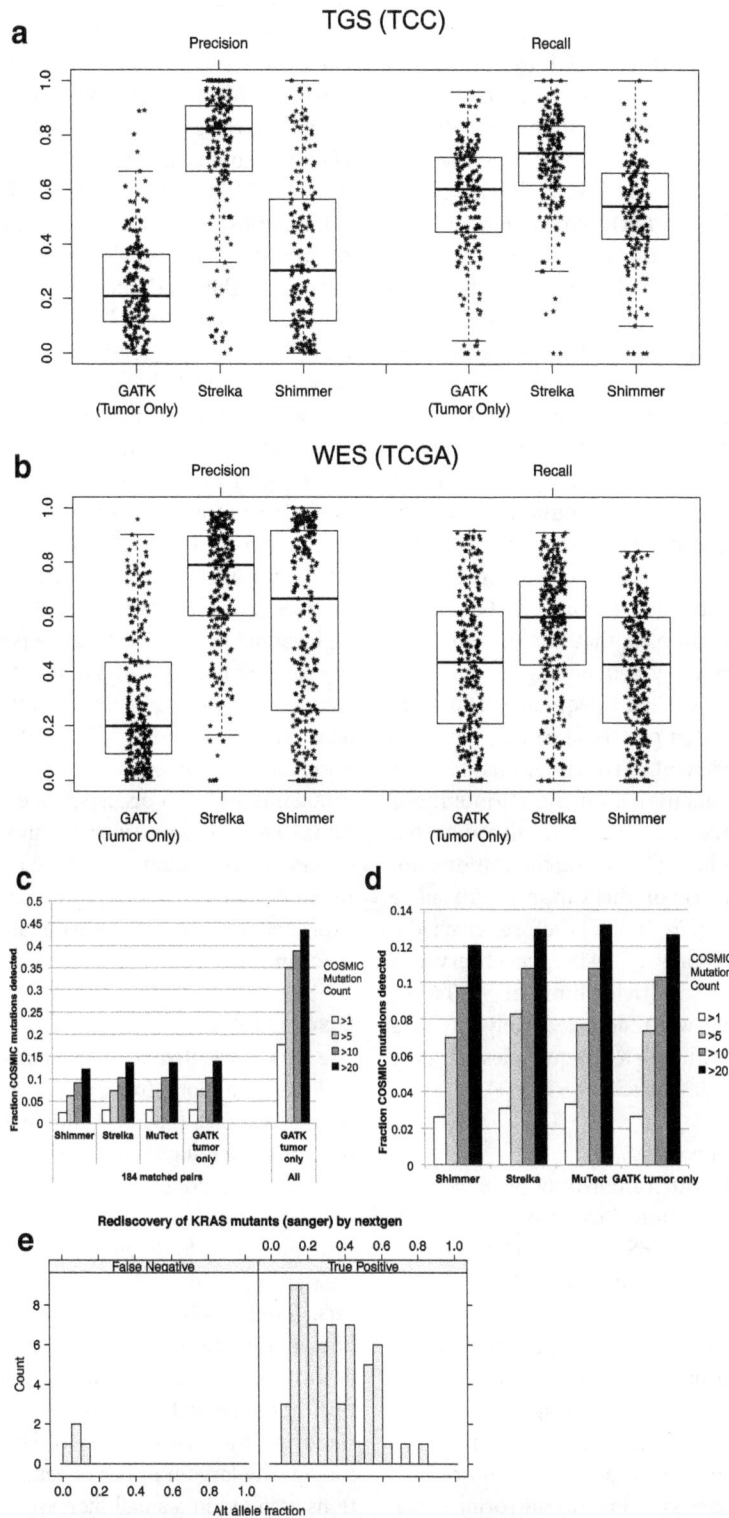

Fig. 3 Recall and precision of tumor-only and matched tumor-normal mutation detection. Recall and precision of methods compared to MuTect in TGS (**a**) and WES (**b**). Distributions are represented with box plots, and individual data points are plotted as asterisks. Fraction of COSMIC mutations detected by **c** matched tumor-normal and tumor-only methods within 182 TGS samples (left) and all TGS samples using tumor-only methods (right). **d** 250 WES samples. Shading indicates the number of times the mutation was observed in the COSMIC v61 database. **e** TGS alternate allele fraction and accuracy of *KRAS* G12/G13/Q61 mutations initially discovered by capillary sequencing. Not shown are the seven mutations detected in the TGS but not capillary sequencing

the more rare mutations as well as false positives (artifacts and common variants) in COSMIC. The fraction of COSMIC mutations detected in 182 TGS tumor/normal pairs was calculated from three different tumor-normal pair mutation detection methods (Shimmer, Strelka, MuTect) as well as from the GATK tumor-only method. The fraction of COSMIC bases observed was highly similar in all methods (Fig. 3c, left). Similar results were observed in the WES cohort: the tumor-only mutation detection method had similar sensitivity as the three different tumor-normal methods (Fig. 3d). This suggests the tumor-only approach has equivalent sensitivity to detect known cancer mutations.

Sample heterogeneity presents a specific challenge for sensitive detection of somatic mutations. The fraction of reads with a mutated base can be lower than expected due to normal sample contamination, mutational heterogeneity within the tumor, or chromosomal amplification. We therefore examined the sensitivity of our final tuned pipeline to detect low-frequency mutations. One hundred ninety of the lung samples that underwent TGS were also subjected to capillary sequencing at the G12/ G13/Q61 KRAS loci. The capillary sequence data were analyzed with both automated genotype calling pipelines and extensive manual review of chromatograms in order to detect low-frequency mutations. Of the 70 mutations detected by capillary sequencing, 66 were also detected using the tumor-only method. Of the four mutations not detected, three had evidence of the variant, with allele frequencies less than 10% (Fig. 3e). Therefore, given the median overall target coverage of 141×, we observed a mutation allele frequency sensitivity limit of ~ 10%. In addition, seven mutations were detected only in TGS data (not in capillary), with allele frequencies ranging from 8 to 29% (mean = 18.0%, median = 15.6%).

Pan-cancer somatic mutation rates

Mutation rates detected by our tumor-only pipeline were calculated across different tumor sites of origin in TGS (sites with ≥ 50 samples) and WES cohorts. The frequencies observed using tumor-only mutation detection were higher than those from a matched tumor/normal large consortium sequencing project [25] (Fig. 4a, b). We observed a high variability in mutation rates in skin, uterus/ endometrium, lung, and large bowel in agreement with the previous large consortium studies. Skin, uterus, and lung have the highest mutation rates in the "tumor-only" analyses; LAML and CLL have the lowest, mirroring other studies. This suggests that somatic mutations can be greatly enriched using tumor-only methods, but not as precisely identified as matched tumor/normal methods. Our observations have reproduced the overall mutation frequency patterns of large global consortium studies in a completely independent cohort.

Molecular associations with high mutation burden

Although the median mutation rate varies across tumor sites, every site has outlier tumors with very high mutation rates. To identify the potential molecular causes of high mutation rates, we examined DNA polymerase epsilon (POLE) exonuclease domain mutations (amino acids 268-471 and R494 in NP_006222). The recurrent POLE mutations almost always occur in the highly mutated outlier samples (Fig. 4c). Singleton POLE mutations fell into two groups: highly and moderately mutated tumors. Highly mutated samples with POLE mutations were primarily observed in tumors originating from the endometrium/ uterus, large bowel, and ovary. One highly mutated sample with a POLE mutation was observed in breast and pancreatic cancers; the POLE-mutated sample was the most highly mutated in each site.

We have recently observed that the presence of homopolymer indels in both TGFBR2 and ACVR2A is highly correlated with microsatellite instability (MSI) in TGS colorectal samples [26]. Here, we demonstrate that these samples have high mutation rates in the large bowel (Fig. 4d), strengthening the link between ACVR2A+TGFBR2 mutation and MSI status. Additionally, several putative MSI samples in stomach (2), endometrium (3), and breast (1) tumors were observed. Notably, ACVR2A+TGFBR2 mutations and POLE mutations only co-occurred once (singleton POLE mutation). These observations confirm and extend previously observed correlations of specific mutations and elevated mutation rates. Many highly mutated samples remained unexplained and require further analysis to identify mutational mechanisms.

Discussion

We have presented an analysis strategy for the detection of somatic mutations from tumor samples without matched normal samples (Fig. 5, Additional file 5). GATK modifications for detecting somatic mutations included (1) limiting putative mutations to targeted regions, (2) using a VQSR training set of known cancer mutations, and (3) tuning of settings (see Additional file 5) These modifications had a greater impact on reducing false negatives in smaller target sets. Tuning GATK also improved the filter quality of known mutations in whole exome data, although fewer false negatives were initially observed. The use of population genomic datasets (1000 Genomes) was effective at removing the vast majority of likely inherited variants, although the large number of remaining false positive mutations resulted in a small increase in precision. Interestingly, the addition of larger population-specific germline datasets (via the Exome Sequencing Project, ExAC, and KAVIAR) each only removed a modest fraction of additional common variants compared to decreases observed after filtering with a normal pool. Indeed, filtering with ExAC and KAVIAR after the normal pool resulted in removal of only

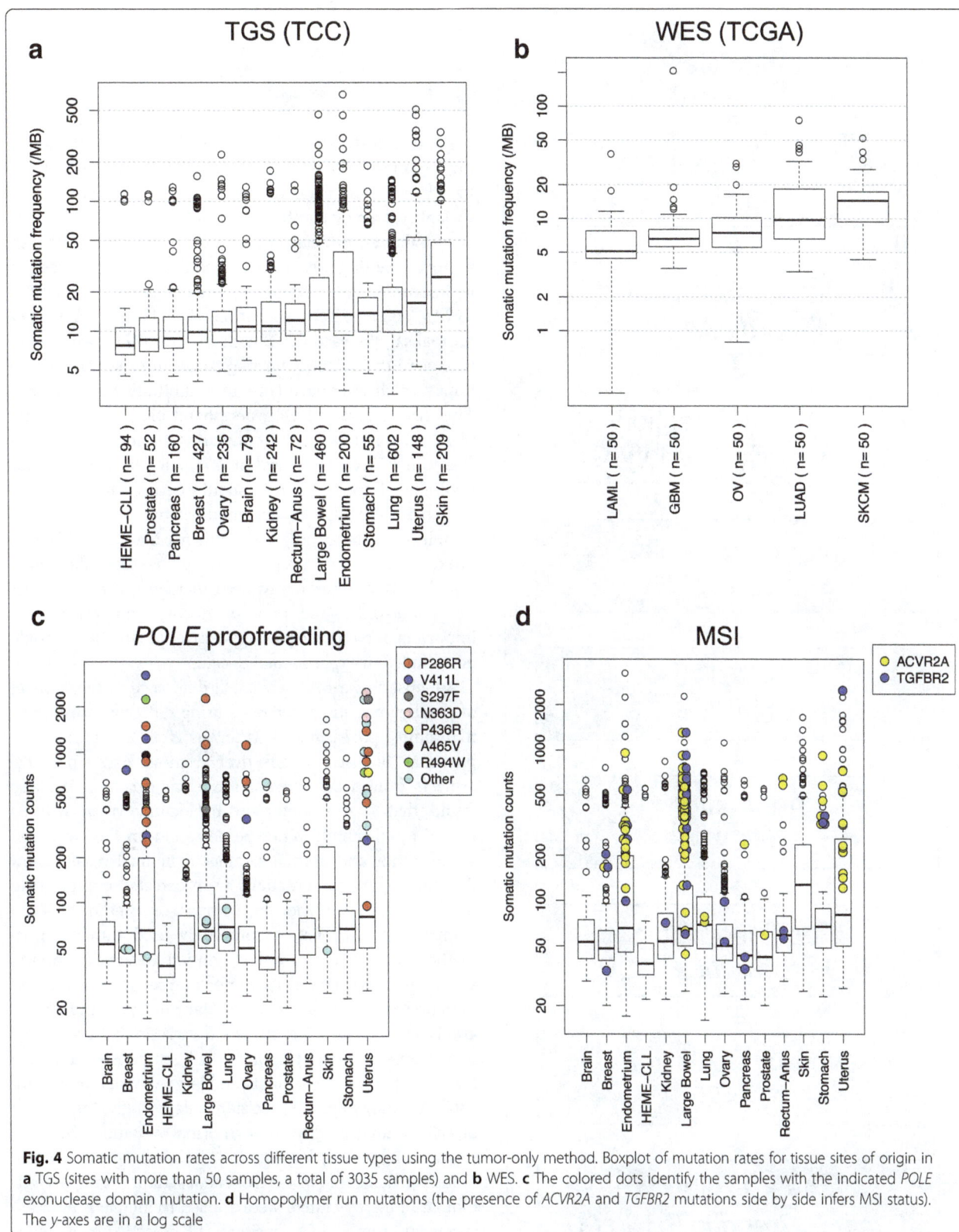

Fig. 4 Somatic mutation rates across different tissue types using the tumor-only method. Boxplot of mutation rates for tissue sites of origin in **a** TGS (sites with more than 50 samples, a total of 3035 samples) and **b** WES. **c** The colored dots identify the samples with the indicated *POLE* exonuclease domain mutation. **d** Homopolymer run mutations (the presence of *ACVR2A* and *TGFBR2* mutations side by side infers MSI status). The *y*-axes are in a log scale

a few variants (Additional file 3: Figure S3). While population databases are helpful in removing inherited variants, they often include overlapping samples and can contain known somatic mutations even when cancer samples have been removed. Therefore, investigators should review population datasets carefully before using them as a filter.

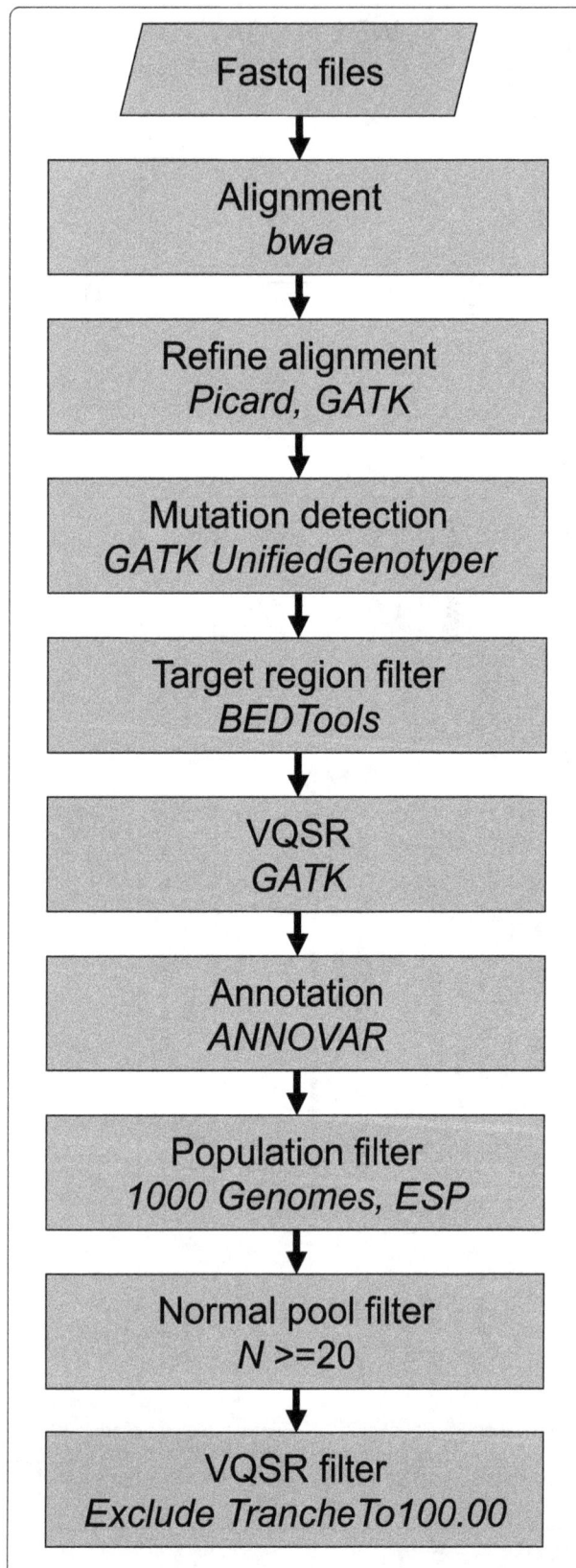

Fig. 5 Schematic of tumor-only mutation calling pipeline. Analytical pipeline overview for tumor mutation calling with a subset of matched normal samples. See Additional file 5 for details of commands, options, and settings

We demonstrated and quantitated the utility of excluding variants observed in a subset pool of normal samples to enrich for somatic mutations. Arbitrary normal pool variant frequency cutoffs of ≥ 5 and ≥ 1% were selected to ensure that known cancer mutations were not erroneously removed. Setting a normal pool allele frequency threshold is important: we observed common cancer mutations (*BRAF* V600E, *PTEN* truncation, *TP53* G245C) in a single normal sample each (TGS cohort). The TGS normal samples were the adjacent normal tissue from surgical resections, which may have contained infiltrating tumor cells. This risk is lessened with peripheral blood normal samples, but observations of circulating tumor cells or cell-free tumor DNA (reviewed in [27]) suggest that a normal pool allele frequency cutoff should be used to avoid false negatives. We also recommend examining the normal sample variants for any well-known cancer mutations to avoid erroneous exclusion. Although we describe mutation detection in tumors without matched normal samples as "tumor-only," the pool of normal samples is very important for reducing false positive variants and should be included in experimental design.

We observed a relatively small difference in the number of putative mutations removed using differently sized normal sample pools. Indeed, as few as 20 to 25 normal samples may be used to effectively remove many potential artifacts from a large tumor sequencing dataset. We also found that it was important to identify variants using GATK multi-sample genotype detection on the combined set of tumor and normal samples. Our final results show that more putative mutations were detected compared to that in three tumor/normal comparison methods. When compared to MuTect, a commonly used tumor/normal method, GATK tumor-only mutation detection, showed similar sensitivity/recall to tumor/normal methods. However, precision was much lower. Many of these "mutations" are likely to be very rare inherited variants that could only be removed by direct tumor/normal comparison, although future method improvements and larger population variant databases may improve precision. Interestingly, the overlap of calls among precise tumor/normal mutation detection was also imperfect, highlighting the challenge of somatic mutation detection in heterogeneous tumor samples. Although numerous filters were applied to increase mutation specificity, tumor-only sensitivity to detect known mutations was equivalent to tumor/normal pair mutation detection. Comparison with manually reviewed capillary sequencing data demonstrated high tumor-only sensitivity (down to 10% mutant allele frequency) in heterogeneous tumor samples. Therefore, tumor-only sequencing supplemented with a normal pool is an effective alternative to paired tumor/normal sequencing, with similar recall but reduced precision.

Recently, Jones et al. [11] described tumor-only sequencing in 58 targeted samples (111 genes) and 100 whole exomes. We have extended their observations by examining 3380 TGS samples (1321 genes) and 250 WES samples (drawn from 5 diseases included in TCGA). Our observations of high sensitivity for known mutations, but lower precision (especially in WES), agree with those of Jones et al.. We have additionally demonstrated significant non-overlap between three different matched tumor/normal methods. This suggests differences between tumor-only and tumor/normal methods may be due to inaccuracies in both analysis strategies. While Jones et al. conclude tumor-only methods may not be sufficient for high accuracy in the clinical setting, we find the high degree of sensitivity may be useful for tumor classification. Finally, we offer detailed methods to enable others to utilize tumor-only mutation detection.

The observed recall and precision of the tumor-only approach with a limited normal pool suggests that this method lends itself to specific use cases. It has been suggested [25] that there are still many cancer genes and mutations to be discovered, requiring sequencing of many more samples. Although the tumor-only approach results in almost half the cost to reach a target sample size (as each tumor no longer needs a matched normal sample), our analysis demonstrated much lower precision that would result in many more false positive mutations. We conclude that tumor-only approaches are not appropriate for novel mutation detection. However, given similar sensitivity to detect known cancer mutations in heterogeneous tumor samples with greatly reduced cost, the tumor-only detection method can be useful for characterization of known mutations. Indeed, we reproduced earlier observations of mutation rate patterns across diseases. We also identified mutations in the exonuclease domain of *POLE* and mutations associated with MSI as two mechanisms explaining highly mutated samples. MSI mutations were observed in large bowel but also occasionally in endometrium and stomach tumors. *POLE* mutations were observed in many tumor types: endometrium/uterus, large bowel, ovary, pancreas, and breast. Sample classification by known recurrent mutations enables the critical next step in cancer genomics: association of genomic alterations with clinical phenotype. The almost doubling of sample size at a given cost gained from omitting matched normal samples can dramatically improve power to associate mutations with phenotype, but researchers must consider the loss of precision that results when matched normal samples are not used.

Conclusions

Detection of somatic mutations using tumor samples and a smaller subset of normal samples is a valid strategy for cancer genomics studies. The use of population datasets (1000 Genomes) reduces the number of inherited variants and artifacts. However, filtering against a pool of normal samples captured and sequenced with the same technology increases precision noticeably and should be considered a required part of a "tumor-only" sequencing experiment. We find that recall across all observed mutations is similar to matched tumor/normal methods, and sensitivity for known cancer mutations is equivalent. However, the precision is lower: many putative mutations detected by the tumor-only method are not observed in matched tumor/normal methods. Therefore, tumor-only detection methods as described here are appropriate for characterization of known mutations in samples. Matched tumor/normal mutation detection is more appropriate for applications requiring high precision such as novel mutation detection and mutation signature analysis and remains the optimal approach, especially as sequencing costs continue to decrease.

Additional files

Additional file 1: Table S1. Sample counts by the site of tumor origin.

Additional file 2: Table S2.

Additional file 3: Figure S1. Large tumor dataset quality control metrics. A. Principal component analysis and B. loadings using sequencing metrics. Colors in A. represent the different tissue sites of origin. C. Ratio of sequence reads aligning to the X and Y chromosome and cutoffs used to infer gender. D. Histogram of average coverage over targeted bases (filtered, aligned reads). **Figure S2:** VQSR filtering effects on tumor-only mutation detection. A. Fraction of total putative TGS mutations falling in each GATK VQSR tranche (PASS being the most specific, SNPto100 being the least specific). B. Fraction of TGS mutations seen in COSMIC more than five times falling into each VQSR tranche. C. Fraction of total putative WES mutations falling in each GATK VQSR tranche (PASS being most specific, SNPto100 being least specific). D. Fraction of WES mutations seen in COSMIC more than five times falling into each VQSR tranche. **Figure S3:** Mutation counts after filtering with additional population databases. Boxplots showing numbers of mutations detected after filtering with KAVIAR, ExAC, or both (excluding AF ≥ 1%) in addition to 1000 Genomes and ESP. The rightmost columns show the minimal effect of filtering with KAVIAR and ExAC after the normal filter has been applied. A. TGS cohort, B. WES cohort. Median counts are indicated by the dark line in the middle of the box. The bottom and top of the box are the first and third quartiles, respectively. The whiskers represent the most extreme points within 1.5 times the interquartile range. The y-axes are in the log scale. **Figure S4:** Normal pool features affect the ability to remove variants. Boxplots showing the putative mutation counts after filtering with titrated sample counts in the normal pool for A. TGS cohort, B. WES cohort. **Figure S5:** Total nonref counts, precision, and recall with subsequent filters. Total nonref counts (left), precision compare to MuTect (middle), and recall compared to MuTect (right) for A. TGS and B. WES. All plots are in a linear scale. **Figure S6:** Precision-recall curve. Plot showing approximate precision vs recall for A. TGS and B. WES. Data point circles are area-proportional to the number of putative mutations at each filter level. Note the largest circle across the middle of the plots corresponds to precision = 0, recall = 1. Also note that data point circle sizes are scaled to fit, and the scaling factors are different for TGS and WES. The red line indicates performance of the random classifier based on positives (median number of MuTect call)/total positions (targeted bases). **Figure S7:** Overlap between mutation calls across four methods. Non-area-proportional Venn diagram showing median mutation counts across samples called by each combination of methods. The bold underlined values are the intersection of all the four methods. The underlined values are the counts unique to each method. A. TGS (TCC) cohort and B. WES (TCGA) cohort. **Figure S8:** Overlap between mutation calls across three matched tumor/normal methods. Non-area-proportional Venn diagram showing median mutation counts across samples called by each combination of methods. The bold underlined values are the intersection of all the three methods. The underlined values are the counts unique to each method. A. TGS (TCC) cohort and B. WES

Additional file 4: Table S3.

Additional file 5: Methods: A detailed description of the analysis methods used for the detection of somatic mutations with an unmatched pool of

Acknowledgements
We thank the many patients who provided the data and tissue to the Total Cancer Care Consortium. Our study received valuable assistance from the Cancer Informatics Core and Collaborative Data Services Core at the H. Lee Moffitt Cancer Center & Research Institute, an NCI-designated Comprehensive Cancer Center, supported under the NIH grant P30-CA76292.

Funding
Total Cancer Care® is enabled, in part, by the generous support of the DeBartolo Family. This study was supported, in part, by the NIH grant P30-CA76292. The sequence data was generated in partnership with Merck & Co.

Authors' contributions
JKT, YZ, SAE, and AEB designed the experiments; JKT, YZ, LC, EAW, and WDC analyzed the data; and JKT, SAE, and AEB wrote and edited the manuscript. All authors read and approved the final manuscript.

Competing interests
The authors declare that they have no competing interests.

Author details
[1]Department of Biostatistics and Bioinformatics, H. Lee Moffitt Cancer Center and Research Institute, Tampa, FL 33612, USA. [2]Department of Molecular Oncology, H. Lee Moffitt Cancer Center and Research Institute, Tampa, FL 33612, USA.

References
1. Stratton MR, Campbell PJ, Futreal PA. The cancer genome. Nature. 2009;458: 719–24.
2. Watson IR, Takahashi K, Futreal PA, Chin L. Emerging patterns of somatic mutations in cancer. Nat Rev Genet. 2013;14:703–18.
3. Koboldt DC, Chen K, Wylie T, Larson DE, McLellan MD, Mardis ER, Weinstock GM, Wilson RK, Ding L. VarScan: variant detection in massively parallel sequencing of individual and pooled samples. Bioinformatics. 2009;25:2283–5.
4. Koboldt DC, Zhang Q, Larson DE, Shen D, McLellan MD, Lin L, Miller CA, Mardis ER, Ding L, Wilson RK. VarScan 2: somatic mutation and copy number alteration discovery in cancer by exome sequencing. Genome Res. 2012;22:568–76.
5. Hansen NF, Gartner JJ, Mei L, Samuels Y, Mullikin JC. Shimmer: detection of genetic alterations in tumors using next-generation sequence data. Bioinformatics. 2013;29:1498–503.
6. Larson DE, Harris CC, Chen K, Koboldt DC, Abbott TE, Dooling DJ, Ley TJ, Mardis ER, Wilson RK, Ding L. SomaticSniper: identification of somatic point mutations in whole genome sequencing data. Bioinformatics. 2012;28:311–7.
7. Saunders CT, Wong WS, Swamy S, Becq J, Murray LJ, Cheetham RK. Strelka: accurate somatic small-variant calling from sequenced tumor-normal sample pairs. Bioinformatics. 2012;28:1811–7.
8. Cibulskis K, Lawrence MS, Carter SL, Sivachenko A, Jaffe D, Sougnez C, Gabriel S, Meyerson M, Lander ES, Getz G. Sensitive detection of somatic point mutations in impure and heterogeneous cancer samples. Nat Biotechnol. 2013;31:213–9.
9. Ewing AD, Houlahan KE, Hu Y, Ellrott K, Caloian C, Yamaguchi TN, Bare JC, P'ng C, Waggott D, Sabelnykova VY, et al. Combining tumor genome simulation with crowdsourcing to benchmark somatic single-nucleotide-variant detection. Nat Methods. 2015;12:623–30.
10. Kroigard AB, Thomassen M, Laenkholm AV, Kruse TA, Larsen MJ. Evaluation of nine somatic variant callers for detection of somatic mutations in exome and targeted deep sequencing data. PLoS One. 2016;11:e0151664.
11. Jones S, Anagnostou V, Lytle K, Parpart-Li S, Nesselbush M, Riley DR, Shukla M, Chesnick B, Kadan M, Papp E, et al. Personalized genomic analyses for cancer mutation discovery and interpretation. Sci Transl Med. 2015;7: 283ra253.
12. Fenstermacher DA, Wenham RM, Rollison DE, Dalton WS. Implementing personalized medicine in a cancer center. Cancer J. 2011;17:528–36.
13. McKenna A, Hanna M, Banks E, Sivachenko A, Cibulskis K, Kernytsky A, Garimella K, Altshuler D, Gabriel S, Daly M, et al. The Genome Analysis Toolkit: a MapReduce framework for analyzing next-generation DNA sequencing data. Genome Res. 2010;20:1297–303.
14. DePristo MA, Banks E, Poplin R, Garimella KV, Maguire JR, Hartl C, Philippakis AA, del Angel G, Rivas MA, Hanna M, et al. A framework for variation discovery and genotyping using next-generation DNA sequencing data. Nat Genet. 2011;43:491–8.
15. Li H, Durbin R. Fast and accurate short read alignment with Burrows-Wheeler transform. Bioinformatics. 2009;25:1754–60.
16. Wang K, Li M, Hakonarson H. ANNOVAR: functional annotation of genetic variants from high-throughput sequencing data. Nucleic Acids Res. 2010;38:e164.
17. Abecasis GR, Auton A, Brooks LD, DePristo MA, Durbin RM, Handsaker RE, Kang HM, Marth GT, McVean GA. An integrated map of genetic variation from 1,092 human genomes. Nature. 2012;491:56–65.
18. Forbes SA, Bhamra G, Bamford S, Dawson E, Kok C, Clements J, Menzies A, Teague JW, Futreal PA, Stratton MR. The Catalogue of Somatic Mutations in Cancer (COSMIC). Curr Protoc Hum Genet. 2008; Chapter 10:Unit 10 11.
19. Quinlan AR, Hall IM. BEDTools: a flexible suite of utilities for comparing genomic features. Bioinformatics. 2010;26:841–2.
20. Durbin RM, Abecasis GR, Altshuler DL, Auton A, Brooks LD, Gibbs RA, Hurles ME, McVean GA. A map of human genome variation from population-scale sequencing. Nature. 2010;467:1061–73.
21. Lek M, Karczewski KJ, Minikel EV, Samocha KE, Banks E, Fennell T, O'Donnell-Luria AH, Ware JS, Hill AJ, Cummings BB, et al. Analysis of protein-coding genetic variation in 60,706 humans. Nature. 2016;536:285–91.
22. Glusman G, Caballero J, Mauldin DE, Hood L, Roach JC. Kaviar: an accessible system for testing SNV novelty. Bioinformatics. 2011;27:3216–7.
23. Ng SB, Buckingham KJ, Lee C, Bigham AW, Tabor HK, Dent KM, Huff CD, Shannon PT, Jabs EW, Nickerson DA, et al. Exome sequencing identifies the cause of a mendelian disorder. Nat Genet. 2010;42:30–5.
24. Church DM, Schneider VA, Graves T, Auger K, Cunningham F, Bouk N, Chen HC, Agarwala R, McLaren WM, Ritchie GR, et al. Modernizing reference genome assemblies. PLoS Biol. 2011;9:e1001091.
25. Lawrence MS, Stojanov P, Mermel CH, Robinson JT, Garraway LA, Golub TR, Meyerson M, Gabriel SB, Lander ES, Getz G. Discovery and saturation analysis of cancer genes across 21 tumour types. Nature. 2014;505:495–501.
26. Schell MJ, Yang M, Teer JK, Lo FY, Madan A, Coppola D, Monteiro AN, Nebozhyn MV, Yue B, Loboda A, et al. A multigene mutation classification of 468 colorectal cancers reveals a prognostic role for APC. Nat Commun. 2016;7:11743.
27. Haber DA, Velculescu VE. Blood-based analyses of cancer: circulating tumor cells and circulating tumor DNA. Cancer Discov. 2014;4:650–61.

5

Early-life adversity and long-term neurobehavioral outcomes: epigenome as a bridge?

Alexander M. Vaiserman[*] and Alexander K. Koliada

Abstract

Accumulating evidence suggests that adversities at critical periods in early life, both pre- and postnatal, can lead to neuroendocrine perturbations, including hypothalamic-pituitary-adrenal axis dysregulation and inflammation persisting up to adulthood. This process, commonly referred to as biological embedding, may cause abnormal cognitive and behavioral functioning, including impaired learning, memory, and depressive- and anxiety-like behaviors, as well as neuropsychiatric outcomes in later life. Currently, the regulation of gene activity by epigenetic mechanisms is suggested to be a key player in mediating the link between adverse early-life events and adult neurobehavioral outcomes. Role of particular genes, including those encoding glucocorticoid receptor, brain-derived neurotrophic factor, as well as arginine vasopressin and corticotropin-releasing factor, has been demonstrated in triggering early adversity-associated pathological conditions. This review is focused on the results from human studies highlighting the causal role of epigenetic mechanisms in mediating the link between the adversity during early development, from prenatal stages through infancy, and adult neuropsychiatric outcomes. The modulation of epigenetic pathways involved in biological embedding may provide promising direction toward novel therapeutic strategies against neurological and cognitive dysfunctions in adult life.

Keywords: Biological embedding, DNA methylation, Early-life adversity, Epigenetics, Neurobehavioral outcomes

Background

A growing body of research in recent years highlights the importance of early-life environmental influences in determining the adult health status. On the base of these findings, the Developmental Origin of Adult Health and Disease (DOHaD) hypothesis was proposed postulating that unfavorable environmental early-life conditions can result in "developmental programming" of later-life chronic disease [1, 2]. This hypothesis has been initially focused on the lifelong outcomes of prenatal and neonatal malnutrition. In recent years, however, it became increasingly apparent that non-nutritional impacts such as psychological stress exposure during development can also greatly affect the health status throughout adult life, and epigenetic regulation is considered as a key mechanism mediating these effects.

Most research evidence for the developmental programming by stressful conditions early in life is obtained in rodent models (for reviews, see references [3–6]). In these studies, convincing evidence has been obtained to indicate that early stressful exposures such as perinatal stresses, maternal separation, and inadequate maternal care can cause marked neuroendocrine perturbations persisting up to adulthood and causing impaired cognitive, behavioral, and social functioning during the adult life. A body of studies has demonstrated that prenatal stress and exposure to excess levels of exogenous glucocorticoids can both be related to unfavorable health outcomes including low birth weight, neuroendocrine pathology, and enhanced risk for cardio-metabolic, infectious, and psychiatric disorders throughout the adult life [7–9]. The neuroendocrine effects triggered by prenatal stress have been reported to be associated with depressive- or anxiety-like behavioral phenotypes, including altered levels of physical activity, enhanced immobility throughout a forced swim test, and lowered exploration of novel environments [10]. These effects were shown to be mediated by changes in both maternal and fetal hypothalamic-pituitary-adrenal (HPA) axes causing intrauterine exposure to glucocorticoid excess [11, 12]. A role for in-utero glucocorticoid exposure

* Correspondence: vaiserman@geront.kiev.ua
Laboratory of Epigenetics, Institute of Gerontology, Vyshgorodskaya st. 67, Kiev 04114, Ukraine

induced by maternal stress in rats is evident from research in adult offspring born to either mothers with an intact corticosterone secretion or to intrauterine-stressed adrenalectomized dams [13]. The maternal stress-induced glucocorticoids can pass the placental barrier and thereby disrupt the development of the fetal brain. The stress-related maternal-placental-fetal endocrine and immune/inflammatory candidate mechanisms were proposed as possible candidate mechanisms for long-term effects of the fetal stress exposures on physiological characteristics of the developing organism [14, 15]. Early postnatal stages are another important sensitive period for developmental programming. In rodent research, it was shown that impaired mother-infant interactions (e.g., maternal deprivation/separation) throughout the postnatal period can substantially impair the neuroendocrine regulation, including upregulation of hippocampal glucocorticoid receptor (GR) and hypothalamic corticotropin-releasing factor (CRF), and also can lead to enhancement of the adrenocorticotropic hormone and corticosterone levels [16–18]. Such early adversity-induced neuroendocrine changes may lead to behavioral issues during adulthood, including the impaired learning, memory, and also depressive- and anxiety-like behaviors [19]. The long-term effects caused by variation in postnatal maternal care in rodents (e.g., low or high levels of licking and grooming, LG) are most studied in this context to date. The offspring of high-LG mothers exhibited lower levels of stress responsivity, better performance on cognitive tasks, and exploratory behavior in a novel environment during adulthood than the offspring that have been reared by low-LG dams [20, 21]. In these studies, the physiological and biochemical changes induced by adversities in early life were accompanied by substantial alterations on the level of epigenetic control of gene expression and related changes in patterns of DNA methylation, histone modifications, and microRNA regulation.

The evidence for long-lasting effects of adversities in early life from human studies are rather scarce and mainly limited to change in DNA methylation level which is thought to be the most stable form of epigenetic modification. This review is mostly focused on the results obtained from human studies highlighting the causative role of epigenetic pathways in mediating the link between the adversity in early development from prenatal stages through infancy and adult neuropsychiatric outcomes.

Search strategy

In this review, we searched the PubMed database (http://www.ncbi.nlm.nih.gov/pubmed/) to find all published studies on the epigenetic links (both at the genome-wide and candidate gene levels) between early-life adversity and long-term neurobehavioral outcomes in humans. In our search, we used combinations of the following search terms: "biological embedding," "early-life adversity," "epigenetic," "epigenome," "DNA methylation," "neurobehavioral," and "neuropsychiatric." The time period of the search covered articles published from 1994 to 2017 with no language restrictions, although only English language studies were eventually included. There was no restriction on the type of study design; therefore, all clinical, epidemiological, and quasi-experimental studies satisfying the search criteria were included. Several relevant experimental studies closely related to the topic under discussion were also eligible for inclusion. We used these papers to determine whether there is a coherence of effects across humans and non-human species and to examine the contribution of epigenetic mechanisms in biological embedding of adverse early-life exposures.

Biological embedding of adverse experiences in early life

Currently, the regulation of gene activity by epigenetic mechanisms (mitotically or meiotically heritable changes in gene expression that occur without any change in DNA sequence) is suggested to be a key player in mediating the link between stressful events early in life and adult neurobehavioral outcomes [22, 23]. DNA is known to maintain stability during the whole life cycle (except for mutations that occur randomly), while the epigenetic marks are dramatically changed throughout the early developmental stages to initiate distinguished patterns of expression among different developing tissues. The main mechanisms of epigenetic regulation in mammals are covalent modification of DNA by methylation, post-translational modifications (including acetylation, phosphorylation, methylation, and ubiquitinion) of the histone proteins, as well as regulation by non-coding RNAs (ncRNAs) [24].

There are numerous lines of evidence indicating that the mammalian epigenome (i.e., the totality of epigenetic marks across the whole genome) is the most labile and, thereby, most sensitive to various environmental and hormonal cues, at specific stages of early development [25]. In mammals, a global demethylation of DNA followed by remethylation was shown to occur throughout the development of germ cells. A second genome-wide demethylation wave takes place in early embryogenesis, and patterns of methylation are re-established after implantation of the blastocyst [26]. The phases of post-fertilization demethylation and remethylation are likely playing a role in the removal of epigenetic information acquired by the parental generation [27, 28]. Once established throughout early development, epigenetic marks are stable maintained through cell division.

The epigenome thereby seems particularly susceptible to unfavorable environmental conditions during the stages of gametogenesis and early embryogenesis [29]. In mammals, including humans, the period of maximal epigenetic plasticity continues from before birth until weaning [30]. Various environmental cues in early life, particularly severe stresses or trauma, can cause lifelong epigenetic modifications which may, in turn, set the organism off on phenotypic trajectories to health or disease [31, 32]. There are numerous evidences from animal studies that environmental adversities and/or psychosocial stresses early in life can trigger epigenetic modifications with significant functional consequences for brain plasticity and behavior and subsequently lead to a variety of cognitive dysfunctions and psychiatric disorders in adult life [33–36]. The crucial role of epigenetic machinery in the biological embedding of stressful exposures in early life has been demonstrated in a number of rodent models, where considerable variations in both DNA methylation and histone modification have been reported in offspring exposed to different prenatal stresses, inappropriate maternal care, maternal deprivation/separation, as well as to juvenile social enrichment/isolation [3–6].

Remarkably, the earlier the organism is affected by stressful experiences during the intrauterine period, the more pronounced long-term consequences are usually observed, suggesting a causative role of epigenetic processes in pathways to adult-life pathological conditions. One good example for that is a mouse study by Mueller and Bale [37], where exposure to various stressful events during fetal development resulted in elevated stress sensitivity in adulthood, which has been manifested in modified expression of GR and corticotropin-releasing hormone, and also in the enhanced responsivity of HPA axis in prenatally affected animals. These effects have been accompanied by changes in methylation levels and in expression of GR and CRF genes. The period of early gestation was identified in this study as a particularly sensitive stage, suggesting a strong evidence for epigenetic involvement in developmental programming of neuroendocrine functions.

Postnatal exposures, such as neonatal handling (an experimental procedure in which animals are briefly separated from the dam and handled for the first 10 postnatal days), were also shown to have a profound impact on epigenetic profiles. This is a widespread experimental procedure used to understand how adversity early in life can affect neurobehavioral development of animals and place them on a pathway to disease. It has been found that neonatal handling can induce a persistent increase in the transcription level of the nuclear receptor subfamily 3, group C, member 1 (NR3C1) gene encoding the GR [38]. The epigenetic changes, such as those triggered by handling, have been observed in offspring raised by high-LG mothers. Among them, there was a reduced level of DNA methylation in the promoter region of the hippocampal NR3C1 gene [39]. These effects occurred throughout the first week of postnatal life, and they have been shown to be reversed by cross-fostering, persisted into adulthood, and associated

with changed histone acetylation and transcription factor (NGFI-A) binding to the GR promoter. Another gene that was found to be expressed in the adult prefrontal cortex in rats in response to an adversity in early life is the brain-derived neurotrophic factor (BDNF) gene playing a crucial role in the neural and behavioral plasticity and in development of various psychiatric disorders related to adversity early in life, such as depression, bipolar disorder, autism, and schizophrenia [40]. These expression changes have been accompanied by corresponding changes in the methylation levels.

Findings from human studies suggesting a role of epigenetic mechanisms in long-lasting effects of adversities in early life are more limited compared to those obtained from animal models due to the restricted access to suitable biological materials, but they clearly demonstrate that these mechanisms can also operate in man. In the succeeding subsections, findings from human studies are summarized and discussed.

Maternal adversity in pregnancy

It has been well documented in many human studies that maternal exposure to adverse conditions during pregnancy, including an unfavorable social environment, anxiety, depression, starvation, and pain (all known to increase the intrauterine level of glucocorticoids), can be linked to a variety of cognitive and behavioral problems during the adulthood [41–43]. There is consistent evidence that antenatal stress or anxiety has a programming effect on the fetus which can persist up to adulthood and result in an elevated risk of psychiatric and behavioral pathological conditions, including autism, schizophrenia and anxiety/depression-related behaviors, and also impaired cognitive performance in later life [44].

Recent studies highlighted the role of epigenetic mechanisms in mediating long-lasting outcomes of maternal adversities during pregnancy. Pre- and early postnatal dysregulation of epigenetic pathways resulted in genome-wide modulating gene expression in different tissues including the brain, by that influencing the functioning and connectivity of neural circuitry and affecting the risk for neurobehavioral impairments in later life [41]. In a methylome-wide association study (MWAS), maternal depression-associated changes in the DNA methylation levels were revealed in neonatal T lymphocytes; these alterations were found to persist to adult age in the hippocampal tissues [45]. A strong association was observed between maternal depressive symptoms during pregnancy and increased level of NR3C1 exon 1F methylation in male infants, and also lowered methylation level of another gene responsible for these associations, BDNF IV, in both male and female infants [46]. Gestational exposure to maternal depressed or anxious mood in the third trimester of prenatal development caused an enhanced methylation in the CpG-rich region of the promoter and exon1F of the GR gene (NR3C1) in the newborn cord blood, and these effects have been demonstrated to be persistent throughout the infancy [47]. Surprisingly, these epigenetic effects were revealed in offspring but not in maternal blood samples. The methylation levels of NR3C1 gene in cord blood have been associated with the levels of stress response in 3-month-old infants (as measured by salivary cortisol levels), assuming functional consequences of these epigenetic variations for the HPA stress responsiveness. Radtke et al. [48] revealed that maternal exposure to intimate partner violence throughout pregnancy affected the methylation level of NR3C1 gene in the whole blood DNA of 10–19-year-old adolescent offspring. As in the case of the maternal depression during pregnancy, these epigenetic effects were observed in affected offspring, but not in maternal blood. The same effects have been seen in cord blood as a result of maternal pregnancy-associated anxiety [49]. Similar findings were also reported on the SLC6A4 gene encoding the serotonin transporter. The methylation levels of SLC6A4 have been shown to be associated with a number of prenatal and postnatal adverse exposures, including maternal depression during pregnancy, as well as childhood trauma and abuse [50]. Prenatal exposure to a maternal depressed mood throughout the 2nd trimester of gestation has been revealed to be associated with a decreased methylation level in promoter region of SLC6A4 gene, in leukocytes from maternal peripheral blood and in umbilical cord leukocytes obtained from neonates at birth, while no such effects regarding the BDNF gene were observed [51].

In several studies, importance of epigenetic regulation of placental genes, playing a crucial role in maternal-fetal interactions, in long-lasting outcomes of maternal adversity has been reported. Prenatal exposure to maternal anxiety and/or depression has been shown to adversely influence the neurobehavioral development of newborns. These unfavorable neurodevelopmental outcomes have been demonstrated to be linked to the increased methylation levels of the NR3C1 and 11β-hydroxysteroid dehydrogenase type 2 (11β-HSD2) placental genes and to significant perturbations of the HPA axis [52]. The expression levels of the placental human SLC6A4 gene were found to be substantially elevated in placentas from mothers who had untreated mood disorders during pregnancy in comparison with control women [53]. An association between the maternal mood throughout the pregnancy and downregulation of placental 11β-HSD2 gene encoding the cortisol-metabolizing enzyme was revealed in the study by O'Donnell et al. [54]. The infants whose mothers were exposed to higher socioeconomic adversity levels in their pregnancy have also been found to have the lowest methylation levels in the placental 11β-HSD2 gene [55]. The authors have suggested that such methylation patterns of this gene indicate that

cues from environment transmitted from mother to fetus during gestation may program the response to potentially unfavorable environment in postnatal life via lesser exposure to cortisol throughout prenatal development. Overall, the findings from these investigations indicate that placental genes can be implicated in intrauterine programming of neurological functioning.

A schematic representation of hypothetical mechanisms linking maternal adversity in pregnancy to neurobehavioral and cognitive dysfunction in offspring is given in Fig. 1.

Adversity in childhood

In addition to in-utero developmental stage, early infancy is another critical stage of epigenetic plasticity. Early postnatal development is characterized by very rapid growth of various organs and organ systems including the brain and the rest of the nervous system, and epigenetic regulation is regarded as a crucial process through which the formation of specific synapses occurs throughout critical developmental periods [56, 57]. Therefore, in addition to adversities throughout the gestational development, early postnatal adversity can also have a potential for long-term epigenetic programming.

There is increasing evidence that unfavorable conditions in early infancy related to maltreatment, poor quality parenting or loss of parents, parental psychiatric disorders, exposures to physical, sexual, psychological, or emotional abuse, etc. can lead a number of adverse neurobehavioral and cognitive outcomes in adulthood [58–60]. Since the central nervous system interacts with the immune system via the HPA axis and autonomic nervous system (ANS), the immune dysregulation is regarded as a core component of these programming effects. Adversity in early life has been shown to be related to alterations in neural development (particularly of the hippocampus, amygdala, and prefrontal cortex), ANS and HPA axis dysregulation [61], and enhanced levels of inflammatory mediators [62]. The impaired neural development is believed to be a central pathway by which adversity early in life can increase the inflammation level and thereby the risk for adverse psychophysical health outcomes. Moreover, the exposure to chronic stressful conditions in infancy can lead to failure or depletion of normal physiologic processes ("allostatic load hypothesis") and thereby impair the physiological response to stress and other health outcomes in adult life through a process called biological embedding [62–65]. Adult subjects having a history of adversity in their childhood showed the decreased volumes of prefrontal cortex and hippocampus, enhanced level of activation of HPA axis in response to stress, and elevated inflammation levels compared to nonmaltreated persons [63].

Long-lasting emotional and cognitive dysfunctions caused by adversities in early life are thoroughly studied in rodent models. Typically, animals exposed to a postnatal

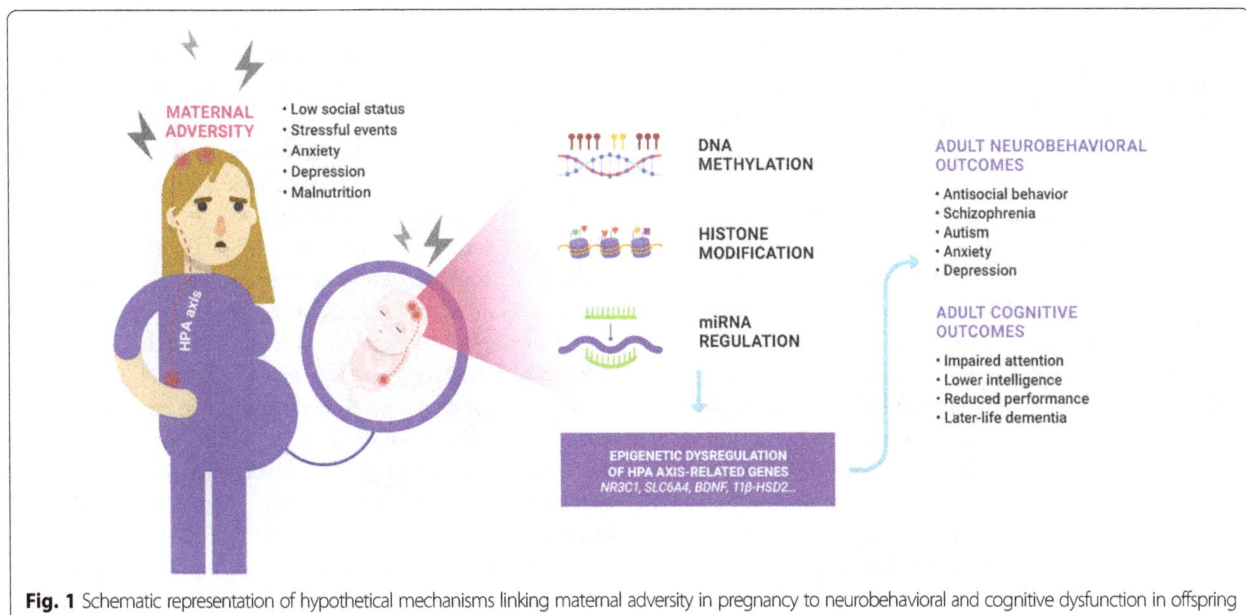

Fig. 1 Schematic representation of hypothetical mechanisms linking maternal adversity in pregnancy to neurobehavioral and cognitive dysfunction in offspring

maternal deprivation demonstrate elevated neuroendocrine response to stress, cognitive impairment, and enhanced levels of anxiety and depressive-like behavior [66–68]. Several phenotypes reported in these models of early-life adversities were likely to share common neurobiological mechanisms. So, there is evidence for impaired glucocorticoid negative-feedback control of the HPA axis, reduced hippocampal neurogenesis, and altered glutamate neurotransmission in both prenatally stressed rats and those animals that experienced inadequate maternal care [68].

These findings from animal models have been extended to humans by highlighting associations between adversities in early life and modified epigenetic patterns in adulthood [69–72]. Substantial epigenetic effects were revealed for the assortment of genes involved in the etiology of conversion disorders, aggressive and suicidal behaviors, and callous-unemotional traits [73, 74]. Among these genes, most are involved in mediating the HPA axis, brain development, immune response, neurotransmission, serotonin synthesis, and other processes. In some studies, psycho-emotional trauma in childhood has been demonstrated to be a potential risk factor for developing depressive symptoms later in life, particularly in response to additional trigger stressful events [75, 76]. For instance, women having a history of childhood abuse and actual diagnosis of major depression showed a sixfold higher level of adrenocorticotropic hormone stress response than the age-matched control individuals, suggesting that there may be permanent changes in set-points for HPA activity in response to stress among those persons who were exposed to early-life stressful conditions [77]. On the basis of these findings, Heim et al. suggested that trauma early in life is related to the sensitization of neuroendocrine stress responses, immune activation,

enhanced central CRF activity, glucocorticoid resistance, and lower hippocampal volume throughout the adult life [75]. These neuroendocrine changes triggered by stresses in early life can likely affect the risk of developing depression in response to stress during adulthood. Data from recent studies highlight the critical role of epigenetic regulation in the linkage between trauma in childhood and depression in adult life [76].

It should be noted, however, that the link between adverse conditions in early life and unfavorable neurobehavioral outcomes in adulthood can be dependent not only on epigenetic processes per se, but also on the genetic background of affected individuals. In particular, different combinations of functional polymorphisms in dopamine and serotonin pathway genes can result in both responder and non-responder phenotypes in the wide range from adverse to advantageous early-life circumstances. For example, a functional polymorphism in the promoter gene of monoamine oxidase A (MAOA), a mitochondrial enzyme that degrades the neurotransmitters including serotonin, norepinephrine, and dopamine, was demonstrated to mediate the association between adversities early in life and enhanced risk for violence and antisocial behavior in adulthood. In the research by Frazzetto et al., the MAOA genotype was found to moderate the link between traumatic events experienced from birth up to the age of 15 years and physical aggression in adult life, as assessed by the Aggression Questionnaire [78]. In this study, scores of physical aggression were shown to be higher in those adult men who have been exposed to traumatic events early in life and who carried the low MAOA activity allele (MAOA-L). These findings were confirmed by later studies. The interaction of

MAOA genotype and childhood adversity on antisocial outcomes was examined in a meta-analysis of 27 studies conducted by Byrd and Manuck [79]. Across 20 male cohorts, adversity in early life has been demonstrated to be a stronger predictor of adult antisocial outcomes for a low-activity, compared to a high-activity, MAOA genotype. Similar, but less consistent, findings were reported in 11 female cohorts studied.

An association between the adversities early in life and long-lasting changes in processes of epigenetic regulation at the whole-genome level was demonstrated repeatedly. Many of such studies used low socioeconomic status (SES) as indicator of early stressful conditions. Low SES, generally accompanied by an enhanced stress load due to a poor quality of nutrimental intake, infections, and higher load of physical work, has been found to strongly predict a number of psycho-emotional pathologies such as schizophrenia and depression in adult life [67]. Disadvantaged early SES was related to profiles of adult blood DNA methylation [80]. Most of the genes differentially methylated in association with low early-life SES are known to be functionally implicated in metabolic and cell signaling pathways. Genome-wide transcriptional profiling demonstrated that in healthy adults with low-SES childhood background, genes bearing response elements for CREB/ATF family of transcription factors transmitting adrenergic signals to leukocytes were substantially upregulated, whereas genes with response elements for the GR, regulating the secretion of cortisol and transducing the anti-inflammatory signals to the immune system, were significantly downregulated [81]. Individuals exposed to low-SES conditions in early life also exhibited raised cortisol levels, elevated expression of pro-inflammatory transcription factor NF-kappaB, as well as increased production of the pro-inflammatory cytokine interleukin 6. On the basis of data obtained, the authors suggested that "low early-life SES programs a defensive phenotype characterized by resistance to glucocorticoid signaling, which in turn facilitates exaggerated adrenocortical and inflammatory responses. Although these response patterns could serve adaptive functions during acute threats to well-being, over the long term, they might exact an allostatic toll on the body that ultimately contributes to the chronic diseases of aging." Chen et al. have revealed that the unfavorable effects of the low-SES conditions in early life on immune system functioning and inflammatory processes in adult life can be at least partly prevented by the high-level maternal warmth [82]. These alterations have been accompanied by changes in genome-wide transcription profiles. Those individuals who had low SES level early in life and whose mothers demonstrated high warmth toward them showed reduced Toll-like receptor-stimulated production of interleukin 6 and lowered activity of immune activating transcription factor (AP-1) and NF-kappaB in comparison with those subjects who had low SES level early

in life but have experienced lower maternal warmth. These findings suggest that disadvantageous effect of low socioeconomic environment in early life might be buffered by a supportive family climate.

Similar lasting effects have been obtained for the unfavorable experiences such as sexual/physical abuse or neglect in early life [83]. Three hundred sixty-two differentially methylated promoters have been identified by a genome-wide analysis in the hippocampal neurons isolated from postmortem brain samples in subjects with a history of heavy abuse throughout infancy in comparison with control persons [84]. Among them, those genes implicated in a cellular or neural plasticity were shown to be the most differentially methylated. Nine hundred ninety-seven gene promoters were identified as being differentially methylated in association with abuse throughout childhood in a whole-blood DNA from adult subjects [85]. Most of these genes are involved in important pathways of cellular signaling associated with development and regulation of transcription. Four hundred forty-eight gene promoters were differentially methylated in T cells from adult male individuals exposed to parental physical aggression in the age of 6 to 15 years relative to a control group [86]. Most these genes are known to play an important role in aggressive behavior.

Long-lasting social and behavioral problems were also observed in persons who experienced parental neglect through the institutionalization in early life [87]. Differential patterns of whole-genome DNA methylation were found in blood samples from institutionalized children and children reared by their biological parents [88]. Most of these differentially methylated genes are related to immune and cellular signaling pathways, including those responsible for development and functioning of the brain as well as in neural communication. One hundred seventy-three genes were differentially methylated among subjects with and without the placement into the foster care system during their childhood [69]. Most of these genes are involved in the ubiquitin-mediated proteolysis pathway, which plays an important role in immune/inflammatory responses, in antigen processing and presentation pathways, and also in some important cellular processes. Moreover, 72 genes known to be related to the control of apoptosis and transcriptional regulation exhibited increased methylation levels in those individuals who had a history of foster care placement, while 101 genes involved in protein catabolic processes and in the control of posttranslational protein modification exhibited lowered levels of methylation in comparison with control subjects. Summary of evidence on the epigenetic link between adverse early-life events and adult-life neurobehavioral outcomes obtained from epigenome-wide association studies (EWAS) is given in Table 1. As we can see from Table 1, most of these EWAS data have been obtained from small samples; therefore, one must use some caution in interpreting these

Table 1 Summary of evidence on the link between adverse early-life events and adult neurobehavioral outcomes from epigenome-wide association studies

Condition /exposure	Stage at exposure	Age at detection	Tissue/cells	Population, sample size (n)	DMRs or up/downregulated genes, n	Function/pathway	Ref.
Maternal depression	Prenatal	Adult	Hippocampal tissue samples	Male postmortem samples with (n = 12) or without (n = 50) a history of maternal depression	294 DMRs associated with 234 genes	Immune system functions	[45]
Low SES	Childhood	45 years	Blood	40 British adults	586 hypermethylated and 666 hypomethylated gene promoters	Cell signaling pathways	[80]
	Childhood	25–40 years	Blood	103 healthy adults	73 upregulated and 37 downregulated genes	Raised cortisol levels; increased IL-6 production	[81]
	Childhood	25–40 years	Blood	53 healthy adults with a history of low early-life SES	330 upregulated and 161 downregulated genes in participants who grew up with high maternal warmth	Immune activation and systemic inflammation; diminishing these outcomes by supportive family climate	[82]
Child neglect /abuse	Childhood	Adult	Hippocampal neurons	25 French-Canadian men with a history of severe childhood abuse and 16 control subjects	248 hypermethylated DMRs; 114 hypomethylated DMRs	Cellular/neuronal plasticity	[84]
	Childhood	45 years	Blood	12 British men with a history of childhood abuse and 28 control subjects	311 hypermethylated and 686 hypomethylated gene promoters	Development, regulation of transcription	[85]
	Childhood	Adult	T lymphocytes	8 subjects with a history of physical aggression from age 6 to 15 years and 57 controls	171 hypermethylated and 277 hypomethylated gene promoters	Aggressive behavior	[86]

DMRs, differentially methylated regions; *SES*, socioeconomic status

results. Further studies with larger samples are clearly required in order to allow more reliable conclusions.

In addition to EWAS, consistent evidence for the importance of epigenetic regulation in mediating long-term effects of early adversity was also provided from some candidate gene research. While a full-genome analysis allows to generate hypotheses on the underlying molecular mechanisms, the candidate gene approach allows to determine whether a specific gene of interest makes a contribution in each particular case. For example, in the McGowan et al. study, epigenetic differences in the brain loci substantially involved in the pathophysiology of suicide have been observed [89]. Specifically, by studying the postmortem hippocampal brain samples from suicidal individuals, the history of neglect/abuse in early childhood was shown to be associated with a lowered hippocampal volume and with severe cognitive impairments. Moreover, the gene encoding ribosomal RNA (rRNA) was significantly hypermethylated throughout the promoter and 5′ regulatory region in the brains of suicide victims, consistent with the decreased level of expression of rRNA gene in the hippocampus. Subsequently, McGowan et al. [90] examined epigenetic differences in a neuron-specific promoter of NR3C1 gene among postmortem hippocampal tissues from suicide completers with or without the child abuse history. The NR3C1 gene was selected for analysis since the decreased level of GRs

within the hippocampus is believed to lead to elevated HPA stress response and thereby might account for an enhanced risk of psychopathology and poorer emotional regulation in those subjects who were abused in childhood. In that study, the levels of expression of NR3C1 gene were considerably decreased in suicide victims having a history of childhood abuse compared to non-abused suicide victims or control individuals; no differences, however, were revealed among non-abused suicide victims and control subjects. The essential effect on the expression of transcripts from the exon 1F NR3C1 promoter has been also observed. Labonté et al. also reported the enhanced methylation levels in the promoter of the 1F NR3C1 and decreased expression of this gene in the hippocampus of suicide completers having a history of abuse compared to either suicide completers with no abuse history or to control subjects [91]. In a more recent research by Bustamante et al., the childhood maltreatment assessed by a retrospective self-report questionnaire has been significantly associated with methylation levels in the NR3C1 promoter region in whole blood of adult persons [92]. Tyrka et al. also demonstrated that adversity in childhood can be linked to the risk for adult psychiatric disorders via epigenetic regulation of glucocorticoid signaling genes such as NR3C1 and gene coding for FK506 binding protein 51 (FKBP5) [93]. In another recent study by the same authors, the reduced methylation levels of NR3C1 gene were significantly associated with maltreatment in childhood and anxiety, depressive and substance-use disorders in adulthood [94]. An enhanced risk for development of stress-associated psychiatric disorders in adulthood was shown to be associated with childhood trauma-dependent, allele-specific demethylation of the functional glucocorticoid response elements of FKBP5 gene playing an important role in regulation of the HPA axis [95]. The demethylation of FKBP5 gene has been associated with elevated stress-dependent gene transcription followed by lasting dysregulation of the stress hormone system and by global effect on immune functioning and areas of the brain related to stress regulation.

One important issue in these studies is limited access to human neural tissues. Thereby, most candidate gene studies examining role of epigenetic variations in developmental programming of adult behavioral and cognitive dysfunctions are based on samples from peripheral tissues. In the above-mentioned study by Bick et al., significant negative correlation was observed between the mothers' parenting reports and methylation levels of NR3C1 gene and also a macrophage migration inhibitory factor gene functionally implicated in the expression of NR3C1 and immune response in offspring blood 5 to 10 years after assessing the maternal caregiving quality [69].

Childhood-adversity caused epigenetic modifications in NR3C1 gene in the human blood samples have also been reported in the Tyrka et al. research [96]. In this study, enhanced levels of NR3C1 methylation were observed in leukocyte DNA from healthy adult individuals exposed to inadequate nurturing or maltreatment during their childhood. The elevated methylation levels of the exon 1F NR3C1 promoter in the peripheral blood of individuals suffering from borderline personality disorder or major depressive disorder have been revealed to be associated with the severity of childhood maltreatment [97]. No such changes have been found, however, in bulimic women exposed to abuse in their childhood [98]. Similar findings have been obtained for a serotonin system playing a crucial role in the brain development (including a region important in stress-regulation such as the hippocampus) and in the etiology of depression [99]. In this study, the childhood trauma, along with male gender and smaller hippocampal volume, has been independently associated with higher levels of peripheral serotonin transporter methylation in adulthood.

In some candidate gene researches, low SES has been used as a reliable indicator of adverse early-life conditions. In the research by Miller and Chen, the adolescent subjects whose families owned homes throughout their early childhood demonstrated higher levels of NR3C1 expression and lower levels of toll-like receptor 4 (TLR4) gene expression in leukocytes from peripheral blood compared to individuals with low SES in early life [100]. Data from this study indicated that low SES early in life may trigger a pro-

inflammatory phenotype in later life. Similar findings have been obtained in African-American men who often have low SES in their childhood. In the study by Witek-Janusek et al., higher levels of childhood trauma and indirect exposure to neighborhood violence have been shown to be related to a greater acute stress-induced IL-6 response and also to a reduced methylation of the IL-6 promoter and lower cortisol response in adulthood [101]. Summary of evidence on the epigenetic link between adverse early-life events and adult-life neurobehavioral outcomes obtained from candidate gene studies is given in Table 2.

Overall, these research findings highlight the mechanisms implicated in early adversity-induced impairment of neuroendocrine pathways associated with stress reactivity and adult social behavior. One of the most significant health outcomes of the childhood adversity is lasting neuroendocrine disturbance caused by adversity-induced alterations in the methylation levels of NR3C1 gene, thereby leading to changed cortisol production and various pathological conditions in adulthood [39, 102].

A schematic representation of hypothetical mechanisms linking childhood adversity to later-life neurobehavioral and cognitive dysfunction is given in Fig. 2.

Natural experiment-based evidence

Causal relationship between stressful events in early life and health problems later in life is evident from a body of quasi-experimental states ("natural experiments"), referring to any kind of naturally occurring circumstances in which subsets of the population have different levels of exposure to a supposed causal factor [103]. Currently, a man-made famine, where dietary insults and chronic stress tend to co-occur in exposed populations, is typically used in quasi-experimental design [104]. The nutritional status might be affected by stressful events at different levels including self-selection of dietary components, intake of calories, and utilization of metabolic wastes for energy production, whereas nutritional factors can, in turn, affect stress response through influencing both peripheral and central mechanisms of stress reactivity [14, 105]. Thereby, famine has numerous features that can be beneficial for its use as a natural experiment in studying lasting outcomes of stressful events in early life [104, 106], although using such research design could confound attempts to distinguish the (intergenerational) effects of nutrition and stress.

In a number of quasi-experimental statues, impaired cognitive and behavioral functioning, as well as psychiatric illness in adulthood, has been reported in cohorts exposed in their early life to natural disasters or stressful historic events, such as World War II [107], Holocaust [108–110], Israeli-Arab war of 1967 [111, 112], Chinese Famine of 1959–1961 [113–117], and Dutch famine of 1944–1945 [118–120]. In some recent quasi-experimental studies, evidence for the epigenetic embedding of stressful historic

Table 2 Summary of evidence on the epigenetic link between adverse early-life events and adult neurobehavioral outcomes from candidate gene studies

Condition/ exposure	Stage at exposure	Age at detection	Tissue/cells	Population, sample size (n)	Function/pathway	Gene/element	Epigenetic outcome	Ref.
Low SES	0–5 years	25–40 years	Saliva	103 adults	Decreased glucocorticoid and increased pro-inflammatory signaling	CREB/ATF gene family NR3C1	Upregulation Downregulation	[81]
Child maltreatment	Early childhood	Adulthood	Postmortem hippocampus	18 male suicide subjects, 12 controls	Impaired ribosomal functioning	RRNa promoter	Hypermethylation	[89]
	Childhood	Adulthood	Postmortem hippocampus	12 abused and 12 non-abused suicide subjects, 12 controls	Impaired stress reactivity	NR3C1	Downregulation	[90]
	Childhood	Adulthood	Postmortem hippocampus	21 abused and 21 non-abused suicide subjects, 14 controls	Impaired stress reactivity	NR3C1 1F	Hypermethylation	[91]
	Childhood	Adulthood	Whole blood	74 maltreated and 73 control subjects	Impaired stress reactivity	NR3C1 1F promoter region	Hypermethylation	[92]
	Childhood	18–59 years	Leukocytes	58 female and 41 male subjects	Impaired stress reactivity	NR3C1 promoter	Hypermethylation	[93]
	Childhood	18–65 years	Leukocytes	213 female and 127 male subjects	Impaired stress reactivity	NR3C1 promoter	Hypomethylation	[94]
	Childhood	19–59 years	Peripheral blood cells	30 subjects with and 46 without the history of child trauma	Immune functioning, stress reactivity	Glucocorticoid response elements of FKBP5 gene	Allele-specific demethylation	[95]
	Childhood	18–59 years	Leukocytes	58 female and 41 male subjects	Impaired stress reactivity	NR3C1 promoter	Hypermethylation	[96]
	Childhood	Adulthood	Peripheral blood	200 subjects with different rate of child maltreatment	Impaired stress reactivity	NR3C1 1F promoter	Hypermethylation	[97]
	Childhood	18–65 years	Peripheral blood	33 maltreated subjects, 36 controls	Stress-related psychopathology	Serotonin transporter gene promoter	Hypermethylation	[99]
	Childhood	18–25 years	Peripheral blood	34 African American men	Higher proinflammatory response to stress	IL-6 gene promoter	Hypomethylation	[101]

events was obtained. Although no relationship between the exposure to the Dutch famine throughout the intra-uterine period and whole-genome DNA methylation level in adulthood was observed [121], an association between the famine exposure during early gestation and changed patterns of methylation at CpG dinucleotides in genes

responsible for growth, development, and metabolism in the whole blood of adult individuals was found in the Tobi et al. study [122]. The gene-specific differences in the patterns of DNA methylation associated with in-utero exposure to the Dutch famine have been indicated in several studies including those of Heijmans et al. [123] and Tobi et al. [124]. The

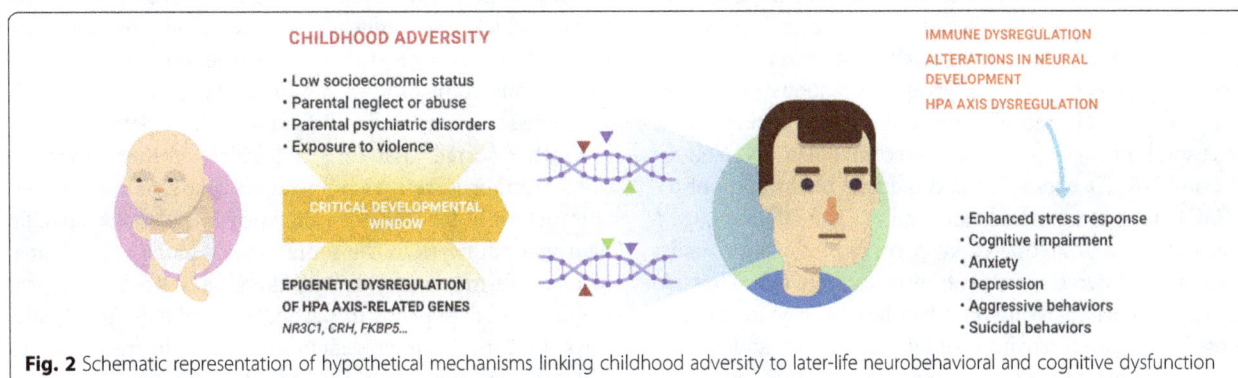

CHILDHOOD ADVERSITY
- Low socioeconomic status
- Parental neglect or abuse
- Parental psychiatric disorders
- Exposure to violence

CRITICAL DEVELOPMENTAL WINDOW

EPIGENETIC DYSREGULATION OF HPA AXIS-RELATED GENES
NR3C1, CRH, FKBP5...

IMMUNE DYSREGULATION
ALTERATIONS IN NEURAL DEVELOPMENT
HPA AXIS DYSREGULATION

- Enhanced stress response
- Cognitive impairment
- Anxiety
- Depression
- Aggressive behaviors
- Suicidal behaviors

Fig. 2 Schematic representation of hypothetical mechanisms linking childhood adversity to later-life neurobehavioral and cognitive dysfunction

differences in DNA methylation levels in HPA axis-associated genes, such as corticotropin-releasing hormone (CRH) and NR3C1 genes, however, were non-significant in the latest study. Importantly, the effect of prenatal famine exposure has been demonstrated to strongly depend on the exposure period, with differences being most pronounced when the famine exposure occurred throughout the periconceptional period rather than throughout the late gestational developmental stage. These findings demonstrate that early intrauterine period is the most sensitive stage in human ontogenesis [125, 126]. Since epigenome is demonstrated to be most plastic during this ontogenetic period, these data are suggestive for the role of epigenetic modifications in driving life-lasting effects of exposures to famine and/or other disasters in early life.

Transgenerational transmission of childhood trauma

Evidence has been also obtained that early adversity-induced neuronal and behavioral effects can be transgenerationally transmitted via epigenetic mechanisms to subsequent generations [45, 127]. In the study by Yehuda et al. [128], the Holocaust survivor offspring were studied which are known to have altered GR sensitivity and vulnerability to psychiatric disorders. In this study, adult offspring with both maternal and paternal Holocaust-induced posttraumatic stress disorder (PTSD) demonstrated decreased levels of the 1F NR3C1 promoter methylation, while offspring with paternal PTSD only exhibited higher methylation levels of 1F NR3C1 promoter in the peripheral blood mononuclear cells compared to participants without parental Holocaust exposure. Similar transgenerational effects were found for another historical event, such as the Tutsi genocide. In the Perroud et al. study [129], mothers exposed to the Tutsi genocide as well as their offspring had higher mineralocorticoid receptor levels and lower cortisol and GR levels in comparison with non-exposed mothers and their children. Furthermore, the exposed mothers and their progeny had higher levels of methylation of the 1F NR3C1 exon than non-exposed subjects.

To examine the mechanisms underlying such transgenerational effects of paternal trauma, Gapp et al. [130] using a mouse model of unpredictable maternal separation and maternal stress have demonstrated that postnatal trauma changes coping behavior in adverse conditions in exposed males when adult and in their adult male offspring. These behavioral changes have been accompanied by elevated levels of NR3C1 expression and reduced methylation of the NR3C1 promoter in the hippocampus. The DNA methylation levels were also lowered in sperm cells of exposed males when adult. Interestingly, the transgenerational transmission of neurobehavioral symptoms has been shown to be prevented by paternal environmental enrichment, and this effect was linked to the reversal of changes in DNA methylation and expression of NR3C1 gene in the hippocampus of the male offspring.

Conclusion

Accumulating evidence assume that adversity early in life can be associated with later neuropsychiatric, cognitive, and behavioral outcomes. Recent findings suggest that childhood adversity can have greater impact on the later health status than stressful exposures in adulthood, as assumed by phenomenon of the biological embedding of early experience. In several studies, credible evidence is obtained that adversity early in life can reach far into the later adulthood partly due to cellular aging, as evident from recent data indicating that severe traumatic and social exposures as well as institutional care history in childhood can be embedded at the molecular level through accelerated telomere shortening [131–133].

It is increasingly clear that epigenetic control of gene expression plays a central role in these effects. Some authors hypothesized that such early-life "epigenetic tuning" may likely prepare particular genes for responses to subsequent triggers [134]. By this mechanism, the functional performance of different tissues and organs may be established well before they are actually challenged. In evolutionary terms, such epigenetic fine-tuning of the expression of responsible genes enables the organism to adapt to varying environmental conditions [135], but it can enhance the risk for disorders, including neuropsychiatric ones, later in life [136]. Thus, epigenetic studies can provide insight into the mechanisms mediating the relationship between early-life adversities, aberrant neuroplastic interactions, and adult health outcomes. The role of particular genes such as hippocampal NR3C1 as well as genes coding arginine vasopressin and CRF in the neurons of the paraventricular nucleus has been demonstrated in mediating the effects of early adversity-associated pathological conditions [70, 137].

In the past decade, significant advances have been achieved in the emerging field of neurobehavioral epigenetics. Some research challenges, however, must be addressed for further progress in the field. For example, it is still not clear how stable are modifications of epigenetic marks which are induced by adversities in early life. Recent findings suggest that such epigenetic modifications can be long-term or even life-long and may persist up to the highest age categories [138–140]. These data, however, are rather scarce; therefore, it requires further investigation. Another issue is that epigenetic patterns can be specific not only for distinct cell types but also for specific neuronal pathways in the same brain regions [141]. Thus, focus of further research will likely be shifted from particular candidate genes to particular candidate gene pathways that may be epigenetically labile in response to adverse conditions in early life. Moreover, as significant epigenetic modifications originate both within and among different types of tissues, one more potentially important issue is applicability of samples from peripheral blood for determining epigenetic modifications in human studies. Indeed, though widespread epigenetic changes might be induced by traumatic experiences in early life, these effects may greatly vary in magnitude and direction in neuronal tissues relative to non-neuronal tissues including peripheral blood. This may limit the opportunity to studying the long-term neurobehavioral impacts of early trauma basing only on peripheral blood samples or buccal swabs. Therefore, animal models, which provide an opportunity to simultaneously measure the epigenetic profiles in both peripheral and brain tissues, can be useful in highlighting epigenetic pathways underlying the biological embedding of early adversity. The use of animal models certainly raises questions concerning the specificity of such pathways across different mammalian species and about similarities and differences among these pathways in various animal species and humans. In addition, the potential impact of subsequent exposure to traumatic events during adolescence and adulthood on the process of epigenetic embedding of early experiences also needs to be considered as the findings from some investigations suggest that epigenome continues to be labile during adulthood [142].

A genuine incorporation of novel knowledge about the mechanisms underlying the process of epigenetic embedding of adverse experiences during sensitive developmental periods into the current paradigm on the causation of adult neurobehavioral and cognitive dysfunction will certainly move the focus of efforts targeted toward prevention of adult psychopathological conditions from the later life stages to early developmental stages from conception to weaning. Indeed, reducing or eliminating risk factors early in life would likely have a potential to prevent neurological dysfunctions and psychopathologies in adult life. In this context, an important point is that epigenetic states, in contrast to the relatively stable genetic information, are reversible and can be modified by environmental factors [143]. Therefore, modulation of epigenetic pathways involved in biological embedding may provide promising new direction toward novel therapeutic strategies against neurological and cognitive dysfunctions in adult life.

Over the last years, the therapeutic potential of pharmaceuticals targeted at chromatin modifying enzymes, such as histone deacetylase (HDAC) inhibitors, in treatment of cognitive and behavioral impairments as well as psychiatric disorders such as anxiety, depression, fear, and schizophrenia has been repeatedly demonstrated [144–146]. In a number of preclinical animal models, the convincing evidence is obtained that treatment with HDAC inhibitors can be effective in the prevention and therapy of experimentally induced cognitive and behavioral abnormalities. Treatment with the HDAC inhibitor sodium butyrate (SB)

reversed the abnormal hyperactive behavior in a rat model of D-amphetamine-induced mania-like behavior [147]. Furthermore, SB and other HDAC inhibitor, valproate, abolished manic-like behaviors and protected the rat brain from metabolic disturbances induced by the metabolic poison, ouabain [148]. These findings were subsequently confirmed in models of depressive- and manic-like behaviors induced by chronic mild stress or maternal deprivation [149]. In the same models, SB treatment improved the recognition memory and reversed the stress-induced decrease of hippocampal neurotrophic factors including BDNF, nerve growth factor, and glial cell line-derived neurotrophic factor [150], and also abolished the maternal deprivation- and chronic mild stress-induced dysfunction in the striatum of rats [151]. In a mouse model of valproic acid (VPA)-induced autism, chronic administration of SB resulted in attenuating the experimentally induced deficits in a novel object recognition and loss of hippocampal dendritic spine, as well as significantly increased level of acetylation of the histone H3 in hippocampus [152]. In the same mouse model of VPA-induced autism, SB attenuated autism-like deficits in social behavior and modified transcription levels of many behavior-associated genes in the prefrontal cortex, in particular, genes implicated in neuronal excitation or inhibition [153]. In a mouse model of isoflurane-induced cognitive deficits, treatment with SB attenuated the repression of contextual fear memory, apparently by promoting histone acetylation and expression of histone acetylation-mediated genes [154]. In the 6-hydroxydopamine-induced Parkinson's disease rat model, administration of SB resulted in a substantial attenuation of motor deficits and also in an increase of striatal dopamine, BDNF, and global H3 histone acetylation levels [155]. The cognition-protective effect of SB was revealed in a rat model of chronic cerebral hypoperfusion; this effect was, at least in part, mediated through enhancing histone acetylation and facilitating the transcription of Nrf2 downstream genes in the hippocampus [156]. HDAC inhibitor phenylbutyrate (PBA) was shown to be able to attenuate hippocampal neuronal loss and reverse the Alzheimer's disease-like phenotype in a mouse model of Alzheimer's disease [157]. In rats with neonatal ventral hippocampal lesions which are commonly used for modeling neurodevelopmental aspects of schizophrenia, treatment with PBA reversed the unfavorable behavioral consequences of these lesions in the ventral hippocampus [158]. In a maternal separation rat model, treatment with another HDAC inhibitor, suberoylanilide hydroxamic acid (SAHA), reversed early-life stress-induced visceral hypersensitivity and anxiety behavior [159]. Taken together, these results suggest that targeting epigenome by specific pharmacological interventions can be a promising therapeutic option in treatment of neuropsychiatric and cognitive impairments, including those related to biological embedding of early life exposures. There are certainly many important issues which need to be addressed before implementation of such interventions in clinical practice, including their effective dose levels, administration frequency, safety, and potential side effects. These issues remain to be addressed in future clinical trials.

Abbreviations

BDNF: Brain-derived neurotrophic factor; CRF: Hypothalamic corticotropin-releasing factor; CRH: Corticotropin-releasing hormone; EWAS: Epigenome-wide association studies; GR: Glucocorticoid receptor; HDAC: Histone deacetylase; HPA: Hypothalamic-pituitary-adrenal; LG: Licking/grooming; MAOA: Monoamine oxidase A; MWAS: Methylome-wide association study; NR3C1: Nuclear receptor subfamily 3 group C member; PBA: Phenylbutyrate; PTSD: Posttraumatic stress disorder; SAHA: Suberoylanilide hydroxamic acid; SB: Sodium butyrate; SES: Socioeconomic status; VPA: Valproic acid

Acknowledgements

The authors would like to thank Oksana Zabuga for the helpful assistance in preparing the manuscript.

Funding

Not applicable.

Authors' contributions

AMV conceived the idea for the manuscript and produced the first draft. AKK was involved in creating the figures and also in the critical review. Both authors read and approved the final manuscript.

Authors' information

AV is a Professor and Head of the Laboratory of Epigenetics, Institute of Gerontology, Kiev, Ukraine. AK is a Research associate of the Laboratory of Epigenetics, Institute of Gerontology, Kiev, Ukraine.

Competing interests

The authors declare that they have no competing interests.

References

1. Hanson MA, Gluckman PD. Developmental origins of health and disease—global public health implications. Best Pract Res Clin Obstet Gynaecol. 2015;29(1):24–31.
2. Eriksson JG. Developmental origins of health and disease—from a small body size at birth to epigenetics. Ann Med. 2016;48(6):456–67.
3. Champagne FA. Interplay between social experiences and the genome: epigenetic consequences for behavior. Adv Genet. 2012;77:33–57.
4. Doherty TS, Roth TL. Insight from animal models of environmentally driven epigenetic changes in the developing and adult brain. Dev Psychopathol. 2016;28:1229–43.
5. Curley JP, Champagne FA. Influence of maternal care on the developing brain: mechanisms, temporal dynamics and sensitive periods. Front Neuroendocrinol. 2016;40:52–66.
6. Kim DR, Bale TL, Epperson CN. Prenatal programming of mental illness: current understanding of relationship and mechanisms. Curr Psychiatry Rep. 2015;17(2):5.
7. Fowden AL, Valenzuela OA, Vaughan OR, Jellyman JK, Forhead AJ. Glucocorticoid programming of intrauterine development. Domest Anim Endocrinol. 2016;56:S121–32.
8. Silberman DM, Acosta GB, Zorrilla Zubilete MA. Long-term effects of early life stress exposure: role of epigenetic mechanisms. Pharmacol Res. 2016;109:64–73.
9. Maccari S, Polese D, Reynaert ML, Amici T, Morley-Fletcher S, Fagioli F. Early-life experiences and the development of adult diseases with a focus on mental illness: the human birth theory. Neuroscience. 2017;342:232–51.
10. Weinstock M. The long-term behavioural consequences of prenatal stress. Neurosci Biobehav Rev. 2008;32:1073–86.
11. Reynolds RM, Jacobsen GH, Drake AJ. What is the evidence in humans that DNA methylation changes link events in utero and later life disease? Clin Endocrinol. 2013a;78:814–22.
12. Reynolds RM, Labad J, Buss C, Ghaemmaghami P, Räikkönen K. Transmitting biological effects of stress in utero: implications for mother and offspring. Psychoneuroendocrinology. 2013b;38:1843–9.
13. Barbazanges A, Piazza PV, Le Moal M, Maccari S. Maternal glucocorticoid secretion mediates long-term effects of prenatal stress. J Neurosci. 1996;16:3943–9.
14. Entringer S, Buss C, Wadhwa PD. Prenatal stress and developmental programming of human health and disease risk: concepts and integration of empirical findings. Curr Opin Endocrinol Diabetes Obes. 2010;17:507–16.
15. Entringer S, Buss C, Wadhwa PD. Prenatal stress, development, health and disease risk: a psychobiological perspective—2015 Curt Richter Award Paper. Psychoneuroendocrinology. 2015;62:366–75.
16. Lippmann M, Bress A, Nemeroff CB, Plotsky PM, Monteggia LM. Long-term behavioural and molecular alterations associated with maternal separation in rats. Eur J Neurosci. 2007;25:3091–8.
17. Nishi M, Horii-Hayashi N, Sasagawa T. Effects of early life adverse experiences on the brain: implications from maternal separation models in rodents. Front Neurosci. 2014;8:166.
18. Tractenberg SG, Levandowski ML, de Azeredo LA, Orso R, Roithmann LG, Hoffmann ES, et al. An overview of maternal separation effects on behavioural outcomes in mice: evidence from a four-stage methodological systematic review. Neurosci Biobehav Rev. 2016;68:489–503.
19. Braun K, Champagne FA. Paternal influences on offspring development: behavioural and epigenetic pathways. J Neuroendocrinol. 2014;26(10):697–706.
20. Korosi A, Baram TZ. Plasticity of the stress response early in life: mechanisms and significance. Dev Psychobiol. 2010;52(7):661–70.
21. Perry R, Sullivan RM. Neurobiology of attachment to an abusive caregiver: short-term benefits and long-term costs. Dev Psychobiol. 2014;56(8):1626–34.
22. Szyf M, Tang YY, Hill KG, Musci R. The dynamic epigenome and its implications for behavioral interventions: a role for epigenetics to inform disorder prevention and health promotion. Transl Behav Med. 2016;6(1):55–62.
23. Cowan CS, Callaghan BL, Kan JM, Richardson R. The lasting impact of early-life adversity on individuals and their descendants: potential mechanisms and hope for intervention. Genes Brain Behav. 2016;15(1):155–68.
24. Canovas S, Ross PJ. Epigenetics in preimplantation mammalian development. Theriogenology. 2016;86(1):69–79.
25. Vaiserman A. Epidemiologic evidence for association between adverse environmental exposures in early life and epigenetic variation: a potential link to disease susceptibility? Clin Epigenetics. 2015;7:96.
26. Vaiserman AM, Koliada AK, Jirtle RL. Non-genomic transmission of longevity between generations: potential mechanisms and evidence across species. Epigenetics Chromatin. 2017;27:38.
27. Lee HJ, Hore TA, Reik W. Reprogramming the methylome: erasing memory and creating diversity. Cell Stem Cell. 2014;14:710–9.
28. Trerotola M, Relli V, Simeone P, Alberti S. Epigenetic inheritance and the missing heritability. Hum Genomics. 2015;9:17.
29. Vickaryous N, Whitelaw E. The role of the early embryonic environment on epigenotype and phenotype. Reprod Fertil Dev. 2005;17:335–40.
30. Hochberg Z, Feil R, Constancia M, Fraga M, Junien C, Carel JC. Child health, developmental plasticity, and epigenetic programming. Endocr Rev. 2011;32:159–224.
31. Feil R, Fraga MF. Epigenetics and the environment: emerging patterns and implications. Nat Rev Genet. 2012;13(2):97–109.
32. Boyce WT, Kobor MS. Development and the epigenome: the 'synapse' of gene–environment interplay. Dev Sci. 2015;18(1):1–23.
33. McGowan PO, Roth TL. Epigenetic pathways through which experiences become linked with biology. Dev Psychopathol. 2015;27(2):637–48.

34. Provencal N, Binder EB. The neurobiological effects of stress as contributors to psychiatric disorders: focus on epigenetics. Curr Opin Neurobiol. 2015;30:31–7.

35. Isles AR. Neural and behavioral epigenetics; what it is, and what is hype. Genes Brain Behav. 2015;14(1):64–72.

36. Halldorsdottir T, Binder EB. Gene × environment interactions: from molecular mechanisms to behavior. Annu Rev Psychol. 2017;68:215–41.

37. Mueller BR, Bale TL. Sex-specific programming of offspring emotionality after stress early in pregnancy. J Neurosci. 2008;28:9055–65.

38. O'Donnell D, Larocque S, Seckl JR, Meaney MJ. Postnatal handling alters glucocorticoid, but not mineralocorticoid messenger RNA expression in the hippocampus of adult rats. Brain Res Mol Brain Res. 1994;26:242–8.

39. Weaver IC, Cervoni N, Champagne FA, D'Alessio AC, Sharma S, Seckl JR, et al. Epigenetic programming by maternal behavior. Nat Neurosci. 2004;7:847–54.

40. Kundakovic M, Gudsnuk K, Herbstman JB, Tang D, Perera FP, Champagne FA. DNA methylation of BDNF as a biomarker of early-life adversity. Proc Natl Acad Sci U S A. 2015;112(22):6807–13.

41. Monk C, Spicer J, Champagne FA. Linking prenatal maternal adversity to developmental outcomes in infants: the role of epigenetic pathways. Dev Psychopathol. 2012;24:1361–76.

42. Lewis AJ, Austin E, Knapp R, Vaiano T, Galbally M. Perinatal maternal mental health, fetal programming and child development. Healthcare (Basel). 2015;3(4):1212–27.

43. Newman L, Judd F, Olsson CA, Castle D, Bousman C, Sheehan P, et al. Early origins of mental disorder—risk factors in the perinatal and infant period. BMC Psychiatry. 2016;16:270.

44. Babenko O, Kovalchuk I, Metz GA. Stress-induced perinatal and transgenerational epigenetic programming of brain development and mental health. Neurosci Biobehav Rev. 2015;48:70–91.

45. Nemoda Z, Massart R, Suderman M, Hallett M, Li T, Coote M, et al. Maternal depression is associated with DNA methylation changes in cord blood T lymphocytes and adult hippocampi. Transl Psychiatry. 2015;5:e545.

46. Braithwaite EC, Kundakovic M, Ramchandani PG, Murphy SE, Champagne FA. Maternal prenatal depressive symptoms predict infant NR3C1 1F and BDNF IV DNA methylation. Epigenetics. 2015;10:408–17.

47. Oberlander TF, Weinberg J, Papsdorf M, Grunau R, Misri S, Devlin AM. Prenatal exposure to maternal depression, neonatal methylation of human glucocorticoid receptor gene (NR3C1) and infant cortisol stress responses. Epigenetics. 2008;3:97–106.

48. Radtke KM, Ruf M, Gunter HM, Dohrmann K, Schauer M, Meyer A, et al. Transgenerational impact of intimate partner violence on methylation in the promoter of the glucocorticoid receptor. Transl Psychiatry. 2011;1:1–6.

49. Hompes T, Izzi B, Gellens E, Morreels M, Fieuws S, Pexsters A. Investigating the influence of maternal cortisol and emotional state during pregnancy on the DNA methylation status of the glucocorticoid receptor gene (NR3C1) promoter region in cord blood. J Psychiatr Res. 2013;47:880–91.

50. Provenzi L, Giorda R, Beri S, Montirosso R. SLC6A4 methylation as an epigenetic marker of life adversity exposures in humans: a systematic review of literature. Neurosci Biobehav Rev. 2016;71:7–20.

51. Devlin AM, Brain U, Austin J, Oberlander TF. Prenatal exposure to maternal depressed mood and the MTHFR C677T variant affect SLC6A4 methylation in infants at birth. PLoS One. 2010;5:e12201.

52. Conradt E, Lester BM, Appleton AA, Armstrong DA, Marsit CJ. The roles of DNA methylation of NR3C1 and 11β–HSD2 and exposure to maternal mood disorder in utero on newborn neurobehavior. Epigenetics. 2013;8:1321–9.

53. Ponder KL, Salisbury A, McGonnigal B, Laliberte A, Lester B, Padbury JF. Maternal depression and anxiety are associated with altered gene expression in the human placenta without modification by antidepressant use: implications for fetal programming. Dev Psychobiol. 2011;53:711–23.

54. O'Donnell KJ, Bugge Jensen A, Freeman L, Khalife N, O'Connor TG, Glover V. Maternal prenatal anxiety and downregulation of placental 11β–HSD2. Psychoneuroendocrinology. 2012;37:818–26.

55. Appleton AA, Armstrong DA, Lesseur C, Lee J, Padbury JF, Lester BM, et al. Patterning in placental 11-B hydroxysteroid dehydrogenase methylation according to prenatal socioeconomic adversity. PLoS One. 2013;8:e74691.

56. Bale TL. Epigenetic and transgenerational reprogramming of brain development. Nat Rev Neurosci. 2015;16(6):332–44.

57. Qiao Y, Yang X, Jing N. Epigenetic regulation of early neural fate commitment. Cell Mol Life Sci. 2016;73(7):1399–411.

58. Varese F, Smeets F, Drukker M, Lieverse R, Lataster T, Viechtbauer W, et al. Childhood adversities increase the risk of psychosis: a meta-analysis of patient-control, prospective- and cross-sectional cohort studies. Schizophr Bull. 2012;38:661–71.

59. Brent DA, Silverstein M. Shedding light on the long shadow of childhood adversity. JAMA. 2013;309:1777–8.

60. Strüber N, Strüber D, Roth G. Impact of early adversity on glucocorticoid regulation and later mental disorders. Neurosci Biobehav Rev. 2014;38:17–37.

61. Chiang JJ, Taylor SE, Bower JE. Early adversity, neural development, and inflammation. Dev Psychobiol. 2015;57(8):887–907.

62. Ehrlich KB, Ross KM, Chen E, Miller GE. Testing the biological embedding hypothesis: is early life adversity associated with a later proinflammatory phenotype? Dev Psychopathol. 2016;28(4pt2):1273–83.

63. Danese A, McEwen BS. Adverse childhood experiences, allostasis, allostatic load, and age-related disease. Physiol Behav. 2012;106:29–39.

64. Remmes J, Bodden C, Richter SH, Lesting J, Sachser N, Pape HC, et al. Impact of life history on fear memory and extinction. Front Behav Neurosci. 2016;10:185.

65. Rubin LP. Maternal and pediatric health and disease: integrating biopsychosocial models and epigenetics. Pediatr Res. 2016;79(1–2):127–35.

66. Meaney MJ, Szyf M, Seckl JR. Epigenetic mechanisms of perinatal programming of hypothalamic–pituitary–adrenal function and health. Trends Mol Med. 2007;13:269–77.

67. Hackman DA, Farah MJ, Meaney MJ. Socioeconomic status and the brain: mechanistic insights from human and animal research. Nat Rev Neurosci. 2010;11:651–9.

68. Maccari S, Krugers HJ, Morley-Fletcher S, Szyf M, Brunton PJ. The consequences of early-life adversity: neurobiological, behavioural and epigenetic adaptations. J Neuroendocrinol. 2014;26(10):707–23.

69. Bick J, Naumova O, Hunter S, Barbot B, Lee M, Luthar SS, et al. Childhood adversity and DNA methylation of genes involved in the hypothalamus-pituitary-adrenal axis and immune system: whole-genome and candidate-gene associations. Dev Psychopathol. 2012;24:1417–25.

70. Vialou V, Feng J, Robison AJ, Nestler EJ. Epigenetic mechanisms of depression and antidepressant action. Annu Rev Pharmacol Toxicol. 2013;53:59–87.

71. Smart C, Strathdee G, Watson S, Murgatroyd C, McAllister-Williams RH. Early life trauma, depression and the glucocorticoid receptor gene–-an epigenetic perspective. Psychol Med. 2015;45(16):3393–410.

72. Turecki G, Meaney MJ. Effects of the social environment and stress on glucocorticoid receptor gene methylation: a systematic review. Biol Psychiatry. 2016;79(2):87–96.

73. DeLisi M, Vaughn MG. The vindication of Lamarck? Epigenetics at the intersection of law and mental health. Behav Sci Law. 2015;33(5):607–28.

74. Frodl T. Do (epi)genetics impact the brain in functional neurologic disorders? Handb Clin Neurol. 2017;139:157–65.

75. Heim C, Newport DJ, Mletzko T, Miller AH, Nemeroff CB. The link between childhood trauma and depression: insights from HPA axis studies in humans. Psychoneuroendocrinology. 2008;33:693–710.

76. Heim C, Binder EB. Current research trends in early life stress and depression: review of human studies on sensitive periods, gene–environment interactions, and epigenetics. Exp Neurol. 2012;233:102–11.

77. Heim C, Newport DJ, Heit S, Graham YP, Wilcox M, Bonsall R, et al. Pituitary-adrenal and autonomic responses to stress in women after sexual and physical abuse in childhood. JAMA. 2000;284:592–7.

78. Frazzetto G, Di Lorenzo G, Carola V, Proietti L, Sokolowska E, Siracusano A, et al. Early trauma and increased risk for physical aggression during adulthood: the moderating role of MAOA genotype. PLoS One. 2007;2(5):e486.

79. Byrd AL, Manuck SB. MAOA, childhood maltreatment, and antisocial behavior: meta-analysis of a gene–environment interaction. Biol Psychiatry. 2014;75(1):9–17.

80. Borghol N, Suderman M, McArdle W, Racine A, Hallett M, Pembrey M, et al. Associations with early-life socio-economic position in adult DNA methylation. Int J Epidemiol. 2012;41:62–74.

81. Miller GE, Chen E, Fok AK, Walker H, Lim A, Nicholls EF, et al. Low early-life social class leaves a biological residue manifested by decreased glucocorticoid and increased proinflammatory signaling. Proc Natl Acad Sci U S A. 2009;106:14716–21.

82. Chen EE, Miller GE, Kobor MS, Cole SW. Maternal warmth buffers the effects of low early-life socioeconomic status on pro-inflammatory signaling in adulthood. Mol Psychiatry. 2011;16:729–37.

83. Hornung OP, Heim CM. Gene–environment interactions and intermediate phenotypes: early trauma and depression. Front Endocrinol (Lausanne). 2014;5:14.

84. Labonté B, Suderman M, Maussion G, Navaro L, Yerko V, Mahar I, et al. Genome-wide epigenetic regulation by early-life trauma. Arch Gen Psychiatry. 2012a;69:722–31.

85. Suderman M, Borghol N, Pappas JJ, Pinto Pereira SM, Pembrey M, Hertzman C, et al. Childhood abuse is associated with methylation of multiple loci in adult DNA. BMC Med Genet. 2014;7:13.

86. Provençal N, Suderman MJ, Guillemin C, Vitaro F, Côté SM, Hallett M, et al. Association of childhood chronic physical aggression with a DNA methylation signature in adult human T cells. PLoS One. 2014;9:e89839.

87. Julian MM. Age at adoption from institutional care as a window into the lasting effects of early experiences. Clin Child Fam Psychol Rev. 2013;16(2):101–45.

88. Naumova O, Lee M, Koposov R, Szyf M, Dozier M, Grigorenko EL. Differential patterns of whole-genome DNA methylation in institutionalized children and children raised by their biological parents. Dev Psychopathol. 2012;24:143–55.

89. McGowan PO, Sasaki A, Huang TC, Unterberger A, Suderman M, Ernst C, et al. Promoter-wide hypermethylation of the ribosomal RNA gene promoter in the suicide brain. PLoS One. 2008;3:e2085.

90. McGowan PO, Sasaki A, D'Alessio AC, Dymov S, Labonté B, Szyf M, et al. Epigenetic regulation of the glucocorticoid receptor in human brain associates with childhood abuse. Nature Neurosci. 2009;12:342–8.

91. Labonté B, Yerko V, Gross J, Mechawar N, Meaney MJ, Szyf M, et al. Differential glucocorticoid receptor exon 1(B), 1(C), and 1(H) expression and methylation in suicide completers with a history of childhood abuse. Biol Psychiatry. 2012b;72:41–8.

92. Bustamante AC, Aiello AE, Galea S, Ratanatharathorn A, Noronha C, Wildman DE, et al. Glucocorticoid receptor DNA methylation, childhood maltreatment and major depression. J Affect Disord. 2016;206:181–8.

93. Tyrka AR, Ridout KK, Parade SH. Childhood adversity and epigenetic regulation of glucocorticoid signaling genes: associations in children and adults. Dev Psychopathol. 2016;28(4pt2):1319–31.

94. Tyrka AR, Parade SH, Welch ES, Ridout KK, Price LH, Marsit C, et al. Methylation of the leukocyte glucocorticoid receptor gene promoter in adults: associations with early adversity and depressive, anxiety and substance-use disorders. Transl Psychiatry. 2016;6(7):e848.

95. Klengel T, Mehta D, Anacker C, Rex-Haffner M, Pruessner JC, Pariante CM, Pace TW, et al. Allele-specific FKBP5 DNA demethylation mediates gene-childhood trauma interactions. Nat Neurosci. 2013;16(1):33–41.

96. Tyrka AR, Price LH, Marsit C, Walters OC, Carpenter LL. Childhood adversity and epigenetic modulation of the leukocyte glucocorticoid receptor: preliminary findings in healthy adults. PLoS One. 2012;7:e30148.

97. Perroud N, Paoloni-Giacobino A, Prada P, Olié E, Salzmann A, Nicastro R, et al. Increased methylation of glucocorticoid receptor gene (NR3C1) in adults with a history of childhood maltreatment: a link with the severity and type of trauma. Transl Psychiatry. 2011;1:e59.

98. Steiger H, Labonté B, Groleau P, Turecki G, Israel M. Methylation of the glucocorticoid receptor gene promoter in bulimic women: associations with borderline personality disorder, suicidality, and exposure to childhood abuse. Int J Eat Disord. 2013;46:246–55.

99. Booij L, Szyf M, Carballedo A, Frey EM, Morris D, Dymov S, et al. DNA methylation of the serotonin transporter gene in peripheral cells and stress-related changes in hippocampal volume: a study in depressed patients and healthy controls. PLoS One. 2015;10(3):e0119061.

100. Miller G, Chen E. Unfavorable socioeconomic conditions in early life presage expression of proinflammatory phenotype in adolescence. Psychosom Med. 2007;69:402–9.

101. Witek-Janusek L, Tell D, Gaylord-Harden N, Mathews HL. Relationship of childhood adversity and neighborhood violence to a proinflammatory phenotype in emerging adult African American men: an epigenetic link. Brain Behav Immun. 2017;60:126–35.

102. Davidson RJ, McEwen BS. Social influences on neuroplasticity: stress and interventions to promote well-being. Nat Neurosci. 2012;15:689–95.

103. Vaiserman A. Early-life origin of adult disease: evidence from natural experiments. Exp Gerontol. 2011;46(2–3):189–92.

104. Mill J, Heijmans BT. From promises to practical strategies in epigenetic epidemiology. Nat Rev Genet. 2013;14:585–94.

105. Entringer S, Wadhwa PD. Developmental programming of obesity and metabolic dysfunction: role of prenatal stress and stress biology. Nestle Nutr Inst Workshop Ser. 2013;74:107–20.

106. Steiger H, Thaler L. Eating disorders, gene–environment interactions and the epigenome: roles of stress exposures and nutritional status. Physiol Behav. 2016;162:181–5.

107. Kesternich I, Siflinger B, Smith JP, Winter JK. The effects of World War II on economic and health outcomes across Europe. Rev Econ Stat. 2014;96:103–18.

108. Yehuda R, Bierer LM. Transgenerational transmission of cortisol and PTSD risk. Prog Brain Res. 2008;167:121–35.

109. Bercovich E, Keinan-Boker L, Shasha SM. Long-term health effects in adults born during the Holocaust. Isr Med Assoc J. 2014;16:203–7.

110. Keinan-Boker L, Shasha-Lavsky H, Eilat-Zanani S, Edri-Shur A, Shasha SM. Chronic health conditions in Jewish Holocaust survivors born during World War II. Isr Med Assoc J. 2015;17(4):206–12.

111. Malaspina D, Corcoran C, Kleinhaus KR, Perrin MC, Fennig S, Nahon D, et al. Acute maternal stress in pregnancy and schizophrenia in offspring: a cohort prospective study. BMC Psychiatry. 2008;8:71.

112. Kleinhaus K, Harlap S, Perrin M, Manor O, Margalit-Calderon R, Opler M, et al. Prenatal stress and affective disorders in a population birth cohort. Bipolar Disord. 2013;15(1):92–9.

113. St Clair D, Xu M, Wang P, Yu Y, Fang Y, Zhang F, et al. Rates of adult schizophrenia following prenatal exposure to the Chinese famine of 1959–1961. JAMA. 2005;294(5):557–62.

114. MQ X, Sun WS, Liu BX, Feng GY, Yu L, Yang L, et al. Prenatal malnutrition and adult schizophrenia: further evidence from the 1959–1961 Chinese famine. Schizophr Bull. 2009;35(3):568–76.

115. Song S, Wang W, Hu P. Famine, death, and madness: schizophrenia in early adulthood after prenatal exposure to the Chinese Great Leap Forward Famine. Soc Sci Med. 2009;68(7):1315–21.

116. Huang C, Phillips MR, Zhang Y, Zhang J, Shi Q, Song Z, et al. Malnutrition in early life and adult mental health: evidence from a natural experiment. Soc Sci Med. 2013;97:259–66.

117. Wang C, An Y, Yu H, Feng L, Liu Q, Lu Y, et al. Association between exposure to the Chinese famine in different stages of early life and decline in cognitive functioning in adulthood. Front Behav Neurosci. 2016;10:146.

118. de Rooij SR, Painter RC, Phillips DI, Osmond C, Tanck MW, Bossuyt PM, et al. Cortisol responses to psychological stress in adults after prenatal exposure to the Dutch famine. Psychoneuroendocrinology. 2006;31(10):1257–65.

119. de Rooij SR, Veenendaal MV, Räikkönen K, Roseboom TJ. Personality and stress appraisal in adults prenatally exposed to the Dutch famine. Early Hum Dev. 2012;88:321–5.

120. Susser E, St Clair D. Prenatal famine and adult mental illness: interpreting concordant and discordant results from the Dutch and Chinese Famines. Soc Sci Med. 2013;97:325–30.

121. Lumey LH, Terry MB, Delgado-Cruzata L, Liao Y, Wang Q, Susser E, et al. Adult global DNA methylation in relation to pre-natal nutrition. Int J Epidemiol. 2012;41:116–23.

122. Tobi EW, Slieker RC, Stein AD, Suchiman HE, Slagboom PE, van Zwet EW, et al. Early gestation as the critical time-window for changes in the prenatal environment to affect the adult human blood methylome. Int J Epidemiol. 2015;44(4):1211–23.

123. Heijmans BT, Tobi EW, Stein AD, Putter H, Blauw GJ, Susser ES, et al. Persistent epigenetic differences associated with prenatal exposure to famine in humans. Proc Natl Acad Sci U S A. 2008;105:17046–9.

124. Tobi EW, Lumey LH, Talens RP, Kremer D, Putter H, Stein AD, et al. DNA methylation differences after exposure to prenatal famine are common and timing- and sex-specific. Hum Mol Genet. 2009;18:4046–53.

125. Heijmans BT, Tobi EW, Lumey LH, Slagboom PE. The epigenome: archive of the prenatal environment. Epigenetics. 2009;4:526–31.

126. Roseboom TJ, Painter RC, van Abeelen AF, Veenendaal MV, de Rooij SR. Hungry in the womb: what are the consequences? Lessons from the Dutch famine. Maturitas. 2011;70:141–5.

127. Gröger N, Matas E, Gos T, Lesse A, Poeggel G, Braun K, et al. The transgenerational transmission of childhood adversity: behavioral, cellular, and epigenetic correlates. J Neural Transm (Vienna). 2016;123(9):1037–52.

128. Yehuda R, Daskalakis NP, Lehrner A, Desarnaud F, Bader HN, Makotkine I, et al. Influences of maternal and paternal PTSD on epigenetic regulation of the glucocorticoid receptor gene in Holocaust survivor offspring. Am J Psychiatry. 2014;171(8):872–80.

129. Perroud N, Rutembesa E, Paoloni-Giacobino A, Mutabaruka J, Mutesa L, Stenz L, et al. The Tutsi genocide and transgenerational transmission of maternal stress: epigenetics and biology of the HPA axis. World J Biol Psychiatry. 2014;15(4):334–45.

130. Gapp K, Bohacek J, Grossmann J, Brunner AM, Manuella F, Nanni P, et al. Potential of environmental enrichment to prevent transgenerational effects of paternal trauma. Neuropsychopharmacology. 2016;41(11):2749–58.

131. Puterman E, Gemmill A, Karasek D, Weir D, Adler N.E, Prather AA, et al. Lifespan adversity and later adulthood telomere length in the nationally representative US Health and Retirement Study. Proc Natl Acad Sci U S A 2016;113(42):E6335–E6342.

132. Humphreys KL, Esteves K, Zeanah CH, Fox NA, Nelson CA 3rd, et al. Accelerated telomere shortening: tracking the lasting impact of early institutional care at the cellular level. Psychiatry Res. 2016;246:95–100.

133. Mitchell C, Hobcraft J, McLanahan SS, Siegel SR, Berg A, Brooks-Gunn J, et al. Social disadvantage, genetic sensitivity, and children's telomere length. Proc Natl Acad Sci U S A. 2014;111(16):5944–9.

134. Scott BR, Belinsky SA, Leng S, Lin Y, Wilder JA, Damiani LA. Radiation-stimulated epigenetic reprogramming of adaptive-response genes in the lung: an evolutionary gift for mounting adaptive protection against lung cancer. Dose-Response. 2009;7:104–31.

135. Barouki R, Gluckman PD, Grandjean P, Hanson M, Heindel JJ. Developmental origins of non-communicable disease: implications for research and public health. Environ Health. 2012;11:42.

136. Godfrey KM, Costello PM, Lillycrop KA. The developmental environment, epigenetic biomarkers and long-term health. J Dev Orig Health Dis. 2015;6(5):399–406.

137. Palma-Gudiel H, Córdova-Palomera A, Leza JC, Fañanás L. Glucocorticoid receptor gene (NR3C1) methylation processes as mediators of early adversity in stress-related disorders causality: a critical review. Neurosci Biobehav Rev. 2015;55:520–35.

138. Turecki G, Ota VK, Belangero SI, Jackowski A, Kaufman J. Early life adversity, genomic plasticity, and psychopathology. Lancet Psychiatry. 2014;1(6):461–6.

139. Vaiserman AM. Early-life nutritional programming of longevity. J Dev Orig Health Dis. 2014;5:325–38.

140. Kundakovic M, Jaric I. The epigenetic link between prenatal adverse environments and neurodevelopmental disorders. Genes (Basel). 2017;8(3):104.

141. McGowan PO. Epigenetic clues to the biological embedding of early life adversity. Biol Psychiatry. 2012;72:4–5.

142. Talens RP, Christensen K, Putter H, Willemsen G, Christiansen L, Kremer D, et al. Epigenetic variation during the adult lifespan: cross-sectional and longitudinal data on monozygotic twin pairs. Aging Cell. 2012;11:694–703.

143. Sen P, Shah PP, Nativio R, Berger SL. Epigenetic mechanisms of longevity and aging. Cell. 2016;166(4):822–39.

144. Penney J, Tsai LH. Histone deacetylases in memory and cognition. Sci Signal. 2014;7(355):re12.

145. Fuchikami M, Yamamoto S, Morinobu S, Okada S, Yamawaki Y, Yamawaki S. The potential use of histone deacetylase inhibitors in the treatment of depression. Prog Neuro-Psychopharmacol Biol Psychiatry. 2016;64:320–4.

146. Qiu X, Xiao X, Li N, Li Y. Histone deacetylases inhibitors (HDACis) as novel therapeutic application in various clinical diseases. Prog Neuro-Psychopharmacol Biol Psychiatry. 2017;72:60–72.

147. Moretti M, Valvassori SS, Varela RB, Ferreira CL, Rochi N, Benedet J, et al. Behavioral and neurochemical effects of sodium butyrate in an animal model of mania. Behav Pharmacol. 2011;22(8):766–72.

148. Lopes-Borges J, Valvassori SS, Varela RB, Tonin PT, Vieira JS, Gonçalves CL, et al. Histone deacetylase inhibitors reverse manic-like behaviors and protect the rat brain from energetic metabolic alterations induced by ouabain. Pharmacol Biochem Behav. 2015, 128:89–95.

149. Resende WR, Valvassori SS, Réus GZ, Varela RB, Arent CO, Ribeiro KF, et al. Effects of sodium butyrate in animal models of mania and depression: implications as a new mood stabilizer. Behav Pharmacol. 2013;24(7):569–79.

150. Valvassori SS, Varela RB, Arent CO, Dal-Pont GC, Bobsin TS, Budni J, et al. Sodium butyrate functions as an antidepressant and improves cognition with enhanced neurotrophic expression in models of maternal deprivation and chronic mild stress. Curr Neurovasc Res. 2014;11(4):359–66.

151. Valvassori SS, Resende WR, Budni J, Dal-Pont GC, Bavaresco DV, Réus GZ, et al. Sodium butyrate, a histone deacetylase inhibitor, reverses behavioral and mitochondrial alterations in animal models of depression induced by early- or late-life stress. Curr Neurovasc Res. 2015;12(4):312–20.

152. Takuma K, Hara Y, Kataoka S, Kawanai T, Maeda Y, Watanabe R, et al. Chronic treatment with valproic acid or sodium butyrate attenuates novel object recognition deficits and hippocampal dendritic spine loss in a mouse model of autism. Pharmacol Biochem Behav. 2014;126:43–9.

153. Kratsman N, Getselter D, Elliott E. Sodium butyrate attenuates social behavior deficits and modifies the transcription of inhibitory/excitatory genes in the frontal cortex of an autism model. Neuropharmacology. 2016;102:136–45.

154. Zhong T, Qing QJ, Yang Y, Zou WY, Ye Z, Yan JQ, et al. Repression of contexual fear memory induced by isoflurane is accompanied by reduction in histone acetylation and rescued by sodium butyrate. Br J Anaesth. 2014; 113(4):634–43.

155. Sharma S, Taliyan R, Singh S. Beneficial effects of sodium butyrate in 6–OHDA induced neurotoxicity and behavioral abnormalities: modulation of histone deacetylase activity. Behav Brain Res. 2015;291:306–14.

156. Liu H, Zhang JJ, Li X, Yang Y, Xie XF, Hu K. Post-occlusion administration of sodium butyrate attenuates cognitive impairment in a rat model of chronic cerebral hypoperfusion. Pharmacol Biochem Behav. 2015;135:53–9.

157. Cuadrado-Tejedor M, Ricobaraza AL, Torrijo R, Franco R, Garcia-Osta A. Phenylbutyrate is a multifaceted drug that exerts neuroprotective effects and reverses the Alzheimer's disease-like phenotype of a commonly used mouse model. Curr Pharm Des. 2013;19(28):5076–84.

158. Sandner G, Host L, Angst MJ, Guiberteau T, Guignard B, Zwiller J. The HDAC inhibitor phenylbutyrate reverses effects of neonatal ventral hippocampal lesion in rats. Front Psychiatry. 2011;1:153.

159. Moloney RD, Stilling RM, Dinan TG, Cryan JF. Early-life stress-induced visceral hypersensitivity and anxiety behavior is reversed by histone deacetylase inhibition. Neurogastroenterol Motil. 2015;27(12):1831–6.

6

A genomic case study of desmoplastic small round cell tumor: comprehensive analysis reveals insights into potential therapeutic targets and development of a monitoring tool for a rare and aggressive disease

Elisa Napolitano Ferreira[1], Bruna Durães Figueiredo Barros[1], Jorge Estefano de Souza[2], Renan Valieris Almeida[1], Giovana Tardin Torrezan[1], Sheila Garcia[1], Ana Cristina Victorino Krepischi[3], Celso Abdon Lopes de Mello[4], Isabela Werneck da Cunha[5], Clóvis Antonio Lopes Pinto[5], Fernando Augusto Soares[5], Emmanuel Dias-Neto[1], Ademar Lopes[4], Sandro José de Souza[6] and Dirce Maria Carraro[1]* [iD]

Abstract

Background: Genome-wide profiling of rare tumors is crucial for improvement of diagnosis, treatment, and, consequently, achieving better outcomes. Desmoplastic small round cell tumor (DSRCT) is a rare type of sarcoma arising from mesenchymal cells of abdominal peritoneum that usually develops in male adolescents and young adults. A specific translocation, t(11;22)(p13;q12), resulting in *EWS* and *WT1* gene fusion is the only recurrent molecular hallmark and no other genetic factor has been associated to this aggressive tumor. Here, we present a comprehensive genomic profiling of one DSRCT affecting a 26-year-old male, who achieved an excellent outcome.

Methods: We investigated somatic and germline variants through whole-exome sequencing using a family based approach and, by array CGH, we explored the occurrence of genomic imbalances. Additionally, we performed mate-paired whole-genome sequencing for defining the specific breakpoint of the EWS-WT1 translocation, allowing us to develop a personalized tumor marker for monitoring the patient by liquid biopsy.

Results: We identified genetic variants leading to protein alterations including 12 somatic and 14 germline events (11 germline compound heterozygous mutations and 3 rare homozygous polymorphisms) affecting genes predominantly involved in mesenchymal cell differentiation pathways. Regarding copy number alterations (CNA) few events were detected, mainly restricted to gains in chromosomes 5 and 18 and losses at 11p, 13q, and 22q. The deletions at 11p and 22q indicated the presence of the classic translocation, t(11;22)(p13;q12). In addition, the mapping of the specific genomic breakpoint of the EWS-WT1 gene fusion allowed the design of a personalized biomarker for assessing circulating tumor DNA (ctDNA) in plasma during patient follow-up. This biomarker has been used in four post-treatment blood samples, 3 years after surgery, and no trace of EWS-WT1 gene fusion was detected, in accordance with imaging tests showing no evidence of disease and with the good general health status of the patient.

(Continued on next page)

---

* Correspondence: dirce.carraro@cipe.accamargo.org.br
[1]International Research Center/CIPE, A.C. Camargo Cancer Center, São Paulo, SP, Brazil
Full list of author information is available at the end of the article

(Continued from previous page)

Conclusions: Overall, our findings revealed genes with potential to be associated with risk assessment and tumorigenesis of this rare type of sarcoma. Additionally, we established a liquid biopsy approach for monitoring patient follow-up based on genomic information that can be similarly adopted for patients diagnosed with a rare tumor.

Keywords: Desmoplastic small round cell tumor, Genomic profiling, Whole-exome sequencing, EWS-WT1 gene fusion, Personalized biomarker, Liquid biopsy

Background

Comprehensive molecular profiling is an especially important tool to gain insights on the biological pathways involved in tumor onset and to improve the management and treatment of rare tumors. Desmoplastic small round cell tumor (DSRCT) is a very rare type of sarcoma, with an age-adjusted incidence rate of 0.3 cases/million [1], which typically arises from the abdominal or pelvic peritoneum and occurs mainly in male adolescents and young adults (peak incidence at 20–24 years of age) [1]. Current therapeutic approaches involve the use of multimodal therapeutic regimen, including aggressive polychemotherapy, debulking surgery, and whole abdominal radiation [2].

A specific translocation, t(11;22)(p13;q12), is detected in DSRCT cases, juxtaposing the Ewing's sarcoma gene (*EWSR1*) to the Wilm's tumor gene (*WT1*). The chimeric transcript containing the 5′ region of the *EWSR1*, which includes the N-terminal transactivation domain of EWS, and the 3′ sequence of *WT1* containing 2–4 zinc finger domains have been shown to upregulate EGR-1 [3] and induce the expression of PDGFA [4] and IGF1R [5].

Apart from this translocation, no other recurrent genomic alteration has been reported in DSRCT cases. Silva et al. [6] detected a somatic amplification involving *AURKB* and *MCL1* genes in one patient, and La Starza et al. [7] found specific genomic imbalances, including gain at chromosome 3 reported in two cases and chromosome 5 polysomy in one case. In terms of point mutations, the data is even scarcer. Variants of unknown clinical significance were reported in *ARID1A* and *RUNX1* genes in one patient [6], whereas in another study, no mutations were detected in a panel of 29 genes evaluated in a cohort of 24 DSRCT cases [8]. This limited genomic information about DSRCT impairs new and more efficient therapeutic opportunities for the young patients affected with this rare tumor.

Here, aiming to contribute with the knowledge of the genomic abnormalities that underlies DSRCT, we performed a comprehensive genomic profiling using a family based approach in one case of DSRCT diagnosed in a young male patient with pelvic tumor, who presented excellent outcome sustained for above 3 years. We identified somatic mutations in a genomic background of rare germline variants either homozygous or

as compound heterozygous inheritance, which can improve the understanding of the genetic basis of this rare tumor. We have also generated the profile of genomic imbalances, which was confirmed by whole-exome sequencing. In addition, as we were able to define the precise genomic breakpoints of the EWS-WT1 translocation by whole-genome and Sanger sequencing, we managed to establish a personalized strategy for tracking DNA tumor traces in plasma, allowing an accurate monitoring of tumor recurrence.

Overall, our analysis revealed potential genes and pathways associated with this rare sarcoma and demonstrated the feasibility of using genomic profiling for the benefit of patients affected by rare tumors by developing a personalized monitoring strategy.

Methods

DNA extraction

Tumor tissues and blood samples were collected following the technical and ethical procedures of A.C. Camargo Tumor Bank, registered at National Council for Ethics in Research by the number B001 [9]. Genomic DNA and plasma DNA were extracted in DNA and RNA Bank [10] using QIASymphony DNA Mini kit (QIAGEN, Hilden, Germany) for tumor and leukocyte DNA and QIAamp DNA blood Midi kit (QIAGEN, Hilden, Germany) for plasma DNA, following standard procedures.

Target sequencing

Target sequencing was performed using the Ion AmpliSeq™ Comprehensive Cancer Panel, which comprises all exons from 409 genes associated with different types of tumors (AmpliSeq, Ion Torrent™). This panel, based on multiplex PCR, was performed with as little as 40 ng of DNA from the tumor sample. Library was prepared based on Ion AmpliSeq™ Library Preparation protocol and sequenced at Ion Proton™ platform (Ion Torrent™), according to the manufacturer's instructions.

Whole-exome sequencing

Whole-exome sequencing of the tumor and leukocyte DNA samples from the patient and his mother were performed using the TargetSeq™ Exome Enrichment Kit (Life Technologies), followed by paired-end sequencing (75 × 50) in SOLiD 5500xl System (Life Technologies). Leukocyte

DNA sample from his father was submitted for whole-exome sequencing using Ion Xpress™ Plus Fragment Library kit and Ion TargetSeq™ Exome Enrichment Kit (Life Technologies), followed by sequencing at Ion Proton™ platform (Ion Torrent™), according to the manufacturer's instructions. Single-end sequencing was performed on an Ion PI™ Chip v2 with 200 pb sequencing kit (Ion Torrent™).

Whole-genome sequencing

Whole-genome sequencing was performed by mate-paired DNA libraries prepared using the 5500 SOLiD™ Mate-Paired Library Construction Kit (Life Technologies), following the manufacturer's instructions. Briefly, genomic DNA from tumor and leukocyte of the patient was sheared with a Covaris sonicator into approximately 2 Kb fragments, circularized with mate-paired adaptors, nick-translated and digested, incorporated with sequencing adaptors and individual barcodes (distinct barcodes were used for the tumor and leukocyte DNA), and submitted to emulsion PCR. Mate-paired sequencing (60×60) was performed in a SOLiD 5500xl System (Life Technologies).

Sanger sequencing

For validation, primers were designed flanking the variants, in order to generate fragments of nearly 400 bp. PCR reactions were performed using GoTaq® Green Master Mix (Promega, Madison, WI, USA), using 15 ng of DNA, with 300 nM of each primer, for a final reaction volume of 20 µL. Approximately 200 ng of PCR-amplified fragments were purified with ExoSAP-IT (USB Corporation, Cleveland, OH, USA) and sequenced in both directions. All alterations were evaluated in all four samples (mother, father, and patient's leukocyte and tumor). Products were analyzed using an ABI 3130xl DNA sequencer (Applied Biosystems, Foster City, CA, USA), and sequences were aligned with the respective gene reference sequence using CLC Genomics Workbench Software (QIAGEN, Hilden, Germany).

Comparative genome hybridization based on microarrays (array CGH)

Comparative genomic hybridization based on microarrays was performed in a commercial whole-genome 180 K platform containing 180,000 oligonucleotide probes (Agilent Technologies; design 22060), using DNA from the tumor sample. Reference DNA was a commercially available human pool of samples from multiple anonymous healthy donors (Promega Corporation). Technical procedures are described in Torrezan et al. [11]. Hybridization and washing were performed as recommended by the manufacturer. Scanned images were processed using Feature Extraction 10.7.3.1 software (Agilent Technologies), and array CGH analysis was conducted with Nexus Copy

Number software 7.0 (Biodiscovery). We used the FASST2 segmentation algorithm, according to the following settings: minimum of five consecutive probes (effective resolution of ~70 Kb for CNA calling), significance threshold set at 10^{-8}, and threshold $\log_2$ Cy3/Cy5 of 0.33 and −0.3 for gains for loss, respectively, and 1.2 and −1.1 for high copy number gains and homozygous losses, respectively. All copy number alterations are reported in the Database of Genomic Variants [12].

Bioinformatics analysis
Comprehensive cancer panel

Sequencing reads from Ion Proton™ were mapped to the reference genome (GRCh37/hg19) with TMAP (torrent mapper 4.2.18). Sequence variants (SNVs and indels) were identified with Torrent Variant Caller 4.0-5, followed by confirmation by GATK protocol vs3.2-2-gec30cee [13]. Variants were annotated using SnpEff version 3.5d (build 2014-03-05) [14].

Whole-exome sequencing

Sequencing reads from SOLiD 5500xl System were mapped to the reference genome (GRCh37/hg19) with Lifescope (LifeScope™ Genomic Analysis Software v2.5.1). Sequencing reads from Ion Proton™ were mapped to the reference genome (GRCh37/hg19) with TMAP (torrent mapper 4.2.18). Sequence variants (SNVs and indels) were identified following the GATK protocol vs3.2-2-gec30cee [13] for SOLiD 5500XL System and with Torrent Variant Caller 4.0-5, followed by GATK protocol vs3.2-2-gec30cee for Ion Proton reads. Variants were annotated using SnpEff version 3.5d (build 2014-03-05) [14] and an in-house developed script. Identified variants were compared to dbNSFP version 2.4 [15, 16]; COSMIC v69 [17]; 1000 Genomes [18]; NHLBI GO Exome Sequencing Project version ESP6500SI-V2 [19]; HapMap [20]; and dbSNP version 138 [21, 22] for further annotation. Somatic variants were defined for regions with a minimum coverage of 10× for both tumor and leukocyte sample from the patient and minimum variant frequency of 20% in the tumor only. De novo variants were defined with a minimum coverage of 10× for leukocyte samples of the patient and his parents and with a minimum variant frequency of 30%. To identify rare polymorphisms inherited in homozygosity, we selected variants with a minimum coverage of 10× for leukocyte samples of the patient and his parents, detected in heterozygosis in both parents and homozygosis in the patient presenting a minor allele frequency ≤10% in the public databases (1000 Genome [18], NHLBI GO Exome Sequencing Project [19], and HapMap [20]). To identify germline compound heterozygosis cases, we identified genes with two distinct heterozygous mutations in the patient, where each variant was exclusively present in one of his parents in heterozygosity and detected in regions with a minimum coverage of 10× for all leukocyte samples. We discarded variants that are detected with a minor allele frequency above 10% in the 1000 Genome Project [18]. Copy number alterations were detected using the bioinformatics packages Excavator (version 2.2) [23] and cn.mops (version 1.8.9) [24] by comparing exome data from the tumor to leukocyte from the patient. For visualization, we used circos 0.67-7 package [25].

Whole-genome sequencing

For detecting structural variations, mate-pair reads obtained by SOLiD 5500xl System were analyzed by svdetect (version r0.8b) [26].

Ingenuity Pathway Analysis

We applied the core analysis of Ingenuity Pathway Analysis (IPA) system (QIAGEN, Germantown, MD, USA) to identify gene interaction networks.

Digital droplet PCR

Digital droplet PCR assays were carried out using the QX200™ Droplet Digital™ (ddPCR™) System (Bio-Rad). A primer-probe assay labeled with FAM was designed for the amplification of wild-type *WT1* gene and a primer-probe assay labeled with HEX was designed for the amplification of the gene fusion event (EWS-WT1). For the amplification reaction, we used 1× ddPCR Supermix, 1× primer-probe assay (FAM), 1× primer-probe assay (HEX), and 4 µl of DNA. Droplet generation, PCR amplification, and droplet counting were performed following the manufacturer's recommendations.

DNA samples from tumor tissue (60 ng–6 pg) and from leukocytes (6 ng) were used as positive and negative controls, respectively. We loaded 4 µl of 30 µl (1/8) of cfDNA samples from the patient. We also used DNA and cell-free DNA extracted from leukocytes and plasma, respectively, from healthy donors as negative controls and performed non-template control. All reactions were performed with at least two replicates.

Results

In this study, we performed a comprehensive genomic profiling of one case of desmoplastic small round cell tumor (DSRCT) by a combination of targeted sequencing, array CGH, whole genome, and whole exome applied in a family based format. The patient studied here is a 26-year-old male, who presented at A.C. Camargo Cancer Center in November, 2011, with a large abdominal mass and a small nodule on the pelvic region. Staging images showed that the disease was limited to the abdominal cavity. He underwent a CT-guided biopsy that revealed a desmoplastic small round cell tumor (DSRCT), showing positivity for EMA, desmin, and nuclear staining for WT1

(carboxy-terminus antibody). FISH analysis was positive for EWS translocation.

The patient started systemic treatment with 4 cycles of vincristine, cyclophosphamide, and doxorubicin (VAC) and alternated with ifosfamide, carboplatin, and etoposide (ICE). After 4 cycles, the best response was stable disease, with minor reduction in the tumor dimensions. He underwent complete surgical cytoreduction, with resection of the large mass and resection of peritoneal implant on the pelvic region, and hyperthermic intra-peritoneal chemotherapy (HIPEC), with cisplatin and doxorubicin. The patient presented a complete recovery from these procedures. After that, the patient received four more cycles of chemotherapy and total abdominal irradiation (total of 30 Gy). After a follow-up of 48 months since surgery, the patient is asymptomatic, with no signs of disease (Additional file 1: Figure S1).

The comprehensive genomic profiling was carried out in multiple fronts. To identify actionable mutations, we carried out targeted sequencing of the most important actionable genes in the tumor sample. Further, to identify genes and mutations possibly involved with tumor onset and predisposition, we performed whole exome sequencing, using the DSRCT tumor sample and blood samples from the patient and his both parents (Additional file 2: Table S1). Array CGH was performed in tumor sample to identify structural rearrangements and copy number imbalances. Whole-genome sequencing defined one tumor marker used to precisely monitor patient after treatment.

Producing a portrait of somatically acquired variants

To identify actionable mutations or pathways related to DSRCT in this patient, we initially performed targeted sequencing using a cancer-oriented gene panel composed of 409 genes in the tumor sample (Comprehensive Cancer Panel – Thermo Scientific). Since no actionable mutation for targeted therapy was detected in the tumor, we investigated the complete landscape of somatic mutations by whole-exome sequencing (WES) the tumor and the patient's leukocyte. The analysis of the tumor revealed 15 somatic acquired mutations, 12 of which were protein-affecting variants (validated by capillary sequencing) including one non-sense mutation in the *ZNF808* gene, one nucleotide change at the 3' splice site of *RIMS4*, and 10 missense mutations considered disease associated by at least one pathogenicity prediction program (Table 1).

Gene ontology enrichment analysis of the 12 genes harboring protein-affecting somatic mutations revealed several biological processes such as muscle tissue/organ development (*ZFPM2* and *MEGF10*), which is related to the mesothelium origin of this tumor, cell adhesion (*DPP4, CDH9, CNTNAP4, MEGF10*), response to mechanic stimulus (*MEIS2, TRPA4*), and response to abiotic

Table 1 Description of somatically acquired point mutations detected in the DSRCT by whole-exome sequencing

Chromosome position	Gene symbol	Variant description	Variant type	Frequency (tumor coverage)	Coverage of leukocyte DNA	dbSNP	PolyPhen	Sift	Mutation taster
chr3:436494	CHL1	c.3033A>G, p.A111A	Synonymous	35% (55×)	53×	–	–	–	–
chr6:134305546	TBPL1	c.315T>G, p.V105V	Synonymous	23% (31×)	28×	–	–	–	–
chr12:34179763	ALG10	c.1335A>T, p.A445A	Synonymous	43% (82×)	66×	–	–	–	–
chr1:45808899	TOE1	c.1058C>T, p.P353L	Missense	20% (15×)	18×	rs145913038	Benign	Damaging	Polymorphism
chr2:162875307	DPP4	c.1352C>T, p.P451L	Missense	37% (41×)	46×	–	Deleterious	Tolerated	Disease causing
chr5:126753368	MEGF10	c.1169G>C, p.G390C	Missense	22% (82×)	39×	–	Deleterious	Damaging	Disease causing
chr5:26915867	CDH9	c.394G>C, p.D132Y	Missense	25% (71×)	75×	–	Deleterious	–	Disease causing
chr6:123319098	CLVS2	c.176G>A, p.R59Q	Missense	40% (25×)	20×	–	Deleterious	Damaging	Disease causing
chr8:106813312	ZFPM2	c.1002T>A, p.S334R	Missense	28% (36×)	44×	–	Deleterious	Tolerated	Disease causing
chr8:72983969	TRPA1	c.245T>C, p.I82T	Missense	36% (45×)	35×	–	Deleterious	Damaging	Disease causing
chr15:37385900	MEIS2	c.521G>A, p.R86Q	Missense	26% (31×)	23×	–	Possible damaging	Damaging	Disease causing
chr16:76495948	CNTNAP4	c.1210G>T, p.A404S	Missense	33% (42×)	43×	–	Benign	Tolerated	Disease causing
chr17:10300120	MYH8	c.4362G>T, p.K1454N	Missense	26% (38×)	33×	–	Deleterious	–	Disease causing
chr19:53057457	ZNF808	c.1288G>T, p.E430Ter	Nonsense	43% (30×)	27×	–	–	Tolerated	Polymorphism
chr20:43385680	RIMS4	c.455-2T>A	3′ splice site	28% (29×)	37×	–	–	–	–

stimulus (*DPP4*, *MEIS2*, *TRPA1*) (Additional file 3: Table S2). Intriguingly, biological network analysis obtained using Ingenuity Pathway Analysis (IPA) interconnected the 15 genes harboring somatic mutations in a single network associated with cell death and survival, cell damage or degeneration, and nervous system development and function (Fig. 1a).

Searching for germline variants associated with DSRCT

In an attempt to identify de novo germline mutations and inherited variants potentially associated with DSRCT, we performed whole-exome sequencing of the leukocyte DNA from the patient's parents (Additional file 2: Table S1). For selecting genetic variants, a minimum coverage of 10× in all samples with at least 30% frequency of the variant allele was considered. Based on these criteria, no de novo variants were found.

Next, we explored the possibility of finding genetic variants associated with DSRCT in an autosomal recessive model of inheritance. First, we searched for polymorphisms (MAF ≤10%) occurring in homozygosity in the patient that were inherited from both heterozygous parents. Four polymorphisms inherited in homozygosis were found in *ADAMTS12*, *RASSF1*, *VEZT*, and *ISX* genes (population frequency ranging from 2.0 to 7.8%). All polymorphisms lead to missense alterations, two of them reported as possibly disease associated by at least one pathogenicity prediction program (Table 2). Interestingly, biological network analysis showed an interconnection between the four genes in a single network from IPA,

showing association with cell cycle and digestive system development and function (Fig. 1b).

Next, to identify candidate genes affected by compound heterozygosity, we looked for genes containing two distinct variants inherited independently from each parent. We could confirm 11 genes affected by germline compound heterozygous mutations, in which one variant allele was inherited from the mother and the other variant allele was inherited from the father (MAF ≤10%) (Table 3). We speculate that these genes could be associated with risk to DSRCT development in an autosomal recessive model of inheritance.

Gene ontology analysis of these 11 genes showed enrichment of biological processes related to muscle tissue development (*LAMB2*, *SYNE1*, and *TTN*), morphogenesis (*C2CD3* and *TTN*), and cell cycle (*RSPH1*, *TTN*, and *SPICE1*) (Additional file 4: Table S4). Functional analysis of IPA revealed that 9 of the 11 genes are interconnected in a single network related to cancer, organismal injury and abnormalities, and gastrointestinal disease.

Copy number alterations

Genomic copy number alterations (CNA) were investigated in the DSRCT tumor sample using array CGH in a 180-K platform. Few copy number alterations were detected (Fig. 2a), including aneuploidies such as gain of chromosomes 5 and 18, and 11p, 13q, and 22q deletions. Only one small focal homozygous deletion was identified in a segment of ~1.3 Mb at 9p22.2 (chr9:17,106,384-18,449,088; hg19), encompassing the *CNTLN* and *SH3GL2* genes.

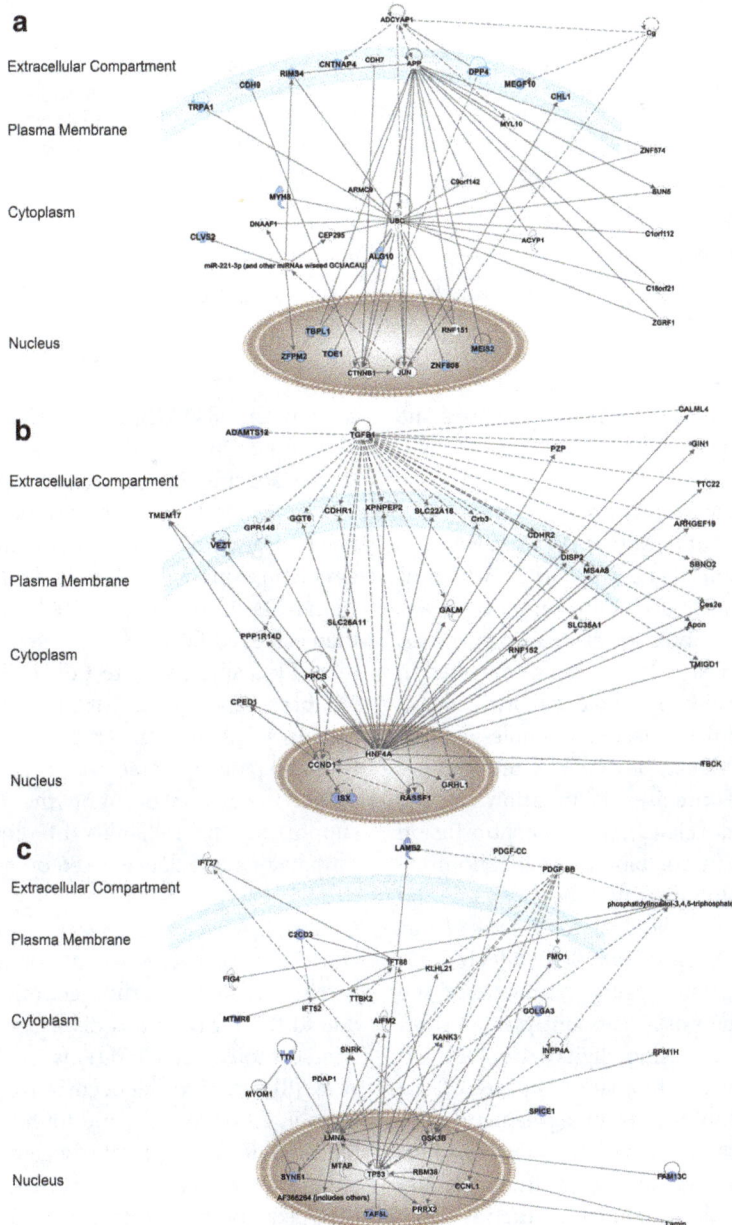

Fig. 1 Network analysis by IPA. **a** Interaction network of genes harboring protein-affecting somatic mutations (network score = 45) is associated with the top disease and functions: cell death and survival, nervous system development and function, cellular compromise. **b** Interaction network of genes harboring rare polymorphisms detected in homozygosis in the patient (network score = 12) is associated with the top disease and functions: cell cycle, digestive system development and function, hair and skin development and function. **c** Interaction network of genes affected by compound heterozygous variants (network score = 25) is associated with the top disease and functions: cancer, organismal injury, abnormalities, and gastrointestinal disease. Continuous and dashed lines indicate direct and indirect interactions between molecules, respectively. Blue molecules represent the genes encountered in our analysis and blank molecules represent other genes automatically included by IPA. Molecules are displayed by various shapes depending on the functional class of the gene product, according to IPA Path designer shapes (Additional file 7)

The detection of copy number losses affecting terminal segments of 11p and 22q suggested the presence of the chromosomal translocation t(11;22)(p13;q12) involving *EWSR1* and *WT1* genes.

Additionally, we used NGS data from the WES of the tumor and patient's leukocyte to search for CNAs, and 98.4% of the events detected by array CGH were validated, demonstrating the efficacy of WES for identification of a

Table 2 Description of rare polymorphisms detected in homozygosity in the DSRCT patient. All variants were validated by sanger sequencing

Gene symbol	cDNA change	Protein change	Type	dbSNP (MAF)	Patient (Frequency/ Coverage)	Mother (Frequency/ Coverage)	Father (Frequency/ Coverage)	Polyphen	Sift	Mutation Taster
VEZT	c.1486G > A	p.V496I	Missense	rs10507051 (0.0302)	100% / 17	17.9% / 28	35.0% / 80	PD	T	DC
ISX	c.248G > A	p.R83Q	Missense	rs8140287 (0.0308)	100% / 13	37.5% / 24	50.0% / 70	PrD	T	DC
RASSF1	c.409G > T	p.A137S	Missense	rs2073498 (0.0711)	83.3% / 12	27.5% / 40	53.1% / 32	B	T	P
ADAMTS12	c.3529 T > C	p.W1177R	Missense	rs3813474 (0.0513)	100% / 51	42.0% / 88	45.0% / 40	B	T	P

MAF Minor allele frequency, *PrD* Probably damaging, *B* Benign, *PD* Possibly damaging, *D* Damaging, *T* Tolerated, *DC* Disease causing, *P* Polymorphism. (*) low confidence prediction

wide range of somatic events, besides point mutations and indels (Fig. 2b; Additional file 5: Table S3).

Establishment of a personalized monitoring strategy based on detection of circulating tumor DNA (ctDNA)

The genomic translocation t(11;22)(p13;q12), which is considered the molecular hallmark of this tumor type, was initially detected by FISH analysis for diagnostic purposes. Furthermore, the same translocation was also detected in the array CGH and confirmed by whole-genome sequencing. The mate-pair approach used for whole-genome sequencing followed by validation by PCR and Sanger sequencing allowed the precise delimitation of the chromosomal breakpoints (Fig. 3). This somatic fusion event was then used as a tumor biomarker for monitoring the patient along the follow-up period using a liquid biopsy-based approach. We searched for traces of circulating tumor DNA in plasma samples collected 17, 36, 42, and 47 months after surgery. No signs of the translocation in any of the post-treatment plasma samples were detected (Fig. 3) using digital droplet PCR (ddPCR). The absence of the biomarker in any of the post-treatment plasma samples is in agreement with favorable clinical response of the patient, showing long-term disease-free survival and no sign of disease recurrence. As a positive control, we confirmed the presence of cell-free circulating DNA by detecting non-rearranged WT1 gene in all plasma samples.

Despite the unavailability of plasma samples at the moment of diagnosis and before treatment (neoadjuvant/ adjuvant chemotherapy and surgery) to be used as a baseline positive control, we carried out stringent control assays. We tested the robustness of the approach by evaluating six different amounts of tumor DNA, ranging from 60 ng to 6 pg, and searched for both the tumor-specific fusion event and for the non-rearranged WT1 gene. We achieved a linear quantification of tumor marker and wild-type DNA, and we were able to discriminate the presence of the fusion event even in extremely low quantity of DNA (6 pg) (Fig. 3d). To test the specificity of the ddPCR assay, we used leukocyte sample of the

patient and also DNA from plasma and leukocyte samples of healthy donors, and the absence of detection of tumor-specific fusion confirmed the assay specificity for tumor DNA, without false positive signals (Additional file 6: Figure S2). Further, we mimicked a situation of circulating tumor DNA in body fluid by mixing 1 part of tumor DNA to 100 and 1000 parts of leukocyte DNA, then screened for the fusion event using 1 ng of this DNA mix. Typically, the detection of circulating tumor DNA has been reported as a fraction between 0.1 and 90% of plasma DNA for cancer patients, depending on tumor type and patient characteristics [27]. Here, we were able to detect the fusion event in the 1.0 and 0.1% fractions, supporting the reliability of our established approach for patient surveillance based on liquid-biopsy screening.

Discussion

DSRCT is an aggressive tumor not yet broadly investigated with the powerful genomic tools available. Mainly due to the rarity of this disease, only a few studies investigated molecular alterations in this tumor type. Shukla et al. [8] screened the occurrence of 275 COSMIC mutations in 29 oncogenes and found no alterations in any of the 24 DSRCT samples investigated. More recently, a study based on targeted exome sequencing of six adult patients with pediatric-type malignancies found AURKB and MCL1 amplifications and variants of unknown clinical significance in ARID1A and RUNX1 genes in one DSRCT [6].

Here, by performing a comprehensive screening of the genomic alterations in a family based approach, we identified somatic and germline variants possibly associated with DSRCT. In our study, the use of a commercially available gene panel did not show to be an adequate strategy. Based on this finding, one can argue that screening by commercially available gene panels is not an effective approach for most cases of rare tumors, since the targeted genes represented in these panels are usually those well characterized in common solid tumors. On the other hand, the use of WES not only revealed mutated genes but also showed robustness for detecting DNA copy number alterations. Concordance rates between WES and

Table 3 Description of compound heterozygous variants detected in the DSRCT patient. Each one of the variants was exclusively inherited by one of the parents. The genotype and variant frequency were obtained by leukocyte DNA sequencing. All variants were validated by Sanger sequencing

Gene	cDNA change	Protein change	dbSNP (MAF)	Mother		Father		Patient		Polyphen	Sift	Mutation Taster
				Genotype	Variant Frequency	Genotype	Variant Frequency	Genotype	Variant Frequency			
C2CD3	c.5653 T > C	p.S1885P	rs142277857 (0.001)	T/C	43.1	T/T	-	T/C	53.57	PrD	D	P
	c.3223A > C	p.S1075R	-	A/A	-	A/C	50.91	A/C	41.67	PrD	D	DC
FAM13C	c.1361G > A	p.R454H	rs369226393	G/A	56.4	G/G	-	G/A	50	B	T	P
	c.439C > T	p.P147S	rs73299227 (0.0092)	C/C	-	C/T	51,43	C/T	36.36	PD	D*	DC
GOLGA3	c.209G > A	p.G70E	rs2291256 (0.0581)	G/A	52.3	G/G	-	G/A	47.06	B	D*	P
	c.3728G > A	p.R1243Q	rs140646528 (0.0134)	G/G	-	G/A	60	G/A	25	B	T	P
LAMB2	c.1424G > A	p.R475Q	rs370565848	G/A	36.4	G/G	-	G/A	60	PrD	T	P
	c.5293G > A	p.A1765T	rs74951356 (0.0130)	G/G	-	G/A	55.81	G/A	41.18	B	T	DC
MTMR6	c.685C > G	p.P229A	rs149526134 (0.0002)	C/G	60.9	C/C	-	C/G	26.32	B	T	P
	c.1795G > A	p.A599T	rs62619824 (0.0571	G/G	-	G/A	35.09	G/A	51.85	B	T	DC
RSPH1	c.742G > A	p.G248R	rs117385282 (0.0839)	G/A	50	G/G	-	G/A	31.25	B	T	P
	c.733G > A	p.G245R	rs151158140 (0.0026)	G/G	-	G/A	50.77	G/A	58.33	PD	T	P
SLC9A9	c.1765A > G	p.I589V	rs2289491 (0.0290)	A/G	31.1	A/A	-	A/G	28	B	T	P
	c.1618A > G	p.I540V	rs16853300 (0.0066)	A/A	-	A/G	48.62	A/G	36.36	B	T	P
SPICE1	c.2470A > C	p.T824P	rs57006145 (0.0313)	A/C	40.4	A/A	-	A/C	62.16	PrD	T	DC
	c.850G > A	p.V284M	rs73239152 (0.0078)	G/G	-	G/A	47.54	G/A	29.27	B	D	DC
SYNE1	c.16277C > T	p.T5426M	rs2306914 (0.0463)	C/T	39.1	C/C	-	C/T	41.07	B	T	P
	c. 12442G > C	p.D4148H	rs117501809 (0.0124)	G/G	-	G/C	49.15	G/C	28.57	PrD	D	P
TAF5L	c.721G > A	p.V241I	rs55655740 (0.0042)	G/A	36.0	G/G	-	G/A	48	B	-	DC
	c.1123A > G	p.T375A	rs41304137 (0.0008)	A/A	-	A/G	20	A/G	40	PrD	T	P
TTN	c.106619 T > C	p.I35540T	rs55880440 (0.0046)	T/C	40.0	T/T	-	T/C	57.69	-	-	P
	c.65147C > T	p.S21716L	rs13021201 (0.0108)	C/C	-	C/T	42.86	C/T	58.14	-	-	P

MAF Minor allele frequency, *PrD* Probably damaging, *B* Benign, *PD* Possibly damaging, *D* Damaging, *T* Tolerated, *DC* Disease causing, *P* Polymorphism. (*) low confidence prediction

array CGH (the gold standard for CNA screening) were above 98% (Fig. 2). Among the CNAs not detected in the WES analysis, two of them were mapped to regions not covered by the library probes and five were low-level mosaic alterations (Additional file 3: Table S2). Thus, if we consider CNAs mapping to WES target regions and non-mosaic CNAs, concordance rates were above 99.8%.

In total, 38 somatically acquired alterations, including point mutations (15) and CNAs (23), were detected. The small number of somatic alterations identified here is in agreement with what is expected for pediatric tumors [28]. Moreover, given the occurrence of the driver EWS-WT1 fusion protein, additional oncogenic mutations for tumor onset is probably less necessary.

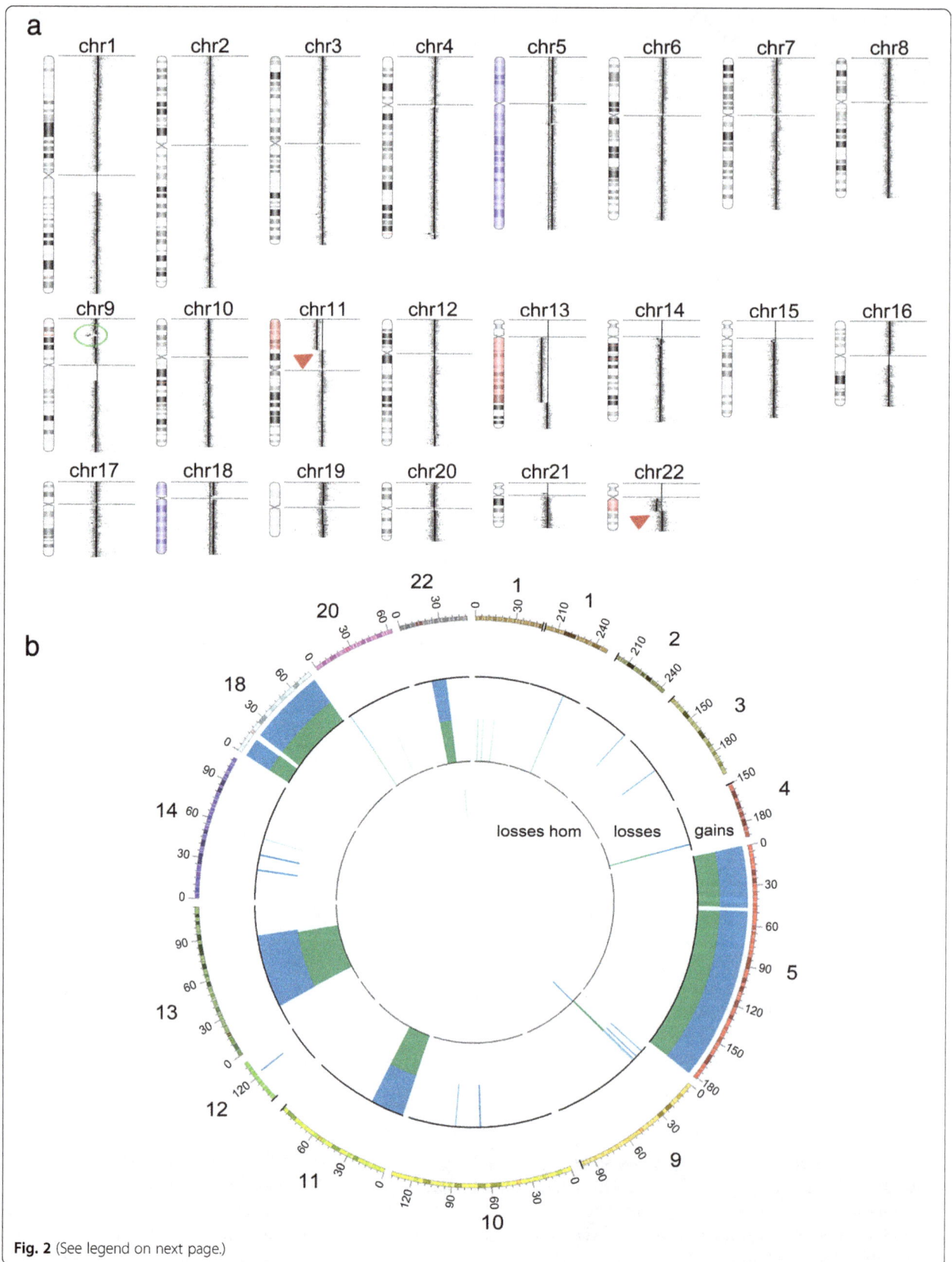

Fig. 2 (See legend on next page.)

(See figure on previous page.)

Fig. 2 Array CGH profile showing the pattern of somatic copy number alterations detected in the DSRCT genome. **a** Copy number alterations detected by array CGH analysis using a 180-K platform with an effective resolution of ~70 Kb: aneuploidy of chromosomes 5 and 18 (gains, *in blue*), and partial losses of chromosome 13q, 11p, and 22q (*in red*). The *green circle* indicates the focal deletion of a segment of 1.3 Mb at 9p24.1. *Arrows* indicate chromosome 11 and chromosome 22 breakpoints, 11p13 and 22q12.2, respectively. **b** *Circus* plot shows the copy number alterations detected by array CGH and WES. Only the genomic regions affected by CNA events are represented. The numbers on each chromosome region are described in megabases. In *blue*, data from array CGH and in *green* data from WES. A great overlap of CNA detection can be observed using both approaches

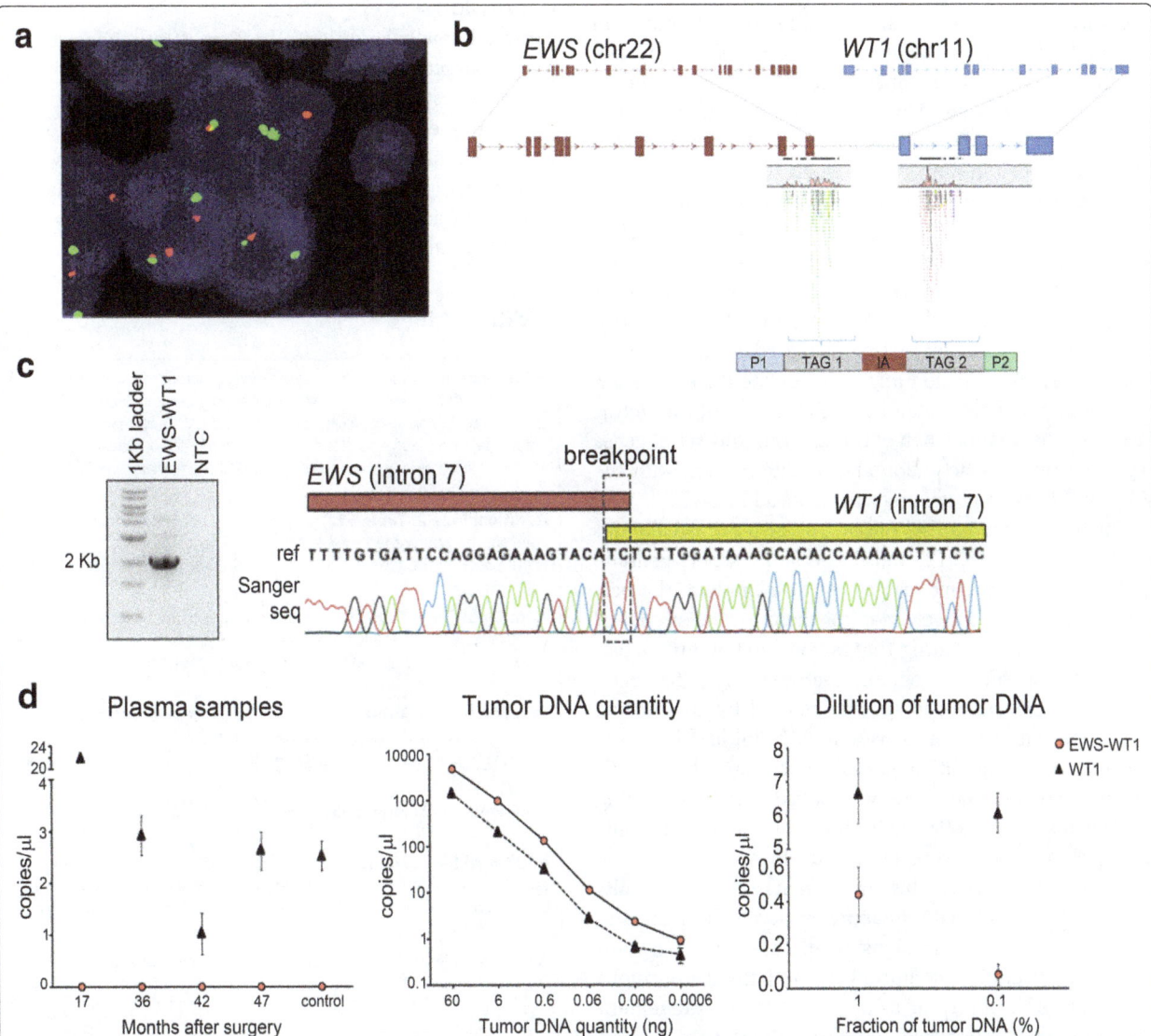

Fig. 3 Use of the chromosomal translocation t(11;22)(p13;q12) as a personalized tool for patient monitoring along follow-up. **a** FISH analysis shows break apart probes for *WT1* gene, indicating the occurrence of the fusion. **b** Mate-pair whole-genome sequencing detected paired reads mapping to *EWS* and *WT1* genes. **c** PCR amplification followed by Sanger sequencing confirmed the breakpoint region involving intronic regions of *EWS* and *WT1* genes. **d** Digital droplet PCR assays for detection of the somatic rearrangement EWS-WT1. *Left panel*—Screening of ctDNA from plasma samples collected serially along patient follow-up by ddPCR. No gene fusion was detected in ctDNA from the patient collected in four different time points after surgery, suggesting no relapse, recurrence, or progression of the disease. Presence of cell-free DNA is shown by detection of non-rearranged WT1 probes in the plasma samples from the patient and from control plasma sample. *Middle panel*—Serial dilutions of tumor DNA to check the sensibility of the approach in detecting the fusion event, starting from 60 ng of input following five dilution series of tenfold as indicated. *Right panel*—Detection of somatic rearrangement in different tumor DNA fractions, 1.0 and 0.1%

We identified 12 genes affected by somatic mutations possibly involved with the disease. These genes are involved with cellular development and morphology that are pathways in which *WT1* gene plays an important role. Similarly, the genes affected by compound heterozygous mutations showed enrichment in biological processes of muscle tissue development and morphogenesis. Altogether, these data suggests that disruption of the embryonic cellular development process is involved with DSRCT onset, which is commonly seen in pediatric tumors.

Another interesting finding is that among the set of somatically mutated genes, 8 showed to be mutated in desmoplastic melanoma samples from TCGA project [29, 30], in frequencies ranging from 5 to 25% of the 20 samples interrogated. This data suggests that mutation in these genes might be involved with the desmoplastic phenotype, seen in both tumor types.

Additionally, 7 out of 15 genes harboring somatic mutations (*CHL1, MEGF10, MEIS2, MYH8, RIMS4, TBPL1,* and *ZFPM2*) are regulated by the same transcription factor, LEF1 ($p < 0.001$ by enrichment analysis), which, in turn, is regulated by WT1 [31]. We therefore postulate that DSRCT tumors presenting increased activity of WT1 due to EWS-WT1 fusion might upregulate the expression of several genes mediated by LEF1 transcription factor. However, the accumulation of mutations in this set of genes regulated by LEF1 activation and its interrelation with the EWS-WT1 fusion protein remains to be addressed.

Finally, the definition of the precise genomic breakpoint of the t(11;22)(p13;q12) translocation by whole-genome and Sanger sequencing enabled the development of a personalized tool to precisely monitor the presence of ctDNA in plasma samples during the patient's follow-up. Detection of tumor-specific genomic rearrangements has been shown as a sensitive and specific method for monitoring of disease status of cancer patients [32–35] and has clear advantages over point mutations concerning the specificity of detection [33]. Here, we applied ctDNA screening in plasma samples collected in three clinical appointments during 3 years after surgery and, up to now, we did not detect the presence of this tumor marker. These results are in agreement with imaging exams (CT scan and PET scan) showing no signs of disease and also with good overall clinical condition of the patient and highlight the applicability of using genomic rearrangement for building personalized tool for patient surveillance. After defining the genomic breakpoint of EWS-WT1 fusion, DSRCT patients can benefit from a highly specific test that has the advantage of a rapid turnaround time and potentially higher sensitivity in detecting disease progression earlier than imaging exams or other cancer antigens measurements, as reported for other tumor types [36, 37]. Monitoring through liquid biopsy is particularly attractive for solid tumors, which cannot be repeatedly sampled without more invasive procedures. Considering the rarity of this subtype of sarcoma and the lack of effective treatment, the detection of specific tumor marker and the monitoring of its persistence can improve the identification of patients with worse prognosis to tailor the treatment more properly. Thus, the perspective is to employ the approach used here for new patients and improve the outcome for those with worse prognosis.

Conclusion

To our knowledge, this is the first comprehensive genomic characterization of one DSRCT case. Continuous efforts to establish the genomic landscape of rare diseases, frequently neglected in large sequencing consortiums, are highly significant to improve the knowledge of defective pathways involved with tumor onset in general, in addition to the strong potential of revealing druggable targets for clinical use.

Additional files

Additional file 1: Figure S1. Patient medical history and sample collection time points. Chemotherapy treatment marked in green consisted of 4 cycles of vincristine, cyclophosphamide, and doxorubicin (VAC) alternated with ifosfamide, carboplatin, and etoposide (ICE). Chemotherapy treatment marked in red consisted of hyperthermic intraperitoneal chemotherapy (HIPEC) with

Additional file 2: Table S1. Statistics of sequencing results. Sequence coverage by Comprehensive Cancer Panel (Thermo Scientific), Whole Exome Sequencing (Thermo Scientific) and Whole Genome Sequencing

Additional file 3: Table S2. Gene Ontology enriched categories of genes affected by somatic mutations. Biological processes with a p-value <0,001 was considered based on Webgestalt annotation tool [38, 39].

Additional file 4: Table S4. Gene Ontology-enriched categories of genes affected by compound heterozygous mutations. Biological processes with a *p* value <0.001 was considered based on WebGestalt anno-

Additional file 5: Figure S3. Copy Number Alterations detected by

Additional file 6: Figure S2. Screening of ctDNA in leukocyte samples. Pre-surgery sample collected at day of surgery. Post-surgery sample collected at 22 months after diagnosis (17 months after

Additional file 7: Description of the functional class of each molecule

Abbreviations

CGH: Comparative genomic hybridization; CNA: Copy number alterations; COSMIC: Catalogue of Somatic Mutations in Cancer; CT: Computed tomography; ctDNA: Circulating tumor DNA; ddPCR: Digital droplet PCR; DSRCT: Desmoplastic small round cell tumor; GATK: Genome Analysis Toolkit; HIPEC: Hyperthermic intraperitoneal chemotherapy; ICE: Ifosfamide, carboplatin, and etoposide; Indel: Small insertions and deletions; IPA: Ingenuity pathway analysis; MAF: Minor allele frequency; PET: Positron emission tomography; SNP: Simple nucleotide polymorphism; TCGA: The cancer genome atlas; VAC: Vincristine, cyclophosphamide, and doxorubicin; WES: Whole-exome sequencing

Acknowledgements
The authors thank the patient and his parents for their collaboration, the A.C. Camargo Cancer Center Biobank for providing the tumor sample, and Louise D. C. Mota for the technical support for plasma DNA collection and extraction.

Funding
This work was supported by São Paulo Research Foundation—FAPESP (2013/23277-8)—and by the National Council of Technological and Scientific Development—CNPq (483775/2012-6).

Authors' contributions
ENF, BDFB, and GTT carried out the sequencing experiments, and BDFB and SG performed the validation experiments. ENF performed and analyzed the ddPCR assays. ACVK performed and analyzed the CGH array experiments and revised the manuscript. JES and RVA conducted the bioinformatics analyses, and SJS supervised the bioinformatics analysis. CCF and AL were responsible for patient treatment and care. IWC, CP, and FAS supervised immunohistochemical reactions and performed the histopathological analyses. SJS and EDN contributed to the analysis of the results and revised the manuscript. DMC and ENF designed the study, analyzed the results, and wrote the initial manuscript. DMC conceived and supervised the study. All authors read and approved the final manuscript.

Competing interests
The authors declare that they have no competing interests.

Author details
[1]International Research Center/CIPE, A.C. Camargo Cancer Center, São Paulo, SP, Brazil. [2]Instituto Metrópole Digital, Federal University of Rio Grande do Norte, Natal, RN, Brazil. [3]Institute of Biosciences, University of São Paulo, São Paulo, SP, Brazil. [4]Departament of Abdominal Surgery, A.C. Camargo Cancer Center, São Paulo, SP, Brazil. [5]Department of Anatomic Pathology, A.C. Camargo Cancer Center, São Paulo, SP, Brazil. [6]Federal University of Rio Grande do Norte, Natal, RN, Brazil.

References
1. Lettieri CK, Garcia-Filion P, Hingorani P. Incidence and outcomes of desmoplastic small round cell tumor: results from the surveillance, epidemiology, and end results database. J Cancer Epidemiol. 2014;2014:680126.
2. Zhang S, Zhang Y, Yu YH, Li J. Results of multimodal treatment for desmoplastic small round cell tumor of the abdomen and pelvis. Int J Clin Exp Med. 2015;8:9658–66.
3. Liu J, Nau MM, Yeh JC, Allegra CJ, Chu E, Wright JJ. Molecular heterogeneity and function of EWS-WT1 fusion transcripts in desmoplastic small round cell tumors. Clin Cancer Res. 2000;6:3522–9.
4. Lee SB, Kolquist KA, Nichols K, Englert C, Maheswaran S, Ladanyi M, Gerald WL, Haber DA. The EWS-WT1 translocation product induces PDGFA in desmoplastic small round-cell tumour. Nat Genet. 1997;17:309–13.
5. Karnieli E, Werner H, Rauscher 3rd FJ, et al. The IGF-I receptor gene promoter is a molecular target for the Ewing's sarcoma-Wilms' tumor 1 fusion protein. J Biol Chem. 1996;271:19304–9.
6. Silva JG, Corrales-Medina FF, Maher OM, Tannir N, Huh WW, Rytting ME, Subbiah V. Clinical next generation sequencing of pediatric-type malignancies in adult patients identifies novel somatic aberrations. Oncoscience. 2015;2:187–92.
7. La Starza R, Barba G, Nofrini V, Pierini T, Pierini V, Marcomigni L, Perruccio K, Matteucci C, Storlazzi CT, Daniele G, Crescenzi B, Giansanti M, Giovenali P, Dal Cin P, Mecucci C. Multiple EWSR1-WT1 and WT1-EWSR1 copies in two cases of desmoplastic round cell tumor. Cancer Genet. 2013;206:387–92.
8. Shukla N, Ameur N, Yilmaz I, Nafa K, Lau CY, Marchetti A, Borsu L, Barr FG, Ladanyi M. Oncogene mutation profiling of pediatric solid tumors reveals significant subsets of embryonal rhabdomyosarcoma and neuroblastoma with mutated genes in growth signaling pathways. Clin Cancer Res. 2012;18:748–57.
9. Campos AH, Silva AA, Mota LD, Olivieri ER, Prescinoti VC, Patrão D, Camargo LP, Brentani H, Carraro DM, Brentani RR, Soares FA. The value of a tumor bank in the development of cancer research in Brazil: 13 years of experience at the A C Camargo hospital. Biopreserv Biobank. 2012;10:168–73.
10. Olivieri EH, Franco Lde A, Pereira RG, Mota LD, Campos AH, Carraro DM. Biobanking practice: RNA storage at low concentration affects integrity. Biopreserv Biobank. 2014;12:46–52.
11. Torrezan GT, da Silva FC, Santos EM, Krepischi AC, Achatz MI, Aguiar Jr S, Rossi BM, Carraro DM. Mutational spectrum of the APC and MUTYH genes and genotype-phenotype correlations in Brazilian FAP, AFAP, and MAP patients. Orphanet J Rare Dis. 2013;8:54.
12. Database of genomic variants. http://projects.tcag.ca/variation/.
13. McKenna A, et al. The genome analysis toolkit: a MapReduce framework for analyzing next-generation DNA sequencing data. Genome Res. 2012;20:1297–303.
14. Cingolani P, Platts A, le Wang L, Coon M, Nguyen T, Wang L, Land SJ, Lu X, Ruden DM. A program for annotating and predicting the effects of single nucleotide polymorphisms, SnpEff: SNPs in the genome of Drosophila melanogaster strain w1118; iso-2; iso-3. Fly (Austin). 2012;6:80–92.
15. Liu X, Jian X, Boerwinkle E. dbNSFP: a lightweight database of human non-synonymous SNPs and their functional predictions. Hum Mutat. 2011;32:894–9.
16. Liu X, Jian X, Boerwinkle E. dbNSFP v2.0: a database of human non-synonymous SNVs and their functional predictions and annotations. Hum Mutat. 2013;34:E2393–402.
17. Forbes SA, Bindal N, Bamford S, Cole C, Kok CY, Beare D, Jia M, Shepherd R, Leung K, Menzies A, Teague JW, Campbell PJ, Stratton MR, Futreal PA. COSMIC: mining complete cancer genomes in the catalogue of somatic mutations in cancer. Nucleic Acids Res. 2011;39:D945–50.
18. 1000 Genomes Project Consortium, Auton A, Brooks LD, Durbin RM, Garrison EP, Kang HM, Korbel JO, Marchini JL, McCarthy S, McVean GA, Abecasis GR. A global reference for human genetic variation. Nature. 2015;526:68–74.
19. Exome Variant Server, NHLBI GO Exome Sequencing Project (ESP), Seattle. http://evs.gs.washington.edu/EVS/. Version: ESP6500SI-V2.
20. International HapMap Consortium. The International HapMap Project. Nature. 2003;426:789–96.
21. Sherry ST, Ward MH, Kholodov M, Baker J, Phan L, Smigielski EM, Sirotkin K. dbSNP: the NCBI database of genetic variation. Nucleic Acids Res. 2001;29:308–11.
22. Database of Single Nucleotide Polymorphisms (dbSNP). Bethesda: National Center for Biotechnology Information, National Library of Medicine. (dbSNP Build ID: 138). Available from: http://www.ncbi.nlm.nih.gov/SNP/.
23. Magi A, Tattini L, Cifola I, et al. EXCAVATOR: detecting copy number variants from whole-exome sequencing data. Genome Biol. 2013;14:R120.
24. Klambauer G, Schwarzbauer K, Mayr A, Clevert DA, Mitterecker A, Bodenhofer U, Hochreiter S. cn.MOPS: mixture of Poissons for discovering copy number variations in next-generation sequencing data with a low false discovery rate. Nucleic Acids Res. 2012;40:e69.
25. Krzywinski M, Schein J, Birol I, Connors J, Gascoyne R, Horsman D, Jones SJ, Marra MA. Circos: an information aesthetic for comparative genomics. Genome Res. 2009;19:1639–45.
26. Zeitouni B, Boeva V, Janoueix-Lerosey I, Loeillet S, Legoix-ne P, Nicolas A, Delattre O, Barillot E. SVDetect: a tool to identify genomic structural variations from paired-end and mate-pair sequencing data. Bioinformatics. 2010;26:1895–6.
27. Taniguchi K, Uchida J, Nishino K, Kumagai T, Okuyama T, Okami J, Higashiyama M, Kodama K, Imamura F, Kato K. Quantitative detection of EGFR mutations in circulating tumor DNA derived from lung adenocarcinomas. Clin Cancer Res. 2011;17:7808–15.
28. Vogelstein B, Papadopoulos N, Velculescu VE, Zhou S, Diaz Jr LA, Kinzler KW. Cancer genome landscapes. Science. 2013;339:1546–58.

29. Gao J, Aksoy BA, Dogrusoz U, Dresdner G, Gross B, Sumer SO, Sun Y, Jacobsen A, Sinha R, Larsson E, Cerami E, Sander C, Schultz N. Integrative analysis of complex cancer genomics and clinical profiles using the cBioPortal. Sci Signal. 2013;6:l1.

30. Cerami E, Gao J, Dogrusoz U, Gross BE, Sumer SO, Aksoy BA, Jacobsen A, Byrne CJ, Heuer ML, Larsson E, Antipin Y, Reva B, Goldberg AP, Sander C, Schultz N. The cBio cancer genomics portal: an open platform for exploring multidimensional cancer genomics data. Cancer Discov. 2012;2:401–4.

31. Gao Y, Toska E, Denmon D, Roberts SG, Medler KF. WT1 regulates the development of the posterior taste field. Development. 2014;141:2271–8.

32. McBride DJ, Orpana AK, Sotiriou C, Joensuu H, Stephens PJ, Mudie LJ, Hämäläinen E, Stebbings LA, Andersson LC, Flanagan AM, Durbecq V, Ignatiadis M, Kallioniemi O, Heckman CA, Alitalo K, Edgren H, Futreal PA, Stratton MR, Campbell PJ. Use of cancer-specific genomic rearrangements to quantify disease burden in plasma from patients with solid tumors. Genes Chromosomes Cancer. 2010;49:1062–9.

33. Leary RJ, Sausen M, Kinde I, Papadopoulos N, Carpten JD, Craig D, O'Shaughnessy J, Kinzler KW, Parmigiani G, Vogelstein B, Diaz Jr LA, Velculescu VE. Detection of chromosomal alterations in the circulation of cancer patients with whole-genome sequencing. Sci Transl Med. 2012;4:162ra154.

34. Donnard ER, Carpinetti PA, Navarro FC, Perez RO, Habr-Gama A, Parmigiani RB, Camargo AA, Galante PA. ICRmax: an optimized approach to detect tumor-specific interchromosomal rearrangements for clinical application. Genomics. 2015;105:265–72.

35. Olsson E, Winter C, George A, Chen Y, Howlin J, Tang MH, Dahlgren M, Schulz R, Grabau D, van Westen D, Fernö M, Ingvar C, Rose C, Bendahl PO, Rydén L, Borg Å, Gruvberger-Saal SK, Jernström H, Saal LH. Serial monitoring of circulating tumor DNA in patients with primary breast cancer for detection of occult metastatic disease. EMBO Mol Med. 2015;7:1034–47.

36. Dawson SJ, Tsui DW, Murtaza M, Biggs H, Rueda OM, Chin SF, Dunning MJ, Gale D, Forshew T, Mahler-Araujo B, Rajan S, Humphray S, Becq J, Halsall D, Wallis M, Bentley D, Caldas C, Rosenfeld N. Analysis of circulating tumor DNA to monitor metastatic breast cancer. N Engl J Med. 2013;368:1199–209.

37. Pereira E, Camacho-Vanegas O, Anand S, Sebra R, Catalina Camacho S, Garnar-Wortzel L, Nair N, Moshier E, Wooten M, Uzilov A, Chen R, Prasad-Hayes M, Zakashansky K, Beddoe AM, Schadt E, Dottino P, Martignetti JA. Personalized circulating tumor DNA biomarkers dynamically predict treatment response and survival in gynecologic cancers. PLoS One. 2015;10:e0145754.

38. Zhang B, Kirov SA, Snoddy JR. WebGestalt: an integrated system for exploring gene sets in various biological contexts. Nucleic Acids Res. 2005;33:W741–8.

39. Wang J, Duncan D, Shi Z, Zhang B. WEB-based GEne SeT AnaLysis Toolkit (WebGestalt): update 2013. Nucleic Acids Res. 2013;41:W77–83.

7

Genome-scale portrait and evolutionary significance of human-specific core promoter tri- and tetranucleotide short tandem repeats

N. Nazaripanah[1], F. Adelirad[1], A. Delbari[1], R. Sahaf[1], T. Abbasi-Asl[2] and M. Ohadi[1*]

Abstract

Background: While there is an ongoing trend to identify single nucleotide substitutions (SNSs) that are linked to inter/intra-species differences and disease phenotypes, short tandem repeats (STRs)/microsatellites may be of equal (if not more) importance in the above processes. Genes that contain STRs in their promoters have higher expression divergence compared to genes with fixed or no STRs in the gene promoters. In line with the above, recent reports indicate a role of repetitive sequences in the rise of young transcription start sites (TSSs) in human evolution.

Results: Following a comparative genomics study of all human protein-coding genes annotated in the GeneCards database, here we provide a genome-scale portrait of human-specific short- and medium-size ($\geq$ 3-repeats) tri- and tetranucleotide STRs and STR motifs in the critical core promoter region between -120 and $+1$ to the TSS and evidence of skewing of this compartment in reference to the STRs that are not human-specific (Levene's test $p < 0.001$). Twenty-five percent and 26% enrichment of human-specific transcripts was detected in the tri and tetra human-specific compartments (mid-$p < 0.00002$ and mid-$p < 0.002$, respectively).

Conclusion: Our findings provide the first evidence of genome-scale skewing of STRs at a specific region of the human genome and a link between a number of these STRs and TSS selection/transcript specificity. The STRs and genes listed here may have a role in the evolution and development of characteristics and phenotypes that are unique to the human species.

Keywords: Short tandem repeat, Core promoter, Human-specific, Trinucleotide, Tetranucleotide

Introduction

Speciation and evolution are, at least in part, due to the plasticity (expansion or contraction) of short tandem repeats (STRs)/microsatellites, which can function as "tuning knobs" in response to the environment or other genes [1–3]. In line with the above, certain STRs are directionally expanded in the human species or co-occur identically in related taxa such as primates [4–8]. Genes that contain STRs in their promoters have higher expression divergence compared to genes with fixed or no

STRs in the gene promoters [9]. Recent reports indicate a role of repetitive sequences in the rise of young transcription start sites (TSSs) in human evolution [10–12].

Preliminary data on the sequencing of a number of "exceptionally long" STRs ($\geq$ 6-repeats), which compose 1–2% of all human core promoter STRs [3], support critical evolutionary adaptive roles for a number of these STRs. Human specificity of the predominant allele of the *RIT2* core promoter STR in the human species, the presence of the shortest allele of this STR (5-repeat) in hunter-gatherer humans (BUSHMAN KB1: rs113265205), the lack of this allele in the agricultural modern humans (Genome Aggregation database: gnomad.broadinstitute. org), and its co-occurrence with schizophrenia provide the

---

* Correspondence: mi.ohadi@uswr.ac.ir; ohadi.mina@yahoo.com
[1]Iranian Research Center on Aging, University of Social Welfare and Rehabilitation Sciences, Tehran, Iran
Full list of author information is available at the end of the article

first indication of STR allele selection in humans [13]. A link between the *CYTH4* core promoter STR (the longest tetranucleotide STR identified in a human gene core promoter) with the Old World monkeys and Apes and evidence of extreme "disease-only" genotypes at this STR with schizophrenia [14] provide the first link between a primate-specific STR and higher-order brain functions in human. The "exceptionally long" CA-repeat in the core promoter of *SCGB2B2* is another example of directional STR expansion in the Old World monkeys and Apes [5]. The *PAXBP1* gene is an extreme example in which expansion of a core promoter CT-repeat occurs in the Old World monkeys and reaches maximum length and complexity in human; OMIM: 617621 [4].

As "exceptionally long" STRs may be subject to natural selection, short- and medium-size alleles ($\geq$ 3-repeats) might have had similar fate. This is indicated by the predominance of specific short- and medium-size penta- and hexanucleotide STRs and their cognate transcription factors (TFs) in the critical core promoter interval [15]. Indeed, shortening of a number of STRs and their identical co-occurrence is linked to the evolution of primates [8]. In line with the above findings, repeats associated with younger human TSSs tend to be shorter than those in older TSSs [10]. In the study reported here, we present genome-scale data on two categories of STRs, i. e., tri- and tetranucleotide STRs, and their implication in human evolution.

Materials and methods

The interval between -120 and $+1$ to the TSS of all human protein-coding genes annotated in the GeneCards database (version 3.0) (www.genecards.org) was screened for tri- and tetranucleotide STRs of $\geq$ 3-repeats, based on the Ensembl database (versions 87-91) (asia.ensembl. org) and using the Microsatellite Repeats Finder at the following link: http://insilico.ehu.es/mini_tools/microsatellites/

The evolutionary status of the identified STRs was analyzed in 25 species (*N*), including primates (*N* = 5), non-primate mammals (*N* = 12), birds and reptiles (*N* = 5), amphibians (*N* = 1), and fish (*N* = 2), based on the Ensembl database.

Human specificity of transcripts was evaluated based on the multiple and pair-wise %identity scoring of the TSS-flanking 5′ untranslated region (UTR), using the sequence alignment program Clustal Omega (https://www. ebi.ac.uk/Tools/msa/clustalo), and the overall composition of the transcript and encoded protein (i.e., length of the transcript, number of exons and amino acids). The threshold of sequence identity was set at 50%, which was based on the comparison of two randomly selected and unrelated sequences in the human genome.

The *p* value for the skewing of the human-specific STR compartment was calculated using Levene's equality of variances test.

The *p* values for transcript enrichment were calculated using the two by two table analysis;

the human-specific tri- and tetranucleotide STR groups were compared against corresponding randomly selected STRs from the non-human-specific STRs. The comparison was set based on the sample size of the human-specific STRs (*n*) and the sample size of the non-human compartments (1.5n).

Results

Overall prevalence of tri- and tetranucleotide STR motifs across human protein-coding core promoter sequences

In total, 56 and 82 STR motifs were detected for the tri- and tetranucleotide repeats, respectively (Figs. 1 and 2). The most prevalent tri- and tetranucleotide STR motifs across the human protein-coding gene core promoters were GGC and GGGC, respectively (Figs. 1 and 2). In the category of non-GC STRs, GGA and TCCC were the most prevalent tri- and tetranucleotides, respectively.

Skewing of the human-specific core promoter tri- and tetranucleotide STRs

A significant skewing of the tri- and tetranucleotide STR distribution was found in the human-specific tri- (Fig. 1) and tetranucleotide (Fig. 2) compartments (Levene's $p < 0.001$). While the most prevalent tri- and tetranucleotide repeats in the non-human-specific category were the GGC- and GGGC-repeats, respectively, the most prevalent human-specific STRs were of the GCC and CTCC motifs, respectively. Disproportionate distribution of human-specific STRs was also detected in other STRs such as CCT, GAA, CTCC, GTTT, and GAAA.

The human-specific tri- and tetranucleotide STRs were of a wide range of motifs, e.g., the CCA motif in *ADCY6*, the TCCC motif in *ARHGEF35*, GCCC in *DRD2*, and GTTT in *MCTP2* (Tables 1 and 2).

In a number of instances, not only the STR, but also the genes containing those STRs, were human-specific (e.g., *ARHGEF35*, *AMY1C*, and *C1orf204*). Furthermore, a number of the tri- and tetranucleotide STRs were found to be unique to the human species at the specified interval of -120 to $+1$ TSS. For example, in the tetranucleotide compartment, CACC, GACA, CCGG, GATA, TCTG, GGCT, and TTTA STRs were detected in human only.

Enrichment of human-specific transcripts at the human-specific STR compartment

Based on sequence comparison and the overall composition of the transcript and encoded protein, 25

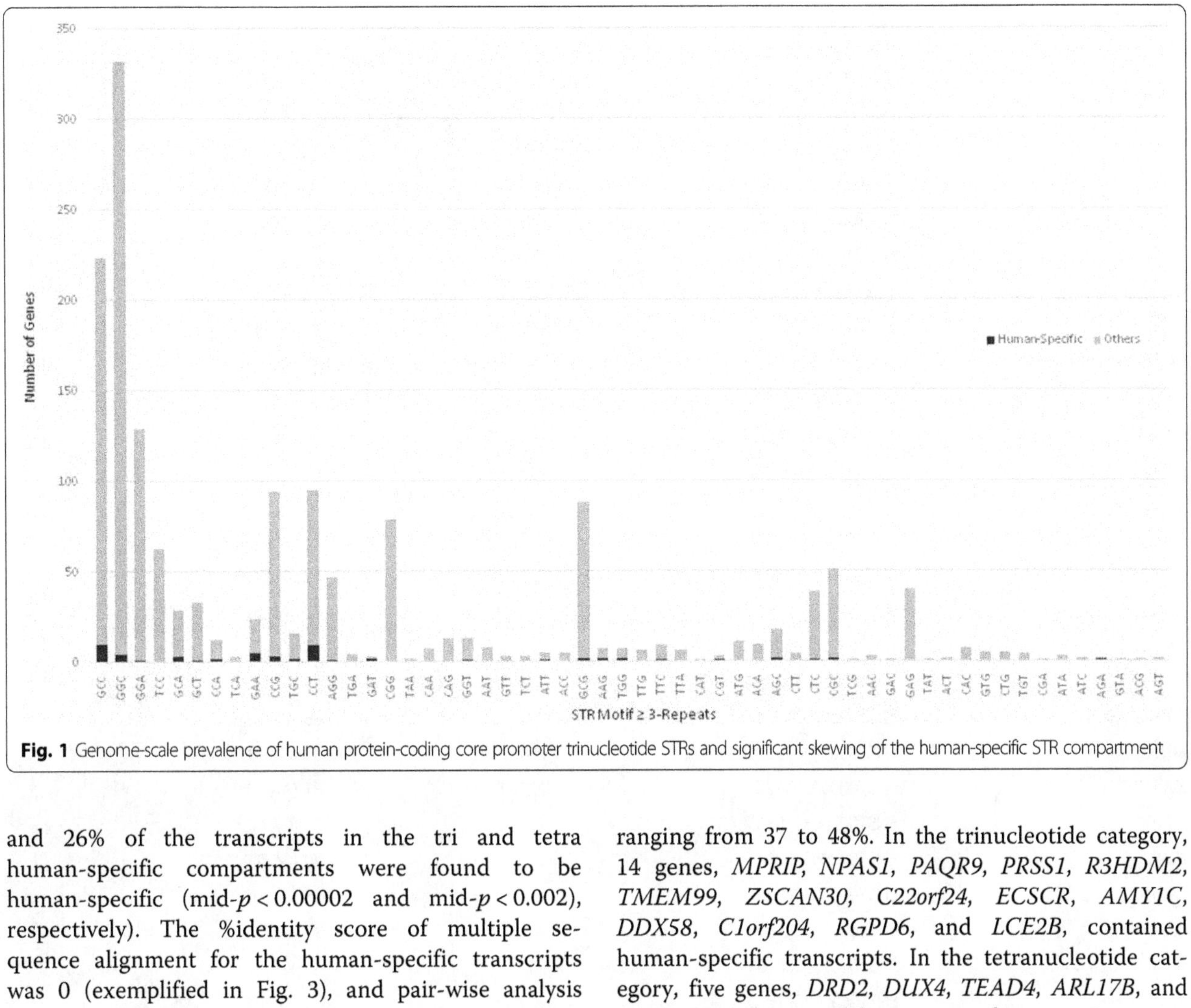

Fig. 1 Genome-scale prevalence of human protein-coding core promoter trinucleotide STRs and significant skewing of the human-specific STR compartment

and 26% of the transcripts in the tri and tetra human-specific compartments were found to be human-specific (mid-p < 0.00002 and mid-p < 0.002), respectively). The %identity score of multiple sequence alignment for the human-specific transcripts was 0 (exemplified in Fig. 3), and pair-wise analysis (exemplified in Fig. 4) resulted in %identity scores

ranging from 37 to 48%. In the trinucleotide category, 14 genes, *MPRIP*, *NPAS1*, *PAQR9*, *PRSS1*, *R3HDM2*, *TMEM99*, *ZSCAN30*, *C22orf24*, *ECSCR*, *AMY1C*, *DDX58*, *C1orf204*, *RGPD6*, and *LCE2B*, contained human-specific transcripts. In the tetranucleotide category, five genes, *DRD2*, *DUX4*, *TEAD4*, *ARL17B*, and *ARHGEF35*, contained human-specific transcripts.

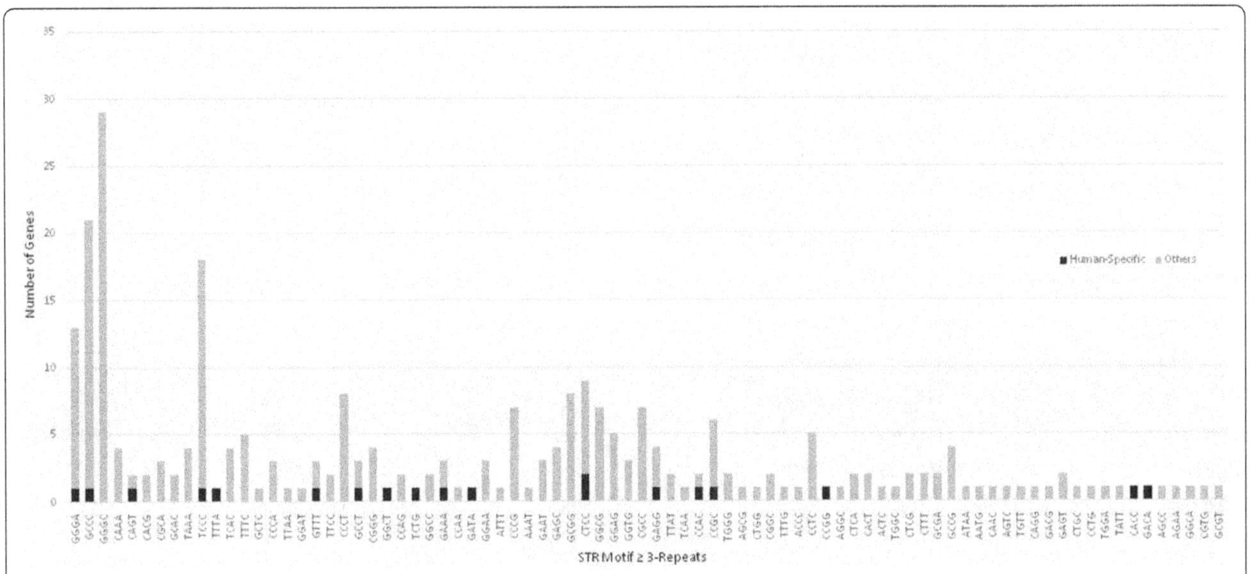

Fig. 2 Genome-scale prevalence of human protein-coding core promoter tetranucleotide STRs and significant skewing of the human-specific STR compartment

Table 1 Genome-scale human-specific core promoter trinucleotide STRs

Human gene symbol	Ensembl transcript ID	Variant no.	STR formula	
ADCY6	ENST00000307885.4	201	− 48 (CCA)3	
AMY1C	ENST00000370079.3	201	− 79 (ATT)3	
APBB1	ENST00000311051.7	202	− 11 (GCC)3	
BRINP2 (FAM5B)	ENST00000361539.4	201	− 26 (GGC)5	
BVES	ENST00000446408.2	203	− 35 (CCT)3	
CCDC178 (C18orf34)	ENST00000300227.12	201	− 79 (AGC)3	− 57 (CGC)5
CDH4	ENST00000543233.2	201	− 31 (CCT)3	
CIAPIN1	ENST00000563341.1	202	− 39 (CCT)3	
CNTNAP2	ENST00000361727.7	201	− 98 (TGC)3	
CST4	ENST00000217423.3	201	− 83 (GGA)3	
CYP4A11	ENST00000310638.8	201	− 86 (CCT)3	
C1orf204	ENST00000368102.5	201	− 11 (AAG)3	
C22orf24	NM_015372.2.1		− 98 (GCA)3	
C3AR1	ENST00000546241.1	202	− 70 (AGA)3	
DDX58	ENST00000379868.5	201	− 33 (CCT)3	
ECSCR	NM_001077693.3.1		− 121 (CCA)3	
GRIN2D	ENST00000263269.3	201	− 67 (GCC)3	
GSDMB	ENST00000394175.6	203	− 55 (GGC)3	
INPP4B	ENST00000503927.5	202	− 88 (CGC)3	
KBTBD12	ENST00000407609.7	204	− 57 (CCT)3	
KIAA1211	ENST00000504228.5	203	− 81 (AAG)3	
KRAS	ENST00000311936.7	202	− 89 (GAA)3	
KTN1	ENST00000395308.5	202	− 70 (GCG)9	
LACTBL1	ENST00000426928.6	201	− 58 (GAA)3	
LCE2B	ENST00000368780.3	201	− 79 (CCT)3	
LCOR (C10orf12)	ENST00000356016.7	202	− 97 (CCT)3	− 108 (GCC)3
MPRIP	ENST00000466186.2	209	− 88 (GCA)11	
MSANTD3 (C9orf30)	ENST00000374885.5	201	− 25 (GCC)7	
NPAS1	ENST00000439365.6	201	− 135 (GAA)9	
OR4X1	ENST00000320048.1	201	− 100 (GAT)3	
PABPC1L2B	ENST00000373521.3	201	− 60 (GCC)3	
PAQR9	ENST00000498470.1	203	− 29 (TGC)3	
PRSS1	ENST00000492062.1	205	− 96 (GAT)3	
RGPD6	ENST00000455695.1	205	− 70 (GGC)5	
RNF215	ENST00000215798.10	201	− 123 (GCT)5	
R3HDM2	ENST00000448732.1	208	− 27 (GCC)3	
SCN3B	ENST00000299333.7	201	− 29 (GGT)3	
SERPINB9	ENST00000380698.4	201	− 12 (GCA)3	
SIGLEC7	ENST00000305628.7	201	− 80 (TTC)3	
SPATC1L (C21orf56)	ENST00000330205.10	202	− 37 (TGG)4	−90 (TGG)4
STUB1	ENST00000219548.8	201	− 91 (GCC)3	
SUMF1	ENST00000272902.9	201	− 102 (AGC)3	
TEX12	ENST00000280358.4	201	− 105 (TGG)3	

Table 1 Genome-scale human-specific core promoter trinucleotide STRs *(Continued)*

Human gene symbol	Ensembl transcript ID	Variant no.	STR formula	
TMEM99	ENST00000301665.7	201	− 32 (CCG)3	− 47 (CCG)3
			− 59 (CCG)3	− 83 (CCG)3
			− 110 (CCG)3	− 125 (CCG)3
			− 48 (GCC)3	− 60 (GCC)3
			− 84 (GCC)3	− 126 (GCC)3
TNNC2	ENST00000372557.1	202	− 53 (GCC)3	
TPTE	ENST00000427445.6	201	− 110 (GCG)3	
TRBJ2-7	ENST00000390419.1	201	− 120 (GGC)3	
TRGV5	NC_000007.14:TRGV5:u_t_1.1		− 48 (CTC)3	
TRIM39	ENST00000376656.8	201	− 58 (CCT)4	
UAP1	ENST00000367926.8	204	− 9 (CGT)3	
VNN2	ENST00000326499.10	201	− 31 (GAA)10	
WRN	NM_000553.4.1		− 67 (GCC)3	− 92 (GCC)3
			− 69 (CCG)4	
WRNIP1	ENST00000618555.4	205	− 67 (CCG)3	
ZDHHC21	XM_006716760.1.1		− 32 (AGG)3	
ZSCAN30	ENST00000639929.1	212	− 57 (GAA)3	

The numbers before the brackets represent the start site of the STR in respect of the corresponding transcription start site. "Variant no" corresponds to the Ensembl isoform number

Table 2 Genome-scale human-specific core promoter tetranucleotide STRs

Human gene symbol	Ensembl transcript ID	Variant no.	STR formula
ARHGAP5	ENST00000345122.7	202	− 110 (GGGA)4
ARHGEF35	ENST00000378115.2	201	− 22 (TCCC)3
ARL17B	ENST00000622877.4	201	− 99 (CTCC)3
ATP7A	ENST00000343533.9	201	− 27 (GAGG)3
DRD2	ENST00000542616.1	207	− 54 (GCCC)3
DUX4	ENST00000565211.1	203	− 144 (GGCT)6
FAM83G	ENST00000388995.10	202	− 80 (TCTG)3
GTF2IRD2B	ENST00000614064.4	206	− 17 (GAAA)3
JCAD (KIAA1462)	ENST00000375377.1	201	− 13 (CCGG)3
MCTP2	ENST00000451018.7	203	− 102 (GTTT)3
METTL21C (C13orf39)	ENST00000267273.6	201	− 69 (CAGT)3
OR10G6	ENST00000307002.3	201	− 123 (GATA)13
PHYHD1	ENST00000308941.9	201	− 107 (TTTA)3
SAMD1	ENST00000269724.5	201	− 75 (CCGC)3
TEAD4	ENST00000540314.1	206	− 51 (CTCC)3
TRAJ49	ENST00000390488.1	201	− 124 (GCCT)7
TRDJ2	ENST00000390475.1	201	− 86 (CCAC)3
TRAV38-1	ENST00000390464.2	201	− 109 (CACC)3
TRAV7	ENST00000390429.3	201	− 111 (GACA)3

The numbers before the brackets represent the start site of the STR in respect of the corresponding transcription start site. "Variant no" corresponds to the Ensembl isoform number

a

NPAS1

```
Prairie      ------------------CACCTGCGACTCCTTCGCGCCTGAAT------------TCTC
Dog          -------------------CGGAGACCTGGGTTCCTGGCCTTGAGGGAGGGCAGCTC
Opossum      ------------------------CTCCTGGGTTCCTG--------------------
Zebrafish    ---CT---------CTTTTACTCTGTGTGCTAATCAGCATT------T---------GA
Human        --AATGGGAGTCATGGCAGCCATGGTGGTCAG--------------------------
Gorilla      -GTCTCCAAGTCTGCGAGGCCGAGGTGG-----GCGCCGAG-------A---------GC
Mouse        GGTCTCAAAGTCTGCGAGGCCGCCGTGG-----GCGCCGAG-------A---------GC
Macaque      --TCTCCAAGTCTGCGAGGCCGAGGTGG-----GCGCCGAG-------A---------GC
Chimpanzee   ----------GGGCGGAGACGCGGCGGGGCGGGGCTCCGGC-------A---------GA
Horse        ----------------------------------------------------------
```

b

DRD2

```
Mouse        -ACGGCTGCCGGAGGGGC------GGCCGTGC----GTGGA-----TGCGGCGGGAGCTG
Anole        GCCGGCTCT-----TGGCGCTTCATGCCAC--TAACTCCTCCA----CCTGCGTGACCTC
Armadillo    ----------------------------------------------CCTCCGTGGGGGCAG
Zebrafish    CGCTG--------CGCCTGG-CATACAGTACGCGCTCCTCTGCTCAC-----------
Chicken      ----------CCGGTGCTGAATCCGCCGC--TCGCTCCGCAGCC--CCGGGG----CGG
Human        -ACTGCTCCCCGCGGGCCAGAGCCGGCCG------AGCTGCTGCCCGCCGGGG----CTC
Dog          ---------CGAAAGCCTCGAGCAGCCGGC--CGCCGTCTCTGCC--CCCGGG----CGC
Bushbaby     -------------CTGG-CCGCCCCG--TGGCTCCGCCGGCC---CCG----------
Gibbon       ----------AGAGCTGGG-CCACCCAG--TGGCTCCACCGCC--CCG----------
Rabbit       ------------AGCCTGG-CCATCCAG--TGGCCCCGCCGCC--CCG----------
```

DDX58

```
Gorilla      -----------------------GCACTTTCGATTTTCCCTTTAGTTATTAAAGTTCCTATGC
Mouse        ----------------------GGCAGTTTCGATTTCCTATGGC--CA--GC--CGGCTAGGC
Human        --------ACAGCCTGCGGGG--AACGTAGCTAGCTGCAAGC--AGAGGC--CGG------
Chimpanzee   --------CTCCAGCTTGGGCAACATAGTGAGAC-----------TC--CGT-----
Prairie      ---------GAACTGTGCGGACTTTA-TAATACAAAC--GC----------------
Horse        GGCTTTAAAGGCAGCGGGGTGCGGGTGAG----------GC--TGGGAC--TCG------
Guinea Pig   -GC---CACCGCGGCCAGTTGCCAGTTTCGGTTTCTCC--TC--TGT------AG------
Rabbit       -----------ATGAAGTGCAGTA-------TATTCAGGC--TGAGAA--AAA------
```

TEAD4

```
Mouse        ---------------------------------------------------GCGAGGCGCGCCCCAC
Human        ---ATTCCAGCGTCCTCCTCGCACACTCGAGGCCAGGGG-GCGGGA-GGGCC-GCAGCTC
Dog          ACAGGTCCAACGGGCGCTCCTC-CAAGCGGAGCCTTGG------AGGGCAA--------
Bushbaby     ----------GTTGGAGCG--CCGGCGGGACTCCTTGGAACTGGCGTAGAG-CACCCAC
Xenopus      -----------GAGCAGAGCTT-TCAGG-AAGCCT---------------
Flycatcher   -----------------CGAATCCTC-----TGTAGTAGCA-GT-----
Chicken      ---------------------AT------TAGATGGGAG-TCCCCTC
Armadillo    -----------------CTC-CCCGCGGGGCCGG-----TGGCGGGGCC-GCCACTC
Gibbon       -------------CAGAGAGA-TCGTCGCGGCCGG------AAGAGTTGGC-GC---T-
Zebrafish    -----------------------TTGGC--------------ATGGA-GC--T-
```

Fig. 3 Multiple sequence alignment of the TSS-flanking 5'UTRs. Examples of ClustAl Omega sequence alignment are represented in the tri- (**a**) and tetranucleotide (**b**) categories. Species inclusion was based on the information available in the Ensembl database

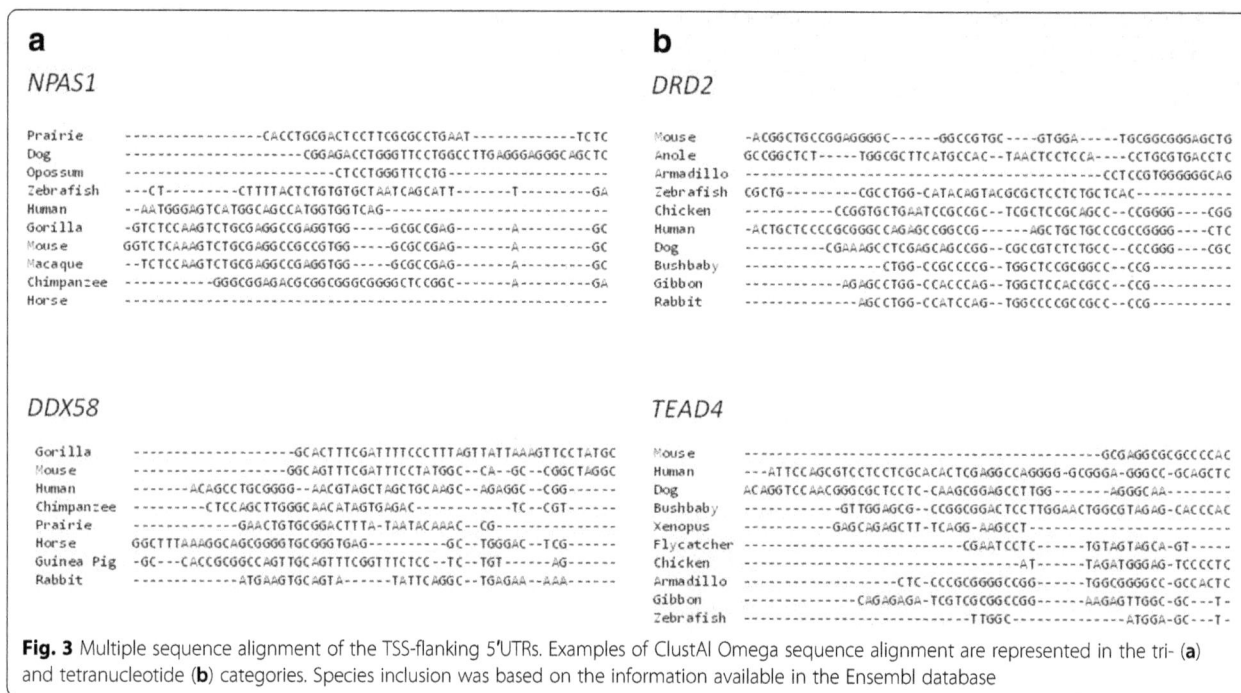

A number of the identified STRs were linked to non-canonical translation in the following genes, *TEAD4*, *ECSCR*, *MPRIP*, *PAQR9*, *PRSS1*, and *ZSCAN30*.

Discussion

There is an ever-growing literature on the biological and pathological implications of STRs at the inter- and intraspecies levels [16–27]. The STRs listed in the present study are genetic codes that are unique to humans and are likely to be responsible for the human-specific regulation of the relevant genes. The significant enrichment of human-specific transcripts at the human-specific STR compartment indicates a link to a mechanism for TSS selection and transcript specificity.

A number of the identified STRs such as GTTT have established repressor activity [6, 28, 29] and are differentially expanded in certain genes in the Old World

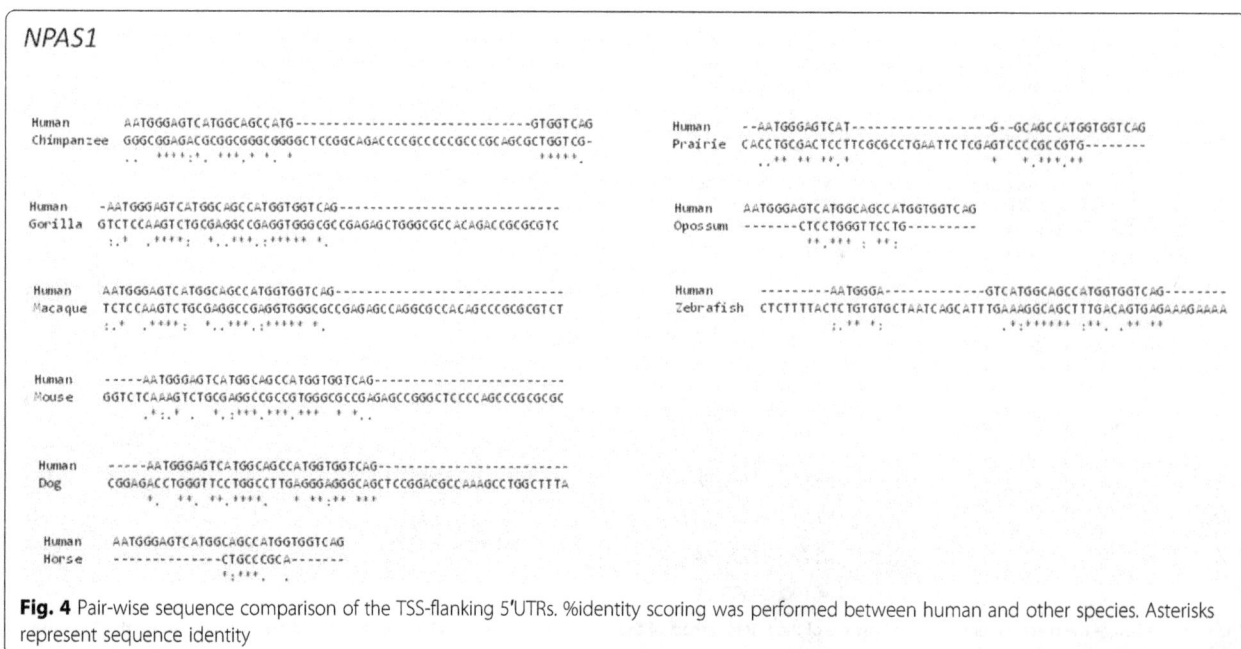

NPAS1

```
Human       AATGGGAGTCATGGCAGCCATG------------------------------GTGGTCAG
Chimpanzee  GGGCGGAGACGCGGCGGGCGGGGCTCCGGCAGACCCCGCCCCCGCCCGCAGCGCTGGTCG-
             ..  ****:*. ***.*.*   *                           *****.

Human       -AATGGGAGTCATGGCAGC-CATGGTGGTCAG-----------------------
Gorilla     GTCTCCAAGTCTGCGAGGCCGAGGTGGGCGCCGAGAGCTGGGCGCCACAGACCGCGCGTC
             :.* ,****:  *.,***.;****** *,

Human       AATGGGAGTCATGGCAGCCATGGTGGTCAG------------------------
Macaque     TCTCCAAGTCTGCGAGGCCGAGGTGGGCGCCGAGAGCCAGGCGCCACAGCCCGCGCGTCT
             :.*  ****:  *,.***,;***** *,

Human       -----AATGGGAGTCATGGCAGCCATGGTGGTCAG--------------------
Mouse       GGTCTCAAAGTCTGCGAGGCCGCCGTGGGCGCCGAGAGCCGGGCTCCCCAGCCCGCGCGC
             .*;.*. *,;***.***.*** *.,

Human       -----AATGGGAGTCATGGCAGCCATGGTGGTCAG--------------------
Dog         CGGAGACCTGGGTTCCTGGCCTTGAGGGAGGGCAGCTCCGGACGCCAAAGCCTGGCTTTA
             *,. **.**.****,   *.**:** ***

Human       AATGGGAGTCATGGCAGCCATGGTGGTCAG
Horse       -------------CTGCCCGCA-------
             *;:***,.
```

```
Human       --AATGGGAGTCAT-----------------G--GCAGCCATGGTGGTCAG
Prairie     CACCTGCGACTCCTTCGCGCCTGAATTCTCGAGTCCCCGCCGTG--------
             ,** ** **,*      *  *,***,**

Human       AATGGGAGTCATGGCAGCCATGGTGGTCAG
Opossum     -------CTCCTGGGTTCCTG--------
             **,***  : **;

Human       ---------AATGGGA-------------GTCATGGCAGCCATGGTGGTCAG-------
Zebrafish   CTCTTTTACTCTGTGTGCTAATCAGCATTTGAAAGGCAGCTTTGACAGTGAGAAAGAAAA
             ;.**,*;      .*;*****,;**.,** **
```

Fig. 4 Pair-wise sequence comparison of the TSS-flanking 5'UTRs. %identity scoring was performed between human and other species. Asterisks represent sequence identity

monkeys and Apes [14]. Purine STRs such as GAAA repeats are also functional in gene expression regulation, and their link to certain diseases unique to humans were previously reported [30, 31]. While the CG-rich STRs (e. g., CCG, GGGC) are subject to DNA methylation and can repress gene expression activity [32], they can also form G4 quadruplex structures, which have significant functions in gene expression regulation [33]. Several other identified STRs can form G4 structures with high overlap fraction (e.g., AGGG/CCCT, GCCC/GGGC).

It is not possible to estimate the number of crucial events that have led to the emergence of the human species. However, only a few genetic changes are needed to spur the evolution of new species in general, exemplified by the highly restricted initial divergence in butterfly hybridization models [34]. Accelerated evolution of a number of the identified genes in the present study (e.g., *DRD2*) has a well-established role in the origin of *Homo sapiens* [35]. Remarkably, a human-specific 7-amino acid transcript of this gene is flanked by a human-specific GCCC-repeat. Human-specific transcripts are increasingly recognized of having a role in the pathogenesis of diseases unique to the human species, such as schizophrenia [25, 36].

In a number of instances, not only the STR and the transcript, but also the gene containing these STRs and transcripts, were unique to humans, e.g., *AMY1C*, which is indicated in the evolution of the human phenotype during the Pleistocene [37].

For a number of the identified genes, sparse literature is available on the relevant function and pathways (e.g., *ARHGEF35*, *CXorf40A*, *C22orf24*, *TMEM99*, and *ARL17B*).

In a number of the identified genes, the STRs were linked to noncanonical (non-AUG) translation. Although the significance of this compartment is unknown for the most part, recent emerging data indicates likely biological functions [38].

The plasticity of STRs confers them unique ability to respond to adaptive evolutionary processes in a more efficient way than the quaternary codes provided by the SNSs. This potential aspect of STRs is vastly unknown at present, and it is expected that identification of STRs that have evolved differentially in humans vs. other species may pave the way for better understanding of the evolutionary implication of these highly mutable motifs.

This study warrants expansion to other vitally important gene regulatory sequences such as the distal promoter, 5′UTR, and 3′UTR. It is also necessary to sequence these STRs in characteristics and diseases that are unique to the human species. The recent reports of mass STR analysis using CRISPR/Cas9 [39] make it particularly more feasible to investigate STRs in the context of human evolution.

Conclusion

Our findings provide the first evidence of genome-scale skewing of STRs at a specific region of the human genome, and support a link between STRs and TSS selection/transcript specificity. The genes and STRs listed here may have a role in the divergence of humans from other species through the development of characteristics and phenotypes that are unique to the human species.

Abbreviations

SNS: Single nucleotide substitution; STR: Short tandem repeat; TF: Transcription factor; TSS: Transcription start site; UTR: Untranslated region

Funding

This research was funded by the University of Social Welfare and Rehabilitation Sciences, Tehran, Iran.

Authors' contributions

NN, FA, and TAA carried out the bioinformatics studies. AD and RS were the advisors of the project and helped in coordination. MO conceived the study, designed the project, supervised the analysis and wrote the manuscript. All authors read and approved the final manuscript.

Competing interests

The authors declare that they have no competing interests.

Author details

[1]Iranian Research Center on Aging, University of Social Welfare and Rehabilitation Sciences, Tehran, Iran. [2]Department of Biostatistics, University of Social Welfare and Rehabilitation Sciences, Tehran, Iran.

References

1. Press MO, Carlson KD, Queitsch C. The overdue promise of short tandem repeat variation for heritability. Trends Genet. 2014;30(11):504–12.
2. King DG. Evolution of simple sequence repeats as mutable sites. Adv Exp Med Biol. 2012;769:10-25.
3. Ohadi M, Mohammadparast S, Darvish H. Evolutionary trend of exceptionally long human core promoter short tandem repeats. Gene. 2012; 507(1):61–7.
4. Mohammadparast S, Bayat H, Biglarian A, Ohadi M. Exceptional expansion and conservation of a CT-repeat complex in the core promoter of PAXBP1 in primates. Am J Primatol. 2014;76(8):747–56.
5. Nikkhah M, Rezazadeh M, Khorshid HK, Biglarian A, Ohadi M. An exceptionally long CA-repeat in the core promoter of SCGB2B2 links with the evolution of apes and Old World monkeys. Gene. 2016;576(1):109–14.
6. Rezazadeh M, Gharesouran J, Mirabzadeh A, Khorshid HK, Biglarian A, Ohadi M. A primate-specific functional GTTT-repeat in the core promoter of CYTH4 is linked to bipolar disorder in human. Prog Neuro-Psychopharmacol Biol Psychiatry. 2015;56:161–7.

7. Namdar-Aligoodarzi P, Mohammadparast S, Zaker-Kandjani B, Kakroodi ST, Vesiehsari MJ, Ohadi M. Exceptionally long 5′ UTR short tandem repeats specifically linked to primates. Gene. 2015;569(1):88–94.

8. Ohadi M, Valipour E, Ghadimi-Haddadan S, Namdar-Aligoodarzi P, Bagheri A, Kowsari A, et al. Core promoter short tandem repeats as evolutionary switch codes for primate speciation. Am J Primatol. 2015;77(1):34–43.

9. Sonay TB, Carvalho T, Robinson MD, Greminger MP, Krützen M, Comas D, et al. Tandem repeat variation in human and great ape populations and its impact on gene expression divergence. Genome Res. 2015;25(11):1591–9.

10. Li C, Lenhard B, Luscombe NM. Integrated analysis sheds light on evolutionary trajectories of young transcription start sites in the human genome. bioRxiv. 2017. https://doi.org/10.1101/192757.

11. Kramer M, Sponholz C, Slaba M, Wissuwa B, Claus RA, Menzel U, et al. Alternative 5′untranslated regions are involved in expression regulation of human heme oxygenase-1. PLoS One. 2013;8(10):e77224.

12. Li Y, Seidel K, Marschall P, Klein M, Hope A, Schacherl J, et al. A polymorphic microsatellite repeat within the ECE-1c promoter is involved in transcriptional start site determination, human evolution, and Alzheimer's disease. J Neurosci. 2012;32(47):16807–20.

13. Emamalizadeh B, Movafagh A, Darvish H, Kazeminasab S, Andarva M, Namdar-Aligoodarzi P, et al. The human RIT2 core promoter short tandem repeat predominant allele is species-specific in length: a selective advantage for human evolution? Mol Gen Genomics. 2017;292(3):611–7.

14. Khademi E, Alehabib E, Shandiz EE, Ahmadifard A, Andarva M, Jamshidi J, et al. Support for "disease-only" genotypes and excess of homozygosity at the CYTH4 primate-specific GTTT-repeat in schizophrenia. Genet Test Mol Biomarkers. 2017;21(8):485–90.

15. Bushehri A, Barez MM, Mansouri S, Biglarian A, Ohadi M. Genome-wide identification of human and primate-specific core promoter short tandem repeats. Gene. 2016;587(1):83–90.

16. Valipour E, Kowsari A, Bayat H, Banan M, Kazeminasab S, Mohammadparast S, et al. Polymorphic core promoter GA-repeats alter gene expression of the early embryonic developmental genes. Gene. 2013;531(2):175–9.

17. Heidari A, Fam ZNS, Esmaeilzadeh-Gharehdaghi E, Banan M, Hosseinkhani S, Mohammadparast S, et al. Core promoter STRs: novel mechanism for inter-individual variation in gene expression in humans. Gene. 2012;492(1):195–8.

18. Bagshaw AT. Functional mechanisms of microsatellite DNA in eukaryotic genomes. Genome Biol Evol. 2017;9(9):2428–43.

19. Bagshaw AT, Horwood LJ, Fergusson DM, Gemmell NJ, Kennedy MA. Microsatellite polymorphisms associated with human behavioural and psychological phenotypes including a gene-environment interaction. BMC Med Genet. 2017;18(1):12.

20. Gymrek M, Willems T, Guilmatre A, Zeng H, Markus B, Georgiev S, et al. Abundant contribution of short tandem repeats to gene expression variation in humans. Nat Genet. 2016;48(1):22–9.

21. Hammock EA, Young LJ. Microsatellite instability generates diversity in brain and sociobehavioral traits. Science. 2005;308(5728):1630–4.

22. Carrat GR, Hu M, Nguyen-Tu M-S, Chabosseau P, Gaulton KJ, van de Bunt M, et al. Decreased STARD10 expression is associated with defective insulin secretion in humans and mice. Am J Hum Genet. 2017;100(2):238–56.

23. Abe H, Gemmell NJ. Evolutionary footprints of short tandem repeats in avian promoters. Sci Rep. 2016;6:19421.

24. Fondon JW, Hammock EA, Hannan AJ, King DG. Simple sequence repeats: genetic modulators of brain function and behavior. Trends Neurosci. 2008; 31(7):328–34.

25. Alizadeh F, Bozorgmehr A, Tavakkoly-Bazzaz J, Ohadi M. Skewing of the genetic architecture at the ZMYM3 human-specific 5′ UTR short tandem repeat in schizophrenia. Mol Gen Genomics. 2018; https://doi.org/10.1007/s00438-018-1415-8.

26. Hannan AJ. Tandem repeats mediating genetic plasticity in health and disease. Nat Rev Genet. 2018; https://doi.org/10.1038/nrg.2017.115.

27. Watts PC, Kallio ER, Koskela E, Lonn E, Mappes T, Mokkonen M. Stabilizing selection on microsatellite allele length at arginine vasopressin 1a receptor and oxytocin receptor loci. Proc Biol Sci. 2017;284(1869):20171896. https://doi.org/10.1098/rspb.2017.1896.

28. Andrioli LPM, Vasisht V, Theodosopoulou E, Oberstein A, Small S. Anterior repression of a Drosophila stripe enhancer requires three position-specific mechanisms. Development. 2002;129(21):4931–40.

29. Andrioli LP, Oberstein AL, Corado MS, Yu D, Small S. Groucho-dependent repression by sloppy-paired 1 differentially positions anterior pair-rule stripes in the Drosophila embryo. Dev Biol. 2004;276(2):541–51.

30. Darvish H, Heidari A, Hosseinkhani S, Movafagh A, Khaligh A, Jamshidi J, et al. Biased homozygous haplotypes across the human caveolin 1 upstream purine complex in Parkinson's disease. J Mol Neurosci. 2013;51(2):389–93.

31. Heidari A, Hosseinkhani S, Talebi S, Meshkani R, Esmaeilzadeh-Gharedaghi E, Banan M, et al. Haplotypes across the human caveolin 1 gene upstream purine complex significantly alter gene expression: implication in neurodegenerative disorders. Gene. 2012;505(1):186–9.

32. Quilez J, Guilmatre A, Garg P, Highnam G, Gymrek M, Erlich Y, et al. Polymorphic tandem repeats within gene promoters act as modifiers of gene expression and DNA methylation in humans. Nucleic Acids Res. 2016; 44(8):3750–62.

33. Sawaya S, Bagshaw A, Buschiazzo E, Kumar P, Chowdhury S, Black MA, et al. Microsatellite tandem repeats are abundant in human promoters and are associated with regulatory elements. PLoS One. 2013;8(2):e54710.

34. Kronforst MR, Hansen ME, Crawford NG, Gallant JR, Zhang W, Kulathinal RJ, et al. Hybridization reveals the evolving genomic architecture of speciation. Cell Rep. 2013;5(3):666–77.

35. Dorus S, Vallender EJ, Evans PD, Anderson JR, Gilbert SL, Mahowald M, et al. Accelerated evolution of nervous system genes in the origin of Homo sapiens. Cell. 2004;119(7):1027–40.

36. Li M, Jaffe AE, Straub RE, Tao R, Shin JH, Wang Y, et al. A human-specific AS3MT isoform and BORCS7 are molecular risk factors in the 10q24. 32 schizophrenia-associated locus. Nat Med. 2016;22(6):649–56.

37. Hardy K, Brand-Miller J, Brown KD, Thomas MG, Copeland L. The importance of dietary carbohydrate in human evolution. Q Rev Biol. 2015;90(3):251–68.

38. Na CH, Barbhuiya MA, Kim MS, Verbruggen S, Eacker SM, Pletnikova O, Troncoso JC, Halushka MK, Menschaert G, Overall CM, Pandey A. Discovery of noncanonical translation initiation sites through mass spectrometric analysis of protein N termini. Genome Res. 2018;28(1):25–36.

39. Shin G, Grimes SM, Lee H, Lau BT, Xia LC, Ji HP. CRISPR–Cas9-targeted fragmentation and selective sequencing enable massively parallel microsatellite analysis. Nat Commun. 2017;8:14291.

8

Ethical frameworks for obtaining informed consent in tumour profiling

Yasmin Bylstra[1,2,3*] (iD), Tamra Lysaght[4], Jyothi Thrivikraman[1], Sangeetha Watson[4] and Patrick Tan[2,5,6]

Abstract

Background: Genomic profiling of malignant tumours has assisted clinicians in providing targeted therapies for many serious cancer-related illnesses. Although the characterisation of somatic mutations is the primary aim of tumour profiling for treatment, germline mutations may also be detected given the heterogenous origin of mutations observed in tumours. Guidance documents address the return of germline findings that have health implications for patients and their genetic relations. However, the implications of discovering a potential but unconfirmed germline finding from tumour profiling are yet to be fully explored. Moreover, as tumour profiling is increasingly applied in oncology, robust ethical frameworks are required to encourage large-scale data sharing and data aggregation linking molecular data to clinical outcomes, to further understand the role of genetics in oncogenesis and to develop improved cancer therapies.

Results: This paper reports on the results of empirical research that is broadly aimed at developing an ethical framework for obtaining informed consent to return results from tumour profiling tests and to share the biomolecular data sourced from tumour tissues of cancer patients. Specifically, qualitative data were gathered from 36 semi-structured interviews with cancer patients and oncology clinicians at a cancer treatment centre in Singapore. The interview data indicated that patients had a limited comprehension of cancer genetics and implications of tumour testing. Furthermore, oncology clinicians stated that they lacked the time to provide in depth explanations of the tumour profile tests. However, it was accepted from both patients and oncologist that the return potential germline variants and the sharing of de-identified tumour profiling data nationally and internationally should be discussed and provided as an option during the consent process.

Conclusions: Findings provide support for the return of tumour profiling results provided that they are accompanied with an adequate explanation from qualified personnel. They also support the use of broad consent regiments within an ethical framework that promotes trust and benefit sharing with stakeholders and provides accountability and transparency in the storage and sharing of biomolecular data for research.

Keywords: Tumour profiling, Informed consent, Genomic data sharing, Germline mutations

Background

Advances in genomic technologies and declining costs of sequencing have expanded opportunities to conduct genetic profiling of diseased cells routinely. In oncology, molecular testing of tumours, such as breast cancer, has been practiced for over 20 years. These tests can define the tumour subtype, which has important implications for the selection of therapeutic options. However, testing has since evolved to differentiate both heritable (germline) and tumour-specific (somatic) mutations in tumours. These developments have revolutionised cancer care and bridged a new era of chemotherapy and targeted treatments.

The value in delineating somatic and germline genomics for therapeutic purposes has already been demonstrated with the efficacy of ADP-ribose polymerase (PARP) inhibitors for patients with a germline BRCA

* Correspondence: yasmin.bylstra@singhealth.com.sg
[1]POLARIS, Genome Institute of Singapore, Agency for Science, Technology and Research, Singapore, Singapore
[2]SingHealth Duke-NUS Institute of Precision Medicine, Singapore, Singapore
Full list of author information is available at the end of the article

mutation [1]. In parallel, next generation sequencing (NGS) platforms are also integral to translational cancer research in identifying and validating promising new biomarkers for the development of cancer treatment. Worldwide collaborative efforts, such as The Cancer Genome Atlas (TCGA) and the International Cancer Genome Consortium (ICGC), have catalogued the genomic landscapes of thousands of tumours. In such settings, germline DNA has been routinely collected for comparative analysis with tumour DNA from the same patient to distinguish unambiguously true somatic mutations from rare germline polymorphisms. However, clinical practice is currently shifting towards a preference of routinely sequencing a patient's tumour tissue alone, to characterise its molecular profile: reasons for this preference include cost reduction and simplifying the logistics of sample collection [2, 3]. Sequencing a patient's tumour tissue alone, in the absence of a matched germline sample, challenges accurate delineation of somatic versus germline mutations due to the heterogeneous nature of mutations observed in tumours.

Until recently, there was no clear guidance on whether or how findings that only imply germline variations from genomic tumour profiling should be returned to patients. International governance bodies, such as the World Health Organization (WHO) and the Organisation for Economic Co-Operation Development (OECD), as well as national regulatory authorities around the world, have issued guidelines on the management of genetic databases; although few have developed explicit guidance on the return of incidental findings [4]. These guidance documents address the return of germline findings known to have health implications for individual participants as well as their genetic relations. However, none address the situation where tumour profiles results in a potential, but unconfirmed germline finding. In response to the increasing utility of tumour-only testing in clinical practice, the American Society of Clinical Oncology (ASCO) updated their policy statement to include recommendations that the patients should be made aware of the possible detection of germline mutations [5]. However, the implications of these recommendations in day-to-day clinical practice have not yet been fully explored, particularly in Asia.

In addition to the uncertainty around managing incidental findings, the need for sharing biomolecular data internationally is increasingly being recognised as critical to understanding the role of genetics in oncogenesis and delivering more effective target therapies for cancer [6]. However, researchers require common guidelines to ensure accountability and ethical oversight for the protection of patient data that is shared between institutions and across international borders [6, 7]. In 2014, the Global Alliance for Genomics and Health (GA4GH) published the *Framework for Responsible Sharing of Genomic and Health-Related Data* that establishes a set of foundational principles for sharing genomic and health-related data [8]. According to this framework, best practices for sharing genomic and health-related data should 'promote and protect respect for the commitment to informed consent' as the foundational principle that underlies the ethical conduct of all research involving human subjects [9]. However, while intended to facilitate compliance with international norms, this framework should also be interpreted in a manner that recognises local cultural practices and the different contexts for storing and sharing data.

In developing an ethical framework that is culturally appropriate and sensitive to local norms, systems and preferences, we initiated a qualitative study in Singapore to explore the understandings, attitudes and preferences that cancer patients and clinicians have towards the return of results of tumour profiling tests as well as the usage and sharing of the data for research purposes. Singapore is an ethnically diverse and multi-cultured country of 5 million situated in South East Asia. As most published studies on patient understandings of genetic testing have focused predominantly on Caucasian populations, there is value in gaining further insights from a diverse Asian perspective. Currently, there are no laws in Singapore to protect patients against employment and insurance discrimination due to their genetic status. Any framework for obtaining informed consent in this context should also take into account local concerns about genetic discrimination and trust in governance mechanisms that oversee the storage and sharing of genome data.

Methods

The study was designed with the aims of exploring and describing the attitudes, understandings and preferences that clinicians and cancer patients have towards participation in tumour profiling research, storage and sharing of tumour genetic data, and the return of tumour profiling results. To achieve these aims, the study design employed qualitative research methods, which are useful for documenting and explaining variation in a wide range of views, needs, values, practices and beliefs [10]. These methods are not designed to estimate proportions in a wider population, quantify relationships between pre-determined variables or provide a single representative or average view or opinion [11]. However, they are particularly useful for policy development and for the design and delivery of health care and are especially well-suited to exploring the understandings and attitudes towards highly complex concepts and subjects that cannot be fully captured with quantitative methodologies.

Evidence for this study was collected from semi-structured qualitative interviews with patients and clinicians at the National Cancer Centre Singapore (NCCS). This method was chosen to provide a contextualised dataset that focused on the specified issues and could generate themes from clearly defined, homogeneous populations within an already known context [10, 12]. Ethics approval for this protocol was obtained from the Domain Specific Research Board (DSRB) of SingHealth on 9 July 2015 to conduct up to 40 semi-structured interviews with SingHealth staff and cancer patients: (2015/2522).

Recruitment

Participants were selected using purposive sampling techniques to allow for greater flexibility in targeting informants and capture a broad range of perspectives [13] until thematic saturation was reached (i.e. no new themes were emerging from the data analysis to justify continued recruitment) [14]. To identify relevant clinicians, clinical members of the research team provided a list of 25 key oncologists at the NCCS. Three emails were sent to these individuals over 3 weeks starting at the end of July 2015. From these emails, six clinicians agreed to be interviewed, resulting in a response rate of 24%. To increase the sample size, a second email invitation was sent to an additional 59 SingHealth oncology staff in early August. Of these, 15 responded and five agreed to participate. This process resulted in a total of 11 participants being recruited from a pool of 74 contacts (a response rate of 14.8%). No further attempts were made to increase the sample size after the data were thematically saturated at 11 interviews. These interviews were conducted between July and September 2015 on the phone and face-to-face based on the preferences of participants.

For the patient group, eligible participants were recruited from the waiting room at the NCCS with the assistance of staff at the registration desk in the public clinic as well as the nurses in the private clinic. Participants were offered a $50 supermarket voucher as fair compensation for their time. Of the 28 patients approached, only three declined to be interviewed resulting in a sample of 25 informants. The much higher response rate of 89.3% in this group was likely due to the support of their treating physician, being present onsite, face-to-face recruitment and compensation. The patient interviews were conducted in October 2015.

Interview protocol

An interview protocol for both groups was developed from the issues identified in a literature review (see Additional file 1). The clinician interviews were structured around three key issues to describe their attitudes and preferences towards (1) how information on the

cancer diagnosis and the role of genetics (if any) is delivered to the patient; (2) delivery of the tumour profiling test results; and (3) the type of informed consent document needed to explain storing, sharing and withdrawal of tumour profile data. The interview protocol for the patient group was designed to explore participant attitudes, understandings and preferences of key issues including the purpose of the test; preferred linguistic labels and options of delivering the informed consent; the test procedures (sharing, storing and re-contact for additional research); perceived benefits and risks; ideas of altruism and solidarity; attitudes towards withdrawal options; and role of family and medical professionals in decision-making. The interview guide was piloted with one patient in the colon cancer clinic before full data collection proceeded.

Data analysis

All interviews were digitally recorded, transcribed verbatim and analysed using qualitative content analysis to identify, categorise and interpret key themes in relation to the consent process for storing and sharing of biomolecular data. Transcripts were read multiple times by the interviewer along with two study team members (YB and TL) to identify major themes and sub-themes. These themes and sub-themes were discussed together by the three study team members to corroborate categories and placement of relevant quotes. A coding frame was developed using these themes, which a fourth research applied to the data using NVivo© software (QSR International). Reliability was checked with two of the team members (YB and TL) independently coding pages of randomly selected interview transcripts. Agreement was measured using Cohen's kappa coefficient [15]. Demographics (age, ethnicity, gender and type of cancer diagnosis) were also collected for each patient and analysed using summative descriptive statistics (averages, median and frequencies).

Results

From August to October 2015, 11 clinicians (7 oncologists, 2 cancer genetic specialists and 3 palliative care doctors) were interviewed at the NCCS. Patients in both the private and public breast cancer clinics were recruited. In total, 25 patients were interviewed (see Table 1 for demographic descriptions of patients).

The average age of those interviewed was 52, with a median age of 54 years (ranging from 27 to 69). The majority were ethnic Chinese (10), with Indian (6) being the next largest group. The process of obtaining informed consent for the tumour profiling tests was discussed to explore patient understandings of consent and their attitudes towards the return of results and sharing of biomolecular data for research. From these discussions,

Table 1 Demographics of breast cancer patients interviewed

Patient ID	Age	Ethnicity	No. of patients
1	43	Bangladeshi	2 (8%)
2	59	Bangladeshi	
3	39	Chinese	10 (40%)
4	46	Chinese	
5	49	Chinese	
6	52	Chinese	
7	52	Chinese	
8	54	Chinese	
9	55	Chinese	
10	59	Chinese	
11	60	Chinese	
12	60	Chinese	
13	58	Filipino	1 (4%)
14	40	Indian	6 (24%)
15	40	Indian	
16	53	Indian	
17	58	Indian	
18	64	Indian	
19	69	Indian	
20	35	Malay	3 (12%)
21	63	Malay	
22	68	Malay	
23	27	Malay-Chinese	1 (4%)
24	50	Pakistani	1 (4%)
25	46	Vietnamese	1 (4%)
Total no. of patients			25

broad themes emerged that described several issues concerning participant understandings of cancer genetics and tumour testing results, therapeutic misconceptions, privacy and confidentiality. Results were supportive of a broad consent model in these contexts.

Current practice for discussing tumour profiling tests
To frame the clinical context of discussions around tumour profiling tests, the communication of this information was explored with both clinicians and patients. Clinicians indicated that their conversations about tumour testing with their patients were heavily simplified and that cancer genetics terms, such as somatic and germline mutations, were not distinguished. Instead, information regarding the test was briefly summarised by explaining that results would clarify treatment options. Clinicians explained that family history was raised if appropriate, or if patients had any concerns, referrals would be made to the cancer genetic clinics for further review.

'And if you tell them that they have this mutation, it means you can receive this drug. It will work on you or not work on you. I think about, that is how we explain it.' (Clinician 1)

Likewise, patients also indicated that discussions around genetics were limited, although some recalled being asked about their family history of cancer. When explored further about the information needs the patients desired, the response ranged widely. Some preferred brief information whereas others wanted to be well-informed. In discussions with patients about cancer genetics and tumour profiling, it became apparent that they had very limited understandings of these concepts and many appeared confused about somatic and germline genetics when raised. Cancer was generally perceived as being primarily hereditary, even by one highly educated patient who had a background in health communications:

'Generally as a lay person we are more inclined to look at family genetics. We would not think about, what you told me. When I say mutations, I was referring to the family genes you mention to me...I know every cancer cell is a mutation... normally when we talk about mutations, we talk about family history.' (Patient 9)

Clinicians interviewed also agreed that patients had limited understandings of genetics, mutations and cancer development. Some suggested that these limitations would even apply to clinicians who did not specialise in cancer genetics:

'It is does not stop at patients. Even physicians. I've had so many...mis...even from physicians referring to me you can understand that their grasp of it is very low between driver and passenger mutations, between actionable and not actionable. So you can't blame patients for not knowing this.' (Clinician 11)

It emerged from both clinicians and patients that the concepts around tumour profiling were complex and would require in depth explanations for an appropriate level of comprehension to be achieved.

Return of tumour profiling results
Current practices were explored regarding the return tumour test results. Some clinicians gave their patients the option of receiving the results as standard practice and others believed that the results should be returned to both the participant and their treating oncologist without any opportunities for either party to opt out. However, not all clinicians agreed with this approach, as with many clinical tests, there can be uncertainty around

the results and their implications for treatment. For example, the pathogenicity of a variant may be unclear (known as 'variant of unknown significance') or a variant may be reported for research opportunities, such as clinical trials, rather than for immediate clinical benefit.

'…if you just give consent and say, "Here are the clinical one and these are research ones", and you just say that, nothing else, no support about possible uncertainty. And the patient comes back and says "What does this mean?", and the doctor says this means "uncertainty". And the patient says "Oh, this is something you never told me, we [didn't] know and I don't really want this.' (Clinician 2)

As the tumour test panels can contain genes that are associated with hereditary conditions, there is the possibility that mutations in these genes derive from germline origin and have familial implications. The prospect of identifying germline incidental findings generated conflicting ideas amongst clinicians. Some clinicians discussed the possibility of discrimination that could follow from germline analyses and suggested that more legal protections, such as the Genetic Information Nondisclosure Act (2008) in the USA, should be in place before these types of tests are introduced widely into precision oncology. Hence, there were stated preferences for tumour profiling tests to exclude analysis of genes that could imply germline mutations until measures were in place. Others felt that patients should know, but should be referred to another healthcare professional trained in discussing germline implications:

'I don't think I can hide this from the patient. You have to tell the patient. Patient's interest for me to tell them to get tested. This has implications for you. I will send you to a trained cancer genetics oncologist or counsellor or whatever to sort this out. It should not be done in my clinic. It has to be someone trained.' (Clinician 10)

Most of the clinicians interviewed were clear about their professional boundaries and limitations. They understood that further evidence would be required to support the origin of a germline finding and that this was usually beyond their role as an oncologist. They also agreed that they did not have sufficient training to counsel and educate patients about germline implications.

Patients, on the other hand, were clearer in their preferences to receive their tumour profiling results. They were informed that this information could include a risk to hereditary conditions, such as breast cancer or cardiac conditions, or new treatments currently under research.

Yet they were clear that they wanted to know about these findings even if they had implications outside their own cancer diagnosis. They indicated that they were open to receiving any information that may help them understand why they were diagnosed with cancer or advance their treatment:

'I'm completely okay with that. So if there is a way that we can receive then why not. We would like to have the information.' (Patient 21)

Many patients interviewed indicated a strong preference to receive results with the provision that their oncologist or another trusted healthcare professional explain the implications of the results. They agreed that receiving such information independent of any explanation could create unnecessary confusion or worry. Therefore, if the option of returning tumour tests is available to patients, the inclusion and management of such incidental findings must also be considered.

Data sharing

Significant to the advancements in research for new therapies is the generation and accessibility of large and diverse genomic data sets. The possibility of sharing the genomic data obtained from the tumour tests with external researchers, both locally and internationally, was discussed with clinicians and patients. Both groups expressed the view that personal information had to be delinked from the stored data before being shared with third parties. Some clinicians also felt that the sociopolitical culture in Singapore would mean that few patients would be overly concerned about the storage and sharing of their results, and that they would likely consent on the basis of assurances that their personal data would be kept confidential in compliance with local laws and regulations:

'We in Singapore are not so worried about big brother or privacy like you in the West. We are used to big brother. We are a democracy, but have an overlay of authoritarianism…we are used to having government know about us and having access to our information. Singaporeans will not be bothered about the storing and sharing of data.' (Clinician 6)

These cultural views were shared amongst some of the patients interviewed who felt that there were sufficient safeguards in Singapore to protect privacy and prevent the data from being disclosed inappropriately and misused, such as the Personal Data Protection Act (2012). However, some patients were concerned about possible misuses, particularly with respect to the potential for discrimination:

'If it is only for the purpose of research it is okay. There is no problem. But if for whatever reason my name will be shown and published in a publically available media, okay then basically I need to see it and basically I need to have a positive consent for myself before it is published.' (Patient 6)

Some of the clinicians interviewed expressed concerns about sharing patient data with research institutions in other countries that lacked the accountability of publicly funded institutions like in Singapore. It was also expressed that sharing participant data for profit-orientated research might create mistrust between oncologists and their patients if such information were revealed at a later point. Such perceptions of 'profit-orientated' institutions being driven towards the commercial development of products for private benefit conflicted with views of genome research as a 'public good'.

On the other hand, the patients interviewed did not draw strong distinctions between public and private goods, although the possibility of commercial products being developed from shared tumour profile data was not raised with these informants either. All patients interviewed appeared to understand that they would not benefit directly from the sharing of tumour profile data. However, their willingness to allow their data to be stored and shared with other institutions was sometimes premised on an understanding that the research was aimed at benefiting future cancer patients:

'I feel very excited that someone can look at this and figure it out. And if they can figure it out here or in Argentina, I don't really care. It is going to be helpful to other people with a similar tumor profile I would actually be very interested in donating my tumor to science.' (Patient 14)

There were also indications amongst clinicians that patients would agree to participate in research altruistically if they believe it had the potential to benefit patients in future as a societal good:

'I think a lot of patients will do it for altruistic reasons.. most patients will do it. But I think they don't want to be made to feel as if they are guinea pigs. And so I think that's the balance you want to strike. I think you might want to say "Look whatever profits we get from these cell lines, we will donate it back to cancer". They don't feel as if they are being taken for granted and they are helping the future.' (Clinician 9)

The reciprocation of indirect benefits back to the cancer community would likely be a strong moral justification for sharing tumour profile data. Most patients

interviewed in this study did not have a family history, many wanted to understand why they had developed cancer, and were trying to make sense of their diagnosis. The possibility of having those questions answered through increased knowledge of the causes and pathology of cancer was highly valued, and patients could view themselves as contributing to that cause as a benefit. Trust in the potential to generate further knowledge around cancer causation may provide the strongest moral justification for consenting to sharing data under a broad consent regiment.

Broad consent as a model

Ensuring that patients understand test outcomes and documenting preferences in both research and clinical settings is conditional for informed consent. The process of obtaining informed consent from patients to take part in the tumour profiling tests was discussed with patients and clinicians. These discussions centred on the length and complexity of the consent form, the management of test results and incidental findings, participation in research and sharing of biomolecular data, the type of preferred consent and withdrawal options. In general, both patients and clinicians preferred that information be provided within a broad or blanket consent regiment with an option to withdraw from the research.

Clinicians were generally familiar with the various types of consent regiments (Table 2), and all but one clinician felt that a blanket or broad consent would be most appropriate in this setting. With respect the usage of tumour profiling data for research, one clinician preferred a categorical consent out of concerns for sharing genetic data outside cancer-related research. However, most of the clinicians felt that documentation with multiple consent tiers would be confusing to patients and cumbersome to manage:

"It would be more easier for scientists or researchers to get the one that the patient already say "Okay, I agree you can use it freely for research" and cover all the parameters with the patient. It is easier for the researcher. For the patient, they will feel "Why I have to consent for so many things?" (Clinician 2)

Patients on the other hand were, at times, confused about the concept of informed consent and the different types of consent needed careful explaining. As discussed above, although most patients preferred to receive any potential incidental findings, this preference still needs to be documented during the consent process.

As patients displayed a limited comprehension of tumour testing and the clinicians expressed they had limited time, additional support such as a dedicated

Table 2 Glossary of terms for informed consent

Types of consent	
Implied consent	Whereby consent is not explicitly sought from participants to use their samples in research.
Blanket consent	Consent that is sought from the participant once, either at or prior to sample collection, for use in any and all future research without the need obtain any further consent.
Broad consent	Consent that is sought from the participant once, either at or prior to sample collection, for use in any and all research without the need obtain further consent from the participant, who then delegates their decision making authority to an IRB (or another institution) for specific research projects.
Categorical consent	Consent that is sought from the participant to use samples in particular categories of research, and may include an option that allows researchers to recontact participants for consent to use samples outside of nominated areas of research.
Specific consent	Consent that is sought from the participant to use samples in specific research projects only, and may include an option that allows researchers to recontact participants for consent to use samples in other projects.
Tiered consent	Provision of multiple options for participants to choose the type of consent they wish to provide.

Types of consent methods	
Opt out	Whereby consent is not explicitly sought for a given action, but participants are informed about the option to withdraw.
Opt in	Whereby verbal or written consent is explicitly sought from the participant to use samples in research.

Types of withdrawal options	
Tiered withdrawal	Whereby participants are given numerous options to withdraw in varying degrees. I.e. to withdraw from further contact while leaving samples and data in the study, or withdraw samples while leaving data, or withdraw all samples, personal information and discontinued use of data
Single withdrawal	Whereby participants are given the option to either continue participation or withdraw completely.

coordinator or counsellor to explain the test in detail and facilitate informed consent was suggested:

'It may be better if someone else that is trained can do it... you just need a trained counsellor or a trained coordinator, research coordinator who is trained to explain it. And then obviously, we have to take the consent, we sort of don't have to go through the details of explaining. We just wrap up and answer any specific questions or concerns.' (Clinician 1)

While some clinicians agreed that a facilitator would be helpful, in contrast others felt that the responsibility to explain the results to participants should lie with the on-cologist who has professional obligations to stay updated on current evidence of best practice:

'They can provide additional information to assist the oncologists, but I think it is incumbent on the individual oncologist to know the information. Because at the end of the day they are physicians; it is their responsibility to keep up to date. Genomics is so much a part of oncology that you have to know.' (Clinician 7)

While patients supported the assistance of a dedicated co-ordinator or counsellor, there were some concerns about a nurse being able to adequately answer questions, given the perceived complexity of content in the consent form:

'Definitely it's not the nurse; doctor should be fine, if they have the time, looking at the patients. So I think a neutral person before this test carried out. I think it would be much better, so that they can understand. But the words are pretty tough here for people to understand.' (Patient 16)

There was recognition from patients and clinicians that support from an additional healthcare professional would allow more time for questions, which may not currently be possible in busy clinical settings. The costs of appointing such a professional in a clinical context were not explored with the informants, although the findings suggest that the existing infrastructure would not be well-equipped to absorb those costs.

Discussion

This paper reports on qualitative research with cancer patients and oncology clinicians in Singapore to explore current practices with tumour profiling tests and con-sent preferences for the return of results and sharing of their tumour profiling data. The results should be inter-preted within the limitations of the study; notably, the small sample size, low response rates from clinicians, and restriction to breast cancer patients interviewed at a single site in Singapore limits the generalisability of re-sults to facilities outside of this context. However, the aim of this study was not to produce generalizable find-ings about patients and clinicians everywhere, but to ex-plore and describe the perspectives, understandings and attitudes of stakeholders who will likely engage and con-tribute to the expansion of tumour profiling tests from within the healthcare settings of Singapore. Thus, find-ings are informative for obtaining consent in these con-texts and may be relevant to other types of genome-related research in Singapore and beyond. From the ana-lysis, three major themes emerged: limited comprehen-sion of cancer genetics and the consent process indicating that decision support is required; the consent preferences regarding the return of test results and usage of tumour profiling data for research; and the issues of trust and accountability in relation to research involvement. These findings are discussed in further detail below.

Decision support for obtaining consent

One significant finding that emerged from the data was the limited comprehension that patients may have of cancer genetics and implications of the tumour profiling results. It was also evident confusion arose around the concept of consent and preferences to obtaining consent. These findings are not limited to Singapore, as previously reported evidence is suggestive of limited comprehension amongst participants in genome research of genomics and cancer genetics [16–19]. In addition, comprehension limits can also be complicated by the multi-lingual context and cultural beliefs within local healthcare settings that may contribute to the varied understandings of genes and inheritance in cancer development [20]. Although cancer healthcare professionals interviewed were aware of the possibility tumour testing panels contained genes associated with hereditary conditions, there was no indication that this was discussed with their patients. In fact, if there were any indications of hereditary implications, clinicians made referrals to inherited cancer services.

Recently, recommendations from both ASCO and National Comprehensive Cancer Network (NCCN) support the view that patients should be informed about the potential of tumour profiling results inferring hereditary conditions, as well as the potential benefits, limitations and risks prior to the test taking place [5, 21]. Clinicians stated that they often lacked the time to explain medical protocols and outcomes in detail with their patients, and indicated that would they would not have time to provide lengthy explanations of the tumour profile tests. This reality of the local healthcare setting suggests that additional resources would be required to support the consent process. In research settings, dedicated co-ordinators are frequently appointed to support the recruitment and consent process. In the context of genomic research, some scholars have recommended the appointment of trained genetic counsellors to deliver the consent documentation and explain to participants the implications of consenting as they are trained to discuss issues related to germline genetic tests [17, 22].

With the significance of tumour profiling panels containing genes associated with hereditary risk, it has been proposed that the role of a genetic counsellor to deliver counselling around such tests should become more predominant in oncology as consultations parallel germline testing [21]. In countries where genetic counselling services are limited, such as Singapore, the involvement of a trained co-ordinator was proposed. With a few exceptions, the clinicians were generally supportive of a dedicated clinical co-ordinator or researcher being available to explain the consent documentation in detail and take the written consent from participants. The additional support to assist with consent will require funding to compensate for the cost of this service. This responsibility may extend to the role of existing hospital employees to assist with the consent or this service could be included in the cost of the tumour profiling test. Institutions will need to consider how the cost of such support can be absorbed.

Consent preferences for returning results and data sharing

Recommendations provided by the ASCO and NCCN also emphasise that patients should be given the opportunity to opt out of receiving possible incidental germline findings. In addition, for those patients interested learning more about germline origin should be further investigated for their pathogenicity [5, 21]. The obligation to return research results and incidental findings to patients in genetics research is contested and currently lacks consensus [4]. In Singapore, there are currently no laws that create legal duties for clinicians or researchers to return results or incidental findings to participants; nor are there any explicit rights 'not to know'. As recommended, results from this study also suggest that participants should be given the option to receive the results of their tumour profiling test, and be made aware of the potential for incidental findings during the consent process.

However, discussions became more complex regarding how incidental findings should be highlighted if patients opted to receive a copy of their tumour profiling results. While one clinician interviewed suggested the removal of those genes with germline implications from the tumour test report, most clinicians and patients were generally comfortable with the inclusion of these genes providing that they were accompanied with an adequate explanation. In recommendations for the delivery of tumour profiling results, it has been suggested that oncologists draw on the expertise of genetics specialists to assist with the interpretation and discussions of those findings with participants [21, 23]. The possibility of incidental germline findings and genetic discrimination also emerged from interview data. As there are currently no laws in Singapore to protect patients against employment and insurance discrimination due to their genetic status this approach also justifies a role for genetics specialists having a role to raise awareness of such issues. Therefore, the possibility of incidental findings being revealed with the return of tumour profiling results should be acknowledged along with ensuring that participants are referred to relevant specialists to validate the findings and take action where appropriate.

There are currently no guidelines or recommendations on how these preferences towards the return of results should be captured. It is also apparent from literature that the consent framework and clinical processes to inform patients and document preferences about the hereditary implications of tumour profiling tests remain uncertain. Results from the present study suggest that clinicians and cancer patients would prefer a simple model where consent is given just once. This model was preferred by clinicians because they lacked the time needed to explain adequately the implications of multiple consent options. Some also felt that participants would not fully comprehend different categories of research and would be happy to provide a one-off consent. They also specified that if testing revealed information beyond somatic implications that this should be captured separately, by including a tick box, to consenting for tumour profiling to be performed.

This view also extended to preferences around the usage of tumour profiling data for research applications. Patients were generally unconcerned about the provision of their data providing it was shared with external researchers in a de-identified format, and in compliance with Singapore laws and regulations. Similar to the many other studies published previously, the findings indicated support for a broad consent model that delegates decision-making authority to an independent oversight body, such as an ethics review committee or institutional review board [24, 25].

Trust and governance

From the results of this study, it is clear that the storage and sharing of tumour profiling data cannot be ethically justified as merely an exercise of personal autonomy when the informed consent of participants is inherently limited. Even with the support of dedicated research staff and a simplified consent process, the degree to which cancer patients can be truly informed of the implications for consenting to the storage and sharing of these data with researchers in Singapore and abroad is uncertain. Thus, it is important to ensure that other measures are in place to protect participants from unnecessary harms and that their data is shared within the morally accepted parameters of the consent. In short, participants must be able to trust that their data will be protected and used for the purposes they consented to.

A lack of trust with clinicians and patients would have significant implications for the value of biomolecular databanks specific to the health needs of the Singaporean population. Storage and sharing these data with external researchers will be key to fostering research and ensuring the widest public health benefits [6]. The potential for these benefits justifies the enormous public resources that are invested in genomic databanks and

their purpose as a public good. Maintaining trust in this public good not only requires security measures to protect the data of participants, but will also require transparency in how the data are accessed and how social and economic benefits are distributed [26]. Any intention to privatise these benefits should be disclosed to participants prior to consenting and policies should be in place to restrict access to the data for purposes participants have consented to.

The results of this study support the adoption of a broad consent model where participants would not consent to specific projects or types of research. However, they also suggest that participants would consent altruistically on the condition that their data is used for research that has the potential to benefit other cancer patients in the future. This finding is supported in the literature with other evidence that solidarity with future patients incentivises participation in research that is unlikely to have direct benefits for participants [27]. The solidarity principle forms the basis of ethical arguments that justify the use of broad consent regiments for genomic research [28] and is strongly advocated by the HUGO Committee on Ethics, Law and Society [29]. Yet, the acceptability of this approach is also attached with provisions for governance mechanisms that ensure transparency and accountability in how data are stored and shared with other researchers and institutions. Such mechanisms may include approval from an ethics review committee for specific projects, or a separate independent body comprised of members with relevant expertise to provide oversight for the release of data to external institutions and the distribution of benefits [7].

While the results of this study indicate that participants would consent to tumour profiling data being shared for the purposes of cancer research, this might not be limited to cancer research only as other types of biomedical research were not discussed in the interviews. However, the consent might not extend to non-medical related research, such as military research or forensic investigations. Concerns over the use of genetic data for these purposes has been raised in the literature [30, 31], and while they are most relevant to germline research rather than somatic tumour profiling, participants are unlikely to understand these differences well enough to assume that they appreciate the risks of sharing these data. In these circumstances, institutions must assume a guardianship role to ensure that the data entrusted to them is not misused or perceived as such.

Finally, the concept of benefit sharing is another principle that has emerged to justify the use of broad consent regiments for genomic research [28] and is also endorsed by HUGO [32] Committee on Ethics, Law and Society. This principle does not imply that participants should benefit directly, as it is important not to promote therapeutic misconception. Rather, the principle prioritises benefits to be shared with *communities*. In the context of this study, the principle implies that mechanisms should be in place for the expedient dissemination of published research results as new discoveries in cancer treatments emerge and the reclassification of variants becomes clinically significant.

Conclusions

As the integration of NGS to inform patient care is continually evolving in oncology practice, this is experience is novel to clinicians, researchers and especially to patients. Therefore, developing a framework for obtaining consent from participants for this type of testing becomes challenging when recommendations specific to tumour profiling worldwide are only emerging and there are no best practice principles explicit to genomic testing in a Singaporean context.

This study has highlighted that there is limited public awareness around cancer causation and genetics as well as an understanding of what informed consent entails. As genomics advances, communication of these concepts will become increasingly complicated, yet highly relevant to ensure realistic expectations of the test outcomes. It has become evident that support is required when tumour profiling tests are offered, from either a clinic co-ordinator or genetic counsellor, so that information and test outcomes are explained, ultimately ensuring that informed consent can be obtained in precision oncology settings.

Abbreviations
ASCO: American Society of Clinical Oncology; DSRB: Domain Specific Research Board; GA4GH: Global Alliance for Genomics and Health; ICGC: International Cancer Genome Consortium; NCCN: National Comprehensive Cancer Network; NCCS: National Cancer Centre Singapore; NGS: Next generation sequencing; OECD: Organisation for Economic Co-Operation Development; PARP: ADP-ribose polymerase; TCGA: The Cancer Genome Atlas; WHO: World Health Organization

Acknowledgements
We would like to acknowledge Dr. Rebecca Dent, Dr. Joanne Ngeow, Dr. Iain Beehuat Tan, Dr. Daniel Tan and their team for their assistance in recruiting our research participants and Professor Alastair Campbell for his support with conceiving this study. We would also like to acknowledge the oncology clinicians and patients for their contributions to our research findings and the POLARIS team members for their support and input.

Funding
This research was funded by the POLARIS program under the Agency for Science, Technology, and Research (A*STAR) Strategic Positioning Fund (SPF) scheme and supported with a Start-Up Grant from the National University of Singapore (WBS: R-171-000-058-133).

Authors' contributions
PT conceived the study. YB, TL and JT contributed to study design, results analysis and manuscript preparation. SJ contributed to results analysis and manuscript preparation. All authors read and approved the final manuscript.

Competing interests
The authors declare that they have no competing interests.

Author details
[1]POLARIS, Genome Institute of Singapore, Agency for Science, Technology and Research, Singapore, Singapore. [2]SingHealth Duke-NUS Institute of Precision Medicine, Singapore, Singapore. [3]Inherited Cardiac Clinic, National University Hospital, Singapore, Singapore. [4]Centre for Biomedical Ethics, Yong Loo Lin School of Medicine, National University of Singapore, Singapore, Singapore. [5]Cancer and Stem Biology, Duke-NUS Medical School, Singapore, Singapore. [6]Biomedical Research Council, Agency for Science, Technology and Research, Singapore, Singapore.

References
1. Farmer H, McCabe N, Lord CJ, Tutt AN, Johnson DA, Richardson TB, Santarosa M, Dillon KJ, Hickson I, Knights C, et al. Targeting the DNA repair defect in BRCA mutant cells as a therapeutic strategy. Nature. 2005;434:917–21.
2. Jones S, Anagnostou V, Lytle K, Parpart-Li S, Nesselbush M, Riley DR, Shukla M, Chesnick B, Kadan M, Papp E, et al. Personalized genomic analyses for cancer mutation discovery and interpretation. Sci Transl Med. 2015;7:283ra253.
3. Catenacci DV, Amico AL, Nielsen SM, Geynisman DM, Rambo B, Carey GB, Gulden C, Fackenthal J, Marsh RD, Kindler HL, Olopade OI. Tumor genome analysis includes germline genome: are we ready for surprises? Int J Cancer. 2015;136:1559–67.
4. Zawati MH, Knoppers BM. International normative perspectives on the return of individual research results and incidental findings in genomic biobanks. Genet Med. 2012;14:484–9.
5. Robson ME, Bradbury AR, Arun B, Domchek SM, Ford JM, Hampel HL, Lipkin SM, Syngal S, Wollins DS, Lindor NM. American Society of Clinical Oncology policy statement update: genetic and genomic testing for cancer susceptibility. J Clin Oncol. 2015;33:3660–7.
6. Knoppers BM, Harris JR, Tasse AM, Budin-Ljosne I, Kaye J, Deschenes M. Zawati MnH: towards a data sharing code of conduct for international genomic research. Genome Med. 2011;3(7):46.
7. Caulfield T, McGruire AL, Cho M, Buchanan JA, Burgess MM, DAnilcyk U, Diaz CM, Fryer-Edwards K, Green SK, Hodosh MA, et al. Research ethics recommendations for whole-genome research: consensus statement. PLoS Biol. 2008;6(3):e73.
8. Knoppers BM. Framework for responsible sharing of genomic and health-related data. HUGO J. 2014;8:1–6.
9. Global Alliance for Genomics and Health: Framework for responsible sharing of genomic and health-related data: development of policies. In 3rd plenary meeting of the global alliance for genomics and health; Leiden, The Netherlands. 2015.
10. Denzin NK, Lincoln YS (Eds.): The SAGE handbook of qualitative research. Thousand Oaks, CA: Sage Publications; 2005.
11. Kuper A, Reeves S, Levinson W. An introduction to reading and appraising qualitative research. BMJ. 2008;337(7666):404–7.
12. Miller WL, Crabtree BF. In: Hesse-Biber SN, Leavy P, editors. Depth interviewing. In approaches to qualitative research: a reader on theory and practice. New York: Oxford University Press; 2004. p. 185–202.
13. Merriam SB: Case study research in education: a qualitative approach. San Francisco, CA: Jossey-Bass Publishers; 1988.
14. Saunders B, Sim J, Kingstone T, Baker S, Waterfield J, Bartlam B, Burroughs H, Jinks C. Saturation in qualitative research: exploring its conceptualization and operationalization. Quality & Quantity. 2017;14:1–15.
15. Berelson B: Content analysis in communication research. Glencose, IL: The Free Press; 1952.

16. Gray SW, Hicks-Courant K, Lathan CS, Garraway L, Park ER, Weeks JC. Attitudes of patients with cancer about personalised medicine and somatic genetic testing. J Oncol Pract. 2012;8(6):329–35.

17. Kaphingst KA, Facio FM, Cheng MR, Brooks S, Eidem H, Linn A, Biesecker BB, Biesecker LG. Effects of informed consent for individual genome sequencing on relevant knowledge. Clin Genet. 2012;82:408–15.

18. McGowan ML, Settersten RA Jr, Juengst ET, Fishman JR. Integrating genomics into clinical oncology: ethical and social challenges from proponents of personalized medicine. Urol Oncol. 2014;32:187–92.

19. Lea DH, Kaphingst KA, Bowen D, Lipkus I, Hadley DW. Communicating genetic and genomic information: health literacy and numeracy considerations. Public Health Genom. 2011;14:279–89.

20. Lim MK. Transforming Singapore health care: public-private partnership. Annals-Academy Med Singapore. 2005;34(7):461–7.

21. Jain R, Savage MJ, Forman AD, Mukherji R, Hall MJ. The relevance of hereditary cancer risks to precision oncology: what should providers consider when conducting tumor genomic profiling? J Natl Compr Cancer Netw. 2016;14:795–806.

22. Levenseller BL, Soucier DJ, Miller VA, Harris D, Conway L, Bernhardt BA. Stakeholders' opinions on the implementation of pediatric whole exome sequencing: implications for informed consent. J Genet Couns. 2014;23:552–65.

23. Raymond VM, Gray SW, Roychowdhury S, Joffe S, Chinnaiyan AM, Parsons DW, Plon SE. Germline findings in tumor-only sequencing: points to consider for clinicians and laboratories. J Natl Cancer Inst. 2016;108(4)

24. Hansson MG. Building on relationships of trust in biobank research. J Med Ethics. 2005;31:415–8.

25. Hansson MG, Dillner J, Bartram CR, Carlson JA, Helgesson G. Should donors be allowed to give broad consent to future biobank research? Lancet Oncol. 2006;7:266–9.

26. Caulfield T, McGuire AL, Cho M, Buchanan JA, Burgess MM, Danilczyk U, Diaz CM, Fryer-Edwards K, Green SK, Hodosh MA, et al. Research ethics recommendations for whole-genome research: consensus statement. PLoS Biol. 2008;6:e73.

27. Felt U, Bister MD, Strassnig M, Wagner U. Refusing the information paradigm: informed consent, medical research, and patient participation. Health (London). 2009;13:87–106.

28. Knoppers BM, Chadwick R. Human genetic research: emerging trends in ethics. Nature Rev Genetics. 2005;6:75–9.

29. Mulvihill JJ, Capps B, Joly Y, Lysaght T, Zwart HAE, Chadwick R. Ethical issues of CRISPR technology and gene editing through the lens of solidarity. Br Med Bull. 2017;122:17–29.

30. Hofmann B. Broadening consent—and diluting ethics? J Med Ethics. 2009;35:125–9.

31. O'Neill O. Autonomy and Trust in Bioethics. Cambridge: Cambridge University Press; 2002.

32. Statement on Benefit Sharing. [http://www.hugo-international.org/Resources/Documents/CELS_Statement-BenefitSharing_2000.pdf].

9

Integrating rare genetic variants into pharmacogenetic drug response predictions

Magnus Ingelman-Sundberg, Souren Mkrtchian, Yitian Zhou and Volker M. Lauschke[*] (iD)

Abstract

Background: Variability in genes implicated in drug pharmacokinetics or drug response can modulate treatment efficacy or predispose to adverse drug reactions. Besides common genetic polymorphisms, recent sequencing projects revealed a plethora of rare genetic variants in genes encoding proteins involved in drug metabolism, transport, and response.

Results: To understand the global importance of rare pharmacogenetic gene variants, we mapped the variability in 208 pharmacogenes by analyzing exome sequencing data from 60,706 unrelated individuals and estimated the importance of rare and common genetic variants using a computational prediction framework optimized for pharmacogenetic assessments. Our analyses reveal that rare pharmacogenetic variants were strongly enriched in mutations predicted to cause functional alterations. For more than half of the pharmacogenes, rare variants account for the entire genetic variability. Each individual harbored on average a total of 40.6 putatively functional variants, rare variants accounting for 10.8% of these. Overall, the contribution of rare variants was found to be highly gene- and drug-specific. Using warfarin, simvastatin, voriconazole, olanzapine, and irinotecan as examples, we conclude that rare genetic variants likely account for a substantial part of the unexplained inter-individual differences in drug metabolism phenotypes.

Conclusions: Combined, our data reveal high gene and drug specificity in the contributions of rare variants. We provide a proof-of-concept on how this information can be utilized to pinpoint genes for which sequencing-based genotyping can add important information to predict drug response, which provides useful information for the design of clinical trials in drug development and the personalization of pharmacological treatment.

Keywords: Pharmacogenetics, Personalized medicine, ADME genes, Genetic variability, Drug response

Background

The response of patients to medical treatment is influenced by a variety of physiological, pathological, environmental, and genetic factors [1]. These inter-individual differences can lower treatment efficacy or manifest in adverse drug reactions (ADRs), which are estimated to cause around 6.5% of all hospital admissions [2]. Overall, the genetic makeup of a patient accounts for 20–30% of the inter-individual variability in drug response [3], but for certain clinically important drugs, such as metoprolol and

torsemide, twin studies suggested genetic contributions to the variability in their pharmacokinetics of up to 90% [4].

Genetic variability in phase I and phase II enzymes, transporters, cytochrome reductases, and nuclear receptors, hereafter jointly termed pharmacogenes, can modulate drug absorption, distribution, metabolism, and excretion (ADME), thereby shaping human drug response and the risk of ADRs. Prominent examples include associations of common *TPMT* variants with hematological toxicity of 6-mercaptopurines, ultrarapid metabolism of CYP2D6 with codeine toxicity, and effects of specific *CYP2C19* polymorphisms on the response to clopidogrel or proton pump inhibitors [5]. Yet, a substantial fraction of the heritable variability in drug response cannot be explained by these common variants, suggesting that other genetic factors are

* Correspondence: volker.lauschke@ki.se
Department of Physiology and Pharmacology, Section of Pharmacogenetics, Karolinska Institutet, SE-171 77 Stockholm, Sweden

important contributors. In recent years, increasing capacities and decreasing costs of next-generation sequencing (NGS) platforms have facilitated large-scale studies of genetic variation and NGS assays are becoming increasingly implemented in clinical diagnostics [6]. Importantly, NGS-based analyses revealed that over 90% of the overall genetic variability in pharmacogenes is allotted to rare genetic variants, but the impact of rare genetic variability on drug pharmacokinetics has not been systematically evaluated (Additional file 1: Table S1) [7–10].

We therefore analyzed the distribution of rare and common gene variants in the 208 clinically most relevant pharmacogenes of 60,706 unrelated individuals and leveraged these genetic variability profiles to predict the relevance of rare SNVs for the pharmacokinetics or ADR risks for several clinically important drugs of diverse therapeutic areas. Based on these analyses, we conclude that the contribution of rare genetic variants is gene- and drug-specific and can account for a substantial part of the unexplained genetic inter-individual variability in drug response. Furthermore, we highlight genes for which comprehensive NGS-based genotyping instead of candidate SNP interrogations can reveal important additional information to personalize pharmacological treatment strategies. The presented data incentivizes the consideration of rare pharmacogenetic variants for the guidance of personalized drug therapy and holds important implications for the design of clinical trials.

Methods

Data sources

Human sequencing data from 60,706 unrelated individuals was obtained from the Exome Aggregation Consortium (ExAC) database [11], a platform that provides summary frequency information of exonic genetic variants from 17 large-scale sequencing projects. Notably, consistency of the individual data sets is assured by reprocessing of all raw data through the same bioinformatic pipelines. We complemented the obtained variants with six non-exonic variants from the 1000 Genomes Project [12] that define *CYP1A2*1C* (rs2069514), *CYP1A2*1F* (rs762551), *CYP2C19*17* (rs12248560), *CYP3A4*22* (rs35599367), *CYP3A5*3* (rs776746), and *UGT1A1*28* (rs8175347). Variants with less than 10,000 called high-quality alleles were not considered. Novel variants were defined relative to dbSNP release 135.

Definitions

Loss-of-function (LoF) intolerance scores were provided by Lek et al. based on the expectation-maximization algorithm [11]. In brief, low scores (< 0.1) indicate that the number of protein-truncating variants is similar to what is expected by chance, whereas high scores (> 0.9) indicate much fewer of such variants are observed than would be

expected, suggesting haploinsufficiency. Aggregated functional variant frequency is defined as the sum of MAFs of all variants predicted to be deleterious. Variants with MAF ≤ 0.01 were considered as rare, and variants with MAF > 0.01 were considered as common.

Variant analyses and computational functionality predictions

Computational algorithms mostly use evolutionary conservation as a metric to predict whether a given variant likely has functional effects. Importantly, we previously evaluated 18 current functionality prediction methods and found that their predictive performance was low for poorly conserved genes, such as cytochrome P450s [13].

Here, we therefore used a functionality prediction method that we previously developed [13]. In brief, using high-quality experimental data for 123 pharmacogenetic alleles, Zhou et al. tailored the parameterization of 18 different algorithms specifically for ADME genes and integrated the results of multiple prediction methods into an ADME-optimized prediction framework [13]. Finally, the model's performance was validated in an independent validation cohort of additional 121 experimentally characterized variants. Overall, the model achieved 92% sensitivity and 95% specificity for loss-of-function and functionally neutral variants, respectively, thereby substantially outperforming previous computational tools on pharmacogenomics data sets.

Results

Analysis of the genetic landscape in 208 human pharmacogenes

We analyzed the genetic variability in 208 genes with importance for drug ADME using exome sequencing data from 60,706 unrelated individuals. In total, we identified 69,923 variants distributed across transporter genes (33,792 variants in 73 genes), genes encoding phase 1 (21,161 variants in 71 genes) and phase 2 enzymes (10,411 variants in 46 genes), nuclear receptors (2338 variants in 9 genes), and other pharmacogenes with miscellaneous functions (2221 variants in 6 genes; Fig. 1a). Notably, 57,773 (83%) of these 69,923 variants we identified were novel as compared to dbSNP release 135 (Fig. 1b).

Evolutionary constraints in transporters as well as in phase 1 and phase 2 drug-metabolizing genes were low as judged by the large numbers of loss-of-function variants identified in these genes (LoF intolerance score = 0.08 ± 0.02 SEM; see the "Methods" section for details). In contrast, nuclear receptors and other selected genes with importance for drug response were highly LoF-intolerant (LoF intolerance score = 0.53 ± 0.11 SEM), comparable to values observed across haploinsufficient genes (LoF intolerance score > 0.5; Fig. 1c) [11]. Importantly, the vast majority of variants were rare (98.5%; MAF < 1%) or very rare (96.2%; MAF < 0.1%) and

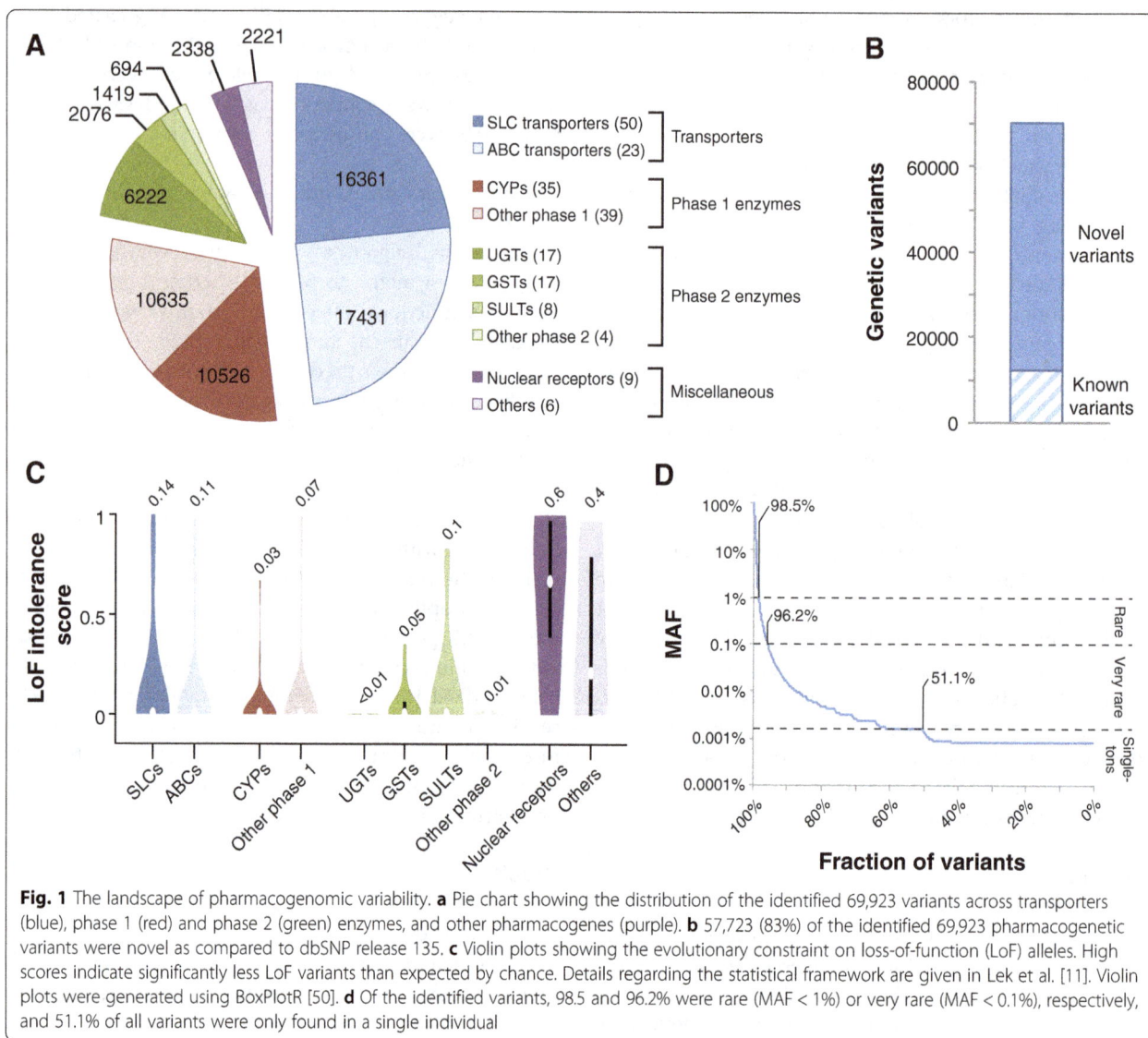

Fig. 1 The landscape of pharmacogenomic variability. **a** Pie chart showing the distribution of the identified 69,923 variants across transporters (blue), phase 1 (red) and phase 2 (green) enzymes, and other pharmacogenes (purple). **b** 57,723 (83%) of the identified 69,923 pharmacogenetic variants were novel as compared to dbSNP release 135. **c** Violin plots showing the evolutionary constraint on loss-of-function (LoF) alleles. High scores indicate significantly less LoF variants than expected by chance. Details regarding the statistical framework are given in Lek et al. [11]. Violin plots were generated using BoxPlotR [50]. **d** Of the identified variants, 98.5 and 96.2% were rare (MAF < 1%) or very rare (MAF < 0.1%), respectively, and 51.1% of all variants were only found in a single individual

more than half (51.1%) of all variants were only detected in a single individual, highlighting the genetic diversity in human pharmacogenes (Fig. 1d).

Rare variants contribute substantially to functional variability

To evaluate the functional importance of rare pharmacogenetic variants, we computed functionality assessments of each SNV using a computational assessment model specifically optimized for the assessment of pharmacogenes (see the "Methods" section for details). We then aggregated frequencies of frameshift, splice, start-lost, stop-gain, and putatively deleterious missense variants and found that the pattern and distribution of genetic variability differed substantially across the 208 pharmacogenes analyzed. Genetic variability with functional impact was governed by few high-frequency variants for some genes, including *ABCB5*, *SLC22A10*, *CYP1A2*,

CYP2C8, or *GSTT2* (Fig. 2a). In contrast, the functionality of the majority of pharmacogenes, including *ABCB1*, *SLC10A1*, and *CYP3A7*, is dominated by rare genetic variants. The frequency of genetic variants predicted to affect the functionality of the gene product differed more than 1000-fold between genes. The most highly variable genes were *SLC22A10* (aggregated functional variant frequency 1.08), *ABCB5* (0.91), and *FMO2* (0.86), whereas the lowest numbers of functional variants were observed for *GSTT1* (0.0006), *RXRA* (0.0007), *PPARD* (0.0011), and *CYP17A1* (0.0014; Fig. 2a).

Notably, rare pharmacogenetic variants were strongly enriched in mutations predicted to cause functional alterations (Fig. 2b), consistent with previous reports [12, 14, 15]. In the 208 pharmacogenes combined, each individual harbored on average a total of 40.6 putatively functional variants (Fig. 2c). Rare variants accounted for 4.4 (10.8%) of these functional variants, of which 1.8, 1.7,

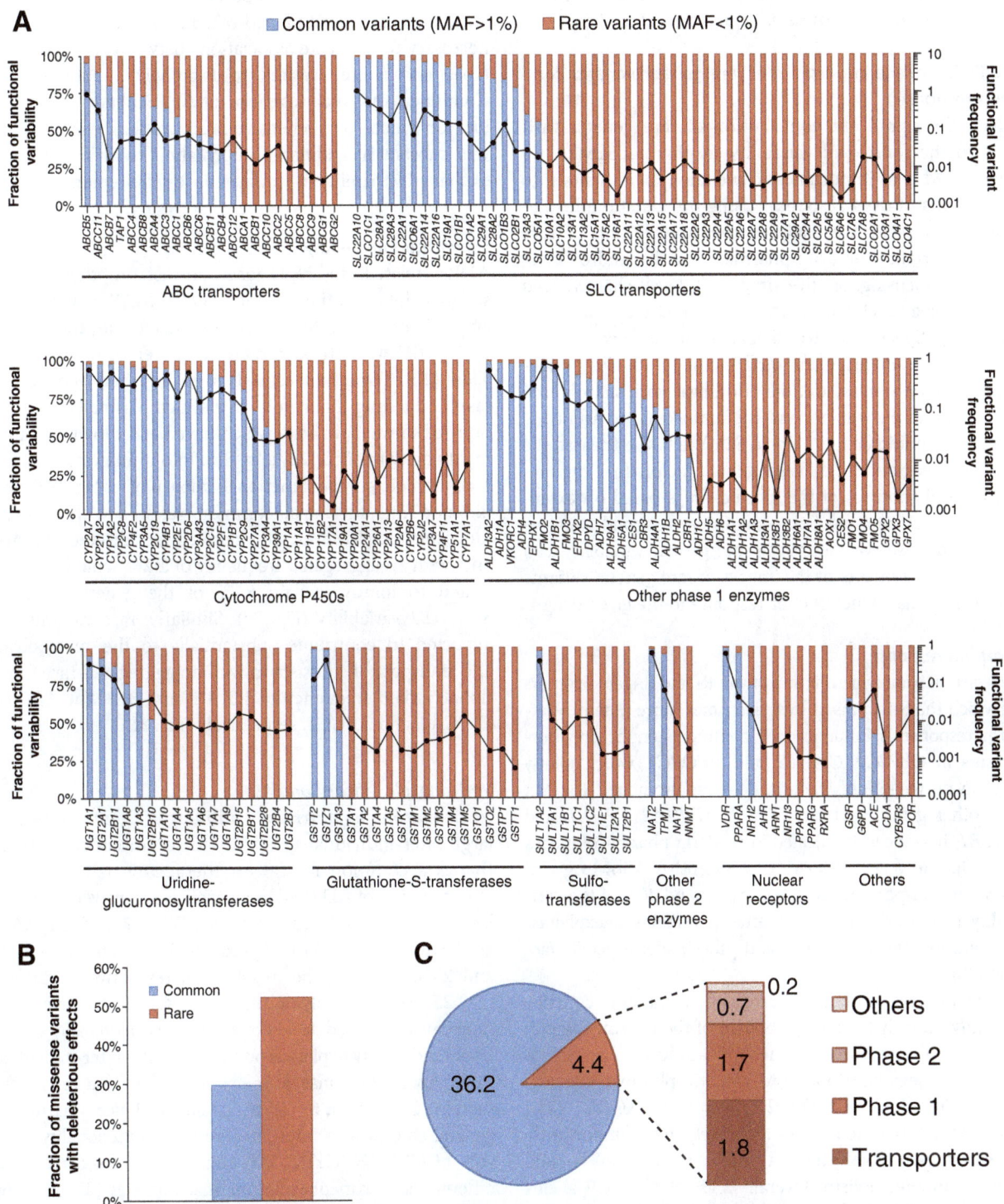

Fig. 2 Rare genetic variants contribute substantially to pharmacogenomic variability. **a** The frequency of putatively functional variants is plotted in log scale and indicated as dots connected by the black line for each of the 208 pharmacogenes analyzed (right y-axis). The fraction of this functional variability that is allotted to common (blue) or rare (red) variants is indicated on the left y-axis. Importantly, overall genetic variability as well as the fraction of functional variation that is allotted to rare variants differs considerably between genes. **b** Rare genetic polymorphisms in pharmacogenes are enriched in variants predicted to cause functional alterations. **c** Across the 208 ADME genes analyzed, each individual was found to harbor on average 4.4 rare functional variants (frameshift, splice, start-lost, stop-gain, and putatively functional missense variants). Of these, 1.8, 1.7, 0.7, and 0.2 are allotted to transporters, phase 1 and phase 2 enzymes, and other pharmacogenes, respectively

0.7, and 0.2 were allotted to transporters, phase 1, phase 2, and other pharmacogenes, respectively (Fig. 2c).

Prediction of the importance of rare genetic variants for drug response

Given the significant contribution of rare genetic variants to the functional variability in pharmacogenes, we considered it of importance to include rare variants into predictions of drug response. Using the genetic information as template, we analyzed the contribution of rare genetic variants for drug pharmacokinetics and/or drug response, focusing on five drugs with well-characterized pharmacology and substantial unexplained inter-individual variability. Specifically, we evaluated the relevance of rare SNVs for the anticoagulant warfarin, the HMG-CoA reductase inhibitor simvastatin, the antifungal voriconazole, the antipsychotic olanzapine, and the antineoplastic agent irinotecan (Additional file 2: Table S2). We first estimated the relative importance of different genetic factors for drug metabolism phenotypes of the specific drugs based on extensive literature analysis. Subsequently in a second step, we integrated these evaluations with our genetic variability data to derive assessments of the impact of rare genetic variants on the pharmacokinetics of or response to the given drug.

Warfarin response

Warfarin is a racemic mixture of the R- and S-stereoisomers of which the S-form is at least five times more potent. Warfarin response is influenced by common genetic polymorphisms in *CYP2C9*, *CYP4F2*, and *VKORC1*, which jointly explain up to 45% of warfarin dose requirements [16]. Yet also other genes, such as *CYP3A4*, *CYP1A2*, *EPHX1*, and *ABCB1*, have been implicated in warfarin pharmacokinetics [17–19]. However, despite this extensive knowledge of warfarin transport and metabolism, around 40% of the variability in warfarin dose requirements remains unexplained by common genetic variants and other patient-specific factors [20].

Our analyses predict that rare genetic variants contribute only minorly to the metabolism of the pharmacologically less potent R-enantiomer of warfarin (Fig. 3a–c). Similarly, their contribution to warfarin pharmacodynamics by alterations in CYP4F2 (3.6%) and VKORC1 (2%) function is expected to be relatively low. Importantly however, rare SNVs have a major impact on hepatic S-warfarin metabolism. Overall, 2.1% of *CYP2C9* alleles are predicted to harbor rare variants with deleterious effects, accounting for 18.4% of the genetically encoded functional differences in CYP2C9 activity (Fig. 3b). Moreover, our analyses predict rare variants with functional consequences in 1.3% of *ABCB1* alleles, encoding the P-gp/MDR1 transporter that is implicated in warfarin clearance, whereas no common deleterious variants were identified (Fig. 3b). However, given the controversy

regarding the functional impacts of common *ABCB1* variants, such as rs1045642 and rs2032582, future research is necessary to delineate associations between *ABCB1* genotypes and factors related to P-gp/MDR1 activity [21]. Combined, our analyses pinpoint *CYP2C9* and *ABCB1* as loci for which comprehensive NGS profiling can likely reveal substantial additional information regarding the unexplained variability in warfarin dose requirements.

Simvastatin myopathy

ADRs related to high-dose simvastatin therapy are strongly linked to the common (12.9% MAF) genetic variant rs4149056 in *SLCO1B1* (encoding the transporter OATP1B1) with an odds ratio of 4.5 per copy of the risk allele [22]. Toxicity is caused by an impaired hepatic uptake of the drug that results in elevated plasma concentrations of simvastatin acid, which have been shown to cause myotoxicity in vitro [23] (Fig. 3d). In our analyses, we correctly predicted the functional impact of rs4149056 and did not find additional common variants with reduced functionality. However, we identified rare deleterious variants with an aggregated frequency of 1.2%, which are estimated to jointly explain 8.7% of the genetic basis of *SLCO1B1* variability (Fig. 3e). Similarly, rare variants are expected to contribute substantially to the metabolism and transport of simvastatin with an aggregated rare functional variant frequency of 1.3, 1.1, and 0.8% for *ABCB1*, *CYP3A4*, and *ABCG2*, respectively (Fig. 3f).

Voriconazole efficacy and ADRs

Voriconazole is a triazole antifungal agent exhibiting large inter-individual variability in serum concentrations that is a common reason for therapeutic failure or the manifestation of ADRs. Voriconazole is extensively metabolized by various CYPs (CYP2C19, CYP2C9, and CYP3A4) and FMOs (FMO1, FMO3, and FMO5) accounting for 75 and 25% of its hepatic metabolism, respectively (Fig. 4a) [24, 25]. Genetic polymorphisms in *CYP2C19* have been reproducibly linked to differences in voriconazole serum levels and jointly explain around 50% of the inter-individual variability in voriconazole metabolism ([26] and references therein). In addition to *CYP2C19* alleles, clinical pharmacogenetic studies also implicated reduced functionality variants of *CYP2C9* (*CYP2C9*2*) and *CYP3A4* (rs4646437) in differences in voriconazole pharmacokinetics [27, 28]. For *CYP2C19*, our analyses identified rare deleterious variants with an aggregated frequency of 1.6%, whereas the common functional *CYP2C19* alleles *CYP2C19*2* and *CYP2C19*17* showed frequencies of 18.5 and 15.3%, respectively (Fig. 4b). Consequently, rare variants are estimated to account for 4.4% of the overall genetic variability of CYP2C19 function. Furthermore, rare alleles contributed substantially to the variability in other genes implicated in voriconazole efficacy

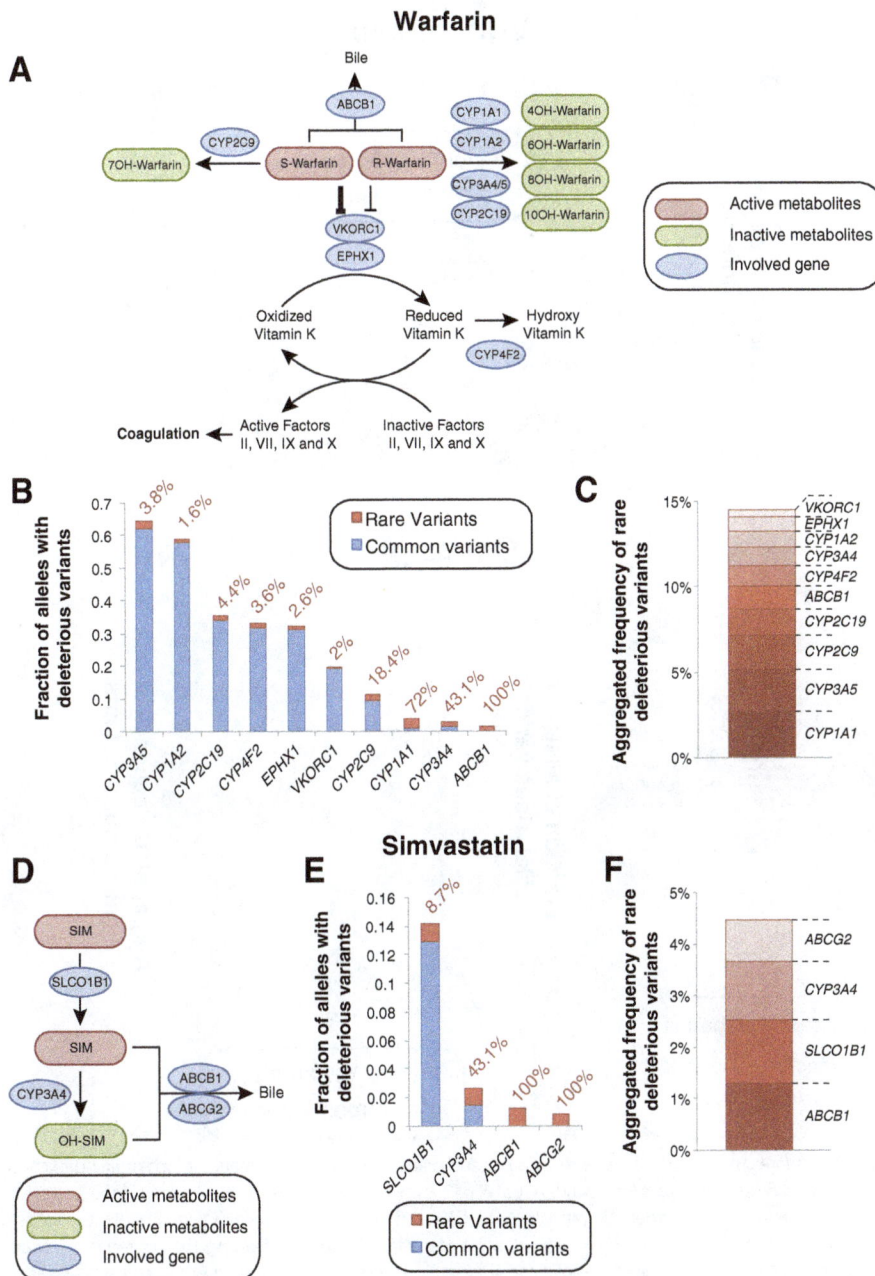

Fig. 3 The relevance of rare genetic variants for warfarin response and simvastatin-related myotoxicity. **a** Scheme depicting the metabolism and therapeutic action of warfarin. The less potent R-enantiomer of warfarin is metabolized by CYP1A1, CYP1A2, CYP3A, and CYP2C19, whereas the more potent S-enantiomer is inactivated by CYP2C9. Warfarin inhibits the VKOR complex, which reduces vitamin K, an essential factor for the formation of functional coagulation factors. See www.pharmgkb.org/pathway/PA145011113 and www.pharmgkb.org/pathway/PA145011114 for further information. **b** Overview of the aggregated frequencies of common (MAF ≥ 1%, blue) and rare deleterious genetic variants (MAF < 1%, red) in genes involved in warfarin pharmacokinetics or pharmacodynamics. Values next to the columns indicate the relative contribution of rare genetic variants. **c** Stacked column plot showing the aggregated frequency of deleterious rare variants of potential relevance for warfarin action. **d** Scheme depicting metabolites and genetic factors involved in the hepatic uptake, metabolism, and excretion of simvastatin. See www.pharmgkb.org/pathway/PA145011109 for further information. **e** Overview of the aggregated frequencies of common (MAF ≥ 1%, blue) and rare deleterious genetic variants (MAF < 1%, red) in genes implicated in simvastatin ADME. Values next to the columns indicate the relative contribution of rare genetic variants. **f** Stacked column plot showing the aggregated frequency of deleterious rare variants of potential relevance for simvastatin pharmacokinetics

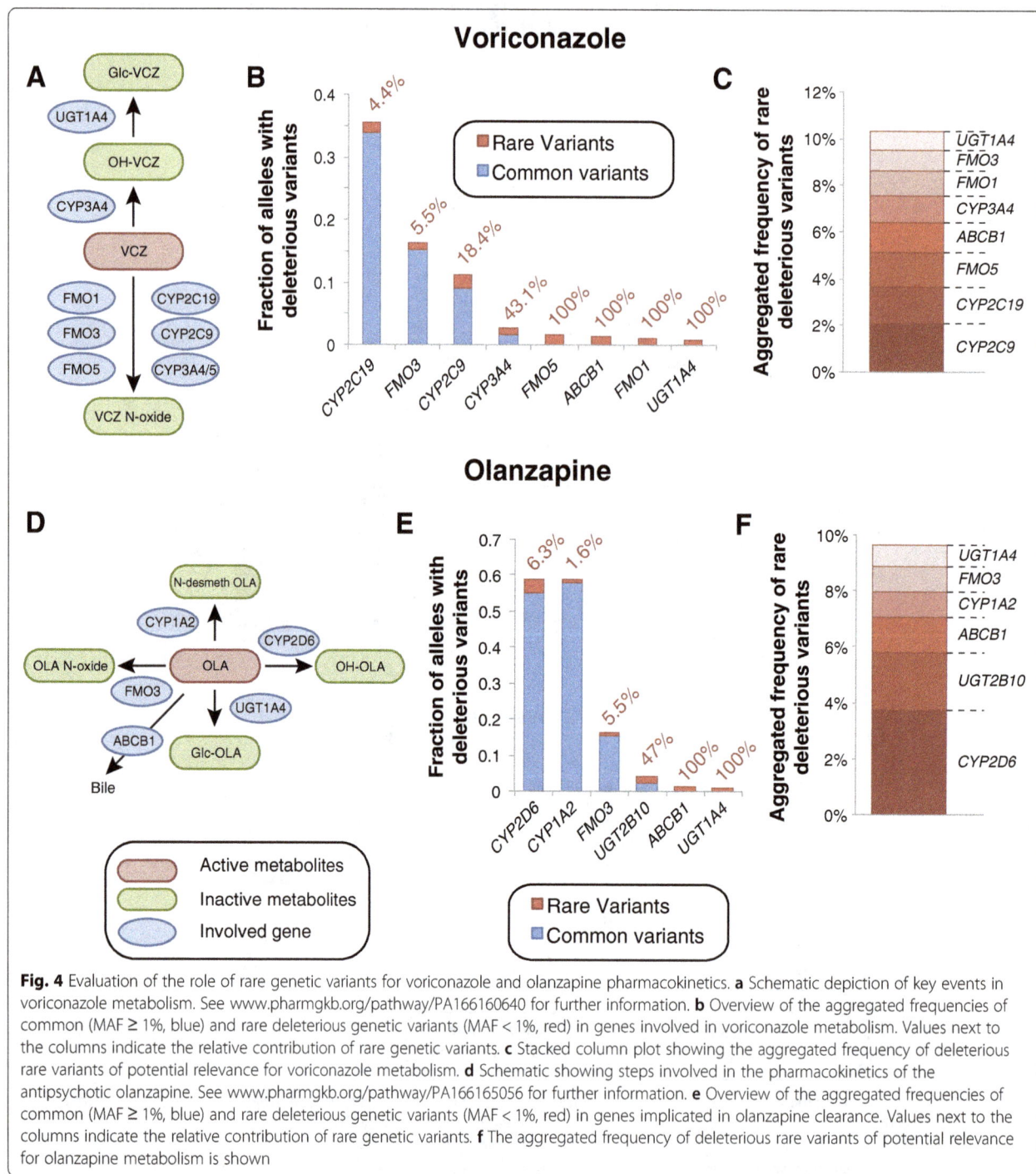

Fig. 4 Evaluation of the role of rare genetic variants for voriconazole and olanzapine pharmacokinetics. **a** Schematic depiction of key events in voriconazole metabolism. See www.pharmgkb.org/pathway/PA166160640 for further information. **b** Overview of the aggregated frequencies of common (MAF ≥ 1%, blue) and rare deleterious genetic variants (MAF < 1%, red) in genes involved in voriconazole metabolism. Values next to the columns indicate the relative contribution of rare genetic variants. **c** Stacked column plot showing the aggregated frequency of deleterious rare variants of potential relevance for voriconazole metabolism. **d** Schematic showing steps involved in the pharmacokinetics of the antipsychotic olanzapine. See www.pharmgkb.org/pathway/PA166165056 for further information. **e** Overview of the aggregated frequencies of common (MAF ≥ 1%, blue) and rare deleterious genetic variants (MAF < 1%, red) in genes implicated in olanzapine clearance. Values next to the columns indicate the relative contribution of rare genetic variants. **f** The aggregated frequency of deleterious rare variants of potential relevance for olanzapine metabolism is shown

and ADRs, including *FMO1* (100% contribution), *FMO5* (100%), *CYP3A4* (43.1%), and *CYP2C9* (18.4%; Fig. 4b, c).

Serum olanzapine levels

The therapeutic benefits for schizophrenic or bipolar patients when treated with the antipsychotic olanzapine are limited by extensive inter-individual variability in olanzapine serum concentrations, which can result in exposure levels outside the therapeutic interval [29]. As

olanzapine serum levels are directly linked to the likelihood of therapeutic success [30] and the risk of ADRs [31, 32], an individualization of dosing regimens promises to increase treatment success rates.

While the metabolism of olanzapine is well characterized, the influence of genetic factors is more controversial (Fig. 4d). CYP2D6 and UGT2B10 hydroxylate or glucuronidate olanzapine, respectively, but so far, no study demonstrated clinically relevant effects of haplotypes of these genes on olanzapine exposure. In contrast, multiple clinical association studies found that genetic variants in *CYP1A2*, *FMO3*, and *UGT1A4* could explain up to 50% of differences in olanzapine serum levels, whereas other studies failed to replicate such associations ([33] and references therein). Rare variants substantially contribute to *UGT1A4* and *UGT2B10* variability and are predicted to account for 100 and 47% of the genetically encoded inter-individual variability in the functionality of these genes (Fig. 4e, f). On the contrary, we estimate that rare variants only explain 6.3, 5.5, and 1.6% of the variability in *CYP2D6*, *FMO3*, and *CYP1A2*, respectively.

Irinotecan toxicity

Irinotecan is a topoisomerase inhibitor prodrug that is used in combination therapy for advanced colorectal, lung, and other cancers. Irinotecan has a narrow therapeutic window and, as a consequence, up to 36% of patients suffer from dose-limiting toxicities [34]. Irinotecan is subjected to a complex interplay of competing metabolic activation and inactivation pathways (Fig. 5a). Around 97% of irinotecan is metabolized by CYP3A4 and CYP3A5 to the pharmacologically inactive metabolites APC and NPC, while only 3% become metabolically activated into SN-38 by the carboxylesterases CES1 and CES2. Subsequently, SN-38 is detoxified by glucuronidation mediated by UGT1A1 and, to a lesser extent, UGT1A9. Irinotecan and its metabolites are excreted into the bile and intestine via multiple transporters of the ABC family. Importantly, the β-glucuronidase enzymes of the intestinal microflora can re-activate glucuronidated SN-38 resulting in diarrhea and damage to all segments of the intestine [35].

Genetic variants in *UGT1A1* have been reproducibly linked to neutropenia and diarrhea toxicity in various ethnicities and dosing regimens [36]. Furthermore, multiple polymorphisms in the transporter genes *ABCB1*, *ABCC1*, *ABCC2*, *ABCG2*, and *SLCO1B1* have been implicated in irinotecan clearance and/or risk of toxicity [37–40]. While associations between *CYP3A* genotype and irinotecan pharmacokinetics are controversial, incorporation of CYP3A activity data into dosing calculations have resulted in reduced incidence of severe neutropenia [41].

Interestingly, our computational analyses of population-scale sequencing data indicate that rare genetic variants are important factors for irinotecan activation and transport (Fig. 5b). The aggregated frequency of rare deleterious alleles in *CES1* and *CES2* were 1.5 and 0.4%, respectively, accounting for 19.6 and 100% of the functional genetic variants in these genes. Similarly, for *SLCO1B1* and *ABCC1*, 8.7 and 40.5% of all deleterious variants were assigned to rare variants, while for *ABCB1*, *ABCC2*, and *ABCG2*, no common variants with functional consequences were identified. Notably though, we do not consider here variants

with functional impacts that do not result in changes of the gene product, such as the synonymous variants rs1045642 (*ABCB1* I1145I) and rs1128503 (*ABCB1* G412G) or the UTR variant rs717620 in *ABCC2*. In contrast, inter-individual variability in UGT1A1 is primarily due to common polymorphisms, such as *UGT1A1*28*, and only an estimated 4.5% are allotted to rare SNVs.

Combined, our evaluations indicate that rare genetic variants in pharmacogenes have the potential to explain a substantial part of the unexplained genetic variability in drug metabolism phenotypes. Examples were selected for which gene-drug interactions were well studied, and we speculate that the relative importance of rare variants is even higher for less extensively characterized drugs. Furthermore, we give indications about the extent of genetically encoded functional variability that would be missed when only considering common genetic variants, thereby providing guidance for the optimal drug-specific choice of genotyping strategy.

Discussion

From a drug development perspective, an appropriate pharmacokinetic profile is of key importance to achieve the desired spatial and temporal exposure pattern of a given drug of interest. However, genetic variants in ADME genes encoding for transporters, drug-metabolizing enzymes, or nuclear receptors modulate drug pharmacokinetics and thus impact treatment efficacy and the risk of ADRs. Consequently, 190 drugs approved by the US Food and Drug Administration (FDA) and 155 drugs approved by EMA currently contain pharmacogenetic information in their labels, of which many are related to drug pharmacokinetics [42, 43]. Besides well-characterized common polymorphisms, ADME genes harbor a plethora of rare genetic variants that are not interrogated by current pharmacogenomic genotyping panels. By leveraging large-scale whole-exome sequencing data from 60,706 individuals, we present here the first analysis in which we systematically integrated information about rare genetic variability into predictions of pharmacokinetic variability (Additional file 2: Table S2).

Individual in silico functionality prediction algorithms distinguish deleterious from neutral variants with sensitivities and specificities between 60 and 90%. Furthermore, by using computational methods optimized for the evaluation of pharmacogenes with low evolutionary constraints, we were able to show that up to 92% sensitivity and 95% specificity can be achieved for loss-of-function and functionally neutral variants, respectively [13]. Furthermore, rare copy number variations in pharmacogenes, accounting for up to 1% of all loss-of-function alleles, are an additional source of genetic variability with relevance for drug metabolism phenotypes that are commonly not considered by computational functionality prediction algorithms [44].

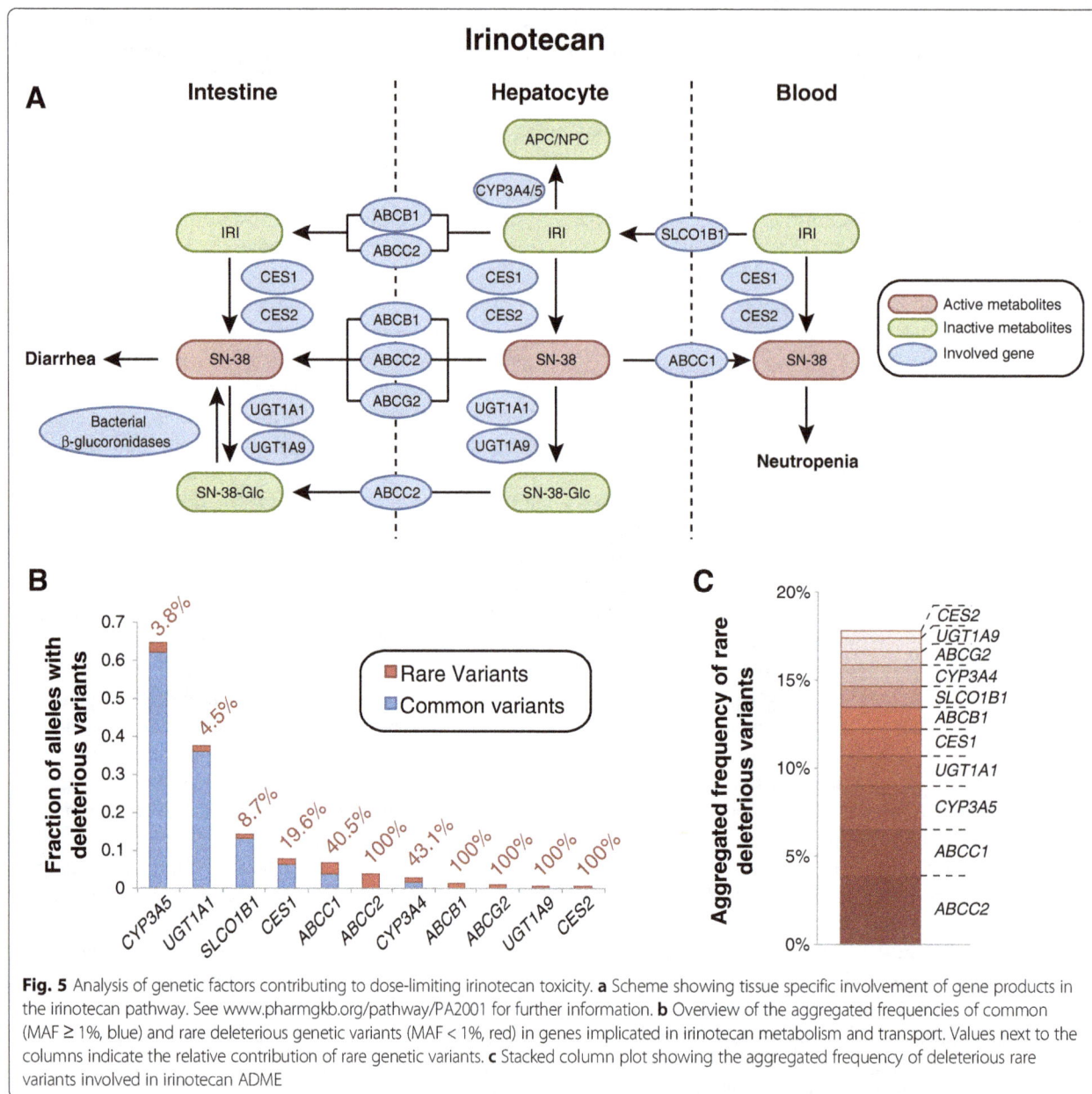

Fig. 5 Analysis of genetic factors contributing to dose-limiting irinotecan toxicity. **a** Scheme showing tissue specific involvement of gene products in the irinotecan pathway. See www.pharmgkb.org/pathway/PA2001 for further information. **b** Overview of the aggregated frequencies of common (MAF ≥ 1%, blue) and rare deleterious genetic variants (MAF < 1%, red) in genes implicated in irinotecan metabolism and transport. Values next to the columns indicate the relative contribution of rare genetic variants. **c** Stacked column plot showing the aggregated frequency of deleterious rare variants involved in irinotecan ADME

Notably, genetic variability in non-coding regions has been demonstrated to have important influence on phenotypic traits [45]. However, while promising progress has been made regarding the prediction of the effects of those variants based on DNA sequence [46], no current prediction framework can reliably predict the functionality of non-coding genetic variation, such as synonymous variants or variants located in UTRs, promoters, or enhancers. With respect to *CYP* alleles, such mutations represent < 1% of all functionally important variant alleles described (https://www.pharmvar.org/genes). We therefore restricted our analyses to the evaluation of LOF variants and variants that directly affect the amino acid sequence of their respective gene products.

Thus, while the predictive power of current functionality prediction methods is still not sufficient to support a recommendation of these tools for genetic counseling of individual patients, our data indicate however that leveraging of NGS technology can yield significant amounts of additional information for pharmacogenomic predictions on a population scale. Accordingly, we advocate for the development of a widened perspective in which conclusions about the functionality of a gene product are not solely based on the interrogation of few common variants. Rather, we recommend that the entire spectrum of genetic variability, including rare or novel variants, should be considered and integrated into gene activity scores. This holistic perspective is especially important as rare polymorphisms are enriched in variants that alter the functionality of the gene product and are the sole genetic factors for variability of more than 50% of the pharmacogenes analyzed (Fig. 2b).

Relating the functional inventory of pharmacogenetic variability to the pharmacology of selected drugs of interest can provide important insights into predicted hotspots of unexplained inter-individual differences in drug metabolism-related phenotypes. In this work, we estimated the relative contribution of rare genetic variants to the variability in pharmacokinetics and/or ADR risk of five clinically important drugs from different therapeutic areas. Rare variants are estimated to contribute significantly to the inter-individual variability of warfarin pharmacokinetics and irinotecan toxicity accounting for 18.4% of deleterious $CYP2C9$ alleles and > 40% of the variability in irinotecan transport (Figs. 3a and 5). In contrast, the relative importance of rare variants is expected to be lower for the metabolism of simvastatin, voriconazole, and olanzapine for which rare variants only contribute between 1.6 and 8.7% of the key metabolic and/or transport processes. Thus, we find that the relevance of rare genetic variants is highly drug-specific, depending on the gene products involved. These findings suggest that it is likely that the inter-individual variability in pharmacokinetics and response for certain drugs is to a large extent determined by rare genetic variability, which is important to consider particularly in drug development. Integrating pharmacological information of the drug of interest with information about the distribution of rare variants in pharmacogenes can guide the design of the genotyping strategy most suitable to reveal important additional genetic factors that improve the prediction of drug metabolism phenotypes.

For many drugs, genetic variability cannot be directly translated into effectiveness or ADR susceptibility due to the interdependency of different metabolic pathways. For instance, genetic or pharmacological inhibition of the major pathway of a given drug can result in a shunt to an alternative otherwise negligible metabolic route, as observed for oxycodone [47]. To date, data regarding the effects of such gene-gene or gene-drug interactions is sparse, which complicates predictions of drug effectiveness or safety even when rare genetic variants are incorporated into the analyses. Thus, while the consideration of pharmacogenomic information including rare genetic variants promises to improve ADME predictions, further work particularly in physiologically based pharmacokinetic (PBPK) modeling is necessary to reliably predict treatment outcomes for the individual patient.

Currently, genotyping is largely based on the interrogation of well-characterized, common polymorphisms. This strategy neglects the impacts of rare variants as experimental in vitro or in vivo data that demonstrate their functional impact is not available. Yet, due to rapidly decreasing sequencing times and costs, we suggest that current NGS technology in combination with more advanced computational prediction methods could already today facilitate the refinement of individualized predictions regarding drug efficacy and its propensity to cause ADRs and thereby to contribute to the implementation of pharmacogenetic markers into routine care [48, 49]. Furthermore, the multitude of ongoing sequencing projects on unprecedented scale, such as the 100K Genomes Project run by the British Department of Health and the 1 Million Genomes project as part of the Chinese Precision Medicine Initiative, will soon provide a wealth of information about non-transcribed, regulatory regions and improve linkage information between variants, which will allow to expand the scope of computational analyses from variants to haplotypes. For the field of pharmacogenomics, these developments hold promise to further increase the predictive power of gene-drug response predictions and to allow more accurate estimates of drug response across more narrowly stratified subpopulations.

Conclusions

We present results suggesting that integration of rare pharmacogenomic variability can improve predictions of drug pharmacokinetics compared to the use of candidate variants. This information is important for drug development and clinical care as well as for future preemptive pharmacogenomic advice. Furthermore, these data incentivize the design of prospective trials using NGS-based genotyping for specific medications, such as warfarin and irinotecan, to assess whether clinical outcomes can be improved.

Acknowledgements
The authors would like to thank the Exome Aggregation Consortium and the groups that provided exome variant data for comparison.

Funding
This study was supported by the European Union's Horizon 2020 research and innovation program U-PGx (grant agreement no. 668353), by the Swedish Research Council (grant agreement numbers 2015-02760, 2016-01153, and 2016-01154), and by the Lennart Philipson Foundation.

Authors' contributions
MI-S and VML designed the study. YZ collected the exome sequencing data. VML devised and conducted the data analysis. SM, MI-S, and VML wrote the manuscript. All authors discussed and agreed on the final version of the manuscript.

Competing interests
The authors declare that they have no competing interests.

References

1. Lauschke VM, Ingelman-Sundberg M. The importance of patient-specific factors for hepatic drug response and toxicity. Int J Mol Sci. 2016;17(10): 1714–27. https://doi.org/10.3390/ijms17101714.

2. Pirmohamed M, James S, Meakin S, et al. Adverse drug reactions as cause of admission to hospital: prospective analysis of 18 820 patients. BMJ. 2004; 329(7456):15–9. https://doi.org/10.1136/bmj.329.7456.15.

3. Sim SC, Kacevska M, Ingelman-Sundberg M. Pharmacogenomics of drug-metabolizing enzymes: a recent update on clinical implications and endogenous effects. Pharmacogenomics J. 2012;13(1):1–11. https://doi.org/10.1038/tpj.2012.45.

4. Matthaei J, Brockmöller J, Tzvetkov MV, et al. Heritability of metoprolol and torsemide pharmacokinetics. Clin Pharmacol Ther. 2015;98(6):611–21. https://doi.org/10.1002/cpt.258.

5. Lauschke VM, Milani L, Ingelman-Sundberg M. Pharmacogenomic biomarkers for improved drug therapy-recent progress and future developments. AAPS J. 2017;20(1):4. https://doi.org/10.1208/s12248-017-0161-x.

6. Singh RR, Luthra R, Routbort MJ, et al. Implementation of next generation sequencing in clinical molecular diagnostic laboratories: advantages, challenges and potential. Exp Rev Precision Med Drug Dev. 2016;1(1):109–20. https://doi.org/10.1080/23808993.2015.1120401.

7. Gordon AS, Tabor HK, Johnson AD, et al. Quantifying rare, deleterious variation in 12 human cytochrome P450 drug-metabolism genes in a large-scale exome dataset. Hum Mol Genet. 2014;23(8):1957–63. https://doi.org/10.1093/hmg/ddt588.

8. Fujikura K, Ingelman-Sundberg M, Lauschke VM. Genetic variation in the human cytochrome P450 supergene family. Pharmacogenet Genomics. 2015;25(12):584–94. https://doi.org/10.1097/FPC.0000000000000172.

9. Kozyra M, Ingelman-Sundberg M, Lauschke VM. Rare genetic variants in cellular transporters, metabolic enzymes, and nuclear receptors can be important determinants of interindividual differences in drug response. Genet Med. 2017;19(1):20–9. https://doi.org/10.1038/gim.2016.33.

10. Bush WS, Crosslin DR, Owusu-Obeng A, et al. Genetic variation among 82 pharmacogenes: the PGRNseq data from the eMERGE network. Clin Pharmacol Ther. 2016;100(2):160–9. https://doi.org/10.1002/cpt.350.

11. Lek M, Karczewski KJ, Minikel EV, et al. Analysis of protein-coding genetic variation in 60,706 humans. Nature. 2016;536(7616):285–91. https://doi.org/10.1038/nature19057.

12. Abecasis GR, Chakravarti A, Donnelly P, et al. A global reference for human genetic variation. Nature. 2015;526(7571):68–74. https://doi.org/10.1038/nature15393.

13. Zhou Y, Mkrtchian S, Kumondai M, et al. An optimized prediction framework to assess the functional impact of pharmacogenetic variants. Pharmacogenomics J. (In review)

14. Nelson MR, Wegmann D, Ehm MG, et al. An abundance of rare functional variants in 202 drug target genes sequenced in 14,002 people. Science. 2012;337(6090):100–4. https://doi.org/10.1126/science.1217876.

15. Tennessen JA, Bigham AW, O'Connor TD, et al. Evolution and functional impact of rare coding variation from deep sequencing of human exomes. Science. 2012;337(6090):64–9. https://doi.org/10.1126/science.1219240.

16. Johnson JA, Cavallari LH. Warfarin pharmacogenetics. Trends Cardiovasc Med. 2015;25(1):33–41. https://doi.org/10.1016/j.tcm.2014.09.001.

17. Kaminsky LS, Zhang Z-Y. Human P450 metabolism of warfarin. Pharmacol Ther. 1997;73(1):67–74. https://doi.org/10.1016/s0163-7258(96)00140-4.

18. Wadelius M, Sörlin K, Wallerman O, et al. Warfarin sensitivity related to CYP2C9, CYP3A5, ABCB1 (MDR1) and other factors. Pharmacogenomics J. 2003;4(1):40–8. https://doi.org/10.1038/sj.tpj.6500220.

19. Pautas E, Moreau C, Gouin-Thibault I, et al. Genetic factors (VKORC1, CYP2C9, EPHX1, and CYP4F2) are predictor variables for warfarin response in very elderly, frail inpatients. Clin Pharmacol Ther. 2009;87(1):57–64. https://doi.org/10.1038/clpt.2009.178.

20. The International Warfarin Pharmacogenetics Consortium, Klein TE, Altman RB, et al. Estimation of the warfarin dose with clinical and pharmacogenetic data. N Engl J Med. 2009;360(8):753–64. https://doi.org/10.1056/NEJMoa0809329.

21. Hodges LM, Markova SM, Chinn LW, et al. Very important pharmacogene summary: ABCB1 (MDR1, P-glycoprotein). Pharmacogenet Genomics. 2011; 21(3):152–61. https://doi.org/10.1097/FPC.0b013e3283385a1c.

22. SEARCH Collaborative Group, Link E, Parish S, et al. SLCO1B1 variants and statin-induced myopathy—a genomewide study. N Engl J Med. 2008;359(8): 789–99. https://doi.org/10.1056/NEJMoa0801936.

23. Kobayashi M, Chisaki I, Narumi K, et al. Association between risk of myopathy and cholesterol-lowering effect: a comparison of all statins. Life Sci. 2008;82(17–18):969–75. https://doi.org/10.1016/j.lfs.2008.02.019.

24. Hyland R, Jones BC, Smith DA. Identification of the cytochrome P450 enzymes involved in the N-oxidation of voriconazole. Drug Metab Dispos. 2003;31(5):540–7.

25. Yanni SB, Annaert PP, Augustijns P, et al. Role of flavin-containing monooxygenase in oxidative metabolism of voriconazole by human liver microsomes. Drug Metab Dispos. 2008;36(6):1119–25. https://doi.org/10.1124/dmd.107.019646.

26. Owusu Obeng A, Egelund EF, Alsultan A, et al. CYP2C19 polymorphisms and therapeutic drug monitoring of voriconazole: are we ready for clinical implementation of pharmacogenomics? Pharmacotherapy. 2014;34(7):703–18. https://doi.org/10.1002/phar.1400.

27. Niwa T, Hata T. The effect of genetic polymorphism on the inhibition of azole antifungal agents against CYP2C9-mediated metabolism. J Pharm Sci. 2016;105(3):1345–8. https://doi.org/10.1016/j.xphs.2016.01.007.

28. He HR, Sun JY, Ren XD, et al. Effects of CYP3A4 polymorphisms on the plasma concentration of voriconazole. Eur J Clin Microbiol Infect Dis. 2014; 34(4):811–9. https://doi.org/10.1007/s10096-014-2294-5.

29. Patel MX, Bowskill S, Couchman L, et al. Plasma olanzapine in relation to prescribed dose and other factors. J Clin Psychopharmacol. 2011;31(4):411–7. https://doi.org/10.1097/JCP.0b013e318221b408.

30. Perry PJ, Lund BC, Sanger T, et al. Olanzapine plasma concentrations and clinical response: acute phase results of the North American Olanzapine Trial. J Clin Psychopharmacol. 2001;21(1):14–20.

31. Perry PJ, Argo TR, Carnahan RM, et al. The association of weight gain and olanzapine plasma concentrations. J Clin Psychopharmacol. 2005;25(3):250–4. https://doi.org/10.1097/01.jcp.0000162800.64378.82.

32. Kinon BJ, Volavka J, Stauffer V, et al. Standard and higher dose of olanzapine in patients with schizophrenia or schizoaffective disorder. J Clin Psychopharmacol. 2008;28(4):392–400. https://doi.org/10.1097/JCP.0b013e31817e63a5.

33. Söderberg MM, Dahl M-L. Pharmacogenetics of olanzapine metabolism. Pharmacogenomics. 2013;14(11):1319–36. https://doi.org/10.2217/pgs.13.120.

34. Fuchs CS, Moore MR, Harker G, et al. Phase III comparison of two irinotecan dosing regimens in second-line therapy of metastatic colorectal cancer. J Clin Oncol. 2003;21(5):807–14. https://doi.org/10.1200/JCO.2003.08.058.

35. Brandi G, Dabard J, Raibaud P, et al. Intestinal microflora and digestive toxicity of irinotecan in mice. Clin Cancer Res. 2006;12(4):1299–307. https://doi.org/10.1158/1078-0432.CCR-05-0750.

36. Campbell JM, Stephenson MD, Bateman E, et al. Irinotecan-induced toxicity pharmacogenetics: an umbrella review of systematic reviews and meta-analyses. Pharmacogenomics J. 2017;17(1):21–8. https://doi.org/10.1038/tpj.2016.58.

37. Han J-Y, Lim H-S, Yoo Y-K, et al. Associations of ABCB1, ABCC2, and ABCG2 polymorphisms with irinotecan-pharmacokinetics and clinical outcome in patients with advanced non-small cell lung cancer. Cancer. 2007;110(1):138–47. https://doi.org/10.1002/cncr.22760.

38. Han J-Y, Lim H-S, Park YH, et al. Integrated pharmacogenetic prediction of irinotecan pharmacokinetics and toxicity in patients with advanced non-small cell lung cancer. Lung Cancer. 2009;63(1):115–20. https://doi.org/10.1016/j.lungcan.2007.12.003.

39. Innocenti F, Kroetz DL, Schuetz E, et al. Comprehensive pharmacogenetic analysis of irinotecan neutropenia and pharmacokinetics. J Clin Oncol. 2009; 27(16):2604–14. https://doi.org/10.1200/JCO.2008.20.6300.

40. Li M, Seiser EL, Baldwin RM, et al. ABC transporter polymorphisms are associated with irinotecan pharmacokinetics and neutropenia. Pharmacogenomics J. 2018;18(1):35–42. https://doi.org/10.1038/tpj.2016.75.

41. van der Bol JM, Mathijssen RHJ, Creemers GJM, et al. A CYP3A4 phenotype-based dosing algorithm for individualized treatment of irinotecan. Clin Cancer Res. 2010;16(2):736–42. https://doi.org/10.1158/1078-0432.CCR-09-1526.

42. https://www.fda.gov/Drugs/ScienceResearch/ResearchAreas/Pharmacogenetics/ucm083378.htm. Accessed 20 May 2017.

43. Ehmann F, Caneva L, Prasad K, et al. Pharmacogenomic information in drug labels: European Medicines Agency perspective. Pharmacogenomics J. 2015; 15(3):201–10. https://doi.org/10.1038/tpj.2014.86.

44. Santos M, Niemi M, Hiratsuka M, et al. Novel copy-number variations in pharmacogenes contribute to interindividual differences in drug pharmacokinetics. Genet Med. 2017; https://doi.org/10.1038/gim.2017.156. [Epub ahead of print]

45. Maurano MT, Humbert R, Rynes E, et al. Systematic localization of common disease-associated variation in regulatory DNA. Science. 2012;337(6099): 1190–5. https://doi.org/10.1126/science.1222794.

46. Lee D, Gorkin DU, Baker M, et al. A method to predict the impact of regulatory variants from DNA sequence. Nat Genet. 2015;47(8):955–61. https://doi.org/10.1038/ng.3331.

47. Samer CF, Daali Y, Wagner M, et al. The effects of CYP2D6 and CYP3A activities on the pharmacokinetics of immediate release oxycodone. Br J Pharmacol. 2010;160(4):907–18. https://doi.org/10.1111/j.1476-5381.2010.00673.x.

48. Lauschke VM, Ingelman-Sundberg M. How to consider rare genetic variants in personalized drug therapy. Clin Pharmacol Ther. 2018;19:20. https://doi.org/10.1002/cpt.976.

49. Lauschke VM, Ingelman-Sundberg M. Precision medicine and rare genetic variants. Trends Pharmacol Sci. 2016;37(2):85–6. https://doi.org/10.1016/j.tips.2015.10.006.

50. Spitzer M, Wildenhain J, Rappsilber J, et al. BoxPlotR: a web tool for generation of box plots. Nat Methods. 2014;11(2):121–2. https://doi.org/10.1038/nmeth.2811.

10

Long non-coding RNAs as novel players in β cell function and type 1 diabetes

Aashiq H. Mirza[1,2,3], Simranjeet Kaur[1] and Flemming Pociot[1,2,3*] (iD)

Abstract

Background: Long non-coding RNAs (lncRNAs) are a sub-class within non-coding RNA repertoire that have emerged as crucial regulators of the gene expression in various pathophysiological conditions. lncRNAs display remarkable versatility and wield their functions through interactions with RNA, DNA, or proteins. Accumulating body of evidence based on multitude studies has highlighted the role of lncRNAs in many autoimmune and inflammatory diseases, including type 1 diabetes (T1D).

Main body of abstract: This review highlights emerging roles of lncRNAs in immune and islet β cell function as well as some of the challenges and opportunities in understanding the pathogenesis of T1D and its complications.

Conclusion: We accentuate that the lncRNAs within T1D-loci regions in consort with regulatory variants and enhancer clusters orchestrate the chromatin remodeling in β cells and thereby act as cis/trans-regulatory determinants of islet cell transcriptional programs.

Keywords: Long non-coding RNAs, Type 1 diabetes, Enhancers, Regulatory elements, 3D genome architecture

Background

Type 1 diabetes (T1D) is a chronic immune-mediated disease resulting from selective destruction of insulin-producing pancreatic islet β cells. A complex interplay between several environmental and genetic risk factors contribute to the onset of T1D [1, 2]. Defects in both immune system and β cells play an active role in T1D pathogenesis [3]. In recent years, efforts have been accelerated to gain insights into the molecular mechanisms of pathogenesis of T1D and to determine how genetic loci contribute to the T1D risk [1, 4]. Based on genome-wide association studies (GWAS), currently more than 50 genomic risk loci have been identified for T1D [2, 5–7]. Approximately, 50% of the genetic risk for T1D is known to reside within the human leukocyte antigen (HLA) region; however, other non-HLA disease susceptibility loci have been identified based on their direct influence on the risk. Some of the well-established candidate genes in the non-HLA risk loci including *INS* (11p15), *CTLA4* (2q33),

PTPN22 (1p13), *PTPN2* (18p11), *ERBB3* (12q13), *IL2RA* (10p15), and *IFIH1* (2q24) have been associated with immune response, insulin expression, and β cell function [1, 4, 8]. The risk alleles for several T1D susceptibility genes are not exclusively confined to T1D but have been shown to confer risk in other prevalent autoimmune disorders, including multiple sclerosis (MS), systemic lupus erythematosus (SLE), and rheumatoid arthritis (RA) [7]. Furthermore, most of these risk variants are located in non-coding genomic regions including long non-coding RNAs (lncRNAs) and are enriched in distal regulatory elements such as enhancers and promoters. Non-coding variants affecting regulatory elements have the potential to perturb chromatin folding leading to mis-expression of the target gene. These facts suggest that the regulatory landscape of human genome plays an important role in pathology of a disease and newer approaches are needed to identify putative regulatory risk variants affecting gene regulation and immune function.

Recent advances in our understanding of lncRNA biology has offered new perspectives on gene regulation and has allowed us to unveil the regulatory potential of these versatile molecules in a spectrum of biological processes and pathologies, including autoimmune and inflammatory disorders. High-throughput technologies such as ChIP-

* Correspondence: flemming.pociot.01@regionh.dk
[1]CPH-DIRECT, Department of Pediatrics, Herlev University Hospital, Herlev Ringvej 75, DK-2730 Herlev, Denmark
[2]Faculty of Health and Medical Sciences, University of Copenhagen, Copenhagen, Denmark
Full list of author information is available at the end of the article

seq and chromosome conformation capture techniques have also opened new possibilities to investigate in detail potential regulatory roles of non-coding genome in gene regulation and 3D chromatin folding. In this review, we discuss the recent discoveries in the field of lncRNAs, regulatory elements, 3D genome architecture, and their implications for T1D and β cell function. We further highlight the role of active enhancers associated with T1D–loci lncRNAs and protein-coding genes in regulating β cell gene expression programs through both *cis*- and *trans*-regulatory mechanisms involving structural remodeling of chromatin in human islets.

Main text

lncRNAs in T1D and other immune-mediated diseases

lncRNAs are non-coding RNAs that are more than 200 nucleotides in length, and are capped, polyadenylated, and spliced like their well-characterized "cousins," protein-coding transcripts, with one exception; lncRNAs do not code for proteins [9]. Most of the lncRNAs are expressed in a cell-specific manner and are usually expressed in lower abundance than the protein-coding transcripts. In terms of genomic location, lncRNAs have been often categorized as long intergenic non-coding RNAs (lincRNAs), intronic lncRNAs, antisense lncRNAs, divergent lncRNAs and enhancer-derived lncRNAs (lncRNAs arising from enhancer-like regions) [10–12] (Fig. 1). lncRNAs have

emerged as important players of gene regulation and have been implicated in various human pathologies [13]. lncRNAs regulate various cellular and biological processes including heterochromatin formation, histone modifications, DNA methylation targeting, and gene silencing [14, 15]. The lncRNA-recruited regulatory complexes orchestrate development and differentiation of various immune cell lineages and actively regulate expression programs within these cells.

Multiple studies have highlighted the potential roles of lncRNAs in pancreatic islets and T1D pathogenesis [10, 16, 17]. Based on transcriptome profiling studies of islets and β cells, more than 1000 islet-specific lncRNAs have been identified in both human and mouse islets [18, 19]. The ability of lncRNAs to regulate gene expression and cell-specific identity provides an exciting opportunity to advance our understanding of T1D pathogenesis. Table 1 lists examples of lncRNAs that have been implicated in β cell function and T1D. lncRNA *MALAT1* has been associated with diabetes-induced microvascular dysfunction in STZ-induced diabetic rats and db/db mice [20]. Knockdown of *MALAT1* prevents the hyper-proliferation of retinal endothelial cells through p38 MAPK signaling and might serve as a potential target for anti-angiogenic therapy for diabetic retinopathy. lncRNA *MEG3* has been associated with paternally inherited risk of T1D [21] and its downregulation affects

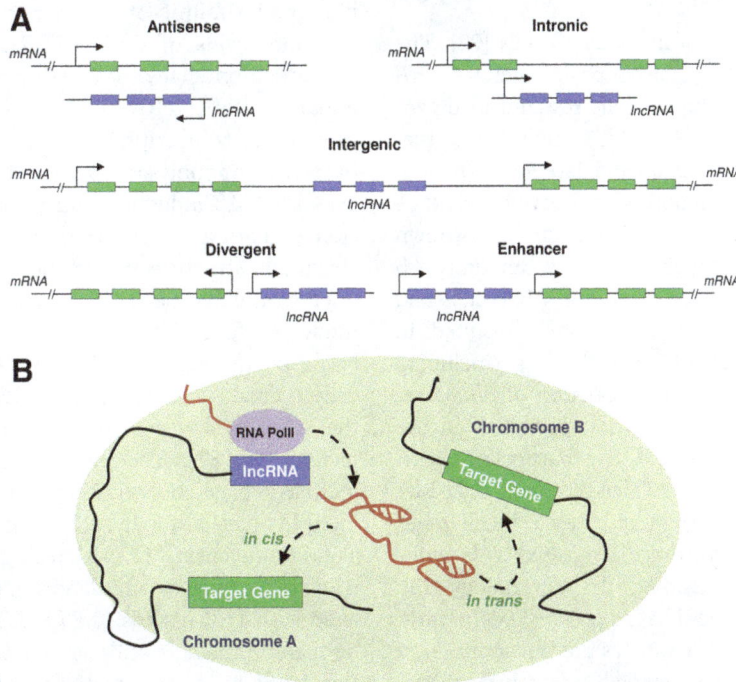

Fig. 1 Bio-types of lncRNAs and enhancer-derived lncRNA function. **a** Different bio-types of lncRNAs based on their genomic location include antisense, intergenic, intronic, divergent and enhancer-derived lncRNAs. lncRNAs are depicted in *blue*, while protein-coding genes are shown in *green*. **b** The postulated role of enhancer-derived lncRNAs for both *cis*- and *trans*-mediated regulation of target genes is shown via chromatin loop formation. Figure modified from Ref. [10, 11]

Table 1 lncRNAs associated with β cell function and type 1 diabetes

lncRNAs	Function	Reference
MEG3	Regulates β cell identity and function via insulin production and apoptosis in mouse MIN6 cells and isolated mouse islets	You et al. 2016 [22]
HI-LNC25	Positively regulates GLIS3 (which contains both T1D and T2D risk variants) in EndoC-βH1 human β cell line	Moran et al. 2012 [18]
βlinc1 (HI-LNC15)	Regulates β cell identity and function in mouse MIN6 cells and EndoC-βH1 human β cell line; also regulates its neighboring gene NKX2.2 (an islet transcription factor).	Arnes et al. 2016 [23]
TUNAR (HI-LNC78)	Knockdown of TUNAR leads to impaired glucose-stimulated insulin secretion in human islets	Akerman et al. 2017 [24]
PLUT (HI-LNC71)	Regulates transcription of PDX1, a key pancreatic β cell transcriptional regulator, in EndoC-βH1 cells, primary islet cells, mouse β cell line MIN6	Akerman et al. 2017 [24]
MALAT1	Upregulation of MALAT1 is associated with microvascular dysfunction (diabetic retinopathy) in STZ-induced diabetic rats and db/db mice	Liu et al. 2014 [20]
TUG1	Downregulation of lncRNA TUG1 expression increased apoptosis and reduced insulin secretion in mouse β cells	Yin et al. 2015 [25]

insulin synthesis and secretion in mouse β cells [22]. The knockdown of *trans*-acting islet-specific lncRNA *HI-LNC25 (LINC01370)* in mature β cells resulted in downregulation of *GLIS3* gene [18]. *GLIS3* encodes an islet transcription factor (TF) and is a candidate gene for both type 1 and type 2 diabetes. Another islet-specific lncRNA *βlinc1* (previously known as *HI-LNC15*) has been shown to be essential for proper specification and function of β cells [23]. Knockdown of *βlinc1* in mouse MIN6 cells and human insulin-producing EndoC-βH1 cells resulted in downregulation of several islet-specific TFs, including Nkx2.2, Pax6, and Mafb [23]. Also, deletion of *βlinc1* resulted in defective islet development and disrupted glucose homeostasis in the adult mice [23]. It is particularly intriguing that *βlinc1* specifically regulates three essential islet TFs (Nkx2.2, Pax6, and MafB) and additional β cell genes on chromosome 2, all of which are associated with endocrine development and maintaining islet morphology [23]. Nuclear-enriched β cell lncRNA *PLUTO (PLUT)* (previously known as *HI-LNC71*) regulates the transcription of *PDX1* gene which is a key pancreatic β cell transcriptional regulator [24]. *PLUT* encompasses a cluster of enhancers that make 3D contacts with the *PDX1* promoter in human islets and in human β cell line EndoC-βH1. Loss of *PLUT* was associated with downregulation of *PDX1* at both

mRNA and protein levels in EndoC-βH1 cells, primary islet cells, and a similar effect was observed for the mouse lncRNA ortholog in mouse β cell line MIN6 [24]. Knockdown of lncRNA *TUNAR (HI-LNC78)* resulted in reduced insulin content and impaired glucose-stimulated insulin secretion in T antigen-excised EndoC-βH3 cells [24]. lncRNA *TUG1* is a highly conserved lncRNA in mammals and is highly expressed in mouse pancreatic tissues [25]. In mouse β cells, downregulation of *TUG1* as a consequence of hyperglycemia resulted in increased apoptosis and reduced insulin synthesis and secretion [25]. These findings suggest that *TUG1* may partially contribute to the impairment of β cell function and could therefore be implicated in diabetes pathogenesis.

In recent years, growing body of evidence has linked dysregulation of lncRNA expression to a spectrum of autoimmune disease [26, 27]. Hrdlickova and colleagues found enrichment of lincRNAs in autoimmune disease-associated loci in a subset of immune cells [28]. A number of studies describe the emerging role of lncRNAs in transcriptional regulation of inflammatory gene expression [29, 30]. For example, in human monocytes, lncRNA *THRIL* has been shown to interact with hnRNP-L and regulate the expression of *TNFα* [31]. Correspondingly, additional examples of lncRNAs involvement in inflammatory signaling cascades and regulation of innate immune responses includes (1) lncRNA *PACER (PACERR)* which has been shown to bind p50 subunit of *NFκB* and control the basal expression levels of *Cox2 (PTGS2)* [32]; (2) in primary human monocytes, knockdown of *NFκB* regulated, enhancer-RNA (eRNA) *IL1β-eRNA* and region of bidirectional transcription (RBT) IL1β-RBT46, mitigated bacterial lipopolysaccharide (LPS) pro-inflammatory cytokine IL1β induction and release [33]; (3) overexpression of natural antisense transcript anti-IL1β alters the chromatin structure around the IL1β promoter and consequently inhibits the IL1β expression [34, 35]. In a murine model, lncRNA *NeST* (Nettoie Salmonella pas Theiler's; *cleanup Salmonella not Theiler's*) was shown to epigenetically regulate the interferon-γ (IFN-γ) locus and control the susceptibility to Theiler's virus and Salmonella infection [36, 37]. Together, these findings indicate that lncRNAs play etiological role in autoimmune diseases. lncRNAs have also been shown to play pivotal roles in the Toll-like receptor (TLR) signaling pathway. For example, when macrophages and dendritic cells (DCs) were stimulated with TLR ligands, the *lincRNA-Cox2A* was found to be highly inducible and also controlled the basal expression levels of interferon-stimulated genes (ISGs) and proinflammatory cytokines [29]. Intriguingly, pseudogenes lncRNAs have been identified to act as functional regulators of inflammatory signaling with their expression being actively regulated. Stimulation of mouse embryonic fibroblast cells by *TNFα* has been found to induce expression of lncRNAs. *Lethe*, a pseudogene lncRNA, has been shown to function as a novel negative regulator of *NF-κB*. *Lethe*, wields its regulatory function by binding directly RelA, a subunit of *NF-κB* heterodimeric complex, preclude *NF-κB* binding to the promoter regions of target genes [38]. Another pseudogene lncRNA Lnc-dendritic cell (*DC*) (*WFDC21P*) has been shown to be involved in monocyte to DC differentiation [39].

Systemic cell-mediated immunity is known to play a central role in the apoptotic β cell destruction that culminates in T1D. The T helper 17 (Th17) cells are known to protect mucosal barriers from opportunistic infections and are also associated with number of autoimmune inflammatory diseases. Like many other autoimmune diseases, T1D is also a T cell-mediated malady, and imbalance between the Th17 cells and T regulatory (Treg) has been implicated in development of the T1D [40, 41]. Recently, Huang et al. [42] demonstrated role of DEAD-box protein 5 (DDX5) as a binding partner of RORγt, a well-known ligand-regulated nuclear receptor that controls the differentiation of Th17 cells. Interestingly, DDX5 coordinates the transcription of selective Th17 genes through its interaction with RORγt, and it is also required for Th17 cell-mediated inflammatory diseases. The interaction between DDX5 and RORγt is dependent on the inherent RNA helicase activity of DDX5 and the binding of Rmrp, an evolutionarily conserved nuclear lncRNA. Furthermore, Rmrp was found mutated in patients with cartilage-hair hypoplasia, and corresponding mutation in Rmrp in mice resulted in altered chromatin interaction, and diminished interaction between the DDX5 and RORγt, and also downregulated expression of selective Th-17 genes [42].

These examples highlight the importance of lncRNAs in regulating gene expression in immune cells and underscore yet another layer of complexity in gene regulation. Future studies should be focused towards elucidating their molecular functions which in turn could provide crucial insights into novel mechanisms of gene regulation, autoimmune and inflammation-mediated disorders, including T1D.

Genome-wide interactions between T1D SNPs, lncRNAs, enhancers, and other distal regulatory elements

More than 90% of disease-associated single-nucleotide polymorphisms (SNPs) are located within the non-coding regions of the genome such as promoters, enhancers, intergenic regions, and ncRNA genes [43]. The disease-associated SNPs have the potential to be regulatory in nature, particularly if they are significantly enriched in functional regulatory elements such as transcription factor binding sites (TFBSs), histone modification marks, DNase-I hypersensitive sites, and expression quantitative

trait loci (eQTLs) [44, 45]. These disease-associated regulatory SNPs are also referred to as "functional SNPs" [44]. Approximately, 10% of the autoimmune disease-associated SNPs are present within lncRNAs and some of these SNPs are also known to act as *cis*-eQTLs [46]. It has been shown that 75% of the lincRNA *cis*-eQTLs specifically alter the expression of lincRNAs in a tissue-dependent fashion but does not affect the nearby protein-coding genes, and many of these *cis*-eQTLs SNPs are known to be associated with complex genetic diseases [47]. Since the expression of protein-coding genes can be regulated by lincRNAs either in *cis* [48] or *trans* [49] manner, this suggests a link between disease-associated SNPs within the non-coding regions with the regulation of protein-coding gene expression.

Distal regulatory elements such as enhancers, locus control regions (LCRs), and insulators are highly abundant in the human genome and play an important role in transcriptional control. These elements represent the primary mechanism by which cell and developmental specific gene expression is accomplished. Enhancers are regulatory sequences that can activate gene expression independent of their proximity to their target genes in a tissue-specific manner [50]. Multiple enhancer elements arrayed over large regions can synergistically regulate the expression of individual genes or gene clusters by altering the TF binding and chromatin states [51, 52]. Additionally, multiple polymorphisms in linkage disequilibrium (LD) impact clusters of enhancer elements active in the same cell type and cooperatively contribute to altered expression of their gene targets [53]. The multiple enhancer variants within a given locus typically target the same gene which results in either gain- or loss-of-function [53]. Additionally, the genes associated with multiple enhancer variants encode proteins that are often functionally related and enriched in common pathways. Recently, several methods have been developed for genome-wide prediction of enhancers primarily based on chromatin marks such as H3K4 monomethyl (H3K4me1) and H3K27 acetyl (H3K27ac) modifications, bi-directional transcription, and binding of p300 [54–57]. The underlying mechanism for enhancer function has been suggested to involve formation of long-range chromatin loops, bringing enhancers and promoters into proximity and allowing interaction of the necessary co-transcriptional factors [58, 59]. Formation of chromatin loops occurs between two distant genomic sequences that are brought in close vicinity by protein complexes and are assumed to be chemically cross-linked. Various chromosomal conformation capture techniques such as 3C (chromosome conformation capture) [60], 4C (circular chromosome conformation capture) [61], 5C (chromosome conformation capture carbon copy) [62], ChIA-PET (Chromatin Interaction Analysis with Paired-End-Tag sequencing)

[63], and Hi-C [64] have been used to detect genome-wide chromosome interactions. Examples of long-range interactions within mammalian gene loci include the locus control region (LCR) and β-globin promoter [65, 66]; the α-globin gene cluster in erythroid cells [67]; the TH2 and MHC loci in T cells [68, 69]; and the imprinted gene clusters Dlx5, Dlx6 [70], and H19-Igf2 [71–73]. Additional example of long-range chromatin loop mediated interaction among regulatory elements on different chromosomes has been observed at the IFNγ and TH2 cytokine loci [74]. The transcriptional regulation of IL-21 gene at the chromatin level was recently uncovered to be mediated through long-range chromatin interaction in CD4+ T cells. IL-21, a pro-inflammatory cytokine with pleiotropic effects, is strongly associated with autoimmunity and inflammation and regulates various immune responses. A study by Park et al. showed that a distal enhancer element within an evolutionary conserved non-coding sequence 49 kb upstream of the IL-21 can upregulate IL-21 gene expression in a STAT3- and NFAT-dependent manner [75]. Stimulation of CD4+ T cells with IL-6 leads to the recruitment of STAT3 to the IL-21 promoter and the distal enhancer region, bringing them in close spatial proximity. As a consequence, this long-range interaction between the promoter and distal enhancer region dependent on IL-6/STAT3 signaling pathway alters the chromatin configuration dynamically, and controls the expression of IL-21 in CD4+ T cells [75].

Based on published genome-wide chromosome conformational capture datasets from various cell-lines and T1D associated SNPs we identified physical interactions between distant regulatory regions in T1D loci. Figure 2 shows an interactive map of T1D loci highlighting the physical interactions between distal regulatory elements and potential functional T1D SNP at each locus. T1D risk SNPs and SNPs in LD (r2 > 0.8, CEU HapMap3 population) were selected and scored based on the original GWAS signal, long range chromosome interactions, overlap with chromatin marks, epigenetic modifications and sequence motifs from various ENCODE cell lines [2, 76–78]. The top most scoring SNP for each region was inferred as the most significant functional SNP and selected for plotting along with the most significant distal chromosomal interaction signal. As an example, in *ERBB3* locus, SNP rs4759229 qualified as the most significant variant. rs4759229 is in perfect LD with T1D risk SNP rs2292239, overlaps a known enhancer region and has a long range interaction signal with an antisense lncRNA *AC008079.1* (Ensembl ID: ENSG00000187979) located at USP18 locus on chromosome 22. In a recent study, we proposed that the *ERBB3* SNP rs2292239 and its proxy SNPs in perfect LD rs3741499 and rs4759229 are putatively functional based on the overlapping open chromatin marks, TFBs and DNase I hypersensitivity peaks [79]. We further showed that SNP rs4759229 overlaps a known enhancer

element and is in the vicinity of several lncRNA transcripts overlapping *ERBB3* locus. The potential functional T1D SNPs within known T1D candidate genes such as *GLIS3*, *ERBB3*, *CTRB1*, *CTSH*, *FUT2*, *IL27*, *SKAP2*, *TNFAIP3* and *PTPN2* had highly significant distal chromosomal interactions including enhancers and lncRNAs that are worthy of specific laboratory investigations (Fig. 2). Intriguingly, the impact of interactions between T1D SNPs and enhancer associated lncRNAs on transcription and ultimately on T1D risk remains to be seen. Based on the above evidence we postulate that the T1D SNPs mapping to enhancer associated lncRNAs could potentially alter the expression of their gene targets through enhancer mediated interactions and thereby significantly impact β cell gene expression.

Many lncRNAs have been reported to be expressed from the enhancer regions that are produced by activity-dependent RNA polymerase II binding of specific enhancers [80]. The expression levels of these enhancer associated lncRNAs positively correlate with the expression of neighboring protein-coding genes, i.e., depletion of enhancer associated lncRNAs led to decreased expression of their neighboring protein-coding genes [48, 80]. In addition, enhancers overlapping lncRNAs have higher H3K4me3/H3K4me1 ratios as compared to enhancers that do not overlap lncRNAs [81]. The enrichment of H3K4me3 marks (which are also associated with active promoters) points towards strong transcriptional capabilities of overlapping lncRNAs. lncRNAs transcribed from active enhancers have been identified as important players in mediating enhancer function [82]. Enhancers associated lncRNA play roles in important physiological processes and influence the activation of protein coding and non-coding genes in both *cis* and *trans* mediated mechanism. For example, lncRNA *NEST* is involved in *cis*-activation of the neighboring interferon γ locus, whereas lncRNA *Jpx* regulates *trans*-activation of another lncRNA, *XIST*, (which is critical for X inactivation) [36, 83]. While acting in *trans*, enhancer associated lncRNAs act over long distances by long range chromatin loop mediated interactions and activate transcription at distal promotors. It has also been suggested that bridging factors such as Mediator/Cohesin complex and enhancer associated lncRNAs are involved in establishment of chromatin looping between the lncRNAs and their regulated distal promotors [84]. Knockdown of either lncRNA or mediator subunits has been shown to abolish the chromosomal interactions [84].

It has been shown that islet-specific lncRNAs and TFs co-regulate genes associated with enhancer clusters [24, 85]. lncRNAs regulating enhancer cluster-associated genes bound by multiple islet-specific TFs include *HI-LNC12*, *HI-LNC15*, *HI-LNC30*, *HI-LNC78*, *HI-LNC80*, *HI-LNC85*, and *PLUT* (*HI-LNC71*) [24]. However, further studies are warranted that employ

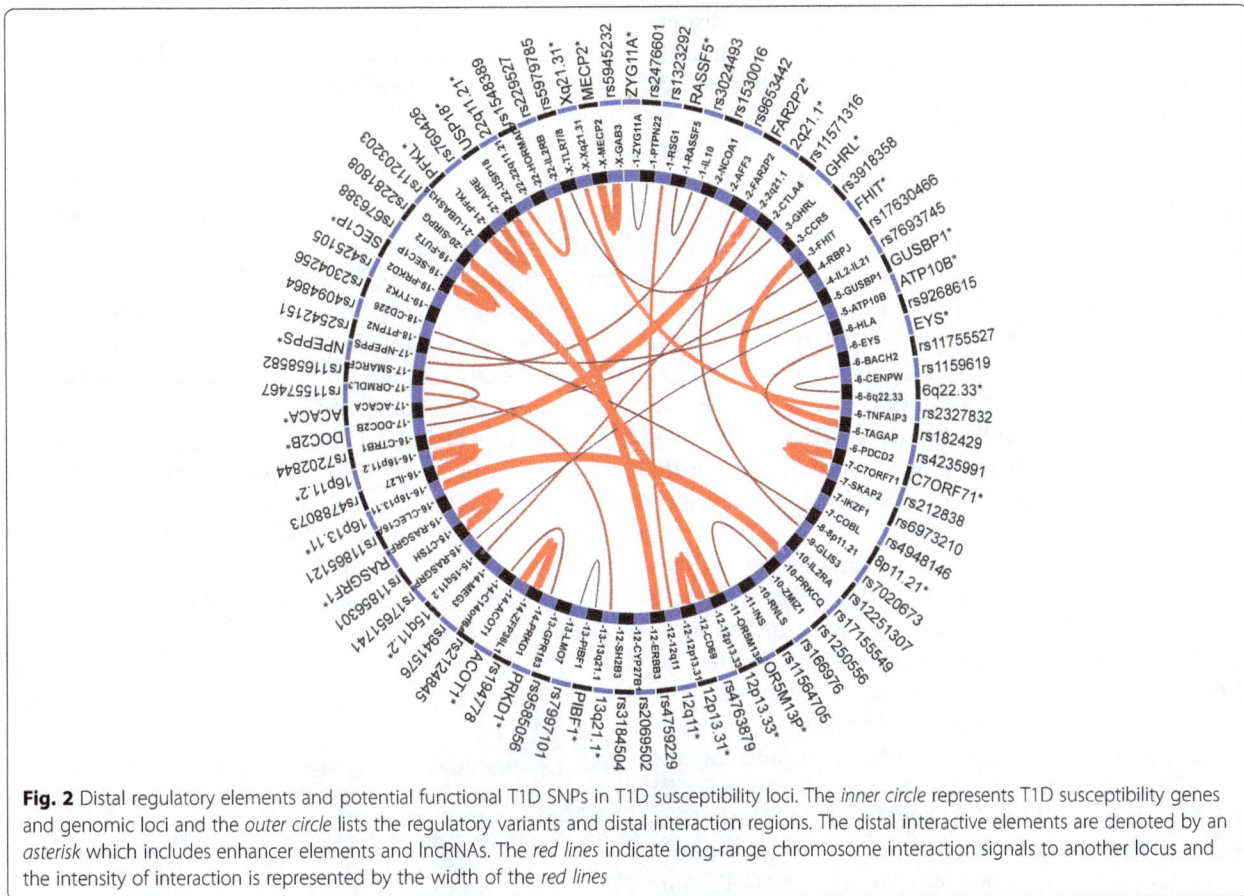

Fig. 2 Distal regulatory elements and potential functional T1D SNPs in T1D susceptibility loci. The *inner circle* represents T1D susceptibility genes and genomic loci and the *outer circle* lists the regulatory variants and distal interaction regions. The distal interactive elements are denoted by an *asterisk* which includes enhancer elements and lncRNAs. The *red lines* indicate long-range chromosome interaction signals to another locus and the intensity of interaction is represented by the width of the *red lines*

chromosomal conformation techniques to identify potential targets of enhancer associated lncRNAs in human islets.

Future challenges and opportunities

Although lncRNAs have achieved formable recognition as key players in gene regulation and disease, there is still a huge gap in our overall understanding of lncRNA regulatory functions and underlying molecular mechanisms, particularly in context of β cell function and development of T1D. The rise of lncRNAs as key regulators of gene expression during normal development and diseases has positioned these pervasive transcripts in the crosshairs of novel disease-specific biomarker discovery. The dysregulation of lncRNA expression not only represents a newfangled layer of intricacy in the molecular architecture of human malady, but it also unveils the potential to use lncRNAs as disease biomarkers. In contrast to their "cousins" mRNA transcripts, the lncRNAs themselves are functional molecules and their expression levels might serve as a better disease indicator. Moreover, expression of lncRNAs is highly tissue-specific and disease-specific which indicates that lncRNA-based expression signatures could effectively be used to accurately diagnose and classify disease. Although, the field of lncRNA-based

diagnostics is still in its infancy, the use of distinct lncRNAs in a clinical diagnostics setting has already taken off. Indeed, lncRNAs have already been suggested as potential biomarkers for a number of diseases, including cancer. For example, *PCA3*, a prostate-specific lncRNA notably overexpressed in prostate cancer, has been developed into diagnostic assay to detect prostate cancer [86]. Nevertheless, there are still many challenges ahead of us that need to be addressed in order to fully appreciate the function of lncRNAs in islet biology and T1D contexts.

Most of the functionally characterized lncRNAs exhibit modular-domain architecture that arises from their well-conserved secondary and tertiary structures and is crucial for their biological functions. This assumes importance as it illustrates the importance of the conservation at secondary and tertiary structure level rather than at primary sequence level [87–89]. Therefore, future studies are needed to identify homologous lncRNAs taking a structure-based evolutionary conservation criterion into consideration rather than relying only on the primary sequence-based conservation in cellular and subclinical models of T1D.

Although, a handful of lncRNAs have been functionally characterized, they have certainly emerged as bona fide players in regulating the gene expression at various levels during all the stages of development and disease. With the advent of next-generation sequencing technologies, thousands of lncRNA genes have already been identified and annotated in human and mouse. According to the recent GENCODE v26 (www.gencodegenes.org), more than 15,000 and 11,000 lncRNA genes have already identified in the human and mouse, respectively. In addition, FANTOM5 cap analysis of gene expression (CAGE) in primary cell types and tissues identified 27,919 human lncRNA genes with accurate 5′ termini [90]. Based on multiple lines of evidence, including genomic, epigenomic features and evolutionary conservation of the lncRNAs, 19,175 were reported as potentially functional in the human genome [90]. Surprisingly, most of the intergenic lncRNAs identified in the FANTOM5 project were transcribed from the enhancers and not from the promoters.

One of the major bottlenecks in studying the lncRNA functions has been their low steady-state levels in the cells [91]. Majority of lncRNAs are expressed at low-levels which makes it more challenging to accurately annotate their gene boundaries. The problem of incomplete annotation of lncRNAs is further compounded by the lack of typical genomic hallmarks of transcription initiation and termination that are often used as primary flag posts for defining the gene boundaries [91]. But, recently many methods have been developed and implemented to improve the annotation of lncRNAs, including RNA Capture Sequencing (CaptureSeq) [92], coupling of rapid amplification of cDNA ends (RACE) technique to long-read sequencing (RACE-Seq) [93], RNA Capture Long Seq (CLS) [94], and genome-scale CRISPR-mediated interference (CRISPRi) [95]. So far, these methods have been used for exploring the transcriptomic structure of lncRNA loci using cell or tissue types that are not relevant to diabetes. Nevertheless, these methods provide an excellent experimental framework for future studies to address the lingering questions regarding the roles and molecular mechanisms of lncRNAs in β cell function and T1D pathogenesis. Therefore, employing methods like CLS, RACE-Seq, CAGE and CRISPRi under the proinflammatory cytokines stimulation and control settings will enable to disentangle the transcriptomic landscape of β cells.

It is known that active β cells exhibit extensive allelic imbalance in gene expression [96]. However, the impact of allelic imbalance on the lncRNA expression has been not studied. A robust reassessment of the regulation of allele-specific gene expression in lncRNA loci overlapping or lying in close proximity of T1D GWAS SNPs in islets and β cells derived from cadaveric pancreas with known genotypes would be highly desirable. This could provide important clues linking disease-associated SNPs with the lncRNA expression. Furthermore, these studies have the potential to unravel the diversity of lncRNA

repertoire, including the enhancer RNAs (eRNAs) [97] and novel rare transcripts and many of which might have important functional roles in modulating the β cell function.

Conclusions

In immune-mediated and inflammatory diseases such as T1D, lncRNA-based transcriptional signatures might open new avenues for lncRNA-based diagnostics, classification or personalized therapeutic regimens in near future. Furthermore, assessment of functional implications of T1D SNPs overlapping lncRNAs and enhancers regions is highly warranted from perspective of β cell function and development of T1D. The precise biochemical characteristics and molecular basis of β- and immune cells expressed lncRNA functions are necessary to elucidate how deregulations of immune cell-specific T1D loci-associated lncRNAs, as well islet-specific lncRNAs, potentially contribute to the development of islet autoimmunity to progression of T1D.

Abbreviations
eQTL: Expression quantitative trait loci; GWAS: Genome-wide association studies; LD: Linkage disequilibrium; lncRNA: Long non-coding RNA; SNP: Single-nucleotide polymorphism; TF: Transcription factor; TFBS: Transcription factor binding site; T1D: Type 1 diabetes

Funding
Not applicable

Authors' contributions
AHM and SK researched the data and drafted and reviewed the manuscript before submission. FP made substantial contribution to discussion of the content and reviewed the manuscript before submission. All authors read and approved the final manuscript.

Authors' information
AHM is a postdoctoral fellow and received predoctoral and postdoctoral training in the laboratories of Professor Flemming Pociot (Copenhagen Diabetes Research Center, Copenhagen, Denmark), Professor Jan Gorodkin (Center for non-coding RNA in Technology and Health, Copenhagen, Denmark), and Professor Francis Barany (Sandra and Edward Meyer Cancer Center, Weill Cornell Medicine, NY, USA). AHM obtained his PhD degree in Cellular and Genetic Medicine from the University of Copenhagen, Denmark, under the supervision of Professor Jan Gorodkin and Professor Flemming Pociot. AHM's research revolves broadly around understanding the role of non-coding RNAs in autoimmune and inflammatory diseases. AHM is currently involved in development of assays and technologies for early detection of tumors using circulating cell-free nucleic acid based genetic and epigenetic biomarkers in collaboration with Professor Francis Barany and Professor Steven Soper (Department of Chemistry, University of Kansas, KS, USA).
SK is a postdoctoral fellow training in the laboratory of Professor Flemming Pociot. SK obtained her PhD degree in Biostatistics and Bioinformatics from University of Copenhagen, Denmark, under the supervision of Professor Flemming Pociot (Copenhagen Diabetes Research Center, Herlev and

Gentofte Hospital, Denmark) and Professor Henrik B. Mortensen (Department of Clinical Medicine, University of Copenhagen, Denmark). SK's research revolves broadly around understanding the role of non-coding RNAs and regulatory elements in β cell function and type 1 diabetes.

FP is a professor of Pediatrics and Clinical Medicine at Herlev and Gentofte Hospital, Denmark and University of Copenhagen, Denmark. FP received his MD from University of Copenhagen and performed his doctoral research at Steno Diabetes Center, Denmark. FP has a strong focus on clinical markers for residual β cell function and to identify early markers for type 1 diabetes risk. FP has been part of the Type 1 Diabetes Genetics Consortium (T1DGC) Steering Group, which published the largest GWAS (genome-wide association study) in T1D. FP has published more than 300 papers in peer reviewed journals accruing >14,000 citations. FP has been ranked no. 21, worldwide by cited papers within the field of Diabetes 1991–2001 and his H-index is 51.

Competing interests

The authors declare that they have no competing interests.

Author details

[1]CPH-DIRECT, Department of Pediatrics, Herlev University Hospital, Herlev Ringvej 75, DK-2730 Herlev, Denmark. [2]Faculty of Health and Medical Sciences, University of Copenhagen, Copenhagen, Denmark. [3]Center for non-coding RNA in Technology and Health, University of Copenhagen, Copenhagen, Denmark.

References

1. Pociot F, Akolkar B, Concannon P, Erlich HA, Julier C, Morahan G, et al. Genetics of type 1 diabetes: what's next? Diabetes. 2010;59:1561–71.
2. Groop L, Pociot F. Genetics of diabetes—are we missing the genes or the disease? Mol Cell Endocrinol. 2014;382:726–39.
3. Soleimanpour SA, Stoffers DA. The pancreatic β cell and type 1 diabetes: innocent bystander or active participant? Trends Endocrinol Metab. 2013;24:324–31.
4. Noble JA, Erlich HA. Genetics of type 1 diabetes. Cold Spring Harb Perspect Med. 2012;2:a007732.
5. Rich SS, Concannon P, Erlich H, Julier C, Morahan J, Nerup J, et al. The type 1 diabetes genetics consortium. Ann N Y Acad Sci. 2006;1079:1–8.
6. Barrett JC, Clayton DG, Concannon P, Akolkar B, Cooper JD, Erlich HA, et al. Genome-wide association study and meta-analysis find that over 40 loci affect risk of type 1 diabetes. Nat Genet. 2009;41:703–7.
7. Onengut-Gumuscu S, Chen W-M, Burren O, Cooper NJ, Quinlan AR, Mychaleckyj JC, et al. Fine mapping of type 1 diabetes susceptibility loci and evidence for colocalization of causal variants with lymphoid gene enhancers. Nat Genet. 2015;47:381–6.
8. Santin I, Eizirik DL. Candidate genes for type 1 diabetes modulate pancreatic islet inflammation and β-cell apoptosis. Diabetes Obes Metab. 2013;15(Suppl 3):71–81.
9. Rinn JL, Chang HY. Genome regulation by long noncoding RNAs. Annu Rev Biochem. 2012;81:145–66.
10. Knoll M, Lodish HF, Sun L. Long non-coding RNAs as regulators of the endocrine system. Nat Rev Endocrinol. 2015;11:151–60.
11. Lam MTY, Li W, Rosenfeld MG, Glass CK. Enhancer RNAs and regulated transcriptional programs. Trends Biochem Sci. 2014;39:170–82.
12. Ulitsky I, Bartel DP. lincRNAs: genomics, evolution, and mechanisms. Cell. 2013;154:26–46.
13. Fitzgerald KA, Caffrey DR. Long noncoding RNAs in innate and adaptive immunity. Curr Opin Immunol. 2014;26:140–6.
14. Khalil AM, Guttman M, Huarte M, Garber M, Raj A, Rivea Morales D, et al. Many human large intergenic noncoding RNAs associate with chromatin-modifying complexes and affect gene expression. Proc Natl Acad Sci U S A. 2009;106:11667–72.

15. Guttman M, Amit I, Garber M, French C, Lin MF, Feldser D, et al. Chromatin signature reveals over a thousand highly conserved large non-coding RNAs in mammals. Nature. 2009;458:223–7.
16. Eliasson L, Esguerra JLS. Role of non-coding RNAs in pancreatic beta-cell development and physiology. Acta Physiol (Oxf). 2014;211:273–84.
17. Motterle A, Gattesco S, Caille D, Meda P, Regazzi R. Involvement of long non-coding RNAs in beta cell failure at the onset of type 1 diabetes in NOD mice. Diabetologia. 2015;58:1827–35.
18. Morán I, Akerman I, van de Bunt M, Xie R, Benazra M, Nammo T, et al. Human β cell transcriptome analysis uncovers lncRNAs that are tissue-specific, dynamically regulated, and abnormally expressed in type 2 diabetes. Cell Metab. 2012;16:435–48.
19. Ku GM, Kim H, Vaughn IW, Hangauer MJ, Myung Oh C, German MS, et al. Research resource: RNA-Seq reveals unique features of the pancreatic β-cell transcriptome. Mol Endocrinol. 2012;26:1783–92.
20. Liu J-Y, Yao J, Li X-M, Song Y-C, Wang X-Q, Li Y-J, et al. Pathogenic role of lncRNA-MALAT1 in endothelial cell dysfunction in diabetes mellitus. Cell Death Dis. 2014;5:e1506.
21. Wallace C, Smyth DJ, Maisuria-Armer M, Walker NM, Todd JA, Clayton DG. The imprinted DLK1-MEG3 gene region on chromosome 14q32.2 alters susceptibility to type 1 diabetes. Nat Genet. 2010;42:68–71.
22. You L, Wang N, Yin D, Wang L, Jin F, Zhu Y, et al. Downregulation of long noncoding RNA Meg3 affects insulin synthesis and secretion in mouse pancreatic beta cells. J Cell Physiol. 2016;231:852–62.
23. Arnes L, Akerman I, Balderes DA, Ferrer J, Sussel L. βlinc1 encodes a long noncoding RNA that regulates islet β-cell formation and function. Genes Dev. 2016;30:502–7.
24. Akerman I, Tu Z, Beucher A, Rolando DMY, Sauty-Colace C, Benazra M, et al. Human pancreatic β cell lncRNAs control cell-specific regulatory networks. Cell Metab. 2017;25:400–11.
25. Yin D, Zhang E, You L, Wang N, Wang L, Jin F, et al. Downregulation of lncRNA TUG1 affects apoptosis and insulin secretion in mouse pancreatic β cells. Cell Physiol Biochem. 2015;35:1892–904.
26. Li J, Xuan Z, Liu C. Long non-coding RNAs and complex human diseases. Int J Mol Sci. 2013;14:18790–808.
27. Hrdlickova B, de Almeida RC, Borek Z, Withoff S. Genetic variation in the non-coding genome: involvement of micro-RNAs and long non-coding RNAs in disease. Biochim Biophys Acta. 1842/2014:1910–22.
28. Hrdlickova B, Kumar V, Kanduri K, Zhernakova DV, Tripathi S, Karjalainen J, et al. Expression profiles of long non-coding RNAs located in autoimmune disease-associated regions reveal immune cell-type specificity. Genome Med. 2014;6:88.
29. Carpenter S, Aiello D, Atianand MK, Ricci EP, Gandhi P, Hall LL, et al. A long noncoding RNA mediates both activation and repression of immune response genes. Science. 2013;341:789–92.
30. Atianand MK, Fitzgerald KA. Long non-coding RNAs and control of gene expression in the immune system. Trends Mol Med. 2014;20:623–31.
31. Li Z, Chao T-C, Chang K-Y, Lin N, Patil VS, Shimizu C, et al. The long noncoding RNA THRIL regulates TNFα expression through its interaction with hnRNPL. Proc Natl Acad Sci U S A. 2014;111:1002–7.
32. Krawczyk M, Emerson BM. p50-associated COX-2 extragenic RNA (PACER) activates COX-2 gene expression by occluding repressive NF-κB complexes. elife. 2014;3:e01776.
33. Ilott NE, Heward JA, Roux B, Tsitsiou E, Fenwick PS, Lenzi L, et al. Long non-coding RNAs and enhancer RNAs regulate the lipopolysaccharide-induced inflammatory response in human monocytes. Nat Commun. 2014;5:3979.
34. Lu J, Wu X, Hong M, Tobias P, Han J. A potential suppressive effect of natural antisense IL-1β RNA on lipopolysaccharide-induced IL-1β expression. J Immunol. 2013;190:6570–8.
35. Carpenter S, Fitzgerald KA. Transcription of inflammatory genes: long noncoding RNA and beyond. J Interf Cytokine Res. 2015;35:79–88.
36. Gomez JA, Wapinski OL, Yang YW, Bureau J-F, Gopinath S, Monack DM, et al. The NeST long ncRNA controls microbial susceptibility and epigenetic activation of the interferon-γ locus. Cell. 2013;152:743–54.
37. Collier SP, Collins PL, Williams CL, Boothby MR, Aune TM. Cutting edge: influence of Tmevpg1, a long intergenic noncoding RNA, on the expression of Ifng by Th1 cells. J Immunol. 2012;189:2084–8.
38. Rapicavoli NA, Qu K, Zhang J, Mikhail M, Laberge R-M, Chang HY. A mammalian pseudogene lncRNA at the interface of inflammation and anti-inflammatory therapeutics. elife. 2013;2:e00762.

39. Wang P, Xue Y, Han Y, Lin L, Wu C, Xu S, et al. The STAT3-binding long noncoding RNA lnc-DC controls human dendritic cell differentiation. Science. 2014;344:310–3.

40. Ryba-Stanisławowska M, Skrzypkowska M, Myśliwiec M, Myśliwska J. Loss of the balance between CD4(+)Foxp3(+) regulatory T cells and CD4(+)IL17A(+) Th17 cells in patients with type 1 diabetes. Hum Immunol. 2013;74:701–7.

41. Ferraro A, Socci C, Stabilini A, Valle A, Monti P, Piemonti L, et al. Expansion of Th17 cells and functional defects in T regulatory cells are key features of the pancreatic lymph nodes in patients with type 1 diabetes. Diabetes. 2011;60:2903–13.

42. Huang W, Thomas B, Flynn RA, Gavzy SJ, Wu L, Kim SV, et al. DDX5 and its associated lncRNA Rmrp modulate TH17 cell effector functions. Nature. 2015;528:517–22.

43. Ricaño-Ponce I, Wijmenga C. Mapping of immune-mediated disease genes. Annu Rev Genomics Hum Genet. 2013;14:325–53.

44. Schaub MA, Boyle AP, Kundaje A, Batzoglou S, Snyder M. Linking disease associations with regulatory information in the human genome. Genome Res. 2012;22:1748–59.

45. Hoffman MM, Ernst J, Wilder SP, Kundaje A, Harris RS, Libbrecht M, et al. Integrative annotation of chromatin elements from ENCODE data. Nucleic Acids Res. 2013;41:827–41.

46. Gong J, Liu W, Zhang J, Miao X, Guo A-Y. lncRNASNP: a database of SNPs in lncRNAs and their potential functions in human and mouse. Nucleic Acids Res. 2015; 43(Database issue):D181–D186.

47. Kumar V, Westra H-J, Karjalainen J, Zhernakova DV, Esko T, Hrdlickova B, et al. Human disease-associated genetic variation impacts large intergenic non-coding RNA expression. PLoS Genet. 2013;9:e1003201.

48. Ørom UA, Derrien T, Beringer M, Gumireddy K, Gardini A, Bussotti G, et al. Long noncoding RNAs with enhancer-like function in human cells. Cell. 2010;143:46–58.

49. Guttman M, Donaghey J, Carey BW, Garber M, Grenier JK, Munson G, et al. lincRNAs act in the circuitry controlling pluripotency and differentiation. Nature. 2011;477:295–300.

50. Visel A, Rubin EM, Pennacchio LA. Genomic views of distant-acting enhancers. Nature. 2009;461:199–205.

51. Sakabe NJ, Savic D, Nobrega MA. Transcriptional enhancers in development and disease. Genome Biol. 2012;13:238.

52. Sanyal A, Lajoie BR, Jain G, Dekker J. The long-range interaction landscape of gene promoters. Nature. 2012;489:109–13.

53. Corradin O, Saiakhova A, Akhtar-Zaidi B, Myeroff L, Willis J, Cowper-Sal lari R, et al. Combinatorial effects of multiple enhancer variants in linkage disequilibrium dictate levels of gene expression to confer susceptibility to common traits. Genome Res. 2014;24:1–13.

54. Visel A, Blow MJ, Li Z, Zhang T, Akiyama JA, Holt A, et al. ChIP-seq accurately predicts tissue-specific activity of enhancers. Nature. 2009;457:854–8.

55. Heintzman ND, Hon GC, Hawkins RD, Kheradpour P, Stark A, Harp LF, et al. Histone modifications at human enhancers reflect global cell-type-specific gene expression. Nature. 2009;459:108–12.

56. Rada-Iglesias A, Bajpai R, Swigut T, Brugmann SA, Flynn RA, Wysocka J. A unique chromatin signature uncovers early developmental enhancers in humans. Nature. 2011;470:279–83.

57. Andersson R, Gebhard C, Miguel-Escalada I, Hoof I, Bornholdt J, Boyd M, et al. An atlas of active enhancers across human cell types and tissues. Nature. 2014;507:455–61.

58. Kadauke S, Blobel GA. Chromatin loops in gene regulation. Biochim Biophys Acta. 1789;2009:17–25.

59. Deng W, Lee J, Wang H, Miller J, Reik A, Gregory PD, et al. Controlling long-range genomic interactions at a native locus by targeted tethering of a looping factor. Cell. 2012;149:1233–44.

60. Dekker J, Rippe K, Dekker M, Kleckner N. Capturing chromosome conformation. Science. 2002;295:1306–11.

61. Zhao Z, Tavoosidana G, Sjölinder M, Göndör A, Mariano P, Wang S, et al. Circular chromosome conformation capture (4C) uncovers extensive networks of epigenetically regulated intra- and interchromosomal interactions. Nat Genet. 2006;38:1341–7.

62. Dostie J, Richmond TA, Arnaout RA, Selzer RR, Lee WL, Honan TA, et al. Chromosome conformation capture carbon copy (5C): a massively parallel solution for mapping interactions between genomic elements. Genome Res. 2006;16:1299–309.

63. Fullwood MJ, Liu MH, Pan YF, Liu J, Xu H, Mohamed YB, et al. An oestrogen-receptor-alpha-bound human chromatin interactome. Nature. 2009;462:58–64.

64. Lieberman-Aiden E, van Berkum NL, Williams L, Imakaev M, Ragoczy T, Telling A, et al. Comprehensive mapping of long-range interactions reveals folding principles of the human genome. Science. 2009;326:289–93.

65. Carter D, Chakalova L, Osborne CS, Dai Y, Fraser P. Long-range chromatin regulatory interactions in vivo. Nat Genet. 2002;32:623–6.

66. Tolhuis B, Palstra RJ, Splinter E, Grosveld F, de Laat W. Looping and interaction between hypersensitive sites in the active beta-globin locus. Mol Cell. 2002;10:1453–65.

67. Vernimmen D, De Gobbi M, Sloane-Stanley JA, Wood WG, Higgs DR. Long-range chromosomal interactions regulate the timing of the transition between poised and active gene expression. EMBO J. 2007;26:2041–51.

68. Spilianakis CG, Flavell RA. Long-range intrachromosomal interactions in the T helper type 2 cytokine locus. Nat Immunol. 2004;5:1017–27.

69. Kumar PP, Bischof O, Purbey PK, Notani D, Urlaub H, Dejean A, et al. Functional interaction between PML and SATB1 regulates chromatin-loop architecture and transcription of the MHC class I locus. Nat Cell Biol. 2007;9:45–56.

70. Horike S, Cai S, Miyano M, Cheng J-F, Kohwi-Shigematsu T. Loss of silent-chromatin looping and impaired imprinting of DLX5 in Rett syndrome. Nat Genet. 2005;37:31–40.

71. Murrell A, Heeson S, Reik W. Interaction between differentially methylated regions partitions the imprinted genes Igf2 and H19 into parent-specific chromatin loops. Nat Genet. 2004;36:889–93.

72. Kurukuti S, Tiwari VK, Tavoosidana G, Pugacheva E, Murrell A, Zhao Z, et al. CTCF binding at the H19 imprinting control region mediates maternally inherited higher-order chromatin conformation to restrict enhancer access to Igf2. Proc Natl Acad Sci U S A. 2006;103:10684–9.

73. Yoon YS, Jeong S, Rong Q, Park K-Y, Chung JH, Pfeifer K. Analysis of the H19ICR insulator. Mol Cell Biol. 2007;27:3499–510.

74. Spilianakis CG, Lalioti MD, Town T, Lee GR, Flavell RA. Interchromosomal associations between alternatively expressed loci. Nature. 2005;435:637–45.

75. Park J-H, Choi Y, Song M-J, Park K, Lee J-J, Kim H-P. Dynamic long-range chromatin interaction controls expression of IL-21 in CD4+ T cells. J Immunol. 2016;196:4378–89.

76. ENCODE Project Consortium, Birney E, Stamatoyannopoulos JA, Dutta A, Guigó R, Gingeras TR, et al. Identification and analysis of functional elements in 1% of the human genome by the ENCODE pilot project. Nature. 2007;447:799–816.

77. Li MJ, Sham PC, Wang J. Genetic variant representation, annotation and prioritization in the post-GWAS era. Cell Res. 2012;22:1505–8.

78. Raychaudhuri S. VIZ-GRAIL: visualizing functional connections across disease loci. Bioinformatics. 2011;27:1589–90.

79. Kaur S, Mirza AH, Brorsson CA, Fløyel T, Størling J, Mortensen HB, et al. The genetic and regulatory architecture of ERBB3-type 1 diabetes susceptibility locus. Mol Cell Endocrinol. 2016;419:83–91.

80. Kim T-K, Hemberg M, Gray JM. Enhancer RNAs: a class of long noncoding RNAs synthesized at enhancers. Cold Spring Harb Perspect Biol. 2015;7:a018622.

81. Murakami S, Gadad SS, Kraus WL. A PreSTIGEous use of LncRNAs to predict enhancers. Cell Cycle. 2015;14:1619–20.

82. Ørom UA, Shiekhattar R. Long noncoding RNAs usher in a new era in the biology of enhancers. Cell. 2013;154:1190–3.

83. Tian D, Sun S, Lee JT. The long noncoding RNA, Jpx, is a molecular switch for X chromosome inactivation. Cell. 2010;143:390–403.

84. Lai F, Orom UA, Cesaroni M, Beringer M, Taatjes DJ, Blobel GA, et al. Activating RNAs associate with mediator to enhance chromatin architecture and transcription. Nature. 2013;494:497–501.

85. Pasquali L, Gaulton KJ, Rodríguez-Seguí SA, Mularoni L, Miguel-Escalada I, Akerman I, et al. Pancreatic islet enhancer clusters enriched in type 2 diabetes risk-associated variants. Nat Genet. 2014;46:136–43.

86. Lee GL, Dobi A, Srivastava S. Prostate cancer: diagnostic performance of the PCA3 urine test. Nat Rev Urol. 2011;8:123–4.

87. Diederichs S. The four dimensions of noncoding RNA conservation. Trends Genet. 2014;30:121–3.

88. Cabili MN, Trapnell C, Goff L, Koziol M, Tazon-Vega B, Regev A, et al. Integrative annotation of human large intergenic noncoding RNAs reveals global properties and specific subclasses. Genes Dev. 2011;25:1915–27.

89. Mercer TR, Mattick JS. Structure and function of long noncoding RNAs in epigenetic regulation. Nat Struct Mol Biol. 2013;20:300–7.

90. Hon CC, Ramilowski JA, Harshbarger J, Bertin N, Rackham OJ, Gough J, et al. An atlas of human long non-coding RNAs with accurate 5′ ends. Nature. 2017;543:199–204.

91. Derrien T, Johnson R, Bussotti G, Tanzer A, Djebali S, Tilgner H, et al. The GENCODE v7 catalog of human long noncoding RNAs: analysis of their gene structure, evolution, and expression. Genome Res. 2012;22:1775–89.

92. Mercer TR, Gerhardt DJ, Dinger ME, Crawford J, Trapnell C, Jeddeloh JA, et al. Targeted RNA sequencing reveals the deep complexity of the human transcriptome. Nat Biotechnol. 2011;30:99–104.

93. Lagarde J, Uszczynska-Ratajczak B, Santoyo-Lopez J, Gonzalez JM, Tapanari E, Mudge JM, et al. Extension of human lncRNA transcripts by RACE coupled with long-read high-throughput sequencing (RACE-Seq). Nat Commun. 2016;7:12339.

94. Lagarde J, Uszczynska-Ratajczak B, Carbonell S, Davis C, Gingeras TR, Frankish A. High-throughput annotation of full-length long noncoding RNAs with capture long-read sequencing (CLS). bioRxiv. 2017;105064. doi: https://doi.org/10.1101/105064.

95. Liu SJ, Horlbeck MA, Cho SW, Birk HS, Malatesta M, He D, et al. CRISPRi-based genome-scale identification of functional long noncoding RNA loci in human cells. Science. 2017;355. doi: 10.1126/science.aah7111.

96. Nica AC, Ongen H, Irminger JC, Bosco D, Berney T, Antonarakis SE, et al. Cell-type, allelic, and genetic signatures in the human pancreatic beta cell transcriptome. Genome Res. 2013;23:1554–62.

97. Li W, Notani D, Rosenfeld MG. Enhancers as non-coding RNA transcription units: recent insights and future perspectives. Nat Rev Genet. 2016;17:207–23.

11

The clinical significance of snail protein expression in gastric cancer

Xiaoya Chen[1], Jinjun Li[1*], Ling Hu[2], William Yang[3], Lili Lu[1], Hongyan Jin[4], Zexiong Wei[4], Jack Y. Yang[5], Hamid R. Arabnia[7], Jun S. Liu[6], Mary Qu Yang[5] and Youping Deng[1,8*]

Abstract

Background: Snail is a typical transcription factor that could induce epithelial-mesenchymal transition (EMT) and cancer progression. There are some related reports about the clinical significance of snail protein expression in gastric cancer. However, the published results were not completely consistent. This study was aimed to investigate snail expression and clinical significance in gastric cancer.

Results: A systematic review of PubMed, CNKI, Weipu, and Wanfang database before March 2015 was conducted. We established an inclusion criterion according to subjects, method of detection, and results evaluation of snail protein. Meta-analysis was conducted using RevMan4.2 software. And merged odds ratio (OR) and 95 % CI (95 % confidence interval) were calculated. Also, forest plots and funnel plot were used to assess the potential of publication bias.
A total of 10 studies were recruited. The meta-analysis was conducted to evaluate the positive rate of snail protein expression. OR and 95 % CI for different groups were listed below: (1) gastric cancer and para-carcinoma tissue [OR = 6.15, 95 % CI (4.70, 8.05)]; (2) gastric cancer and normal gastric tissue [OR = 17.00, 95 % CI (10.08, 28.67)]; (3) non-lymph node metastasis and lymph node metastasis [OR = 0.40, 95 % CI (0.18, 0.93)]; (4) poor differentiated cancer, highly differentiated cancer, and moderate cancer [OR = 3.34, 95 % CI (2.22, 5.03)]; (5) clinical stage TI + TII and stage TIII + TIV [OR = 0.38, 95 % CI (0.23, 0.60)]; (6) superficial muscularis and deep muscularis [OR = 0.18, 95 % CI (0.11, 0.31)].

Conclusions: Our results indicated that the increase of snail protein expression may play an important role in the carcinogenesis, progression, and metastasis of gastric cancer. And this result might provide instruction for the diagnosis, therapy, and prognosis of gastric cancer.

Keywords: Gastric cancer, Snail, Meta-analysis

Background

Epithelial-mesenchymal transition (EMT), a developmental process whereby epithelial cells reduce intercellular adhesion and acquire myofibroblastic features, is critical to tumor progression [1–3]. Meanwhile, the dissolution of intercellular adhesions and the acquisition of a more motile mesenchymal phenotype as part of epithelial-to-mesenchymal transition (EMT) are crucial capacities of invading cancer cells [4]. Snail can induce EMT partly by suppressing the expression of E-cadherin. Reduced expression of E-cadherin may lead to the loss of cell-cell adhesion and cancer progression [5]. In recent years, snail was found to be highly expressed in several carcinomas, including non-small cell lung carcinomas, ovarian carcinomas, urothelial carcinomas, breast cancer, and hepatocellular carcinoma [6–10]. Studies of immunohistochemical analyses suggest that snail is highly expressed in gastric cancer and significantly associated with tumor progression and metastasis [11–13].

* Correspondence: entry2003@126.com; Youpingd@gmail.com
[1]Medical College, Wuhan University of Science and Technology, Wuhan 430065, China
[8]Department of Internal Medicine and Rush University Cancer Center, Rush University Medical Center, Chicago, IL 60612, USA
Full list of author information is available at the end of the article

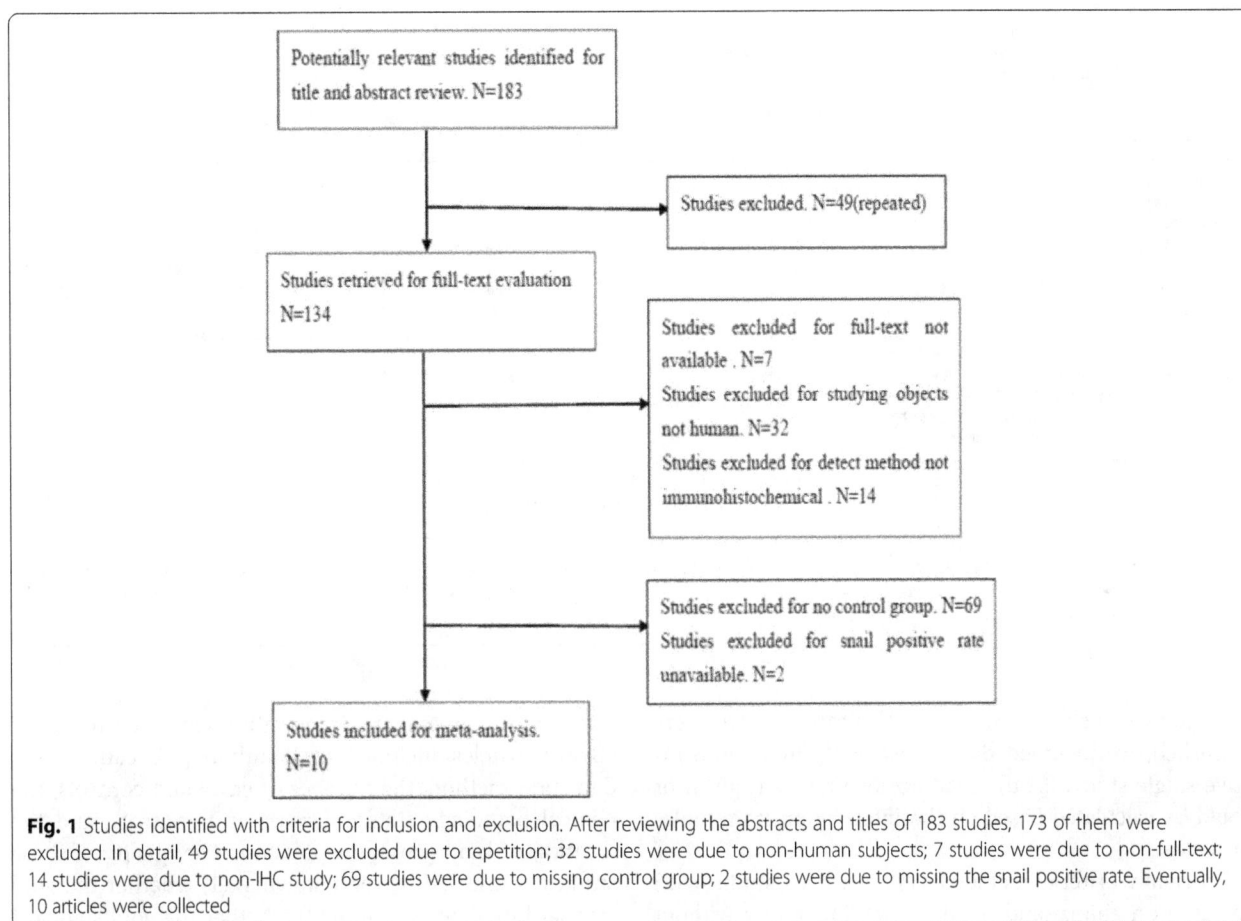

Fig. 1 Studies identified with criteria for inclusion and exclusion. After reviewing the abstracts and titles of 183 studies, 173 of them were excluded. In detail, 49 studies were excluded due to repetition; 32 studies were due to non-human subjects; 7 studies were due to non-full-text; 14 studies were due to non-IHC study; 69 studies were due to missing control group; 2 studies were due to missing the snail positive rate. Eventually, 10 articles were collected

Methods

Study search protocol

A total of 10 studies were identified by primary search strategies using the keywords "snail" combined with "gastric cancer" and synonyms in PubMed, CNKI, Weipu, and Wanfang database.

Inclusion criteria and exclusion criteria

Studies that were included in this meta-analysis met the following criteria: (1) the official published literature or master's and doctoral dissertation in both Chinese and English before March 2015; (2) the detection method used immunohistochemical and the results experienced

Table 1 Main characteristics of the studies included in this meta-analysis

First author	Year	Positive rate											
		Cancer tissue	Adjacent tissue	Normal tissue	Low differentiation	Highly + moderate	TI + TII	TIII + TIV	Superficial	Deep	No metastasis	Metastasis	Quality
Yingfeng Zhu	2007	80/96	33/80	–	56/62	24/34	21/29	59/67	10/16	70/80	23/32	57/64	D
Zhifeng Tang	2010	159/189	26/54	6/32	82/100	61/89	29/46	114/143	–	–	49/73	94/116	D
Yaqin Hao	2011	41/54	22/54	9/30	20/22	21/32	–	–	4/9	17/19	5/11	16/17	D
Shengxi Wang	2011	92/112	28/79	–	66/75	26/37	–	–	15/23	77/89	29/42	63/70	E
Li Jin	2011	78/87	–	7/24	–	–	–	–	–	–	–	–	E
Lina Wang	2011	32/60	16/60	3/20	26/42	6/18	–	–	2/9	30/51	4/7	28/53	D
Wude Zhang	2012	41/48	15/48	–	32/34	9/14	23/27	18/21	22/29	19/19	24/30	7/18	E
Xiaoli Cao	2013	32/45	5/20	–	24/27	8/18	11/20	21/25	9/19	23/26	10/20	22/25	E
Qianjun Li	2013	38/65	–	0/65	–	–	–	–	–	–	–	–	D
Limin Liu	2014	57/80	24/80	–	–	–	6/14	51/66	6/15	51/65	11/24	46/56	C

Review: The clinical significance of snail protein expression in Gastric Cancer : A Meta-analysis
Comparison: 02 The positive expression rate of snail in different gastric tissues
Outcome: 01 Gastric cancer and para-carcinoma tissue

Study or sub-category	Gastric cancer n/N	para-carcinoma n/N	OR (fixed) 95% CI	Weight %	OR (fixed) 95% CI	Year
Yingfeng Zhu	80/96	33/80		14.24	7.12 [3.55, 14.30]	2007
Zhifeng Tang	159/189	26/54		15.24	5.71 [2.95, 11.06]	2010
Lina Wang	32/60	16/60		17.72	3.14 [1.46, 6.75]	2011
Shengxi Wang	92/112	28/79		13.92	8.38 [4.30, 16.34]	2011
Yaqin Hao	41/54	22/54		12.57	4.59 [2.01, 10.49]	2011
Wude Zhang	41/48	15/48		5.19	12.89 [4.71, 35.29]	2012
Xiaoli Cao	32/45	5/20		4.75	7.38 [2.22, 24.52]	2013
Limin Liu	57/80	24/80		16.38	5.78 [2.93, 11.42]	2014
Total (95% CI)	684	475		100.00	6.15 [4.70, 8.05]	

Total events: 534 (Gastric cancer), 169 (para-carcinoma)
Test for heterogeneity: Chi²= 6.68, df = 7 (P = 0.46), I²= 0%
Test for overall effect: Z = 13.20 (P < 0.00001)

```
        0.01    0.1      1      10    100
           Gastric cancer   para-carcinoma
```

Fig. 2 Meta-analysis for the expression of snail protein in gastric cancer and para-carcinoma. Eight of the ten studies compared the expression of snail protein in gastric cancer tissues and the adjacent tissues, including 684 gastric cancer samples and 475 para-carcinoma samples. The I2 value was 0 % and less than 50 %; thus, we chose fixed-effect Mantel-Haenszel model for further analysis. The overall effect was $Z = 13.20$. The odds ratio (OR) was 6.15 with 95 % CI = (4.70, 8.05), and $P < 0.001$

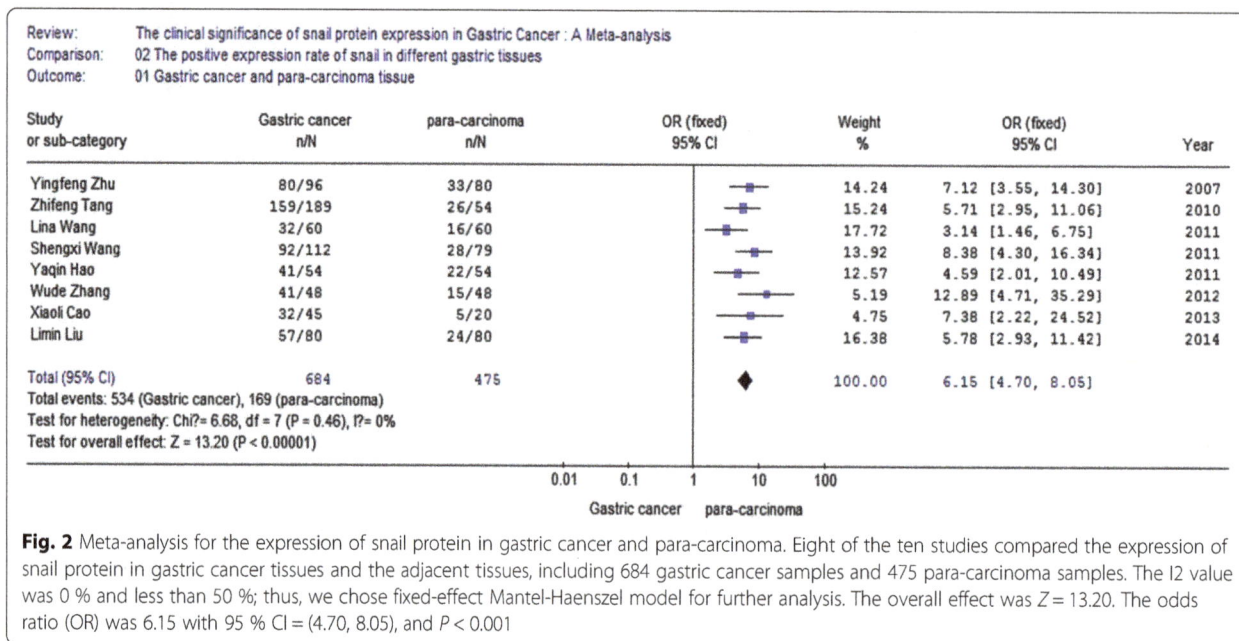

quantitative analysis; (3) when duplicate articles were published, we included the newest or the most informative single study; (5) the snail positive rate was given or could be calculated based on the information from tables or figures.

Exclusion criteria included (1) repetitive studies; (2) research on animal and cellular level; (3) studies without reviews, letters, abstracts and editorials; and (4) the studies without control group.

Data extraction and quality assessment

Two reviewers screened the titles and abstracts according to the inclusion and exclusion criteria listed above independently. Then, they cross-checked the articles and

removed disagreements. Information extracted from the eligible articles included first author, publication year, detection method, the number of cases and controls, the clinical pathology states of cases and controls, and the location of snail protein expression. The quality of these studies is assessed by the following: (1) whether the gold standard method is set up; (2) whether the gold standard test stayed is independent of the evaluation test; (3) whether the blind method is used; (4) whether quantitative data is given or is able to be calculated; (5) whether the definition and diagnosis of the case are correct, independent, and standard; (6) whether the diagnostic steps are detailed; (7) whether the case has a good representation; (8) whether cases and controls are selected and

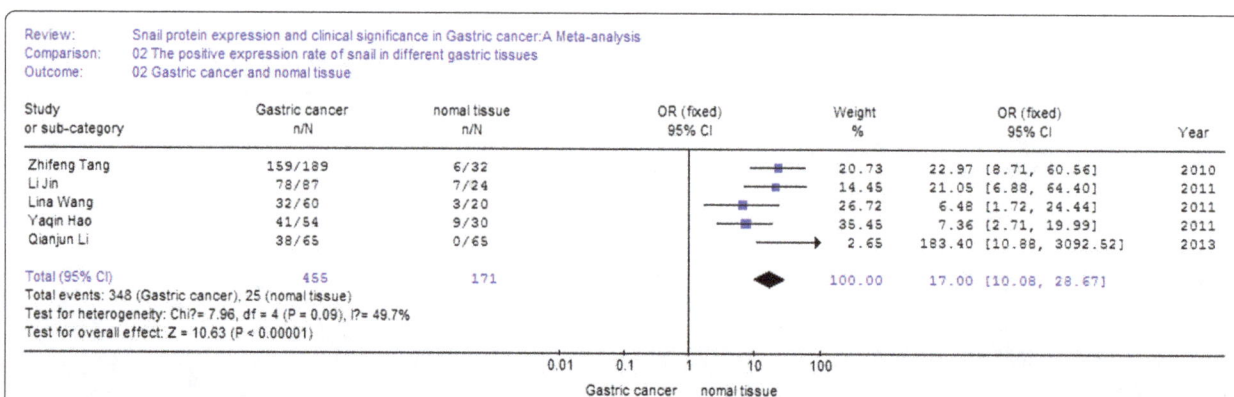

Review: Snail protein expression and clinical significance in Gastric cancer:A Meta-analysis
Comparison: 02 The positive expression rate of snail in different gastric tissues
Outcome: 02 Gastric cancer and nomal tissue

Study or sub-category	Gastric cancer n/N	nomal tissue n/N	OR (fixed) 95% CI	Weight %	OR (fixed) 95% CI	Year
Zhifeng Tang	159/189	6/32		20.73	22.97 [8.71, 60.56]	2010
Li Jin	78/87	7/24		14.45	21.05 [6.88, 64.40]	2011
Lina Wang	32/60	3/20		26.72	6.48 [1.72, 24.44]	2011
Yaqin Hao	41/54	9/30		35.45	7.36 [2.71, 19.99]	2011
Qianjun Li	38/65	0/65		2.65	183.40 [10.88, 3092.52]	2013
Total (95% CI)	455	171		100.00	17.00 [10.08, 28.67]	

Total events: 348 (Gastric cancer), 25 (nomal tissue)
Test for heterogeneity: Chi²= 7.96, df = 4 (P = 0.09), I²= 49.7%
Test for overall effect: Z = 10.63 (P < 0.00001)

```
        0.01    0.1      1      10    100
           Gastric cancer   nomal tissue
```

Fig. 3 Meta-analysis for the expression of snail protein in gastric cancer and normal tissue. Five of the ten studies compared the positive expression of snail protein in gastric cancer tissues with that in normal tissues, including 455 gastric cancer tissue samples and 171 normal samples. The I2 value was 49.7 % and less than 50 %; thus, we chose fixed-effect Mantel-Haenszel model for further analysis. The overall effect was $Z = 10.63$, OR = 17, 95 % CI = (10.08, 28.67), and $P < 0.001$

Review: Snail protein expression and clinical significance in Gastric cancer:A Meta-analysis
Comparison: 03 The relationship between the characteristics of Snail expression and clinical pathology
Outcome: 01 The relationship between snail and lymph node metastasis

Study or sub-category	no metastasis n/N	metastasis n/N	OR (random) 95% CI	Weight %	OR (random) 95% CI	Year
Yingfeng Zhu	23/32	57/64		13.68	0.31 [0.10, 0.94]	2007
Zhifeng Tang	49/73	94/116		16.09	0.48 [0.24, 0.94]	2010
Lina Wang	4/7	28/53		10.84	1.19 [0.24, 5.84]	2011
Shengxi Wang	29/42	63/70		14.16	0.25 [0.09, 0.69]	2011
Yaqin Hao	5/11	16/17		7.41	0.05 [0.01, 0.54]	2011
Wude Zhang	24/30	7/18		12.47	6.29 [1.71, 23.14]	2012
Xiaoli Cao	10/20	22/25		11.40	0.14 [0.03, 0.61]	2013
Limin Liu	11/24	46/56		13.95	0.18 [0.06, 0.53]	2014
Total (95% CI)	239	419		100.00	0.40 [0.18, 0.93]	

Total events: 155 (no metastasis), 333 (metastasis)
Test for heterogeneity: Chi²= 27.29, df = 7 (P = 0.0003), I²= 74.4%
Test for overall effect: Z = 2.14 (P = 0.03)

0.01 0.1 1 10 100
no metastasis   metastasis

Fig. 4 Meta-analysis for the relationship between snail expression and lymph node metastasis. Eight studies analyzed the relationship between snail expression and lymph node metastasis. The results indicated that the I2 value was 74.4 % and greater than 50 %; thus, we chose random-effect model for further analysis. The overall effect was $Z = 2.14$, OR = 0.40, 95 % CI = (0.18, 0.93), and $P < 0.001$

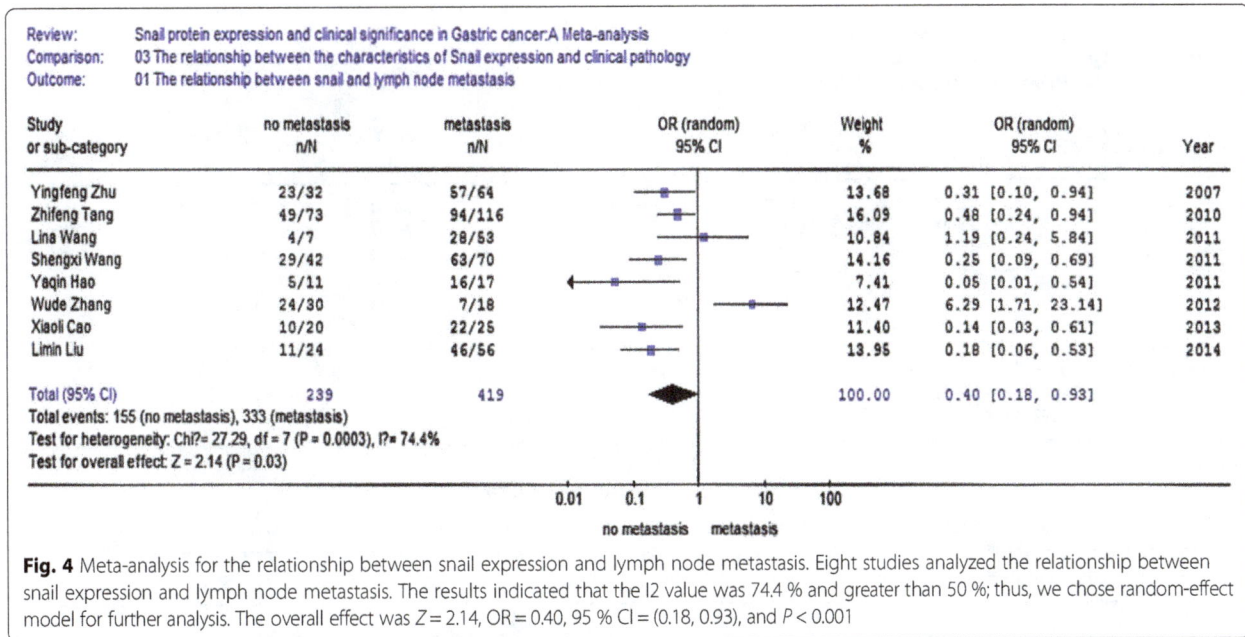

analyzed based on the most important factor. Based on the above standards, we classified the qualities of the research into five grades: (A) meets all 8 quality standards; (B) meets 7 standards; (C) meets 6 standards; (D) meets 5 standards; (E) meets 4 standards.

Statistical analysis

Meta-analysis was conducted with RevMan4.2 software. Odds ratio (OR) with 95 % confidence interval was calculated. Heterogeneity between studies was examined using the I2 statistic [14, 15]. When I2 value was greater than 50 %, we considered that heterogeneity was significant. Fixed-effect Mantel-Haenszel model was chosen as

the main analysis method when the heterogeneities were not confirmed statistically significant. Otherwise, random-effect model was adopted. Funnel plots were used to check for the potential of publication bias. All the P values were two-sided, and statistically significant difference was defined as $P < 0.05$.

Results

Literature search and study characteristics

After reviewing the abstracts and titles of 183 studies, 173 of them were excluded. In detail, 49 studies were excluded due to repetition; 32 studies were due to non-human subjects; 7 studies were due to non-full-

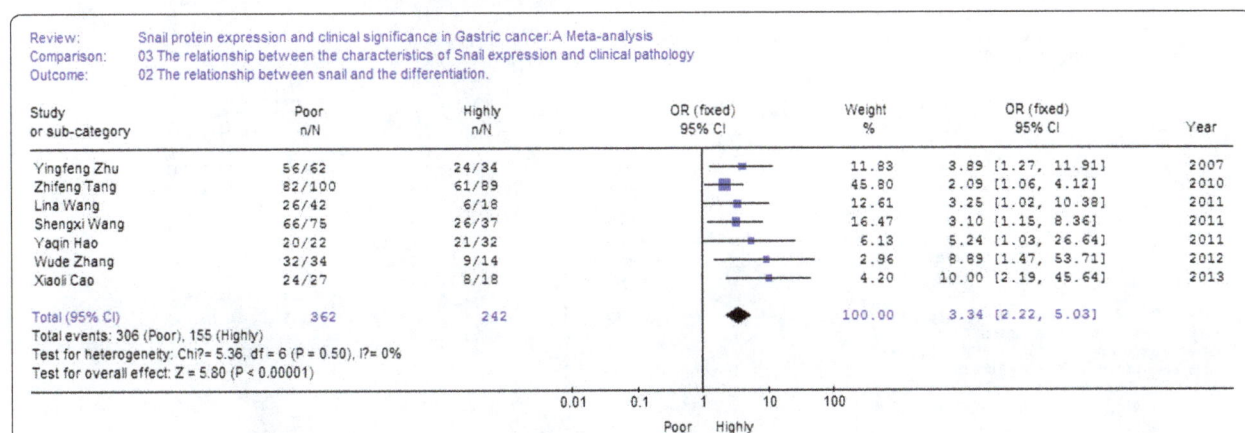

Review: Snail protein expression and clinical significance in Gastric cancer:A Meta-analysis
Comparison: 03 The relationship between the characteristics of Snail expression and clinical pathology
Outcome: 02 The relationship between snail and the differentiation.

Study or sub-category	Poor n/N	Highly n/N	OR (fixed) 95% CI	Weight %	OR (fixed) 95% CI	Year
Yingfeng Zhu	56/62	24/34		11.83	3.89 [1.27, 11.91]	2007
Zhifeng Tang	82/100	61/89		45.80	2.09 [1.06, 4.12]	2010
Lina Wang	26/42	6/18		12.61	3.25 [1.02, 10.38]	2011
Shengxi Wang	66/75	26/37		16.47	3.10 [1.15, 8.36]	2011
Yaqin Hao	20/22	21/32		6.13	5.24 [1.03, 26.64]	2011
Wude Zhang	32/34	9/14		2.96	8.89 [1.47, 53.71]	2012
Xiaoli Cao	24/27	8/18		4.20	10.00 [2.19, 45.64]	2013
Total (95% CI)	362	242		100.00	3.34 [2.22, 5.03]	

Total events: 306 (Poor), 155 (Highly)
Test for heterogeneity: Chi²= 5.36, df = 6 (P = 0.50), I²= 0%
Test for overall effect: Z = 5.80 (P < 0.00001)

0.01 0.1 1 10 100
Poor   Highly

Fig. 5 Meta-analysis for the relationship between snail expression and the differentiation. Seven studies analyzed the relationship between snail expression and the differentiation. The result indicated that the I2 value was 0 % and less than 50 %; thus, we chose fixed-effect Mantel-Haenszel model for further analysis. The overall effect was $Z = 5.80$, OR = 3.34, 95 % CI = (2.22, 5.03), and $P < 0.001$

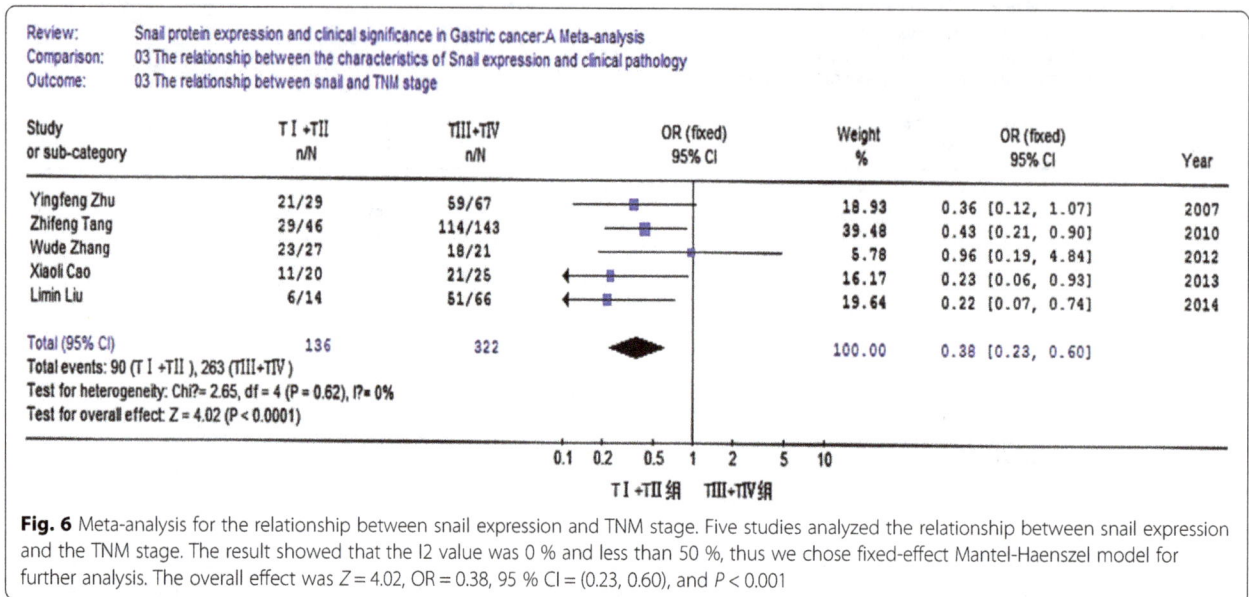

Fig. 6 Meta-analysis for the relationship between snail expression and TNM stage. Five studies analyzed the relationship between snail expression and the TNM stage. The result showed that the I2 value was 0 % and less than 50 %, thus we chose fixed-effect Mantel-Haenszel model for further analysis. The overall effect was $Z = 4.02$, OR = 0.38, 95 % CI = (0.23, 0.60), and $P < 0.001$

text; 14 studies were due to non-IHC study; 69 studies were due to missing control group; 2 studies were due to missing the snail positive rate. Eventually, 10 articles were collected [16–25] (Fig. 1). Detailed characteristics of these 10 eligible studies are summarized in Table 1. A total of 756 gastric cancer tissue samples, 346 para-carcinoma tissue samples, and 171 normal tissue samples were used in these 10 studies. Eight of them reported the relationship between the snail expression and clinical pathology, enrolled the degree of differentiation, the lymph node metastasis, TNM stage, and invasion depth.

Stratification analysis

Eight of the ten studies compared the expression of snail protein in gastric cancer tissues and the adjacent tissues, including 684 gastric cancer samples and 475 para-carcinoma samples. The I2 value was 0 % and less than 50 %; thus, we chose fixed-effect Mantel-Haenszel model for further analysis. The overall effect was $Z = 13.20$. The odds ratio (OR) was 6.15 with 95 % CI = (4.70, 8.05), and $P < 0.001$ (Fig. 2).

Five of the ten studies compared the positive expression of snail protein in gastric cancer tissues with that in normal tissues, including 455 gastric cancer tissue samples and 171 normal samples. The I2 value was 49.7 % and less than 50 %; thus, we chose fixed-effect Mantel-Haenszel model for further analysis. The overall effect was $Z = 10.63$. The odds ratio was 17 with 95 % CI = (10.08, 28.67), and $P < 0.001$ (Fig. 3).

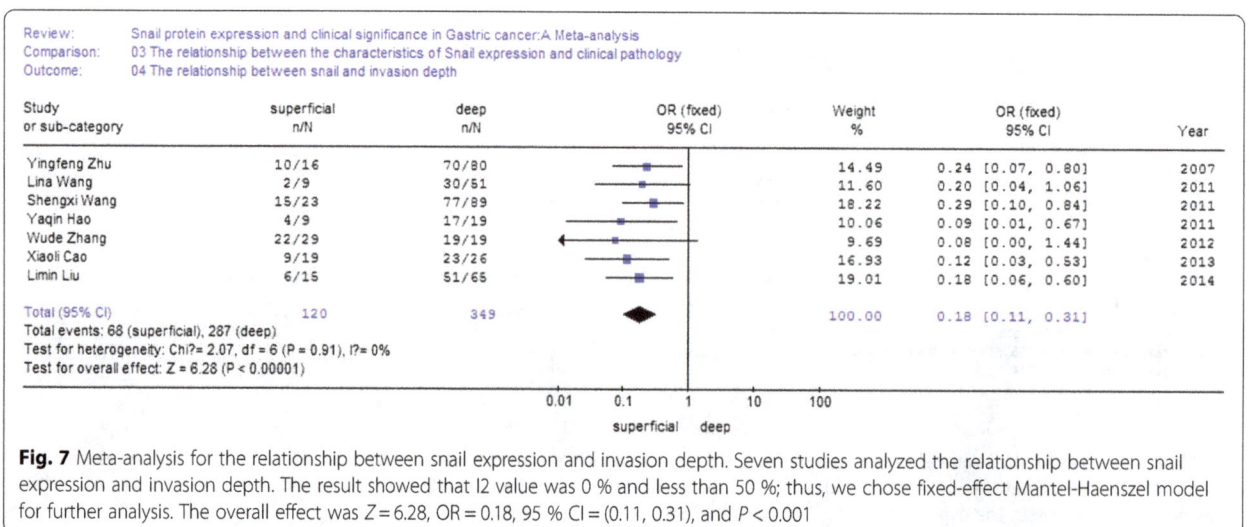

Fig. 7 Meta-analysis for the relationship between snail expression and invasion depth. Seven studies analyzed the relationship between snail expression and invasion depth. The result showed that I2 value was 0 % and less than 50 %; thus, we chose fixed-effect Mantel-Haenszel model for further analysis. The overall effect was $Z = 6.28$, OR = 0.18, 95 % CI = (0.11, 0.31), and $P < 0.001$

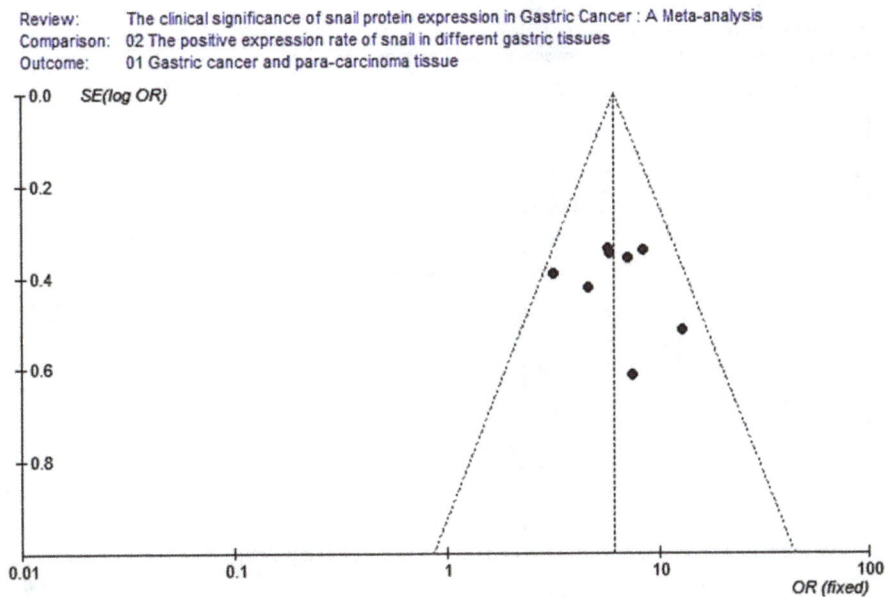

Fig. 8 Funnel plot analysis for the expression of snail protein in gastric cancer and para-carcinoma. Funnel plot analysis for publication bias indicated a low likelihood of publication bias

The relationship between the expression of snail protein and the characteristics of clinical pathology

Eight studies analyzed the relationship between snail expression and lymph node metastasis. The results indicated that the I2 value was 74.4 % and greater than 50 %; thus, we chose random-effect model for further analysis. The overall effect was $Z = 2.14$, OR = 0.40, 95 % CI = (0.18, 0.93), and $P < 0.001$ (Fig. 4). Seven studies

analyzed the relationship between snail expression and the differentiation. The result indicated that the I2 value was 0 % and less than 50 %; thus, we chose fixed-effect Mantel-Haenszel model for further analysis. The overall effect was $Z = 5.80$, OR = 3.34, 95 % CI = (2.22, 5.03), and $P < 0.001$ (Fig. 5). Five studies analyzed the relationship between snail expression and the TNM stage. The result showed that the I2 value was 0 % and less than 50 %;

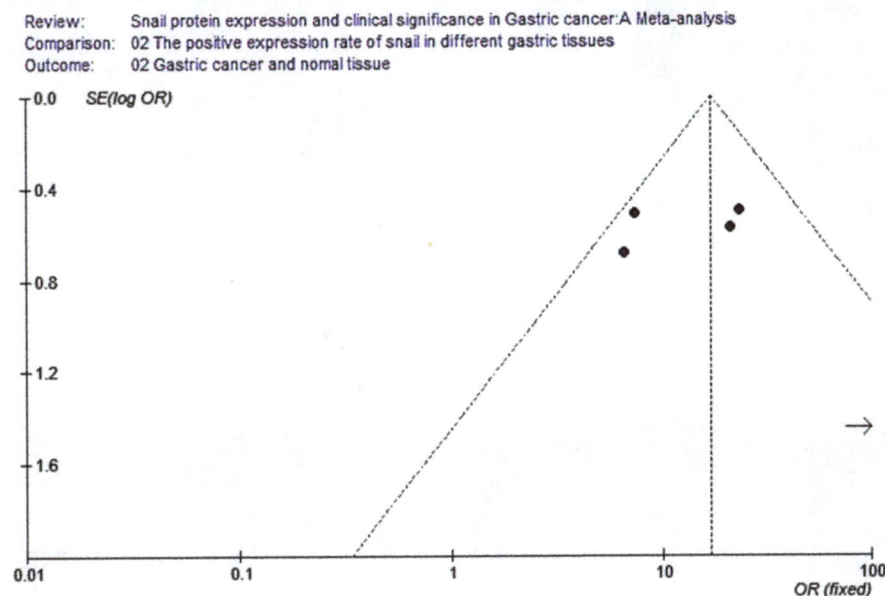

Fig. 9 Funnel plot analysis for the expression of snail protein in gastric cancer and normal tissue. Funnel plot analysis for publication bias indicated a low likelihood of publication bias

Review: Snail protein expression and clinical significance in Gastric cancer:A Meta-analysis
Comparison: 03 The relationship between the characteristics of Snail expression and clinical pathology
Outcome: 01 The relationship between snail and lymph node metastasis

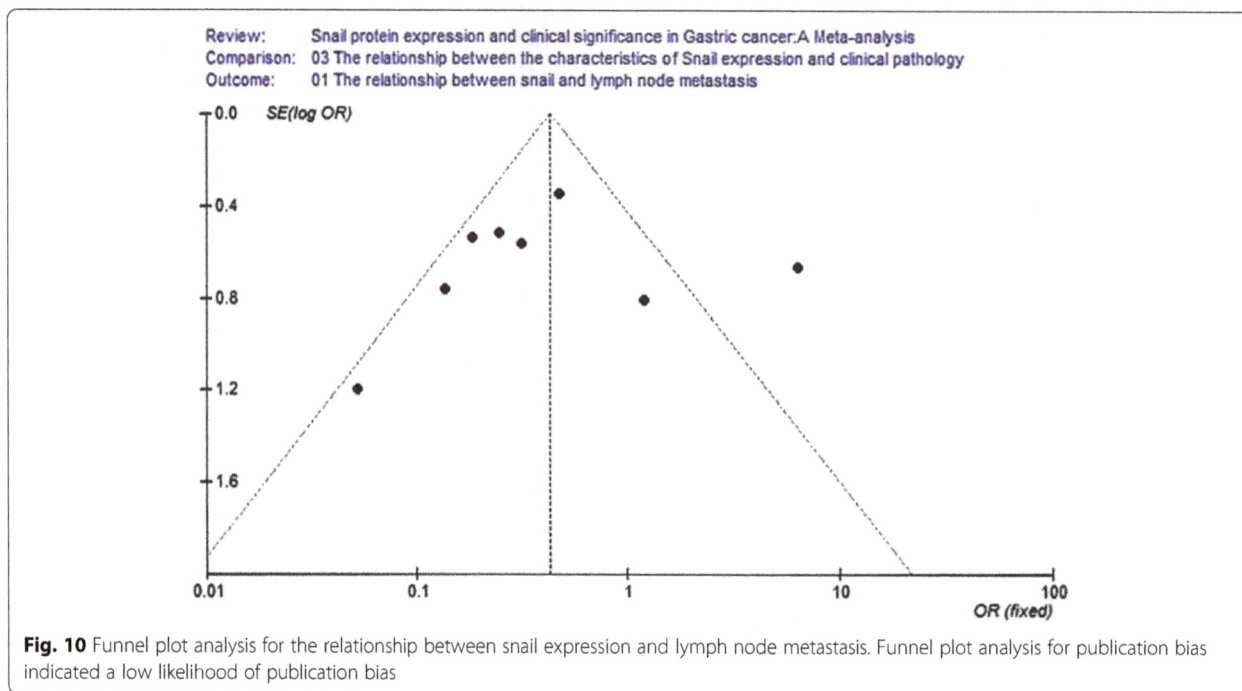

Fig. 10 Funnel plot analysis for the relationship between snail expression and lymph node metastasis. Funnel plot analysis for publication bias indicated a low likelihood of publication bias

thus, we chose fixed-effect Mantel-Haenszel model for further analysis. The overall effect was $Z = 4.02$, OR = 0.38, 95 % CI = (0.23, 0.60), and $P < 0.001$ (Fig. 6). Seven studies analyzed the relationship between snail expression and invasion depth. The result showed that I2 value was 0 % and less than 50 %; thus, we chose fixed-effect Mantel-Haenszel model for further analysis. The overall

effect was $Z = 6.28$, OR = 0.18, 95 % CI = (0.11, 0.31), and $P < 0.001$ (Fig. 7).

Publication bias analysis

Funnel plot analysis for publication bias of these analytical studies (as shown in Figs. 8, 9, 10, 11, 12, and 13) indicated a low likelihood of publication bias.

Review: Snail protein expression and clinical significance in Gastric cancer:A Meta-analysis
Comparison: 03 The relationship between the characteristics of Snail expression and clinical pathology
Outcome: 02 The relationship between snail and the differentiation.

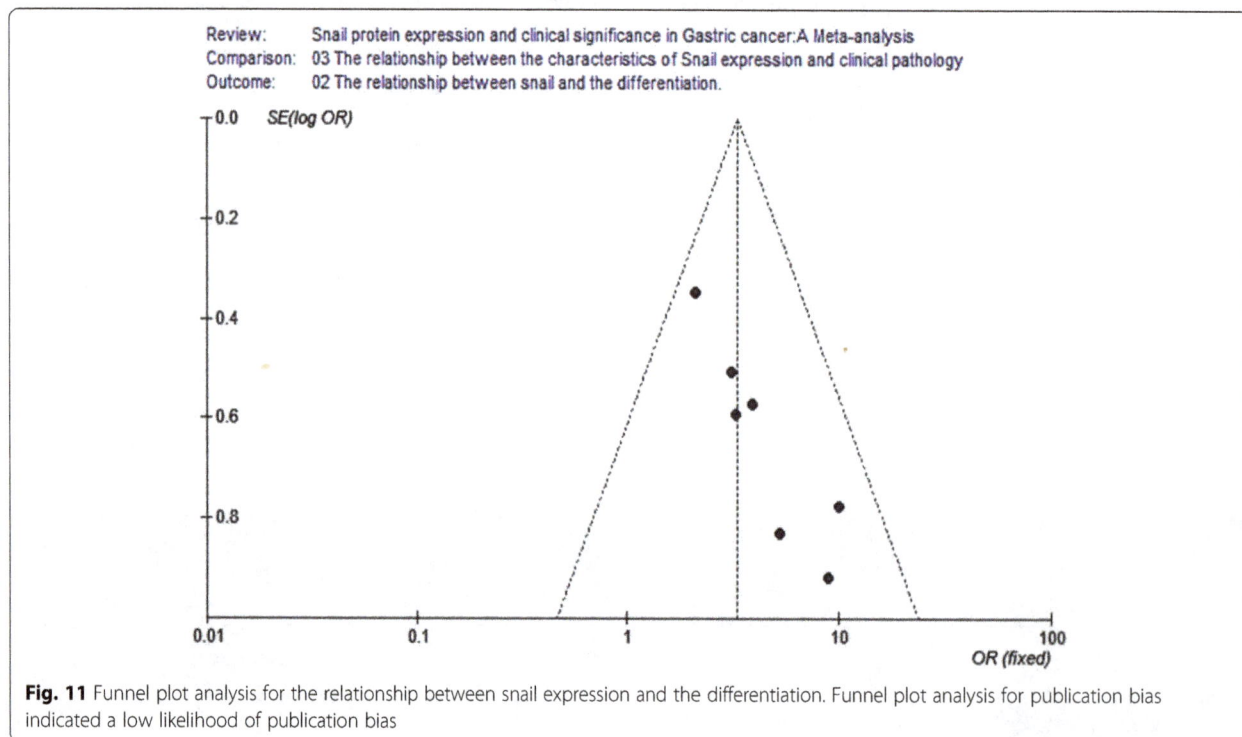

Fig. 11 Funnel plot analysis for the relationship between snail expression and the differentiation. Funnel plot analysis for publication bias indicated a low likelihood of publication bias

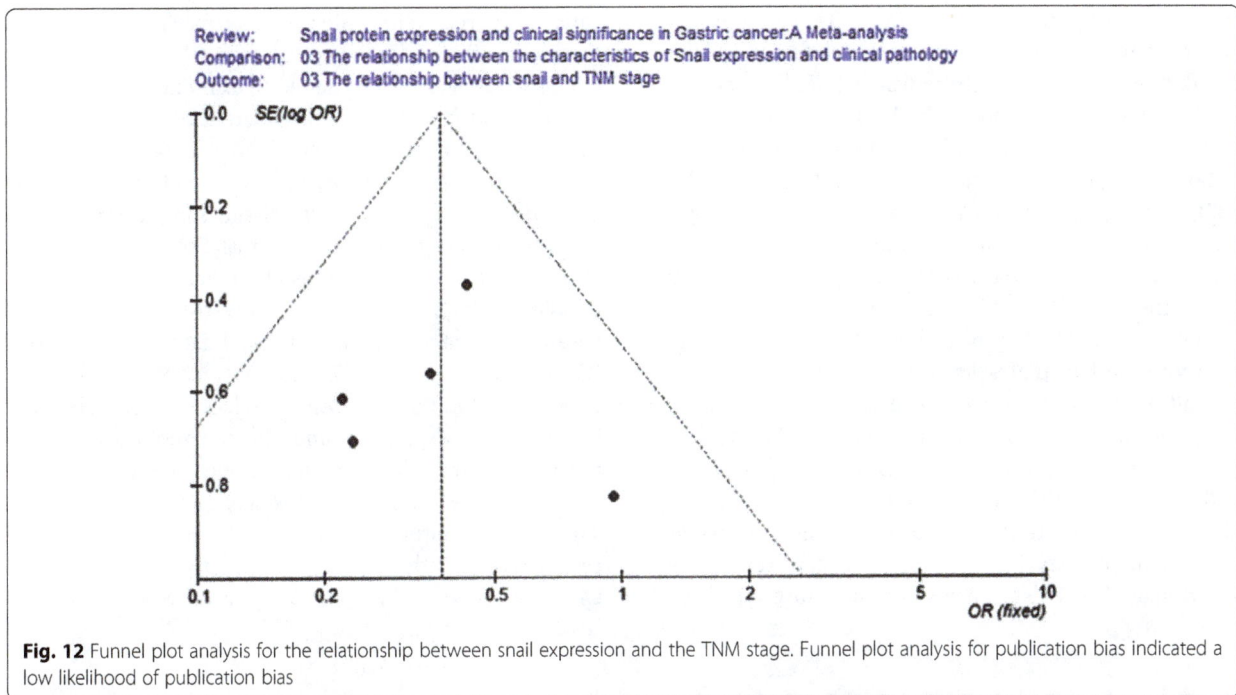

Fig. 12 Funnel plot analysis for the relationship between snail expression and the TNM stage. Funnel plot analysis for publication bias indicated a low likelihood of publication bias

Discussion and conclusions

The emerging roles of some key, EMT-related proteins in cancer progression and their close relationship with clinical pathology parameters make them attractive for developing diagnostic biomarkers and therapies [26]. The transcriptional repression of E-cadherin is mediated mainly by zinc finger transcription factors related to the snail family (SNAIL1), zinc finger E-box binding homeobox-2 (ZEB2), and basic helix-loop-helix family (TWIST) [27, 28]. Network analysis (Fig. 14) revealed that snail expression was significantly correlated with the expression of ZEB2, TWIST (Twist1 and Twist2), and N-cadherin (CDH2). These gene expressions may be regulated by snail at transcriptional level, and they also interact with each other. N-cadherin, encoded by the CDH2 gene, mediates cell-cell adhesion and renders

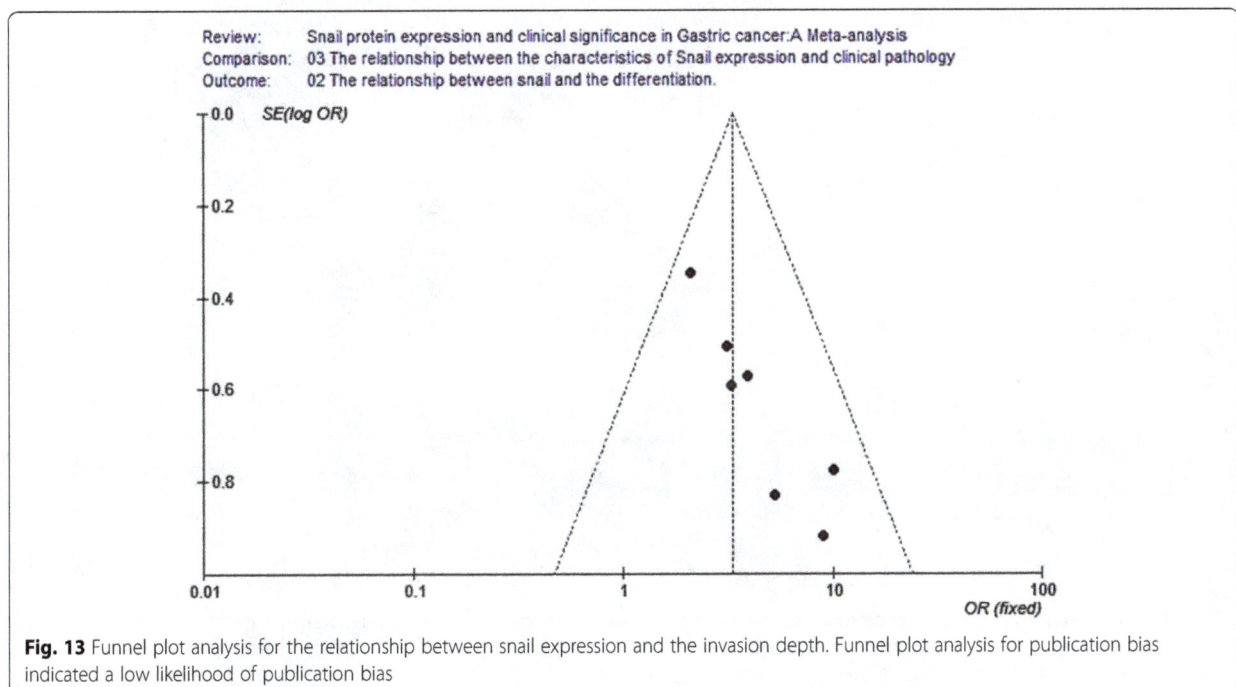

Fig. 13 Funnel plot analysis for the relationship between snail expression and the invasion depth. Funnel plot analysis for publication bias indicated a low likelihood of publication bias

tumor cell migration and invasion [29]. N-cadherin was reported to be a prognostic marker [30], and the up-regulation correlated with advanced TNM stage and poor survival [31]. In addition, TWIST can modulate N-cadherin expression through directly interacting with an E-box, a regulatory element within intron 1 of CDH2 [32], and expression of TWIST appears to be indispensable for the entry of tumor cells into the bloodstream, a significant early step towards metastasis [33]. ZEB2 is also known as SIP1, which interacts through its COOH-terminal region with E-box element of E-cadherin gene promoter and mediates its transcriptional repression by recruiting corepressor complexes [34, 35]. These transcription factors form signaling networks that could initiate and sustain the mesenchymal phenotypes of tumor cells; therefore, the expression of these proteins could define EMT occurrence in a tumor setting. For example, a study in primary human gastric cancers revealed elevated snail and twist expressions in diffuse-type gastric

cancer, whereas ZEB2/SIP1 was primarily expressed in the intestinal type [36] (Fig. 14).

This meta-analysis was aimed to examine the expression of transcription factor snail in different tissue samples and the relationship between increased snail expression and clinicopathological features of gastric cancer. This study combined 756 gastric cancer tissue samples, 346 para-carcinoma samples, and 171 normal tissue samples from 10 individual studies. The results indicated that snail expression is higher in gastric cancer tissues than that in para-carcinoma tissues and normal tissues, respectively (OR = 6.15, 95 % CI = 4.70, 8.05; OR = 17, 95 % CI = 10.08, 28.67). Furthermore, closed correlations were observed between snail expression and clinicopathological characteristics that included the lymph node metastasis, the degree of differentiation, TNM stage, and invasion depth. The positive expression rate of snail was higher in gastric cancer tissues with lymphatic metastasis, OR = 0.40, 95 % CI = (0.18, 0.93). The higher positive rate of snail is

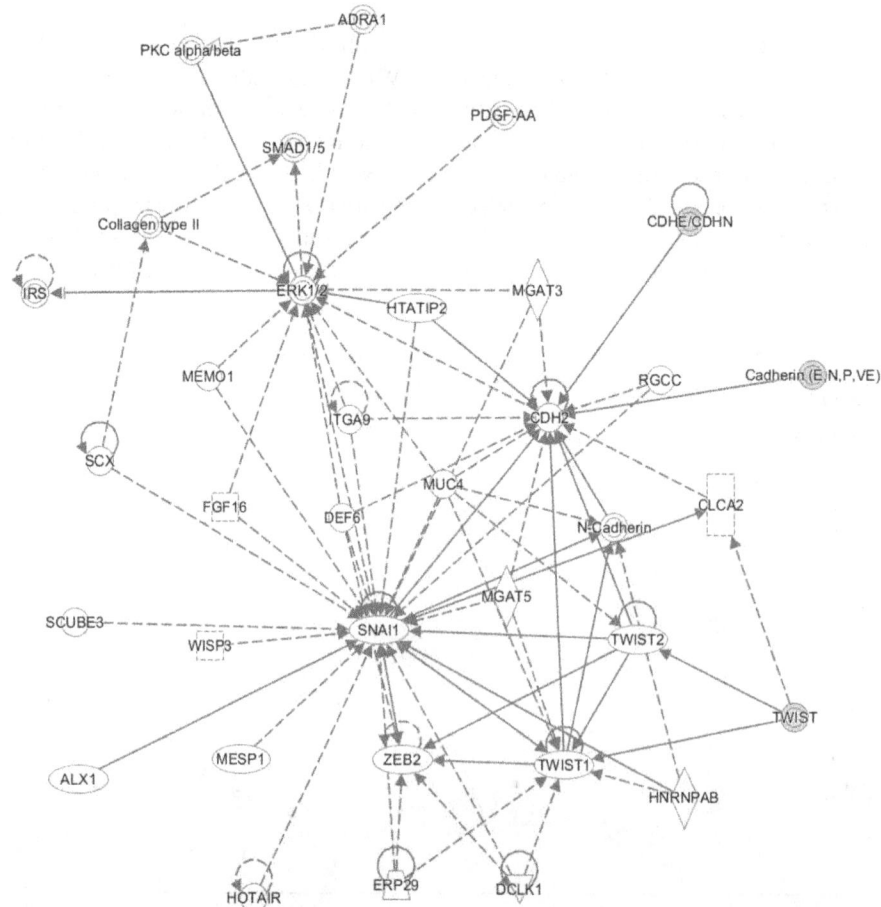

Fig. 14 Gene network analysis. The target genes of cancer-induced differentially expressed protein were used to run the IPA tool for gene network analysis. These genes around *triangles* highlighted genes that are involved in immunity system development function. The network score described in the "Methods" section for the network is 39. The *solid lines* connecting the molecules here represent a direct relation and *dotted lines* an indirect relation

connected with the lower differentiation degree, OR = 3.34, 95 % CI = (2.22, 5.03). The positive expression of snail was higher at late clinical stage, OR = 0.38, 95 % CI = (0.23, 0.60). Moreover, it appeared that the deeper the infiltration was, the higher the expression of snail was, OR = 0.18, 95 % CI = (0.11, 0.31).

The result of funnel plot indicated an imminent possibility of publication bias. Two potential biases might be introduced. First, the languages in collected papers were used in both Chinese and English, which may lead to a language bias. Second, the majority of collected studies did not use blind method, which might result in a measurement bias. Hence, the large-scale samples and double blind statistical tests will be investigated in the future study. Additionally, our review only collected the publications that have full text, since data that can be used for the methodology assessment and meta-analysis were only available in these publications with full text.

Our meta-analysis indicated that snail was highly expressed in gastric cancer. In addition, the overexpression of snail is significantly associated with tumor progression and metastasis.

Competing interests
The authors declare that they have no competing interests.

Authors' contributions
YC, YD, and JL envisioned the project. YC and LL designed the work. YC and LH constructed and validated the pathway models and performed the data analysis, with assistance from WY. YC, ZW, and HJ screened the data. YC, MY, WG, and HRA wrote the manuscript. YL polished the English. All authors read and approved the final manuscript.

Declarations
The research and publication of the research were supported by the Natural Science Foundation Hubei Province of China (2011CDB236 and 2012FFB04903). This article has been published as part of *Human Genomics* Volume 10 Supplement 2, 2016: From genes to systems genomics: human genomics. The full contents of the supplement are available online at http://humgenomics.biomedcentral.com/articles/supplements/volume-10-supplement-2.

Author details
[1]Medical College, Wuhan University of Science and Technology, Wuhan 430065, China. [2]Department of Anesthesiology, Tianyou Hospital, Wuhan University of Science and Technology, Wuhan 430064, China. [3]Texas Advanced Computing Center, University of Texas at Austin, 10100 Burnet Road, Austin, TX 78758, USA. [4]Puren Hospital, Wuhan University of Science and Technology, Wuhan 430081, China. [5]MidSouth Bioinformatics Center, Department of Information Science, George Washington Donaghey College of Engineering and Information Technology and Joint Bioinformatics Graduate Program, University of Arkansas at Little Rock and University of Arkansas for Medical Sciences, 2801 S. University Avenue, Little Rock, AR 72204, USA. [6]Department of Statistics and Harvard School of Public Health, Harvard University, One Oxford St., Cambridge 02138 Massachusetts, USA. [7]Department of Computer Science, University of Georgia, Athens, GA 30602, USA. [8]Department of Internal Medicine and Rush University Cancer Center, Rush University Medical Center, Chicago, IL 60612, USA.

References
1. Polyak K, Weinberg RA. Transitions between epithelial and mesenchymal states: acquisition of malignant and stem cell traits. Nat Rev Cancer. 2009;9:265–73.
2. Thompson EW, Newgreen DF, Tarin D. Carcinoma invasion and metastasis: a role for epithelial-mesenchymal transition. Cancer Res. 2005;65:5991–5.
3. Thiery JP, Sleeman JP. Complex networks orchestrate epithelial-mesenchymal transitions. Nat Rev Mol Cell Biol. 2006;7:131–42.
4. Sanchez-Tillo E, Liu Y, de Barrios O, Siles L, Fanlo L, Cuatrecasas M, et al. EMT-activating transcription factors in cancer: beyond EMT and tumor invasiveness. Cell Mol Life Sci. 2012;69:3429–56.
5. Iwatsuki M, Mimori K, Yokobori T, Ishi H, Beppu T, Nakamori S, et al. Epithelial-mesenchymal transition in cancer development and its clinical significance. Cancer Sci. 2010;101:293–9.
6. Jin H, Yu Y, Zhang T, Zhou X, Zhou J, Jia L, Wu Y, Zhou BP, Feng Y. Snail is critical for tumor growth and metastasis of ovarian carcinoma. Int J Cancer. 2010;126:2102–11.
7. Yanagawa J, Walser TC, Zhu LX, Hong L, Fishbein MC, Mah V, Chia D, Goodglick L, Elashoff DA, Luo J, Magyar CE, Dohadwala M, Lee JM, St John MA, Strieter RM, Sharma S, Dubinett SM. Snail promotes CXCR2 ligand dependent tumor progression in non-small cell lung carcinoma. Clin Cancer Res. 2009;15:6820–9.
8. Kosaka T, Kikuchi E, Mikami S, Miyajima A, Shirotake S, Ishida M, Okada Y, Oya M. Expression of snail in upper urinary tract urothelial carcinoma: prognostic significance and implications for tumor invasion. Clin Cancer Res. 2010;16:5814–23.
9. Muenst S, Daester S, Obermann EC, Droeser RA, Weber WP, von Holzen U, et al. Nuclear expression of snail is an independent negative prognostic factor in human breast cancer. Dis Markers. 2013;35:337–4.
10. Yang MH, Chen CL, Chau GY, Chiou SH, Su CW, Chou TY, Peng WL, Wu JC. Comprehensive analysis of the independent effect of twist and snail in promoting metastasis of hepatocellular carcinoma. Hepatology. 2009;50:1464–74.
11. Kim MA, Lee HS, Lee HE, Kim JH, Yang HK, Kim WH. Prognostic importance of epithelial-mesenchymal transition-related protein expression in gastric carcinoma. Histopathology. 2009;54:442–51.
12. Ryu HS, do Park J, Kim HH, Kim WH, Lee HS. Combination of epithelial-mesenchymal transition and cancer stem cell-like phenotypes has independent prognostic value in gastric cancer. Hum Pathol. 2012;43:520–8.
13. Shin NR, Jeong EH, Choi CI, Moon HJ, Kwon CH, Chu IS, et al. Overexpression of snail is associated with lymph node metastasis and poor prognosis in patients with gastric cancer. BMC Cancer. 2012;12:521.
14. Higgins JPT, Thompson SG, Deeks JJ, Altman DG. Measuring inconsistency in meta-analyses. Br Med J. 2003;327(7414):557–60.
15. Ioannidis JPA, Patsopoulos NA, Evangelou E. Uncertainty in heterogeneity estimates in meta-analyses. Br Med J. 2007;335(7626):914–6.
16. Zhu Y, Wu J, et al. Expression of TGF-β1, snail, E-cadherin and N-cadherin in gastric cancer and its significance. Chin J Clin Oncol. 2007;4(6):384–9.
17. Tang Z, Zhou Y, et al. Expression and clinical significance of transcriptional factor Snail and adhesion factor E-cadherin in gastric cancer. China J Emerg Resuscitat Disaster Med. 2010;5(8):696–9.
18. Hao Y, Ouyang X, et al. Combined detection of Shh, GliI, snail and E-cadherin expression in gastric cancer and its significance. Chin J Clin Oncol. 2011;38(7):382–5.
19. Wang S, Jiang R, Song W. The expression and significance of snail, E-cadherin protein in gastric carcinoma. Shandong Med. 2011;51(38):48–50.
20. Wang L et al. Expression and significance of Cox-2, snail and E-cadherin in gastric cancer. Lanzhou: Master degree thesis of Lanzhou university; 2011. p. 69.
21. Jin L et al. Expression of Snail, CK18 and Fn in gastric carcinoma and their relations with epithelial-mesenchymal transformation. J Hebei Med Univ. 2011;32(3):313–6.
22. Wu D et al. Expression and clinical significance of snail in gastric cancer. Henan. J Surg. 2012;18(4):26–7.
23. Cao X et al. Expression and significance of snail and E-cadherin in gastric cancer. Acta Acad Med Weifang. 2013;35(1):45–8.
24. Li Q et al. Snail, a zinc-finger transcriptional factor, induces gastric carcinoma invasion and metastasis via suppression of E-cadherin expression. Chin J Biomed Eng. 2013;19(6):433–7.
25. Liu L, Li J. Expression and clinical significance of E-cadherin, snail and twist in gastric cancer tissue and lymph node metastases. J Clin Med Pract. 2014;18(21):71–4.

26. Peinado H, Olmeda D, Cano A. Snail, ZEB and bHLH factors in tumor progression: an alliance against the epithelial phenotype. Nat Rev Cancer. 2007;7(6):415–28.

27. Drasin DJ, Robin TP, Ford HL. Breast cancer epithelial-to-mesenchymal transition: examining the functional consequences of plasticity. Breast Cancer Res. 2011;13:226.

28. Peng Z, Wang CX, Fang EH, Wang GB, Tong Q. Role of epithelial-mesenchymal transition in gastric cancer initiation and progression. World J Gastroenterol. 2014;20:5403–10.

29. Shirakihara T, Saitoh M, Miyazono K. Differential regulation of epithelial and mesenchymal markers by deltaEF1 proteins in epithelial mesenchymal transition induced by TGF-beta. Mol Biol Cell. 2007;18:3533–44.

30. Lascombe I, Clairotte A, Fauconnet S, Bernardini S, Wallerand H, Kantelip B, et al. N-cadherin as a novel prognostic marker of progression in superficial urothelial tumors. Clin Cancer Res. 2006;12:2780–7.

31. Hui L, Zhang S, Dong X, Tian D, Cui Z, Qiu X. Prognostic significance of twist and N-cadherin expression in NSCLC. PLoS One. 2013;8:e62171.

32. Alexander NR, Tran NL, Rekapally H, Summers CE, Glackin C, Heimark RL. N-cadherin gene expression in prostate carcinoma is modulated by integrin-dependent nuclear translocation of Twist1. Cancer Res. 2006;66:3365–9.

33. Yang J, Mani SA, Donaher JL, Ramaswamy S, Itzykson RA, Come C, Savagner P, Gitelman I,Richardson A, Weinberg RA. Twist, a master regulator of morphogenesis, plays an essential role in tumor metastasis. Cell. 2004;117:927–39.

34. Fabregat I, Malfettone A, Soukupova J. New Insights into the Crossroads between EMT and Stemness in the Context of Cancer. Edel MJ, ed. J Clin Med. 2016;5(3):37.

35. Vandewalle C, Van Roy F, Berx G. The role of the ZEB family of transcription factors in development and disease. Cell Mol Life Sci. 2009;66:773–87.

36. Rosivatz E, Becker I, Specht K, Fricke E, Luber B, Busch R, Hofler H, Becker KF. Differential expression of the epithelial-mesenchymal transition regulators snail, SIP1, and twist in gastric cancer. Am J Pathol. 2002;161:1881–91.

12

Forward and reverse mutations in stages of cancer development

Taobo Hu[1†], Yogesh Kumar[1†], Iram Shazia[1†], Shen-Jia Duan[2†], Yi Li[3], Lei Chen[4], Jin-Fei Chen[5], Rong Yin[6], Ava Kwong[7], Gilberto Ka-Kit Leung[7], Wai-Kin Mat[1], Zhenggang Wu[1], Xi Long[1], Cheuk-Hin Chan[1], Si Chen[1], Peggy Lee[1], Siu-Kin Ng[1], Timothy Y. C. Ho[1], Jianfeng Yang[1], Xiaofan Ding[1], Shui-Ying Tsang[1], Xuqing Zhou[1], Dan-Hua Zhang[2], the International Cancer Genome Consortium, En-Xiang Zhou[2], Lin Xu[6], Wai-Sang Poon[3], Hong-Yang Wang[4] and Hong Xue[1,8*]

Abstract

Background: Massive occurrences of interstitial loss of heterozygosity (LOH) likely resulting from gene conversions were found by us in different cancers as a type of single-nucleotide variations (SNVs), comparable in abundance to the commonly investigated gain of heterozygosity (GOH) type of SNVs, raising the question of the relationships between these two opposing types of cancer mutations.

Methods: In the present study, SNVs in 12 tetra sample and 17 trio sample sets from four cancer types along with copy number variations (CNVs) were analyzed by AluScan sequencing, comparing tumor with white blood cells as well as tissues vicinal to the tumor. Four published "nontumor"-tumor metastasis trios and 246 pan-cancer pairs analyzed by whole-genome sequencing (WGS) and 67 trios by whole-exome sequencing (WES) were also examined.

Results: Widespread GOHs enriched with CG-to-TG changes and associated with nearby CNVs and LOHs enriched with TG-to-CG changes were observed. Occurrences of GOH were 1.9-fold higher than LOH in "nontumor" tissues more than 2 cm away from the tumors, and a majority of these GOHs and LOHs were reversed in "paratumor" tissues within 2 cm of the tumors, forming forward-reverse mutation cycles where the revertant LOHs displayed strong lineage effects that pointed to a sequential instead of parallel development from "nontumor" to "paratumor" and onto tumor cells, which was also supported by the relative frequencies of 26 distinct classes of CNVs between these three types of cell populations.

Conclusions: These findings suggest that developing cancer cells undergo sequential changes that enable the "nontumor" cells to acquire a wide range of forward mutations including ones that are essential for oncogenicity, followed by revertant mutations in the "paratumor" cells to avoid growth retardation by excessive mutation load. Such utilization of forward-reverse mutation cycles as an adaptive mechanism was also observed in cultured HeLa cells upon successive replatings. An understanding of forward-reverse mutation cycles in cancer development could provide a genomic basis for improved early diagnosis, staging, and treatment of cancers.

Keywords: Single-nucleotide variation, Copy number variation, Interstitial loss of heterozygosity, Precancer mutations, Clonal evolution

* Correspondence: hxue@ust.hk
†Taobo Hu, Yogesh Kumar, Iram Shazia and Shen-Jia Duan contributed equally to this work.
[1]Division of Life Science, Applied Genomics Centre and Centre for Statistical Science, Hong Kong University of Science and Technology, Clear Water Bay, Kowloon, Hong Kong, China
[8]School of Basic Medicine and Clinical Pharmacy, China Pharmaceutical University, Nanjing, China
Full list of author information is available at the end of the article

Background

The progressive development of cancer has been investigated extensively at the cytochemical and genetic levels, leading to the recognition of early premalignant stages characterized by precancerous changes in DNA sequence, gene expression, protein structure, and microscopic rearrangement [1–14]. Genomic analysis also has played an increasingly important role in this regard [15, 16]. In a recent study, we have reported the finding of not only the commonly encountered single-nucleotide variations (SNVs) in the form of gain of heterozygosities (GOHs), but also massive SNVs in the form of interstitial loss of heterozygosities (LOHs) in various types of cancers [17]. This raises the question of the interrelations between the LOH and GOH mutations along with the copy number variations (CNVs) as the most abundant mutational elements of cancer cells. Because cancer cells at different stages of development are known to harbor different mutations, the aim of the present study was to track both GOHs mutating germline homozygous sequence positions to heterozygous ones and LOHs mutating germline heterozygous sequence positions to homozygous ones, through precancer stages to their final allelic forms in the cancer genome.

While forward mutations converting wildtype sequences into mutant forms and reverse mutations restoring the wildtype sequences from the mutant forms have been compared in microbial studies regarding their differential sensitivities to various mutagens [18–20], such studies have not been performed with cancer cells. In this study, a mutation from the original homozygous or heterozygous genotype at a base position in the individual's germline genome to a different genotype constitutes a forward mutation, and its mutation back to the germline original genotype constitutes a reverse mutation. With the large numbers of GOH and LOH occurrences in cancer cells, it becomes useful to examine whether forward GOHs occurring at one stage of cancer development could be reversed by LOHs during a subsequent stage, and vice versa, during cancer development and enquire into the significance of such reversals. Since premalignant cells have been detected in various instances in the vicinity of tumor cells [2–7, 11, 13], one possible experimental approach would be to analyze and compare solid tumors with their vicinal tissues that might be enriched in precancerous cells in terms of the mutations they harbor. A residue-by-residue analysis of the GOHs and LOHs observed in the tumor and its vicinal tissues relative to the white blood cell genome sequence as a control would reveal GOH-to-LOH and LOH-to-GOH reversals between the germline genotype, any precancerous genotypes, and the cancerous genotype. The same applies to the forward and reverse changes in CNVs.

Accordingly, in the present study, "nontumor" tissue isolated at > 2 cm from the tumor, "paratumor" tissue isolated at ≤ 2 cm from the tumor, and tumor from different types of cancers were compared with same-patient white blood cell controls based on massively parallel sequencing. Somatic mutations in both directions, i.e., GOH and LOH types of SNVs and CNV gains and losses, were examined residue-by-residue and window-by-window in order to detect the presence of mutation reversals during the development of cancer cells and to assess their biological significance. The results obtained from both clinical cancer samples and cultured HeLa cells indicated that forward-reverse (FR) mutations together with directional selection constitute important determinants of the mutation profiles of stage-specific cell populations in cancer development.

Methods

Tumor purity and histology

Tumor purity in all B-N-P-T tetra and B-N-T trio samples was estimated using VarScan software [21] and "absCNseq" R package [22]. The "my.res.list" function of absCNseq was applied with the following parameters: alpha.min = 0.2, alpha.max = 1, tau.min = 1.5, tau.max = 5, min.sol.freq = 0, min.seg.len = 0, qmax = 7, and lambda = 0.5.

For histological and immunohistochemical staining (Fig. 1c and Additional file 1: Table S1), the samples were taken from the tumor, the adjacent paratumor region (≤ 2 cm from a tumor), and the nontumor region (> 2 cm from a tumor) of a breast invasive carcinoma (BRCA) patient. The samples were fixed in 4% paraformaldehyde, dehydrated, embedded in paraffin, sectioned, and subjected to standard hematoxylin and eosin (HE) staining. Immunohistochemical staining for estrogen receptor (ER), progesterone receptor (PR), and human epidermal growth factor receptor-2 (HER2) were conducted following the conventional procedures as described [23].

Genomic DNA from clinical samples for AluScan sequencing

DNA extraction and AluScan sequencing library preparation were performed as described previously [17, 24]. White blood cells were treated as representative of germline controls in keeping with the recommendation by The Cancer Genome Atlas (TCGA) project [25]. The N- and P-stage tissues included and subjected to AluScan sequencing in this study were obtained as follows: N-stage tissue was collected at > 2 cm from the edge of the tumor in the vicinity of the tumor, and P-stage tissue was collected at ≤ 2 cm from the edge of the tumor. In line with the published research practices [5, 6, 26], 2 cm was chosen as the cutoff between N- and P-stage tissues. The AluScan cancer cases, designated as B-N-P-T, B-N-T, or N-T-M sample

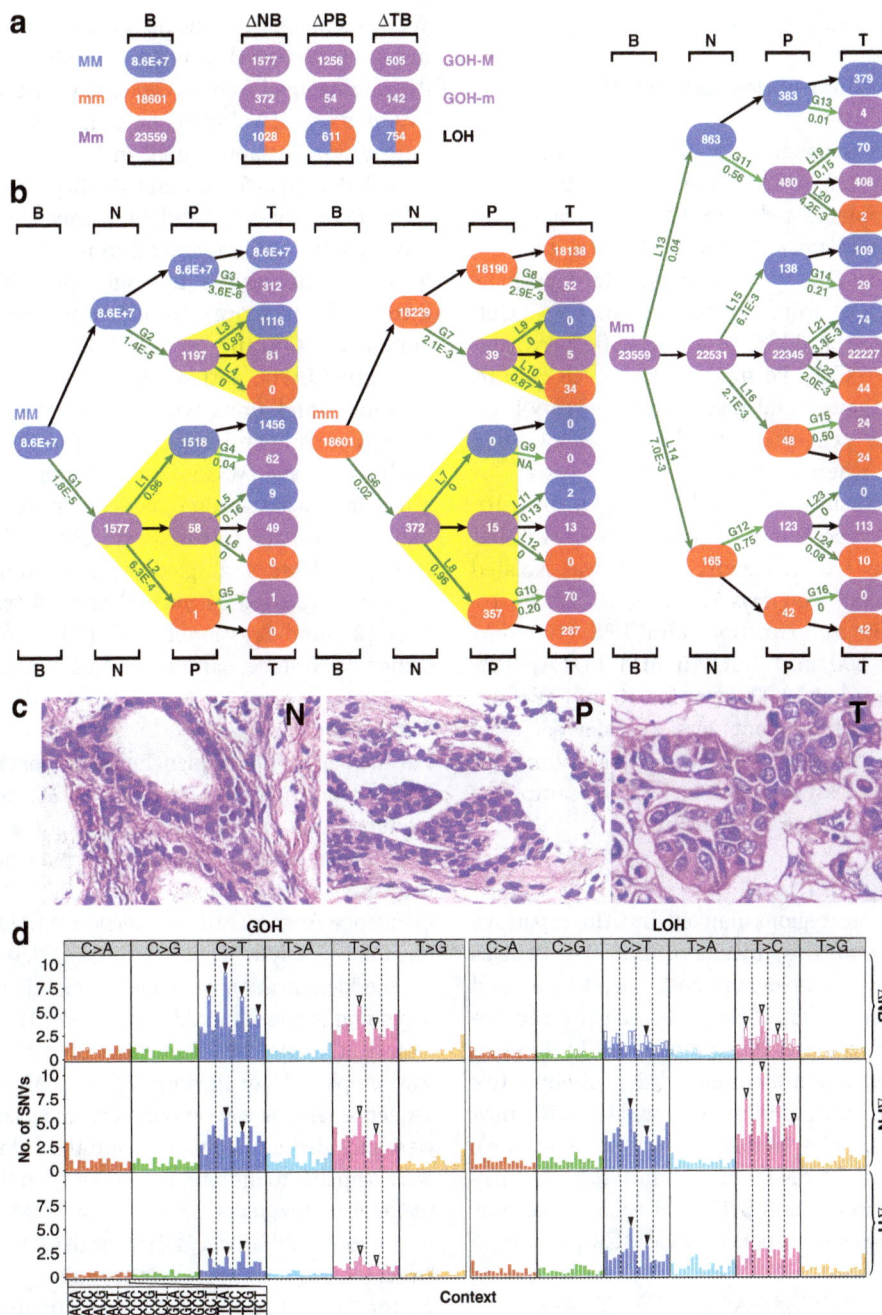

Fig. 1 SNV mutations in B-N-P-T tetra samples. **a** Genotypic changes at N-, P-, or T-stage of the samples. The numbers of genotypic changes in N-, P-, or T-stage sequences relative to B-stage sequences are represented by ΔNB, ΔPB, and ΔTB, respectively. LOH represents the sum of LOH-M and LOH-m changes. The 12 B-N-P-T cases consisted of 4 breast carcinomas (BRCA), 5 stomach adenocarcinomas (STAD), and 3 hepatocellular carcinomas (LIHC) analyzed using AluScan sequencing (Additional file 1: Table S1). **b** Patch diagrams tracing SNVs between the B-, N-, P-, and T-samples originating from MM, mm, or Mm genotypes in B-samples. Mutation rate is indicated below each LOH step (L1, L2, etc.) or GOH step (G1, G2, etc.). **c** Micrographs of N-stage tissue (left), P-stage tissue (middle), and T-stage tissue (right) in one of the representative BRCA B-N-P-T tetra samples. Magnification in each instance was ×400. **d** Mutational profiles for the ΔNB, ΔPN, and ΔTP SNV changes as numerically indicated in the patch diagrams in part **b**. The profiles are separated into the C>A, C>G, C>T, T>A, T>C, and T>G types, where C>A includes both the C-to-A and the complementary G-to-T mutations, etc. Within each type, the 16 possible kinds of sequence contexts are indicated on an expanded scale on the x-axis, and the total number of SNVs observed for each kind of trinucleotide sequence contexts is represented by a vertical bar. In each vertical bar in the ΔNB tier, the solid segment represents the SNVs that were reversed in the next ΔPN tier, e.g., C>T GOHs being reversed by T>C LOHs, whereas the open segment represents the unreversed SNVs. Subgroups of contexts are compartmentalized by vertical dashed lines. M, major allele; m, minor allele; GOH-M, MM-to-Mm mutation; GOH-m, mm-to-Mm mutation; LOH-M, Mm-to-MM mutation; LOH-m, Mm-to-mm mutation

sets, were listed in Additional file 1: Table S1 with demographical and clinical information.

Genomic DNA from cultured HeLa cells for AluScan sequencing

HeLa cell line was obtained from American Type Culture Collection (ATCC, USA). Cells were cultivated in DMEM media supplemented with 10% heat-inactivated fetal bovine serum (Sigma-Aldrich, USA), and medium pH was adjusted to 7.4 by 3-(N-morpholino) propane sulfonic acid (MOPS) from Sigma-Aldrich, USA. Cultures were incubated at 37 °C in a humidified environment containing 5% CO_2. To start the HeLa cell culture, frozen cells were thawed and plated at a density of approximately 4×10^5 cells per Petri dish and allowed to reach confluence whereupon they were harvested by treatment with trypsin-EDTA (Gibco, USA), and 10^5 cells were replated every 2 to 3 days on fresh Petri dishes at intervals of 2 to 3 days. Genomic DNA was isolated from the cells harvested on days 1, 3, 5, 8, 10, 12, 14, 16, 21, 25, 27, and 29 by extraction with TES (100 mM Tris-HCl pH 7.4, 200 mM NaCl, 5 mM EDTA, 0.2% SDS), and centrifuged at 12,000 rpm for 10 min at room temperature. The supernatant was transferred to a new vial and precipitated with an equal volume of ethanol. These successive HeLa cell DNA samplings were subjected to AluScan sequencing.

AluScan sequencing

AluScans of genomic regions flanked by Alu repetitive sequences were obtained by means of inter-Alu PCR as described [17, 24], employing both head-type and tail-type Alu consensus-based primers to ensure capture of a vast number of inter-Alu amplicons. In brief, a 25-μl PCR reaction mixture contained 2 μl Bioline 10× NH4 buffer (160 mM ammonium sulfate, 670 mM Tris-HCl, pH 8.8, 0.1% stabilizer; www.bioline.com), 3 mM $MgCl_2$, 0.15 mM dNTP mix, 1 unit Taq polymerase, 0.1 μg DNA sample, and 0.075 μM each of the four following Alu consensus sequence-based PCR primers:

AluY278T18 (5′-GAGCGAGACTCCGTCTCA-3′);
AluY66H21 (5′-TGGTCTCGATCTCCTGACCTC-3′);
R12A/267 (5′-AGCGAGACTCCG-3′);
L12A/8 (5′-TGAGCCACCGCG-3′).

PCR was carried out at 95 °C, 5 min for DNA denaturation, followed by 30 cycles each of 30 s at 95 °C, 30 s at 50 °C, and 5 min at 72 °C, plus finally another 7 min at 72 °C. Amplicons were purified with ethanol precipitation, sequenced on the Illumina HiSeq platform at Beijing Genomics Institute (Shenzhen, China) and mapped to the hg19 reference human genome for downstream bioinformatic analysis.

WGS and WES raw data

Whole-genome sequencing (WGS) data generated from tumor-blood paired samples with the Illumina system by the International Cancer Genome Consortium (ICGC) and TCGA were downloaded in bam format with permission (https://www.synapse.org/#!Synapse:syn2887117). These included the Pilot-63 set and 86 hepatocellular carcinoma (LIHC), 75 non-small-cell lung cancer (NSCLC), and 22 intrahepatic cholangiocarcinoma (ICC) cases with information accessible through the ICGC Data Portal (https://dcc.icgc.org). In addition, raw WGS data generated by Ouyang et al. [27] from four hepatitis B-positive LIHC patients having pulmonary metastasis were obtained along with data from same-patient liver tissue controls and included in the N-T-M trio sample analysis as the WGS-Liver-M subset. Moreover, the raw data of whole-exome sequencing (WES) from 67 brain metastatic cancer patients were obtained from Brastianos et al. [28]. Tissues sampled at > 2 cm from the edge of the tumors were used as normal control tissues in Ouyang et al. [27] and Brastianos et al. [28], and treated as non-tumor or N-stage, samples in this study.

SNV calling

For the paired-end sequencing reads generated on the Illumina platform by the AluScan, WGS, or WES methods, bioinformatics analysis including alignment, sorting, recalibration, realignment, and removal of duplicates using BWA (Burrows-Wheeler Aligner, version 0.6.1) [29], SAMtools (Sequence Alignment/Map, version 0.1.18) [30] and GATK (Genome Analysis Tool-Kit, version 3.5) were performed for the identification of single nucleotide variations (SNVs) according to the standard framework [31] as described previously [17, 24]. The "UnifiedGenotyper" module of GATK was employed for genotyping of SNVs. Only genomic sequence regions with enough coverage, i.e., read depth > 8, were included in the analysis, and the following parameters were applied to filtrate for SNVs of different genotypes: major allele frequency ≥ 95% for the "MM" loci; major allele frequency ≥ 30% and ≤ 70% and QD ≥ 4 for "Mm" or "mn" loci; and minor allele frequency ≥ 95% and QD ≥ 20 for "mm" loci. Strand bias estimated using Fisher's exact test (FS) was employed to ensure FS value ≤ 20 for both heterozygous "Mm" or "mn" loci and homozygous "MM" or "mm" loci.

For cancer cases with more than two samples from each patient, i.e., the B-N-P-T tetra sample set of 12 cases, the B-N-T trio sample set of 17 cases, and the N-T-M trio sample set of 23 cases, the abovementioned calling of SNVs was first performed for each sample of each case in the multiple sample sets. For each of the multiple-sample cases, only nucleotide positions conformed to all the above SNV calling criteria in every sample of the same patient were included in further analysis. Sites not covered in the further analysis were arising from either lack of sequencing reads or failure to meet the filtering criteria in any one of the samples of the same patient.

Mutational profiles of SNVs

Mutational profiles of SNVs were analyzed following the procedure developed by Alexandrov et al. [32]. For each SNV site, the SomaticSignatures package [33] under R environment was employed to determine its preceding and following bases. The results were unnormalized for the observed trinucleotide frequencies in the human genome. The resulting mutation frequency profiles were illustrated in three different graphical presentations, i.e., the alteration-group plot, context-group plot, and mutation-rate diagram. Custom R scripts for drawing the three different presentations are available at GitHub website (https://github.com/hutaobo/ProfilePlots).

CNV calling and identification of recurrent CNVs

From AluScan data, the AluScanCNV software [34] was employed to call paired CNVs between B- and N-stage (ΔNB), between N- and P-stage (ΔPN), between P- and T-stage (ΔTP), between B- and P-stage (ΔPB), and between B- and T-stage (ΔTB) samples of the same patient in the B-N-P-T tetra sample sets of 12 cases, using fixed window sizes ranging from 50 to 500 kb. The ΔNB, ΔPB, and ΔTB were arranged sequentially to yield the 26 possible serial orders shown in Fig. 8a, b. To identify the recurrent CNVs, all CNVs found in any sequence window of the 12 tetra sample cases at any two of the stages, including ΔNB, ΔPB, ΔTB, ΔPN, and ΔTP, were aggregated. Only the sequence windows where CNV was detected in 6 or more of the 12 patients were considered to harbor a recurrent CNV. CNVs located in the recently identified distal zones [35] were removed from further analysis to reduce background noise introduced by less informative windows in the human genome.

Co-localization of CNVT with CpGe and MeMRE

CpGe and MeMRE entries were downloaded from UCSC Genome Browser as described [35], and somatic CNV (CNVT) entries classified as "copy number variants" were downloaded from the COSMIC database (http://grch37-cancer.sanger.ac.uk/cosmic/download). The human genome was divided into tandem 2000 bp windows, and the average densities of CNVT breakpoints and base pairs in CpGe or MeMRE in each window were calculated. Thereupon, the windows with zero CpGe or MeMRE density were removed to avoid error caused by missing data, and the remaining windows were separated into ten groups based on the percentile of CpGe or MeMRE density. Finally, the average CNVT breakpoint densities in the groups were plotted against the percentile CpGe or MeMRE density.

Mutation enrichment in genes and pathways

The results of variant analysis of AluScan data of the 12 tetra sample cases were uploaded to BioMart of the Ensembl database to generate a list of their gene contents under R environment using the "biomaRt" R package [36]. For the "getBM" function, "chromosome_name," "start_position," "end_position," "external_gene_name," "ensembl_gene_id." and "description" were selected as attributes, with "chromosomal_region" filter type, "sublist" filter value, "ENSEMBL_MART_ENSEMBL" biomart type, and "grch37.ensembl.org" host. The resultant gene list was uploaded to DAVID Bioinformatics Resources 6.7 [37] using "Functional Annotation Tool" to obtain three lists of mutation enriched functional groups and pathways as annotated in the three databases GOTERM, InterPro, and KEGG, respectively, with mutated genes specified for each group and pathways. Only those functionally annotated groups and pathways yielding Bonferroni-corrected p value, Benjamini-corrected p value, and FDR q value all less than 0.05 were considered statistically significant.

Statistical analysis and data visualization

Statistical analyses were performed using R software (http://www.r-project.org). The significance probability (p) values were calculated by the two-tailed t test or chi-square test functions in R, and the Pearson correlation coefficients (r) were calculated by the cor function in R. Figures were drawn using the ggplot2, lattice, or ellipse package under R environment, except for Fig. 8b which was drawn using the Circos program [38].

Results

Genotypic changes in nontumor and paratumor tissues

White blood cells (B), tumor tissue (T), paratumor tissue (P) immediately adjacent to the tumor, and more remote nontumor tissue (N) were collected in 12 same-patient tetra sample cases consisted of four breast carcinomas (BRCA), five stomach adenocarcinomas (STAD), and three hepatocellular carcinomas (LIHC) (Additional files 1 and 2: Tables S1 and S2) and subjected to DNA analysis using the AluScan platform based on inter-Alu polymerase chain reaction (PCR) followed by massively parallel sequencing as described in the "Methods" section. The genotype of a base residue was referred to as a major allele (M) when it matches the sequence of human reference genome hg19 or as a minor allele (m) when there was no match, thereby enabling the identification of changes in the form of MM-to-Mm GOH ("GOH-M"), mm-to-Mm GOH ("GOH-m"), Mm-to-MM LOH ("LOH-M"), or Mm-to-mm LOH ("LOH-m") [17]. Figure 1a, b show the total number of residue-by-residue changes in the N-, P-, or T-sample genomes relative to B-sample, viz. ΔNB, ΔPB, or ΔTB respectively in terms of GOH-M, GOH-m, and LOH (sum of instances of LOH-M and LOH-m). Since the numbers of GOH-M, GOH-m, and LOH mutations were higher in ΔNB than in ΔTB, and comparable in ΔPB and ΔTB, both the N-sample and P-sample cells had to be regarded as premalignant or early malignant cells despite their normal morphology and expression of immunohistochemistry (IHC) markers, in contrast with T-sample cells showing enlarged nuclei (Fig. 1c) and reduced expression of IHC markers (Additional file 1: Table S1). Since the residues of minor bases different from "m" were rare in the samples analyzed, mutations involving them are listed in Additional files 3 and 4: Tables S3 and S4 but not shown in Fig. 1a, b. Notably, 96% of the B-to-N-stage forward GOH mutations were reversed in P-stage via steps L1 and L8, and 56% and 75% of the B-to-N-stage forward LOHs were reversed via steps G11 and G12, respectively. On the other hand, only 16% and 0% of the B-to-N-stage forward GOH mutations were reversed in T-stage via steps L5 and L12, and only 1% and 0% of the B-to-N-stage LOH mutations were reversed in T-stage via steps G13 and G16.

Moreover, the LOH mutations partitioned Mm genotypes between MM and mm products on a non-random basis. Thus, the ratio of MM/mm products from the L1 and L2 steps was 1518/1, whereas the ratio of MM/mm products from the L7 and L8 steps was 0/357. Likewise, the ratio of MM/mm products from the L3 and L4 steps was 1116/0, and the ratio of MM/mm products from the L9 and L10 steps was 0/34. Therefore, the partition of LOH products in each of these instances was biased by strong lineage effect in favor of restoring the original germline genotype that gave rise to the Mm residue in the first place (as highlighted by yellow triangles in Fig. 1b).

Notably, in Fig. 1b right panel, the partition of the germline Mm genotypes via LOH steps L13 and L14 yielded a greater MM/mm product ratio than the partition via LOH steps L15 and L16, and greater still than the partition via LOH steps L21 and L22, although in each instance, MM products exceeded mm products (Fig. 2a). Since all these three successive partitions emanated from the germline Mm genotypes, their diminishing MM/mm ratios could not be the consequence of lineage effects. Instead, because MM genotypes in the genome have been optimized in general for growth in the course of human evolution, they tended to be favored over mm genotypes. The finding of [L13/L14 = 5.7] > [L15/L16 = 2.9] > [L21/L22 = 1.7] could be the result of the N-stage cells having gone through a more prolonged period of positive selection for MM genotypes than the P-stage cells, and the P-stage cells in turn have gone through a more prolonged period of positive selection than T-stage cells.

When the trinucleotide-based mutational profile method [32] was employed to classify the GOHs and LOHs observed in the B-N-T-P tetra samples into the C>A, C>G, C>T, T>A, T>C, and T>G groups, the results showed that C>T and T>C mutations were particularly prominent among both GOHs and LOHs, in keeping with the expectation that transitions would exceed transversions in SNVs (Fig. 1d). The C>T GOHs among the ΔNB changes displayed peak frequencies at the four NCG triplets, conforming to the "signature 1A" (marked by four solid arrowheads) common to cancers, and likely ascribable to the contribution of spontaneous deamination of 5-methylcytosine at methylated CpG to form thymidine [32, 39]. These deaminations would also explain the ~ 50% greater occurrence of CG>TG GOHs than TG>CG GOHs in the ΔNB changes. In support of this, Fig. 2b shows that although there were less CG dimers than other dimers among AluScan captured as well as whole-genome sequences (Additional file 5: Figure S1), more CG dimers underwent SNV mutations than any other dimers. In Fig. 1d, all SNV frequency columns in the ΔNB tier were represented by a solid segment and an open segment; the mutations in the solid segments were reversed in the next ΔPN tier, whereas the open segments were unreversed. Both the C>T and T>C GOHs show large solid segments indicating their extensive reversals in the ΔPN changes; since the T>C LOHs in the ΔPN tier were mostly reversals of the C>T GOHs in the ΔNB tier, these T>C LOHs were likewise more abundant than ΔPN C>T LOHs and showed four NTG peaks (marked by open arrows), which may be referred to as a "signature 1A"-like LOH feature.

Figure 2c summarizes the forward and reverse mutation occurrences in the B-N-P-T samples; more SNVs and CNVs occurred in N-stage (viz. sum of types II, III, IVa, and IVb patterns) than in P- and T-stages combined (viz. type I). Reversals of N-stage SNVs and CNVs (viz. sum of types IVa and IVb patterns) were common, amounting to ~ 70% of N-stage SNVs or ~ 40% of N-stage CNVs, and far more of such reversals took place in P-stage (type IVa) than in T-stage (type IVb), see Additional files 3 and 6: Tables S3 and S5 for detailed numbers of the SNVs and CNVs at different stages.

When another 17 B-N-T trio sample sets consisted of 1 BRCA, 2 LIHC, and 14 non-small cell lung cancers (NSCLC) were analyzed with respect to the GOH and LOH changes in the N- and T-stage cells relative to B-stage cells (Fig. 3, Additional files 7 and 8: Tables S6 and S7), the results obtained showed the same regularities as the B-N-P-T tetra samples: the B genomes displayed much higher LOH (L5, L6) rates and GOH-m (G3, G4) rates than GOH-M (G1, G2) rates, strong lineage effects in LOH partitions between MM and mm products (highlighted by yellow triangles), and prominent

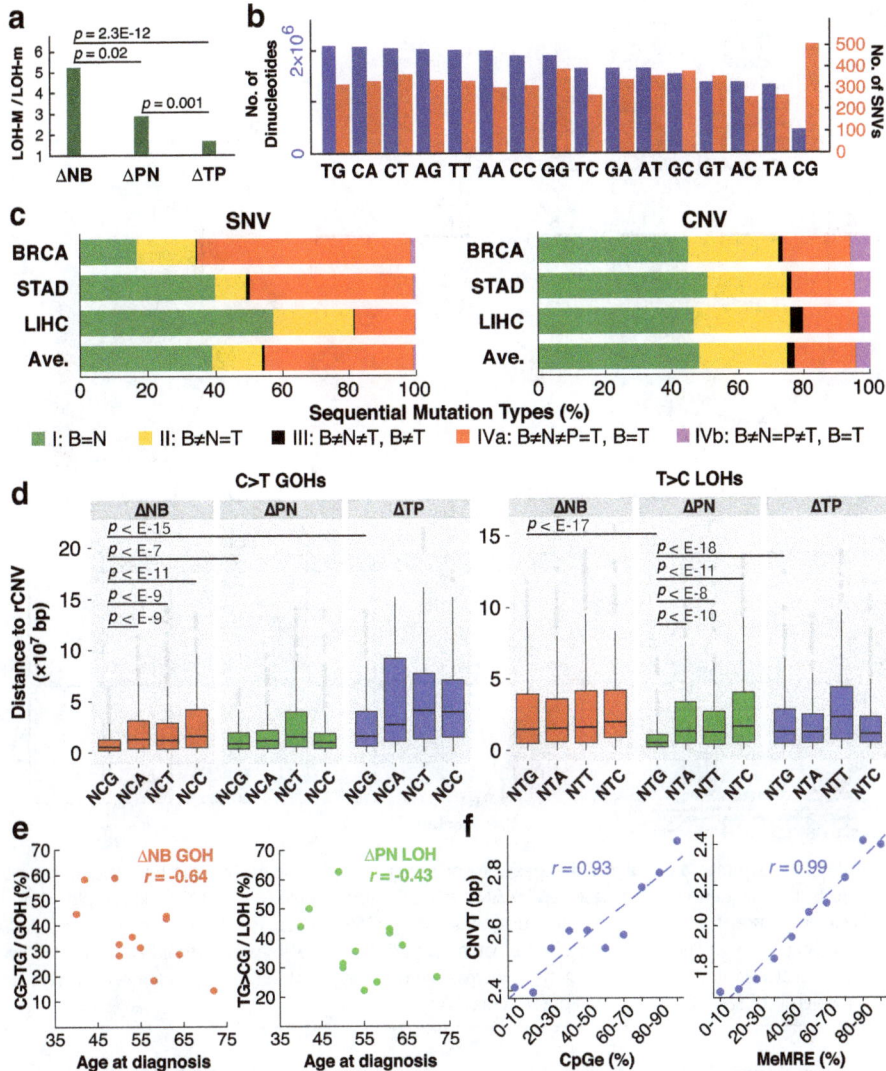

Fig. 2 Properties of mutations in B-N-P-T tetra samples. **a** M over m preference in LOHs. LOH-M/LOH-m ratios for LOHs arising at germline Mm positions are shown for N-, P-, and T-stages (data from Fig. 1b, right panel). **b** Dinucleotides in genomic sequences captured by AluScan (blue bars) and SNVs found at the first base of dinucleotides (red bars). **c** Percentile of different types of sequential SNV and CNV changes in 12 tetra sample cases of BRCA, STAD, and LIHC. Type I (green) B=N, viz. no SNV (or CNV) found in ΔNB. Type II (yellow) B ≠ N = T, viz. same SNV (or CNV) found in ΔNB and ΔTB. Type III (blue) B ≠ N ≠ T and B ≠ T, viz. altered in ΔNB and ΔTN and also in ΔTB. Type IVa (red) B ≠ N ≠ P = T and B = T, viz. altered in ΔNB and ΔPN but not in ΔTP or ΔTB. Type IVb (purple) B ≠ N=P ≠ T and B = T, viz. altered in ΔNB and ΔTP but not in ΔPN or ΔTB. **d** Average distances between GOHs (left) or LOHs (right) and their nearest recurrent CNVs (rCNVs). The left panel shows that on average, CG>TG GOHs in ΔNB were closer to their nearest rCNVs than it was the case with 11 other kinds of C>T GOHs; the right panel shows that on average, TG>CG LOHs in ΔPN were closer to their nearest rCNVs than it was the case with 11 other kinds of LOHs, with the horizontal bars indicating how much closer in terms of p values. **e** Correlation between patient's age at diagnosis and percentage of CG>TG GOHs among all GOHs for ΔNB (left) or percentage of TG>CG LOHs among all LOHs for ΔPN (right). **f** Correlation of numbers of somatic CNV breakpoints found in tumors (CNVT) from the COSMIC database with either evolutionarily conserved CpG-rich regions (CpGe) (left panel) or unmethylated CpG-rich regions (MeMRE) (right panel) from UCSC Table Browser database [35]. p, significance probability; r, Pearson correlation coefficient (see Fig. 1 for abbreviations)

FR-mutations, viz. L1 reversing G1, L4 reversing G3, G5 reversing L5, and G6 reversing L6.

Genotypic changes in cultured HeLa cells

When frozen HeLa cells were restarted in culture and sequentially sampled for AluScan sequencing, the results obtained also showed a wave of forward mutations followed by reverse mutations. Figure 4a shows the changes in the genotypes of base residues between day 10 and day 5 (viz. Δ10−5) and between day 14 and day 5 (viz. Δ14−5), and these changes are indicated in the patch diagrams in Fig. 4b. Notably, of the 273 MM residues that mutated to Mm via the G1 step, 263 of them were reverted to MM by day 14, and none was mutated to mm.

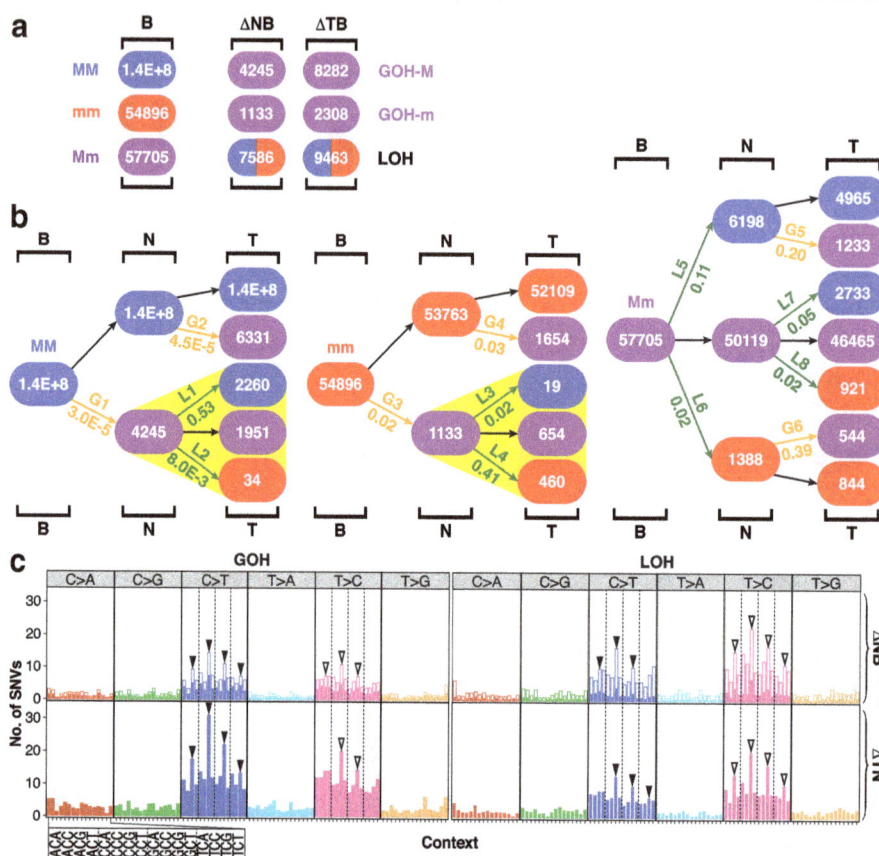

Fig. 3 SNV mutations in B-N-T trio samples. **a** Genotypic changes in N- or T-stage of the samples. The numbers of genotypic changes in N- or T-stage sequences relative to B-stage sequences are represented by ΔNB and ΔTB, respectively. The 17 B-N-T trio samples consisted of 1 BRCA, 2 LIHC, and 14 non-small cell lung cancer (NSCLC) cases. **b** Patch diagrams tracing SNVs between the B-, N-, and T-samples. **c** Mutational profiles for the ΔNB and ΔTN SNV changes as numerically indicated in the patch diagrams in part **b**. In each vertical bar in the ΔNB tier, the solid segment represents the SNVs that were reversed in the ΔTN tier, whereas the open segment indicates the unreversed SNVs (see Additional files 7 and 8: Tables S6 and S7 for details of SNVs, and Fig. 1 for abbreviations)

Similarly, of the 95 mm residues that mutated to Mm via the G3 step, 83 of them were reverted to mm, and none was mutated to MM. Thus, the ratio of MM/mm products from the yellow-highlighted L1 and L2 LOH steps was 263/0 and that for the L3 and L4 LOH steps was 0/83, displaying striking lineage effects in both instances comparable to the lineage effects displayed by the N-stage cells in Fig. 1b that were also yellow-highlighted. Since HeLa cells were transformed cells, the forward-reverse mutation cycles formed by the G1-L1 steps, or by the G3-L4 steps, in Fig. 4b could not be related to the oncogenic transformation. Instead, they likely represented a mechanism employed by the cells in the process of adapting to replating and growth.

Figure 4c shows the mutational profiles of GOHs (left panel) and LOHs (right panel) observed in the transitions between day 5 and day 10 (viz. Δ10–5, upper tier) and between day 10 and day 14 (viz. Δ14–10, lower tier), where the solid or open segments in the Δ10–5 tier represent the mutations that were reversed or unreversed

respectively in the Δ14–10 tier. As in the case of the profiles for the ΔNB and ΔPN changes in Fig. 1d, both the CG>TG (blue) and TG>CG (pink) GOH peaks in the Δ10–5 tier were extensively reversed in the Δ14–10 tier, giving rise to the prominent TG>CG (pink) and CG>TG (blue) LOH peaks respectively in the Δ14–10 tier. The G1, L1, L2, G3, L3, and L4 rates in Fig. 4b were also similar to their counterpart G1, L1, L2, G6, L7, and L8 rates in Fig. 1b.

Genotypic changes in primary and metastatic tumors

Figures 5 and 6 compare the mutations observed in five cancer groups based on same-patient N-stage, T-stage, and metastatic stage (M-stage) samples: (i) AluScan group of 2 N-T-M trio sets analyzed with AluScan sequencing, (ii) WGS-Liver-M group of 4 trio sets of liver-to-lung metastasis analyzed by Ouyang et al. [27] using WGS, and 67 trio sets involving brain metastases analyzed with WES by Brastianos et al. [28], which were separated into (iii) 38 WES-Non-Lung cancers, (iv) 6

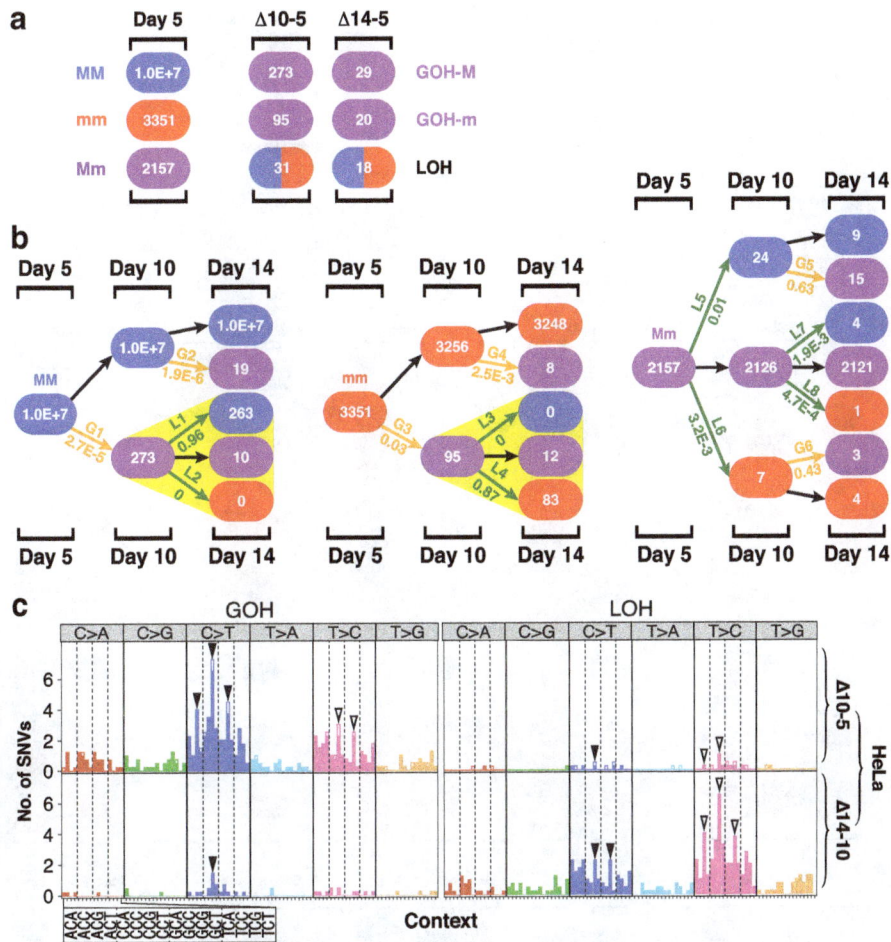

Fig. 4 SNV mutations in HeLa cells. **a** Numbers of base positions of different genotypes on day 5, and their changes observed on day 10 relative to day 5 (Δ10–5), and on day 14 relative to day 5 (Δ14–5). **b** Patch diagrams tracing the mutated changes of MM, mm, and Mm residues of day 5 DNA in day 10 DNA and day 14 DNA. LOHs showing large lineage effects are highlighted by yellow triangles. **c** Mutational profiles for the changes indicated in part **b** between day 5 and day 10 DNAs (Δ10–5) and between day 10 and day 14 DNAs (Δ14–10). For each vertical bar in the Δ10–5 tier, the solid segment represents SNVs that were subsequently reversed in the Δ14–10 tier, and the open segment represents the unreversed SNVs

WES-NSCLC-L (L = low in C>A GOHs) cancers, and (v) 23 WES-NSCLC-H (H = high in C>A GOHs) cancers. Although the five N-T-M trio groups compared in Fig. 5a were analyzed using variously the AluScan, WES, and WGS platforms, the ratios of the [ΔTN]/N and [ΔMN]/N counts both indicated that the rates of LOH far surpassed the rates of GOH-m, which in turn far surpassed the rates of GOH-M (Additioanl files 9 and 10: Tables S8 and S9). All five groups also displayed pronounced lineage effects in Fig. 5b in the partitions of LOH mutations of Mm genotypes between MM and mm products (highlighted by yellow triangles).

In Fig. 6a, the relative prominences of ΔTN GOHs, ΔTN LOHs, ΔMT GOHs, and ΔMT LOHs varied among the five different cancer groups. This could arise in part from biological dissimilarities between the sequences analyzed on the different platforms on account of their varied sequence coverages of the genome. The SNV sites

observed in the five groups displayed non-identical distri-butions among the genic, proximal, and distal sequence zones [35], as well as non-identical replication timings during the cell cycle (Fig. 6b). The proportion of ΔTN GOHs that became reversed in the ΔMT changes, marked by solid segments of the GOH frequency bars in the ΔTN tiers, was highest in the AluScan group, also quite high in the WES-NSCLC-L group, modest in the WES-Non-Lung group, and lowest in the WGS-Liver-M and WES-NSCLC-H groups, even though the WES-NSCLC-L, WES-Non-Lung, and WES-NSCLC-H groups were all analyzed based on the WES platform [28].

The WES-NSCLC-H group was unique in its display of particularly eminent C>A GOHs. Previously, C>A trans-versions were linked to polycyclic aromatic hydrocarbons [40] and acrolein [41] in tobacco smoke. The 23 WES-NSCLC-H samples were derived entirely from smokers, in accord with smoking being a significant factor

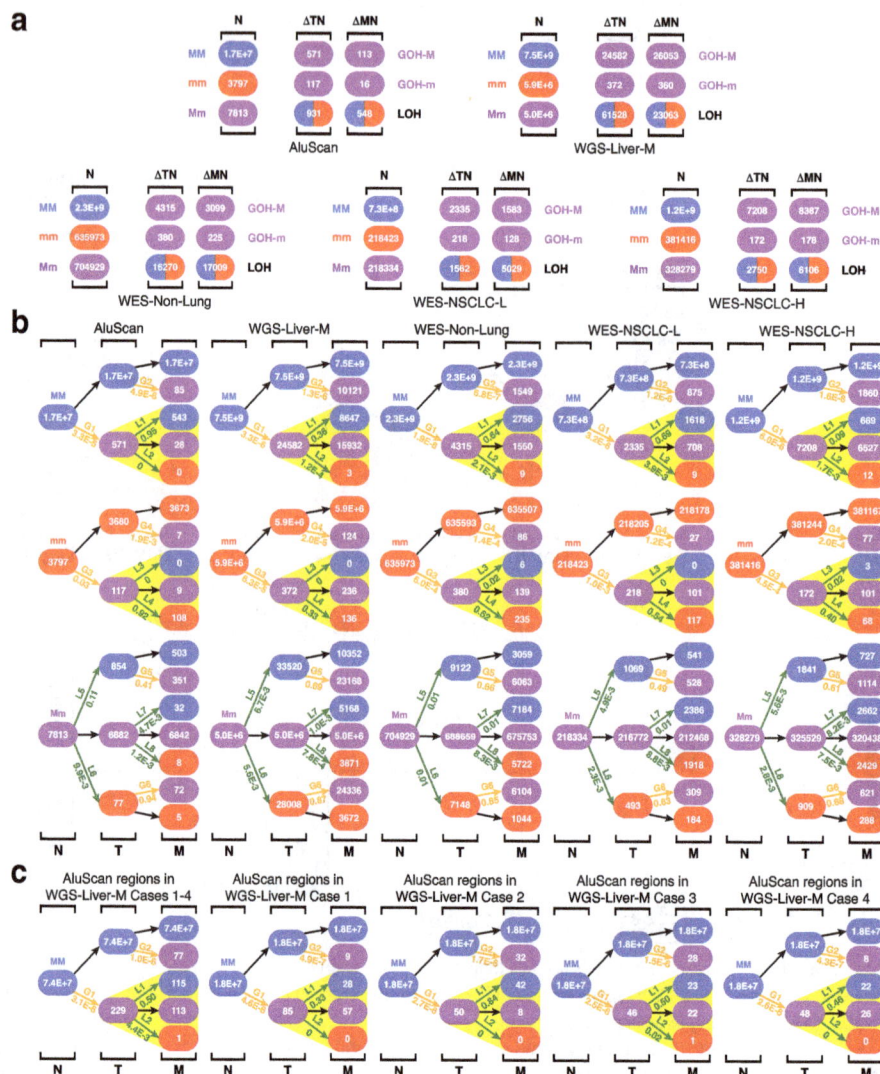

Fig. 5 SNV mutations in N-T-M trio samples. **a** Genotypic changes in T- or M-stage sequences. The numbers of genotypic changes in T- or M-stage sequences relative to N-stage sequences in each of the five case groups are represented by ΔTN and ΔMN, respectively. The five case groups include AluScan group of 2 N-T-M trio sets analyzed with AluScan sequencing, WGS-Liver-M group of 4 trio sets of liver-to-lung metastasis analyzed by whole-genome sequencing (WGS), and 67 trio sets involving brain metastases analyzed with whole-exome sequencing (WES) which were separated into 38 WES-Non-Lung cancers, 6 WES-NSCLC-L (L = low in C>A GOHs) cancers, and 23 WES-NSCLC-H (H = high in C>A GOHs) cancers. In the trio sets of WGS-Liver-M, WES-Non-Lung, WES-NSCLC-L, and WES-NSCLC-H, because nontumor tissues were sampled at > 2 cm from tumor's edge as controls instead of blood cells, the samples were designated as "N-stage" for comparability with Figs. 1a and 3a. **b** Patch diagrams tracing SNVs between the N, T, and M samples (see Additional files 9 and 10: Tables S8 and S9 for details of SNVs). M, metastatic tumor. (liver = hepatocellular carcinoma; NSCLC = non-small-cell lung cancer; non-lung = all 12 types of solid tumors in Reference [27] except lung adenocarcinomas and lung squamous carcinomas, see Fig. 1 for abbreviations). **c** Patch diagrams tracing the SNVs in the fraction of the four WGS sequences in the WGS-Liver-M group that corresponded to all the AluScan-captured regions analyzed in Fig. 1

for their elevated C>A GOHs. However, the WES-NSCLC-L samples with much more subdued C>A GOHs included two non-smokers and four smokers, suggesting that smoking or high C>A GOHs could play a less important carcinogenic role in a minority of smokers.

When the AluScan-capturable regions were extracted from the four N-T-M trio samples in the WGS-Liver-M group and analyzed with respect to their genotypic changes,

the results obtained were similar to those obtained from the entire WGS sequences for the same samples: (a) among the ΔTN changes, the LOH/GOH-M ratios of 2.5 for the WGS-based samples (Fig. 5a), and 2.1 for the AluScan-based samples (Additional file 11: Figure S2a), were both substantially greater than unity; (b) among the ΔMN changes, the LOH/GOH-M ratios of 0.89 for the WGS-based samples, and 1.1 for the AluScan-based

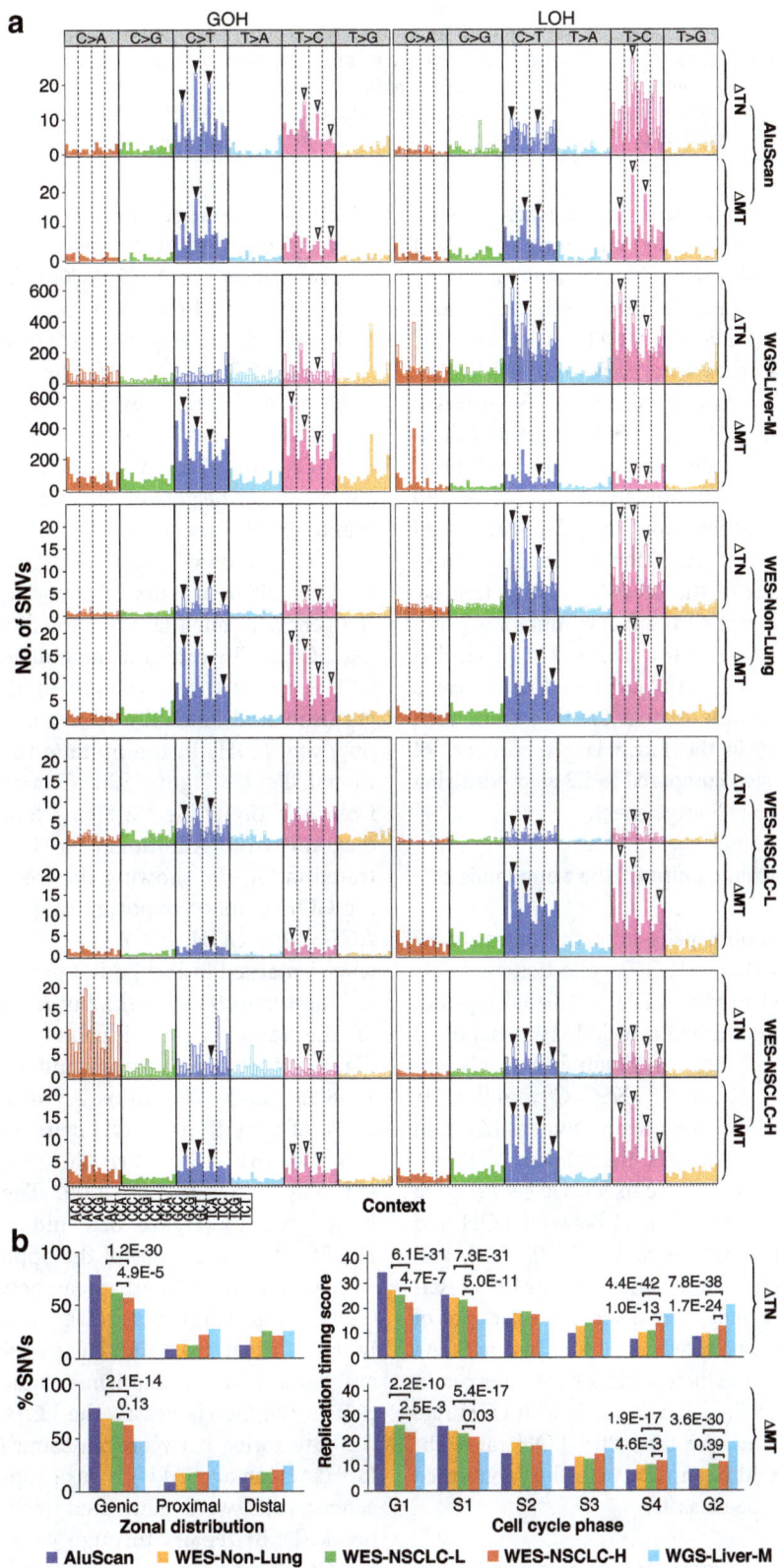

Fig. 6 (See legend on next page.)

(See figure on previous page.)
Fig. 6 Properties of SNVs in N-T-M trio samples. **a** Mutational profiles for the ΔTN and ΔMT SNV changes as numerically indicated in the patch diagrams in Fig. 5b. In each vertical bar in the ΔTN tier, the solid segment represents the SNVs that were reversed in the ΔMT tier, whereas the open segment indicates the unreversed SNVs. **b** Zonal distribution and replication timing of the SNVs in the ΔTN tier and the ΔMT tier in the five case groups. Left panels: zonal classification of SNV (GOH and LOH) sites determined as described [35]. Right panels: replication timing scores derived from ENCODE at UCSC based on the "Repli-chip" method [52] (see Figs. 1 and 5 for abbreviations)

samples, were both close to unity; (c) in the patch diagram for the total WGS-based mutations originating from MM residues in the four samples (Fig. 5b), the rates for the L1 and L2 steps were 0.36 and 1.2E–4, respectively. In the total AluScan-based samples (Additional file 11: Figure S2b), the rates for the L1 and L2 steps were 0.50 and 4.4E-3 respectively. Thus, both WGS-based and AluScan-based analyses yielded a high L1/L2 > 100 rate ratio indicative of strong lineage effects in the LOH mutations that reversed the GOH mutation in the G1 step; and (d) the mutational profiles for the AluScan-based ΔTN and ΔMT changes (Additional file 11: Figure S2c) were highly similar to the WGS-based ones (Fig. 6a, WGS-Liver-M) with respect to the major mutation peaks in both the N-to-T and T-to-M transitions. The patch diagrams for the four individual AluScan-based cases (cases 1–4, Fig. 5c) were all similar to that for their sum total (WGS-Liver-M, Fig. 5c) in the much larger numbers of LOHs arising from L1 step compared to L2 step, testifying in each instance to a strong lineage effect.

Whole-genome sequencing confirmed the abundance of interstitial LOHs

A total of 246 tumor-control pairs from the International Cancer Genome Consortium (ICGC) collection of WGS data [42] were analyzed to yield LOH and GOH types of SNVs in each paired samples. These included a panel of 63 pan-cancer cases (pilot-63) (Fig. 7a), 22 intrahepatic cholangiocarcinoma (ICC), 86 LIHC, and 75 NSCLC cases (Fig. 7b, Additioanl file 12: Table S10), showing prominent LOHs in each instance. In the Pilot-63 dataset, the different ΔTB mutation counts in T-stage cells relative to B-stage cells (Fig. 7a left panel) yielded a rate ratio of 4300 between LOH and GOH-M, which was comparable to the 5400, 2700, and 5300 rate ratios observed in Figs. 1 and 3 and earlier in Reference [17], respectively, indicating a vastly greater rate of LOH than GOH in the cancer cells in all four instances. As well, in all four instances, the three mutation rates remain in the same order of $R_{LOH} > R_{GOH-m} > R_{GOH-M}$, with LOH rate being the highest. The massive interstitial LOH rates observed earlier based on AluScan data were thus confirmed by the ICGC Pilot-63 WGS dataset.

Evidence from mutational profiles for gene conversions in LOH production

For the ΔTB SNVs of Pilot-63 WGS dataset, Fig. 7c shows the alteration-group plots of mutational profiles,

which are rearranged in Fig. 7d so that opposing GOH pairs or opposing LOH pairs are placed side-by-side, e.g., by pairing the ATG>ACG GOH (pink bar) with the ACG>ATG GOH (blue bar) in section 3 of the left panel and similarly pairing the ATG>ACG LOH (pink bar) with the ACG>ATG LOH (blue bar) in section 3 of the right panel (marked by arrowheads). Figure 7d shows the strikingly similar heights of the opposing C>T (blue) or T>C (pink) LOH bars in the right panel, but the generally dissimilar heights of the opposing C>T (blue) or T>C (pink) GOH bars in the left panel. The context-group plots in Additional file 13: Figure S3a show comparable rates for different pairs of opposing LOHs in contrast to the generally unequal rates for different pairs of opposing GOHs. The rates for the individual pairs of opposing GOHs are further displayed in the mutation-rate diagrams in Additional file 13: Figure S3a and those for the opposing LOHs in the mutation-rate diagrams in Additional file 13: Figure S3b. One of the GOH diagrams from Additional file 13: Figure S3a and one of the LOH diagrams from Additional file 13: Figure S3b are illustrated in Fig. 7e, showing the frequencies for all opposing GOH pairs or opposing LOH pairs, e.g., the rates of ACG>ATG GOH and ATG>ACG GOH changes (arrowhead-marked in Fig. 7d left panel) were dissimilar (229 in blue versus 95 in pink), but the rates of LOH changes of the same triplet duplexes (arrowhead-marked in Fig. 7d right panel) were similar (1617 in blue versus 1558 in pink). The ratios between the frequencies (or rates) of the different LOH pairs were 192/183, 150/141, 713/704, 1617/1558, 204/200, and 178/174, which varied only between 1.01–1.06. The results from Additional file 13: Figure S3a and b are summarized in Fig. 7f, where over 61% of the opposing pair frequencies were greater than 2 and spread between 1 and 14 for the GOHs (blue bars), but 100% between 1 and 2 for the LOHs (striped red bars), clearly indicative of the different mutational mechanisms employed for the production of the GOHs versus the LOHs. This divergence of the rate ratios between opposing GOHs and opposing LOHs was in accord with our proposal that the LOHs in cancer cells were generated mainly by double-strand break (DSB) repairs through gene conversion, whereas the GOHs were produced by more diverse mechanisms including mutations due to the highly error-prone nature of the DNA polymerase employed for interhomolog recombination [17] and deaminations that accounted

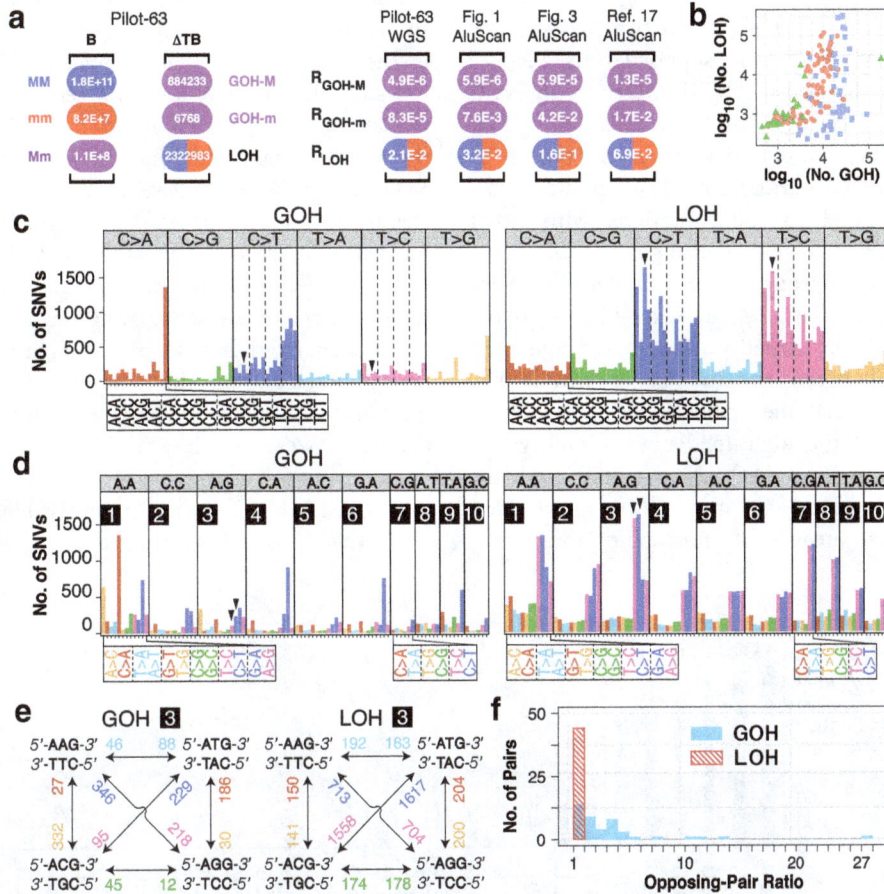

Fig. 7 Properties of ICGC whole-genome sequencing of tumor (T)-blood (B) pairs. **a** Left panel: numbers of different genotypic changes between T- and B-stage sequences (ΔTB) in ICGC Pilot-63 pan-cancer samples. Right panel: rates of different types of SNV mutations. For Pilot-63 samples, the rates were derived from WGS ΔTB/B values in the left panel; for B-N-P-T AluScan samples, from ΔTB/B values in Fig. 1a; for B-N-T AluScan samples, from ΔTB/B values in Fig. 3a; for Reference [17] samples, from AluScan results on six types of cancers [17]. **b** Scatter plot of the numbers of GOHs and LOHs in 22 intrahepatic cholangiocarcinoma (ICC, green triangles), 86 hepatocellular carcinomas (LIHC, red circles), and 75 non-small cell lung cancer (NSCLC, blue squares) pairs of samples (Additional file 12: Table S10). **c** Alteration-group plots of mutational profiles for GOHs and LOHs between B- and T-stages in Pilot-63 samples. Each plot was grouped using the six alteration types: C>A, C>G, C>T, T>A, T>C, and T>G. **d** Context-group plots of mutational profiles for GOHs and LOHs. Each plot is arranged by the ten context groups: A.A, C.C, A.G, C.A, A.C, G.A, C.G, A.T, T.A, and G.C, designating the different immediate 5′ and 3′ flanking nucleotides. The opposing GOH mutations (left panel) or opposing LOH mutations (right panel) are placed side-by-side (color-coded as in part **c**). **e** Representative mutation-rate diagrams, GOH-3 (left panel) and LOH-3 (right panel), were generated from the ICGC Pilot-63 dataset (see additional nine pairs of diagrams in Additional file 13: Figure S3). In these diagrams based on triplet duplexes, the rates of opposing mutations from part **d** were paired and labeled on bidirectional arrowheads with same color-codes as in part **d**. **f** Distribution of the observed rate ratios between opposing GOH pairs (the blue columns) and LOH pairs (the striped red column) (see Fig. 1 for abbreviations)

for the ~ 50% greater occurrence of CG>TG GOHs than TG>CG GOHs in the ΔNB changes (Fig. 1d). In a DSB at a heterozygous C/T, LOH by gene conversion could yield either a C/C or T/T homozygous position at comparable rates, depending on which homologous chromatid bears the DSB. On the other hand, because GOHs depend on point mutations rather than gene conversions, this comparable-rate constraint would not apply to GOHs.

Moreover, for the B-N-P-T tetra samples, 95.5% of the forward LOHs in the B-to-N transition (steps L13 and

L14, Fig. 1b), 98.7% of the reverse LOHs in the N-to-P transition (steps L1 and L8, Fig. 1b), and 95.2% of the reverse LOHs in the P-to-T transition (steps L3 and L10, Fig. 1b) occurred within the copy number neutral regions (Additional file 14: Figure S4), suggesting that both the forward LOHs and the reverse LOHs were mostly brought about by gene conversion.

Distances between SNVs and recurrent CNVs

That the N-stage SNVs and CNVs in the B-N-P-T tetra samples both underwent active reversions, and more in P-stage than in T-stage (Fig. 2c) suggest some form of possible correlation between these two types of mutations. This was supported by Fig. 2d which shows that the sites of C>T GOHs with NCG context occurring in the ΔNB changes, and T>C LOHs with NTG context occurring in the ΔPN changes, were located particularly close to the recurrent CNVs compared to the mutations with other contexts or in other stages of change, $p < 10^{-7}$. Furthermore, these two groups of SNVs declined with the age at diagnosis (Fig. 2e), in resemblance to the decrease of global DNA methylation in old age [43]. The correlation between somatic CNVs with CpGe and MeMRE (Fig. 2f), the increased SNVs at CpG sites (Fig. 2b), and the high tendency of methylated CpG conversion to TpG [44] also pointed to some SNV-CNV relationships in the CNV production process, such as breakpoint misrepair and merit investigation.

Frequency classes of serial CNV changes

In the B-N-P-T tetra sample cases, the status of any CNV in the N-, P-, and T-stages could be CN-unaltered (U), CN-gain (G), or CN-loss (L) relative to its status in B-stage. Arranging in serial order, the CN-status found in the N-P-T stages (Additional file 6 and 15: Tables S5 and S11) yielded 26 different serial orders, and their frequencies fell into three classes (Fig. 8a, b). In the LUG order, for example, each CNV site was CN-loss in N-stage, CN-unaltered in P-stage, and CN-gain in T-stage, and the total number of sequence windows in the B-N-P-T sequences analyzed that exhibited such an LUG order made up the frequency on the y-axis of Fig. 8a. The three frequency classes separated by vertical dashed lines in the figure were:

I.   Class I (U = 2)—comprising six different orders, where a U status occurred in two of the N-, P-, and T-stages.

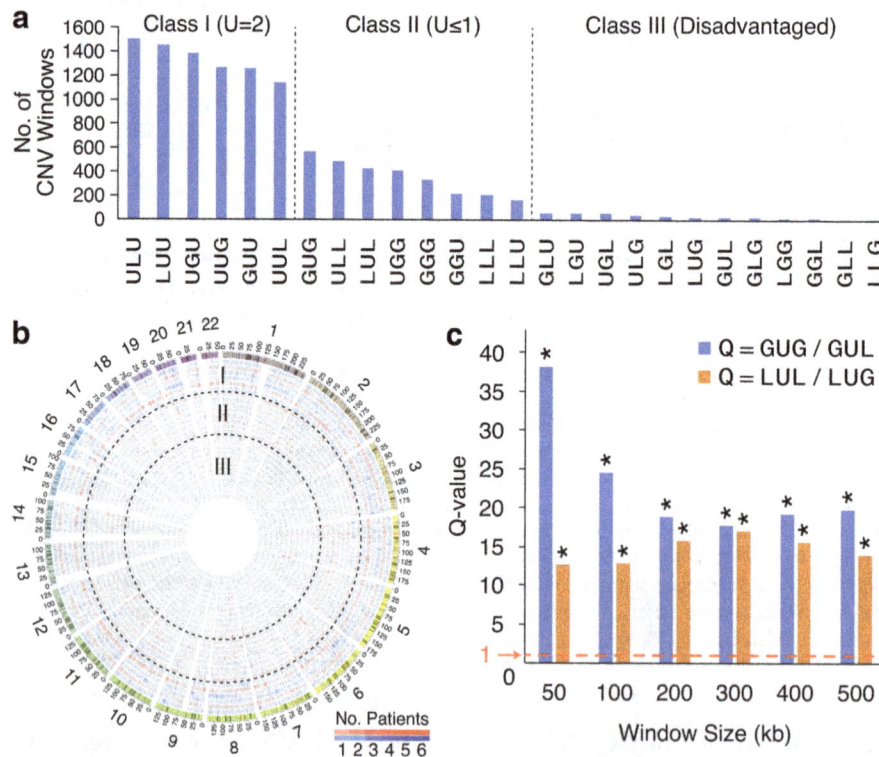

Fig. 8 Serial orders of copy number (CN) changes in B-N-P-T tetra samples. **a** Frequencies of three classes of sequential orders of CN changes. Total numbers of CNV windows conformed to each serial order of changes are plotted out for all 26 possible orders. The CN status of 500 kb windows of N-, P-, or T-stage was determined relative to B-stage for 12 B-N-P-T tetra samples as described in the "Methods" section. The total numbers of windows that conformed to the different possible serial orders of CN changes (Additional file 15: Table S11) provided the basis for their partition into three frequency classes (separated by two vertical dashed lines). U stands for CN-unaltered, G for CN-gain, and L for CN-loss. **b** Circos diagram showing the chromosomal distribution of different CNV serial orders. The 26 different orders are arranged from the rim, showing chromosome banding, inward in accordance to their left-to-right arrangement in part **a**, viz. ULU (blue) in the outermost ring followed by LUU (red), UGU (blue), etc., where orders with a CN-status of U at N-stage are colored blue, and orders with a CN-status of G or L at N-stage are colored red. Classes I–III are separated by dashed circles in black. **c** GUG/GUL and LUL/LUG frequency ratios determined using different window sizes. Without lineage effects, these ratios would be expected to yield Q = 1 (as represented by the red dashed line). In contrast, all the Q values of GUG/GUL (blue) and LUL/LUG (red) observed in sequence windows varying from 50 to 500 kb significantly exceeded unity (*$p < 10^{-16}$) (see Fig. 1 for abbreviations)

II. Class II (U ≤ 1)—comprising eight different orders, where the U status occurred in no more than one of the N-, P-, and T-stages.

III. Class III (disadvantaged)—comprising 12 different orders, where 10 of them (viz. outside of LUG and GUL) included an abrupt double-dose change directly from G to L, or L to G in the order.

The plausible basis for these different classes could be straightforward; the CNV orders in class I entailed minimal copy-number departures from the starting B-stage and were therefore well tolerated; in comparison, the class II of CNV orders incurred greater departures from U and were less well tolerated. Every CNV order in class III involved at least one double-dose change jumping either from G to L or from L to G between two successive stages of cancer development, a distinct disadvantage that led to their lowest frequencies.

The double-dose disadvantage explained the low frequencies of GLU, LGU, UGL, ULG, LGL, GLG, LGG, GGL, GLL, and LLG, but not the low frequencies of LUG and GUL which fell into class III even though they did not incur any double-dose copy number changes, in contrast to GUG and LUL which belonged to the more abundant class II. The contrast indicates that lineage effects were important not only to LOH partitions (Figs. 1b, 3b, and 5b) but also to the frequencies of different CNV orders. In GUG, the G status of T-stage cells constituted a reversion to the G status of N-stage cells. In LUL, the L status of T-stage cells likewise constituted a reversion to the L status of the N-stage cells. Thus, both these reversions were favored by lineage effects, allowing GUG and LUL to join class II even though they each incurred two CNV status changes. In contrast, lineage effects acted against LUG and GUL, because the CNV status of the T-stage cells in these cases was not a restoration of the CNV status of the N-stage cells, thereby explaining their diminished frequencies. These lineage effects were observable when different sizes of sequence windows were employed for CNV identification: as shown in Fig. 8c, both the quotients (Q value) of GUG/GUL and LUL/LUG greatly exceeded unity (marked by dashed red line), yielding significant lineage effects of $p < 10^{-16}$ for all sizes of sequence windows ranging from 50 to 500 kb.

Discussion

Premalignant and precancer cells have been observed in a variety of cancers [1–14]. The clonal evolution hypothesis of tumor cell populations postulates that a common progenitor normal cell gives rise to both precancer cells and tumor cells through stepwise genetic variations in cancer evolution [1]. Within this conceptual framework, the relationship between a precancer stage cell and the

tumor cell may vary between an "inverted pyramid" mode where there exists a large degree of interdependence between successive mutations such that the early mutations provide internal selection pressures for later mutations to result in a linear selection of mutations and a "nexus" mode where the mutations are not interdependent and there are no selection pressures, and the emergence of precancer cells and tumor cells would proceed largely in parallel [45]. In the present study, genomic sequence analysis employing the AluScan platform revealed that the nontumor tissue isolated at > 2 cm from the tumor and P-stage tissue isolated at ≤ 2 cm from tumor's edge (see the "Methods" section) both contained numerous GOHs and LOHs along with CNVs, thus pointing to these tissue regions as premalignant or early malignant stages despite their apparently normal cell morphologies. Three lines of evidence support a largely sequential relationship between the stages of cancer genome development, leading from the germline B-stage genome to the N-stage genome, then the P-stage genome, and finally the T-stage genome, and beyond that in certain instances to an M-stage genome:

a. Residue-by-residue tracing of these mutations through the B-, N-, P-, and T-stages pointed to much higher LOH rates and GOH-m rates than GOH-M rates (Fig. 1a), in accord with our earlier findings [17]. In addition, LOH reversals of the forward GOH mutations with strong lineage effects on the partition of LOH products of heterozygous residues between the homozygous MM and mm genotypes were prevalent, favoring the restoration of the homozygous germline genotypes that gave rise to the heterozygous residues in the first place. These lineage effects, observable not only in the aggregate for the B-N-P-T samples (highlighted by yellow triangles in Fig. 1b) but also for individual B-N-P-T samples (Additional file 3: Table S3), were in accord with the linear inverted pyramid relationship, with GOH mutations occurring at the N-stage exerting substantial influence on the outcome of LOH mutations occurring at the P-stage and GOHs occurring at the P-stage exerting substantial influence on the outcome of LOH mutations occurring at the T-stage. In contrast, such effects would be difficult to explain based on the nexus-type relationship arising from parallel developments of the N-, P-, and T-stage cells from the common progenitor normal cell.

b. The diminishing LOH-M/LOH-m ratios from L13/L14 = 5.7 to L15/L16 = 2.9 and on to L21/L22 = 1.7, again also observable with both aggregate (Fig. 1b) and individual (Additional file 3: Table S3) B-N-P-T samples, might stem from the longer period of positive selection for revertant mutations the N-stage cells were subjected to compared to P-stage cells and P-stage cells compared to T-stage cells. In any event, the sequential change in the LOH-M/LOH-m ratio from N to P and then to T was readily explicable in terms of the inverted pyramid mode of sequential selection but not in terms of the nexus mode of parallel selection.

c. While the steeply unequal CNV frequencies between GUG and GUL and between LUL and LUG (Fig. 8c) were again in accord with the sequential inverted pyramid mode of development from N to P and then to T, they would be incompatible with a parallel nexus mode.

Accordingly, these convergent lines of evidence derived from the B-N-P-T tetra samples, and also supported by those from the B-N-T trio samples (Fig. 3), the N-T-M trio samples based on AluScan, WES, and WGS (Figs. 5 and 6), and ICGC B-T-paired samples based on WGS (Fig. 7), pointed to a linear cancer development sequence between the B-N-P-T stages, as represented in the stage-specific population (SSP) model in Fig. 9a. In this SSP model, while each of the N-, P-, and T-stage cell populations could comprise multiple cell clones, a majority of the cell clones within the same stage would display largely similar mutational and morphological characteristics.

Figure 9b shows that although the 12 B-N-P-T tetra sample cases were derived from the three types of solid tumors, they all displayed a largely similar mutational trend; the SNVs found at N-stage (σ_N) comprised different proportions of GOHs (red) and LOHs (orange) and underwent substantial reversions in P-stage cells (light green), followed by a much smaller number of additional reversions occurring in the T-stage cells (dark green). Altogether, that more N-stage SNVs were reversed in P-stage than in T-stage in all 12 samples amounted to a highly non-random observation ($p = 3.1 \times 10^{-12}$), in confirmation of the stage-specific difference in mutational activities between P- and T-stage cells. The LOH/GOH ratios in tumor tissues relative to same-patient white blood cell samples as controls were different for different cancer types: 0.32 for BRCA, 1.16 for STAD, and 4.29 for LIHC (data from Additional file 4: Table S4), in accordance with Fig. 7b which showed more LOHs in LIHC than in NSCLC or ICC. Importantly, as shown by a comparison of Additional file 11: Figure S2 with Figs. 5a–b and 6a, WGS sequences and their AluScan-capturable subsets of the N-T-M trio samples in the WGS-Liver-M group were in substantial accord with respect to the finding of forward-reverse mutation cycles (FR-cycles) between different cancer developmental stages, the greater LOH rates than GOH rates in the N-to-T transition, the strong lineage effects observed in the LOH-reversals in

the T-to-M transition, and the mutational profiles of both the N-to-T and T-to-M transitions. These results provide useful validation for the application of the AluScan platform for mutation analysis.

Earlier, comparison of different cancer-control pairs indicated that the LOH rates were greater than GOH-m rates, which were in turn greater than GOH-M rates in different types of cancers, pointing to widespread inter-homolog chromosomal gene conversions arising from defective DNA double-strand break repair in cancers to cause massive LOHs and tag-along GOHs [17]. In addition, the prominence of "signature 1A" in Fig. 1d suggests that N-stage cells acquired substantial numbers of GOHs through deamination of 5-methylcytosine. In Fig. 1b, likewise, the LOH rate of 0.04 in the L13 step exceeded the GOH-m rate of 0.02 in the G6 step, and even more so the GOH-M rate of 1.8E–5 in step G1. This high propensity of N-stage cells toward LOH mutations suggest that they already resembled mature cancer cells in the possession of a defective DSB repair that allowed massive gene conversions, thus establishing the gene conversion-enhancing DSB defect as a very early event in cancer development and a key departure of N-stage cells from normal B-stage cells. The major consequence of this defect was massive forward LOHs and tag-along GOHs. On the one hand, these large numbers of LOHs and GOHs would increase the probability of generating essential mutations needed by the developing cancer cells to advance toward full-fledged malignancy. On the other hand, they could also bring about excessive mutation load that would slow down the growth of the increasing propagation-unconstrained cells. Accordingly, to reduce the mutation load, mutations of the N-stage genome that served to reverse the forward LOHs and GOHs would be positively selected resulting in high reversal rates of 0.96 for L1 and L8 steps, 0.56 for G11 step, and 0.75 for G12 step, thereby conferring on the P-stage cells their outstanding characteristics of highly active reversals. Notably, in the B-N-P-T tetra samples, a great majority of both the forward and reverse LOHs occurred within the copy number neutral regions (Additional file 14: Figure S4), suggesting that both the forward LOHs and the reverse LOHs were mostly caused by DSB repair through gene conversion. While the different types of cancers analyzed showed similar N- and P-stage mutational properties, different cancers varied with respect to the abundance of LOH relative to GOH in both the AluScan results (Fig. 9b) and the WGS results (Fig. 7b), exemplified by the higher LOH frequencies in LIHC compared to other types of cancers and suggesting that LOH/GOH ratios could be useful for cancer subtyping. The finding of high rates of SNVs in the N-stage cells despite their normal morphology was consistent with the elevated SNV

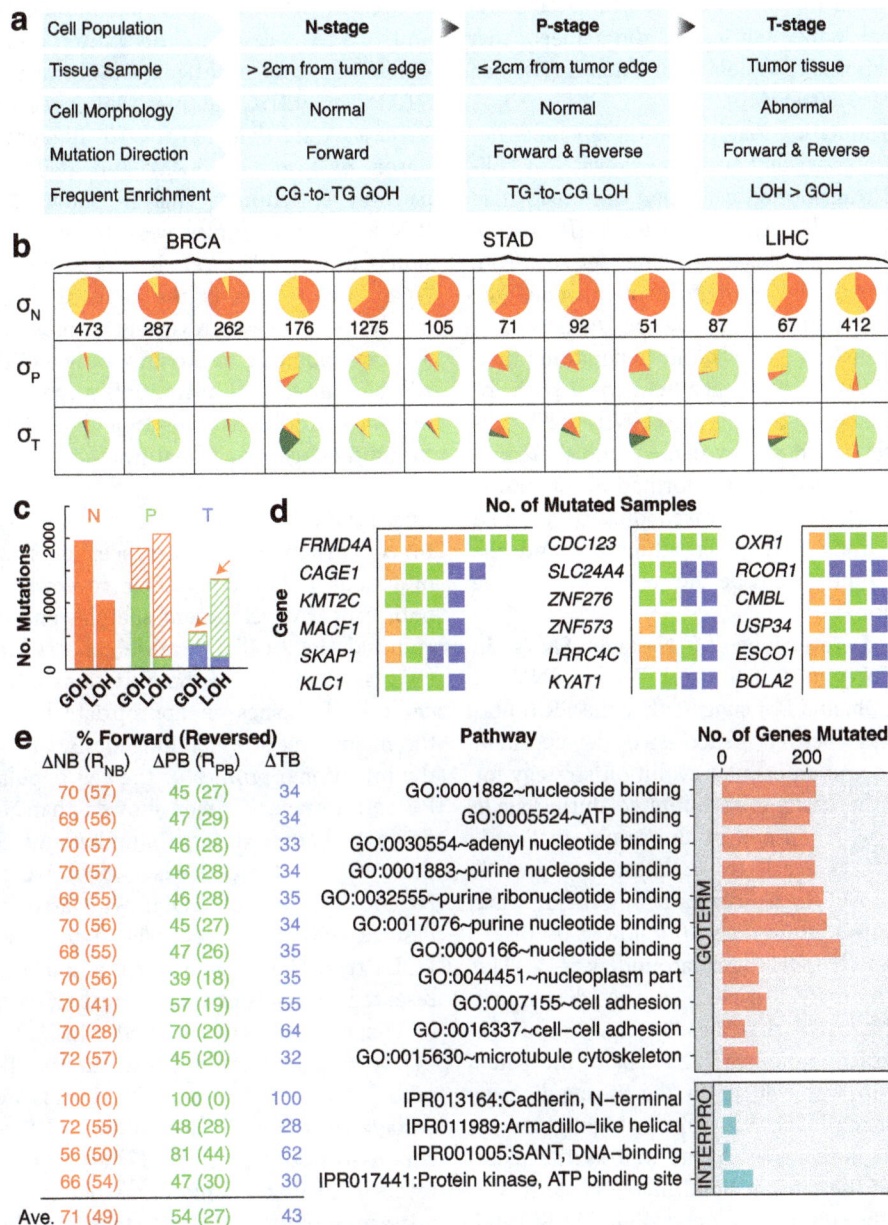

Fig. 9 Mutational features of different stages of cancer development. **a** stage-specific population (SSP) model of cancer development. **b** Reversal of N-stage SNVs at P- and T-stages in 12 tetra sample cases of BRCA, STAD, and LIHC. Colored sectors represent N-stage GOHs (red), N-stage LOHs (orange), P-stage reversals of N-stage SNVs (light green), and T-stage reversals of N-stage SNVs (dark green), respectively. σ_N shows the total number of SNVs occurred at N-stage compared to B-stage cells with relative proportions of GOH and LOH shown by colored sectors. σ_P and σ_T show the proportions of N-stage SNVs unreversed and reversed at P-stage and T-stage, as color-coded sectors. **c** Forward and reverse SNVs in N-, P-, and T-stage samples. Left: N-stage SNVs comprising forward GOHs and LOHs (solid red). Middle: P-stage SNVs comprising forward GOHs and LOHs (solid green) and GOHs and LOHs that reversed N-stage LOHs and GOHs, respectively (striped red). Right: T-stage SNVs comprising forward GOHs and LOHs (solid blue) and GOHs and LOHs that reversed P-stage LOHs and GOHs (striped green) and N-stage LOHs and GOHs (striped red highlighted by arrows), respectively. **d** Frequently mutated genes in the 12 tetra sample cases. Each mutation found in a BRCA (orange), STAD (green), or LIHC (blue) sample is represented by a square listed with the gene. **e** Pathway enrichments of mutations in the 12 tetra sample cases. The horizontal bars showing the numbers of mutated genes are arranged from top down in the order of increasing Bonferroni-corrected p values. The percentage of genes in the pathway that displayed one or more forward SNVs at N-, P-, or T-stage is indicated under ΔNB, ΔPB, and ΔTB, respectively. The percentage of N-stage SNVs that were reversed subsequently at P- or T-stage was indicated by (R_{NB}). The percentage of P-stage SNVs that were reversed subsequently at T-stage was indicated by (R_{PB}) (see Fig. 1 for abbreviations)

prevalences by 27-fold ($p < 0.001$) or 36-fold ($p < 0.0001$) observed in normal kidney cortices of the subjects that were smokers or exposed to the environmental carcinogen aristolochic acid, respectively [46].

The necessity of mutation load reduction in cancer development was also consistent with the slower multiplication of cultured transformed cells than untransformed cells at low population density, e.g., upon transformation of a C3H/10T1/2CL8 fibroblast cell line derived from C3H mouse embryos by 3-methylcholanthrene, the transformed cells exhibited a saturation density 2–3 times that of untransformed cells, but generation times of 22 and 27 h, viz. 40–70% longer than the 15.5 h for the untransformed cells [47]. Likewise, NIH 3T3 cells displayed retarded growth at low density and increased saturation density preceding the formation of transformed loci [48], while the increased density attained might stem from reduced contact inhibition, and the longer generation times could be the result of excessive deleterious mutations.

The pronounced reversions of N-stage SNVs in P-stage, P-stage SNVs in T-stage, and T-stage SNVs in M-stage (Figs. 1b, 3b, and 5b) suggest that the FR mutations, or FR-cycles, between successive development stages could be a common cellular evolution strategy for the adaptation to the changes encountered during stage transitions. This was confirmed by the results in Fig. 4, where adaption of HeLa cells to replating and growth likewise gave rise to FR-cycles comprising a major wave of CG>TG rich GOHs around day 10 followed by reversions via TG>CG rich LOHs later around day 14. The similarity between the FR-cycles of the developing cancer cells in the patch diagrams of Fig. 1 and the FR-cycles of the serially sampled HeLa cells in the patch diagrams of Fig. 4b was evident in the strong lineage effects of the reverting LOH mutations as highlighted by yellow triangles in both instances, as well as the close agreement between the rates of both the GOH steps (G1 and G6 in Fig. 1b, the equivalent G1 and G3 in Fig. 4b) and the ensuing LOH steps (L1, L2, L7, and L8 in Fig. 1b, and the equivalent L1, L2, L3, and L4 in Fig. 4b) observed in the two sets of patch diagrams. Since the HeLa samples were taken from the time series of cell populations on days 5, 10, and 14, the similarity of the FR-cycles between the N-P-T stages and those between different HeLa cell samplings suggest that, in both cases, a wave of GOH mutations was followed subsequently by extensive reversions. Moreover, it is notable that, when a deviant *Drosophila melanogaster* population induced by extreme starvation was allowed to readapt to the ancestral culture environment, reversions of SNPs back to ancestral allele genotypes over 50 generations of evolution amounted to about 50% [49], comparable to the average ~ 39% level of SNV reversions exhibited by P-stage cells in the form of type IVa changes in Fig. 2c.

The *FRMD4A* gene [50] was mutated in 4 BRCA cases and 3 STAD cases in the 12 tetra sample cases, and *CAGE1* for cancer antigen 1 [51] was mutated in BRCA, STAD, and LIHC samples. SNVs recurrent in 4 out of 12 cases were detected for 16 different genes (Fig. 9d). Based on the GOTERM and INTERPRO databases, pathway enrichment analysis shows that SNVs in the B-N-P-T tetra samples were frequent in the cell adhesion pathway (Fig. 9e). It was striking that all of the N-stage mutations in the cadherin N-terminal domain family persisted unreversely throughout the P- and T-stages, pointing to the importance of this family of cell adhesion molecules at multiple stages of cancer development, see Additional files 16 and 17: Tables S12 and S13 for mutated genes and pathways.

Conclusion

In conclusion, the occurrences of a wave of forward mutations followed by their reversals are observed in both cancer development samples and serial samples of cultured HeLa cells. Because cancers are driven by mutations, the nature of the mutations in the evolving cancer cells furnishes an appropriate basis for delineating the major stages of carcinogenesis. In the present study, the mutational profiles of the cell populations in the N-, P-, and T-stage samples showed that N-stage cells surprisingly harbored large numbers of SNV mutations, more GOHs than LOHs, which were enriched with NCG>NTG type of GOHs with associated CNVs. The P-stage cells displayed, relative to N-stage cells, more LOHs than GOHs. A major fraction of their LOHs represented reversals of the forward GOH mutations found in N-stage and was enriched with NTG>NCG type of LOHs with associated CNVs. In the T-stage cells, the ratio between LOHs and GOHs was even higher than P-stage cells (Fig. 9c, see Additional file 3: Table S3 for data used in this plot). At T-stage, there were numerous reversals of P-stage mutations but far fewer reversals of N-stage mutations. The extents of these reversals of N-stage mutations in P-stage and P-stage mutations in T-stage were unexpectedly large. Moreover, as shown by the AluScan, WGS, and WES results in Fig. 5b, the uniformly high rates of the revertant L1, L4, G5, and G6 steps in the different groups of cancers indicated that T-stage mutations were likewise subjected to extensive reversals in M-stage cells, which confirmed the importance of FR mutations as a cellular mechanism for regulating the mutation load. Accordingly, the N-, P-, and T-stage cell populations represented different developmental stages of cancer development, each with its own mutational characteristics that best fulfilled the role of that particular developmental stage. The identification of the intermediate N- and P-stages not only provides a basis for facilitating early diagnosis, subtyping, and staging of cancers, but also suggests that the early N-stage cells, which have not yet accomplished their requisite mutation reversals and hence mutation load reduction, might be relatively deficient in growth and replication vigor, in which case it could be advantageous to target therapeutic interventions at these early stages of pre-cancer and cancer cells before they have accomplished their mutation reversals to become fully malignant, therapy-resistant cancers.

Additional files

Additional file 1: Table S1. Information on 103 samples analyzed by

Additional file 2: Table S2. Tumor purities of B-N-P-T tetra and B-N-T

Additional file 3: Table S3. Summary of SNV mutations in B-N-P-T tetra

Additional file 4: Table S4. The exact residue-by-residue SNV mutations

Additional file 5: Figure S1. Total numbers of different dinucleotide sites in the human genome. Numbers of CG as well as other 15 types of dinucleotides in human reference genome hg19 are plotted

Additional file 6: Table S5. Summary of CNV mutations in B-N-P-T tetra

Additional file 7: Table S6. Summary of SNV mutations in B-N-T trio

Additional file 8: Table S7. The exact residue-by-residue SNV mutations in each sample of the B-N-T trio sample cases.

Additional file 9: Table S8. Summary of SNV mutations in N-T-M trio samples. (A) AluScan, (B) WES-Non-Lung, (C) WES-NSCLC-L, (D) WES-

Additional file 10: Table S9. The exact residue-by-residue SNV mutations in each sample of the AluScan N-T-M trio sample cases.

Additional file 11: Figure S2. SNV mutations in the AluScan-capturable regions of WGS samples in the WGS-Liver-M group. In this figure, AluScan-capturable sequences, corresponding to all the AluScan-captured sequences analyzed in Fig. 1, were extracted from the four N-T-M trio sets in WGS-Liver-M group and analyzed. **a** Genotypic changes in T-stage and M-stage cells. The numbers of genotypic changes in T- or M-stage sequences relative to N-stage sequences are represented by ΔTN and ΔMN, respectively. **b** Patch diagrams tracing SNVs between the N-, T-, and M-samples. **c** Mutational profiles of the ΔTN and ΔMT SNV changes as numerically indicated in the patch diagrams in part b. In each vertical bar in the ΔTN tier, the solid segment represents the SNVs that were reversed in the ΔMT tier, whereas the open segment indicates the unreversed

Additional file 12: Table S10. Numbers of GOHs and LOHs in 22 ICC,

Additional file 13: Figure S3. Mutation-rate diagrams of Pilot-63 samples from ICGC analyzed by WGS. **a** Mutation-rate diagrams for GOHs. Each of the ten diagrams of triplet duplexes corresponds to a context group, labeled 1–10 as in Fig. 7d. The mutation rates of opposing GOH mutations are labeled on double-headed arrows, except for the single-headed curved arrows in groups 7–10, where the two sequences are identical in a triple duplex. Each double-headed arrows is accompanied by two color-coded mutation rates that correspond to the heights of color-coded bars in Fig. 7d, e.g., in context group 1, the conversion of double-stranded ACA/TGT to AAA/TTT is associated with a mutation rate of 162, colored red to correspond to the red C>A bar with A.A context in

the left panel of Fig. 7d; whereas the opposing conversion of AAA/TTT to ACA/TGT is associated with a mutation rate of 641, colored orange to correspond to the orange A>C bar with A.A context in the left panel of Fig. 7d. **b** Mutation-rate diagrams for LOHs. The arrows employed are similar to those in part a. All arrows in parts a and b are shown as dashed lines for transitions (TSs) or solid lines for transversions (TVs). In the ten diagrams in part a or part b, the boxed TS/TV ratio given for each diagram represents the ratio pertaining to all the TS and TV mutations in the diagram, e.g., in diagram 1 of part a, TS equals the sum of the four TS rates in the diagram, and TV the sum of the eight TV rates, yielding TS/TV = 1430/2804 = 0.51. The different rates in the diagrams in parts a and b are color-coded as in Fig. 7d

Additional file 14: Figure S4. Most of the LOHs observed in the course of cancer development occurred in copy-neutral regions of the genome. **a** Upper panel: reverse LOHs occurring in the N-to-P transition (viz. ΔPN). Pie chart indicates that 1850 out of 1875 (98.7%) of the reverse LOHs via L1 and L8 steps analyzed in Fig. 1b occurred in copy-neutral regions. **b** Upper panel: reverse LOHs occurring in the P-to-T changes (viz. ΔTP). Pie chart indicates that 1095 out of 1150 (95.2%) of the reverse LOHs via L3 and L10 steps occurred in copy-neutral regions. **c** Upper panel: forward LOHs occurring in the B-to-N transition (viz. ΔNB). Pie chart indicates that 986 out of 1028 (95.9%) of the forward LOHs via L13 and L14 steps occurred in copy-neutral regions. In parts **a**–**c**, the lower panels show for reference the proportions of CN-neutral, CN-gain, and CN-loss in the course of the B-to-N, N-to-P, and P-to-T transitions, respectively.

Additional file 15: Table S11. The exact window-by-window CNV

Additional file 16: Table S12. List of genes harboring SNV mutations in

Additional file 17: Table S13. SNV mutations enriched pathways and

Abbreviations

AluScan: Genome-wide scanning using Alu-based primers; B: White blood cell; BRCA: Breast invasive carcinoma; CNV: Copy number variation; CNVT: Somatic copy number variation; CpGe: Evolutionary conserved CpG doublets; GOH: Gain of heterozygosity; LIHC: Liver hepatocellular carcinoma; LOH: Loss of heterozygosity; M: Metastatic tumor; MeMRE: Unmethylated CpG; N: Nontumor; NSCLC: Non-small cell lung cancer; P: Paratumor; rCNV: Recurrent copy number variation; SNV: Single-nucleotide variation; STAD: Stomach adenocarcinoma; T: Primary tumor; TCGA: The Cancer Genome Atlas; WES: Whole-exome sequencing; WGS: Whole-genome sequencing

Acknowledgements

We thank the whole group of the International Cancer Genome Consortium http://icgc.org/committees-and-working-groups). Y. Kumar was a recipient of International Ph.D. Studentship from Hong Kong University of Science and Technology. X. Long was a recipient of Hong Kong Ph.D. Fellowship from the Government of Hong Kong SAR. F.W. Pun was a recipient of Research Fellowship from HKUST Jockey Club Institute of Advanced Study. Hututa Technologies Limited assisted with the computation facilities.

Funding

The study was supported by grants to H. Xue from the University Grants Committee (VPRDO09/10.SC08, VPRDO14SC01, DG14SC02, SRFI11SC06, SRFI11SC06PG, and SBI16SC03) and Innovation and Technology Fund (ITS/113/15FP) of Hong Kong SAR and grants to J. F. Chen from the National 973 Basic Research Program of China (2013CB911300), National Natural Science Foundation of China (81272469), and Natural Science Foundation of Jiangsu Province special clinical project (BL2012016). The funders had no role in the study design, data collection and analysis, decision to publish, or preparation of the manuscript.

Authors' contributions

HX conceived and initiated the study. SJD, YL, LC, JFC, RY, AK, GKKL, DHZ, EXZ, LX, WSP, and HYW organized and collected the clinical samples and data. IS performed the HeLa cell-based experiments. TH, YK, IS, WKM, ZW, XL, CHC, SC, PL, SKN, TYCH, JY, XD, SYT, and XZ analyzed the samples and data. HX, TH, and SYT wrote the paper. The International Cancer Genome Consortium (ICGC) which led a worldwide cancer genomics collaboration including a project on pan-cancer analysis of whole genomes (PCAWG) contributed tumor-control sample pairs collected and sequenced by PCAWG to the present study. All authors read and approved the final manuscript.

Competing interests

The authors declare that they have no competing interests.

Author details

[1]Division of Life Science, Applied Genomics Centre and Centre for Statistical Science, Hong Kong University of Science and Technology, Clear Water Bay, Kowloon, Hong Kong, China. [2]Department of General Surgery, The Second Xiangya Hospital, Central South University, Changsha, Hunan, China. [3]Department of Surgery, The Chinese University of Hong Kong, Shatin, Hong Kong, China. [4]Eastern Hepatobiliary Surgery Institute, Second Military Medical University, Shanghai, China. [5]Department of Oncology, Nanjing First Hospital, Nanjing Medical University, Nanjing, China. [6]Jiangsu Key Laboratory of Cancer Molecular Biology and Translational Medicine, Jiangsu Cancer Hospital, Nanjing, China. [7]Division of Neurosurgery, Department of Surgery, Li Ka Shing Faculty of Medicine, Queen Mary Hospital, The University of Hong Kong, 102 Pokfulam Road, Pokfulam, Hong Kong, China. [8]School of Basic Medicine and Clinical Pharmacy, China Pharmaceutical University, Nanjing, China.

References

1. Nowell PC. The clonal evolution of tumor cell populations. Science. 1976; 194:23–8.
2. Roncalli M, Borzio M, Brando B, Colloredo G, Servida E. Abnormal DNA content in liver-cell dysplasia: a flow cytometric study. Int J Cancer. 1989;44: 204–7.
3. Fearon ER, Vogelstein B. A genetic model for colorectal tumorigenesis. Cell. 1990;61:759–67.
4. Libbrecht L, Desmet V, Van Damme B, Roskams T. The immunohistochemical phenotype of dysplastic foci in human liver: correlation with putative progenitor cells. J Hepatol. 2000;33:76–84.
5. Shen LJ, Zhang HX, Zhang ZJ, Li JY, Chen MQ, Yang WB, Huang R. Detection of HBV, PCNA and GST-pi in hepatocellular carcinoma and chronic liver diseases. World J Gastroenterol. 2003;9:459–62.
6. Wang GS, Wang MW, Wu BY, You WD, Yang XY. A novel gene, GCRG224, is differentially expressed in human gastric mucosa. World J Gastroenterol. 2003;9:30–4.
7. Gorgoulis VG, Vassiliou LV, Karakaidos P, Zacharatos P, Kotsinas A, Liloglou T, Venere M, Ditullio RA Jr, Kastrinakis NG, Levy B, et al. Activation of the DNA damage checkpoint and genomic instability in human precancerous lesions. Nature. 2005;434:907–13.
8. Oosterhuis JW, Looijenga LH. Testicular germ-cell tumours in a broader perspective. Nat Rev Cancer. 2005;5:210–22.
9. Bateman CM, Colman SM, Chaplin T, Young BD, Eden TO, Bhakta M, Gratias EJ, van Wering ER, Cazzaniga G, Harrison CJ, et al. Acquisition of genome-wide copy number alterations in monozygotic twins with acute lymphoblastic leukemia. Blood. 2010;115:3553–8.
10. Ding L, Ley TJ, Larson DE, Miller CA, Koboldt DC, Welch JS, Ritchey JK, Young MA, Lamprecht T, McLellan MD, et al. Clonal evolution in relapsed acute myeloid leukaemia revealed by whole-genome sequencing. Nature. 2012;481:506–10.
11. Cooper CS, Eeles R, Wedge DC, Van Loo P, Gundem G, Alexandrov LB, Kremeyer B, Butler A, Lynch AG, Camacho N, et al. Analysis of the genetic phylogeny of multifocal prostate cancer identifies multiple independent clonal expansions in neoplastic and morphologically normal prostate tissue. Nat Genet. 2015;47:367–72.
12. Andor N, Graham TA, Jansen M, Xia LC, Aktipis CA, Petritsch C, Ji HP, Maley CC. Pan-cancer analysis of the extent and consequences of intratumor heterogeneity. Nat Med. 2016;22:105–13.
13. Yadav VK, DeGregori J, De S. The landscape of somatic mutations in protein coding genes in apparently benign human tissues carries signatures of relaxed purifying selection. Nucleic Acids Res. 2016;44:2075–84.
14. McGranahan N, Swanton C. Clonal heterogeneity and tumor evolution: past, present, and the future. Cell. 2017;168:613–28.
15. Beerenwinkel N, Antal T, Dingli D, Traulsen A, Kinzler KW, Velculescu VE, Vogelstein B, Nowak MA. Genetic progression and the waiting time to cancer. PLoS Comput Biol. 2007;3:e225.
16. Kuhner MK, Kostadinov R, Reid BJ. Limitations of the driver/passenger model in cancer prevention. Cancer Prev Res (Phila). 2016;9:335–8.
17. Kumar Y, Yang J, Hu T, Chen L, Xu Z, Xu L, Hu XX, Tang G, Wang JM, Li Y, et al. Massive interstitial copy-neutral loss-of-heterozygosity as evidence for cancer being a disease of the DNA-damage response. BMC Med Genet. 2015;8:42.
18. Lieb M. Forward and reverse mutation in a histidine-requiring strain of Escherichia coli. Genetics. 1951;36:460–77.
19. Skopek TR, Liber HL, Kaden DA, Thilly WG. Relative sensitivities of forward and reverse mutation assays in Salmonella typhimurium. Proc Natl Acad Sci U S A. 1978;75:4465–9.
20. Ruiz-Rubio M, Hera C, Pueyo C. Comparison of a forward and a reverse mutation assay in Salmonella typhimurium measuring L-arabinose resistance and histidine prototrophy. EMBO J. 1984;3:1435–40.
21. Koboldt DC, Zhang Q, Larson DE, Shen D, McLellan MD, Lin L, Miller CA, Mardis ER, Ding L, Wilson RK. VarScan 2: somatic mutation and copy number alteration discovery in cancer by exome sequencing. Genome Res. 2012;22:568–76.
22. Bao L, Pu M, Messer K. AbsCN-seq: a statistical method to estimate tumor purity, ploidy and absolute copy numbers from next-generation sequencing data. Bioinformatics. 2014;30:1056–63.
23. Chen Z, Chen X, Zhou E, Chen G, Qian K, Wu X, Miao X, Tang Z. Intratumoral CD8(+) cytotoxic lymphocyte is a favorable prognostic marker in node-negative breast cancer. PLoS One. 2014;9:e95475.
24. Mei L, Ding X, Tsang SY, Pun FW, Ng SK, Yang J, Zhao C, Li D, Wan W, Yu CH, et al. AluScan: a method for genome-wide scanning of sequence and structure variations in the human genome. BMC Genomics. 2011;12:564.
25. Cancer Genome Atlas Research N, Weinstein JN, Collisson EA, Mills GB, Shaw KR, Ozenberger BA, Ellrott K, Shmulevich I, Sander C, Stuart JM. The cancer Genome Atlas Pan-Cancer analysis project. Nat Genet. 2013;45:1113–20.
26. Qiu X, Zheng J, Guo X, Gao X, Liu H, Tu Y, Zhang Y. Reduced expression of SOCS2 and SOCS6 in hepatocellular carcinoma correlates with aggressive tumor progression and poor prognosis. Mol Cell Biochem. 2013;378:99–106.
27. Ouyang L, Lee J, Park CK, Mao M, Shi Y, Gong Z, Zheng H, Li Y, Zhao Y, Wang G, et al. Whole-genome sequencing of matched primary and metastatic hepatocellular carcinomas. BMC Med Genet. 2014;7:2.
28. Brastianos PK, Carter SL, Santagata S, Cahill DP, Taylor-Weiner A, Jones RT, Van Allen EM, Lawrence MS, Horowitz PM, Cibulskis K, et al. Genomic characterization of brain metastases reveals branched evolution and potential therapeutic targets. Cancer Discov. 2015;5:1164–77.
29. Li H, Durbin R. Fast and accurate short read alignment with burrows-wheeler transform. Bioinformatics. 2009;25:1754–60.
30. Li H, Handsaker B, Wysoker A, Fennell T, Ruan J, Homer N, Marth G, Abecasis G, Durbin R. Genome Project Data Processing S: the sequence alignment/map format and SAMtools. Bioinformatics. 2009;25:2078–9.
31. McKenna A, Hanna M, Banks E, Sivachenko A, Cibulskis K, Kernytsky A, Garimella K, Altshuler D, Gabriel S, Daly M, DePristo MA. The Genome Analysis Toolkit: a MapReduce framework for analyzing next-generation DNA sequencing data. Genome Res. 2010;20:1297–303.
32. Alexandrov LB, Nik-Zainal S, Wedge DC, Aparicio SA, Behjati S, Biankin AV, Bignell GR, Bolli N, Borg A, Borresen-Dale AL, et al. Signatures of mutational processes in human cancer. Nature. 2013;500:415–21.
33. Gehring JS, Fischer B, Lawrence M, Huber W. SomaticSignatures: inferring mutational signatures from single-nucleotide variants. Bioinformatics. 2015; 31:3673–5.
34. Yang JF, Ding XF, Chen L, Mat WK, Xu MZ, Chen JF, Wang JM, Xu L, Poon WS, Kwong A, et al. Copy number variation analysis based on AluScan sequences. J Clin Bioinforma. 2014;4:15.

35. Ng SK, Hu T, Long X, Chan CH, Tsang SY, Xue H. Feature co-localization landscape of the human genome. Sci Rep. 2016;6:20650.

36. Durinck S, Spellman PT, Birney E, Huber W. Mapping identifiers for the integration of genomic datasets with the R/bioconductor package biomaRt. Nat Protoc. 2009;4:1184–91.

37. Huang da W, Sherman BT, Lempicki RA. Systematic and integrative analysis of large gene lists using DAVID bioinformatics resources. Nat Protoc. 2009;4: 44–57.

38. Krzywinski M, Schein J, Birol I, Connors J, Gascoyne R, Horsman D, Jones SJ, Marra MA. Circos: an information aesthetic for comparative genomics. Genome Res. 2009;19:1639–45.

39. Helleday T, Eshtad S, Nik-Zainal S. Mechanisms underlying mutational signatures in human cancers. Nat Rev Genet. 2014;15:585–98.

40. Pfeifer GP, Denissenko MF, Olivier M, Tretyakova N, Hecht SS, Hainaut P. Tobacco smoke carcinogens, DNA damage and p53 mutations in smoking-associated cancers. Oncogene. 2002;21:7435–51.

41. Feng Z, Hu W, Hu Y, Tang MS. Acrolein is a major cigarette-related lung cancer agent: preferential binding at p53 mutational hotspots and inhibition of DNA repair. Proc Natl Acad Sci U S A. 2006;103:15404–9.

42. International Cancer Genome Consortium, Hudson TJ, Anderson W, Artez A, Barker AD, Bell C, Bernabe RR, Bhan MK, Calvo F, Eerola I, et al. International network of cancer genome projects. Nature. 2010;464:993–8.

43. Tsang SY, Ahmad T, Mat FW, Zhao C, Xiao S, Xia K, Xue H. Variation of global DNA methylation levels with age and in autistic children. Hum Genomics. 2016;10:31.

44. Poole A, Penny D, Sjoberg BM. Confounded cytosine! Tinkering and the evolution of DNA. Nat Rev Mol Cell Biol. 2001;2:147–51.

45. Ilyas M, Straub J, Tomlinson IP, Bodmer WF. Genetic pathways in colorectal and other cancers. Eur J Cancer. 1999;35:1986–2002.

46. Hoang ML, Kinde I, Tomasetti C, McMahon KW, Rosenquist TA, Grollman AP, Kinzler KW, Vogelstein B, Papadopoulos N. Genome-wide quantification of rare somatic mutations in normal human tissues using massively parallel sequencing. Proc Natl Acad Sci U S A. 2016;113:9846–51.

47. Reznikoff CA, Bertram JS, Brankow DW, Heidelberger C. Quantitative and qualitative studies of chemical transformation of cloned C3H mouse embryo cells sensitive to postconfluence inhibition of cell division. Cancer Res. 1973;33:3239–49.

48. Rubin H, Yao A, Chow M. Heritable, population-wide damage to cells as the driving-force of neoplastic transformation. Proc Natl Acad Sci U S A. 1995; 92:4843–7.

49. Teotonio H, Chelo IM, Bradic M, Rose MR, Long AD. Experimental evolution reveals natural selection on standing genetic variation. Nat Genet. 2009;41: 251–7.

50. Goldie SJ, Mulder KW, Tan DW, Lyons SK, Sims AH, Watt FM. FRMD4A upregulation in human squamous cell carcinoma promotes tumor growth and metastasis and is associated with poor prognosis. Cancer Res. 2012;72: 3424–36.

51. Kunze E, Schlott T. High frequency of promoter methylation of the 14-3-3 sigma and CAGE-1 genes, but lack of hypermethylation of the caveolin-1 gene, in primary adenocarcinomas and signet ring cell carcinomas of the urinary bladder. Int J Mol Med. 2007;20:557–63.

52. Hansen RS, Thomas S, Sandstrom R, Canfield TK, Thurman RE, Weaver M, Dorschner MO, Gartler SM, Stamatoyannopoulos JA. Sequencing newly replicated DNA reveals widespread plasticity in human replication timing. Proc Natl Acad Sci U S A. 2010;107:139–44.

13

A novel RLBP1 gene geographical area-related mutation present in a young patient with retinitis punctata albescens

Concetta Scimone[1,2], Luigi Donato[1,2], Teresa Esposito[3], Carmela Rinaldi[1*], Rosalia D'Angelo[1] and Antonina Sidoti[1,2]

Abstract

Background: Autosomal recessive forms of retinitis punctata albescens (RPA) have been described. RPA is characterized by progressive retinal degeneration due to alteration in visual cycle and consequent deposit of photopigments in retinal pigment epithelium. Five loci have been linked to RPA onset. Among these, the retinaldehyde-binding protein 1 gene, RLBP1, is the most frequently involved and several founder mutations were reported. We report results of a genetic molecular investigation performed on a large Sicilian family in which appears a young woman with RPA.

Results: The proband is in homozygous condition for a novel *RLBP1* single-pair deletion, and her healthy parents, both heterozygous, are not consanguineous. Thenovelc.398delC (p.P133Qfs*258) involves the exon 6 and leads to a premature stop codon, resulting in a truncated protein entirely missing of CRAL-TRIO lipid-binding domain.
Pedigree analysis showed other non-consanguineous relatives heterozygous for the same mutation in the family. Extension of mutation research in the native town of the proband revealed its presence also in healthy subjects, in a heterozygous condition.

Conclusions: A novel *RLBP1* truncating mutation was detected in a young girl affected by RPA. Although her parents are not consanguineous, the mutation was observed in a homozygous condition. Being them native of the same small Sicilian town of Fiumedinisi, the hypothesis of a geographical area-related mutation was assessed and confirmed.

Keywords: Retinitis punctata albescens, RLBP1, Frameshift mutation, Population study, Geographical-area related mutation, RP mutation spectrum

Background

Retinitis pigmentosa (RP) includes more than 70 different forms of inherited eye disorders characterized by progressive vision loss due to photoreceptors degeneration. This heterogeneity is caused by the high number of genes involved in disease's development. Therefore, each RP form differs from another for causative gene, inheritance pattern, symptomatology, age onset, and clinical features. About genetics, more than 50% of cases are affected by autosomal recessive forms due to mutations in almost 50 loci [1]. Among these, the *retinaldehyde-binding protein 1 (RLBP1)* mutations are cause of retinitis punctata albescens

(RPA, OMIM#136880) [2]. RPA is a progressive retinal degeneration belonging to the group of rod-cone dystrophies and has an early onset characterized by night blindness. At diagnosis, fundus appears with punctate white–yellow deposits. Progressive macular atrophy is the main cause of visual acuity loss, and narrowing of the visual field may occur in late teen-age [3]. RPA has an incidence of 1/800000 people worldwide, and mutations at RLBP1 gene were reported only in about 1% of patients affected by autosomal recessive forms [2]. However, RPA cases associated with *Rhodopsin (RHO)*, *Retinol Dehydrogenase 5 (RDH5)*, *Peripherin 2 (PRPH2)*, and *Lecithin Retinol Acyltransferase (LRAT)* genes were also reported [4–6]. About RLBP1 gene, different mutations are linked to a wider spectrum of phenotype as Bothnia retinal dystrophy (BD), Newfoundland rod-cone dystrophy (NFRCD), and fundus albipunctatus (FA). These forms differ for age of

---
* Correspondence: crinaldi@unime.it
[1]Department of Biomedical and Dental Sciences and Morphofunctional Imaging, Division of Molecular Genetics and Preventive Medicine, University of Messina, via C. Valeria 1, I-98125 Messina, Italy
Full list of author information is available at the end of the article

onset, progression, and for severity [7]. A founder effect was proven for mutation p.R234W, causing Bothnia phenotype [8], as well as for splice-junctions mutations detected in NFRCD cases [9]. So, different clinical manifestations are tightly linked to the effects of mutations on protein's structure. *RLBP1* is expressed in retinal pigment epithelium (RPE) and encodes for the cellular retinaldehyde-binding protein 1, CRALBP, involved in visual cycle. Particularly, CRALBP binds 11-cis-retinol which needs to be oxidized in 11-cis-retinal; 11-cis-retinal is carried into photoreceptors where it combines with opsin, resulting in visual pigments formations [10]. This process is common in both cones and rods.

We describe a novel *RLBP1* frameshift mutation, detected in a homozygous condition in a young 31-years-old woman, affected by RPA, certainly with no consanguineous parents up to the 4th generation ancestor, and native in Fiumedinisi, a small Sicilian town in province of Messina. Fiumedinisi is entered in a valley of Nebrodi mountains, at a height of about 200 above sea level. Homozygous condition for a novel mutation is a rare event in patients whose parents are not consanguineous; however, in this case, parents are both native of Fiumedinisi. This leads us to hypothesize that detected mutation is a geographical area-related variant.

Methods
Case analysis
Case description
Here we present a case of a 31-years-old woman (Fig. 1, IV:7), born in Fiumedinisi, a small Sicilian (Italy) town. Her parents, also native of Fiumedinisi, are not consanguineous. About the proband, at the age of five, myopia was diagnosed; two years later, she began suffering from night vision disturbance. Fundus revealed the typical

"salt and pepper" aspect (Fig. 2a), without macula involvement; additionally, optical coherent tomography (OCT) examination showed the presence of numerous well-demarcated homogenous dome-shaped lesions, originating from the RPE layer (Fig. 2b). One year later, fundus analysis confirmed the progressive kind of phenotype, so RPA was diagnosed. Thereafter, she has report continuous worsening with also reduction of the visual field due to "retinal-tapetum" degeneration (Fig. 2c). No evidences of eye diseases were reported neither for her parents nor for younger sister.

Molecular analysis
DNA was extracted from peripheral blood. Exons and exon-intron bourdaries of *RLBP1*, *PRPH2*, *RHO*, *LRAT*, and *RDH5* genes were amplified by polymerase chain reaction (PCR). Primers sequences and PCR conditions are available upon request. Direct sequencing was performed using BigDye Terminator v3.1 chemistry and sequencing was ran on a 3500 Genetic Analyzer (Applied Biosystems). Molecular screening of all genes was performed in the proband; then, detected variants were also searched in the other family members.

In-silico prediction
Effects of the novel mutation on CRALBP tertiary structure were predicted by RaptorX (http://raptorx.uchicago.edu/) prediction tool.

Population study
Samples collection
To test the frequency of novel c.398delC variant, two groups made up by 300 and 600 subjects, respectively, heterogeneous for age and gender, were collected. The first one was recruited in Fiumedinisi and sampling criteria include Fiumedinisi native ancestors by at least

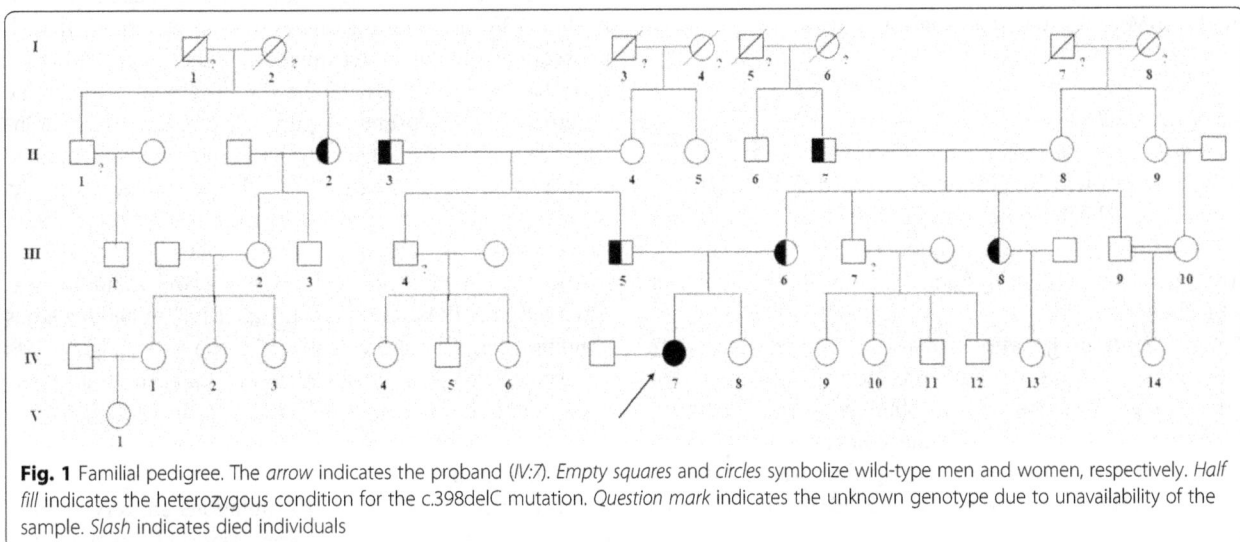

Fig. 1 Familial pedigree. The *arrow* indicates the proband (*IV:7*). *Empty squares* and *circles* symbolize wild-type men and women, respectively. *Half fill* indicates the heterozygous condition for the c.398delC mutation. *Question mark* indicates the unknown genotype due to unavailability of the sample. *Slash* indicates died individuals

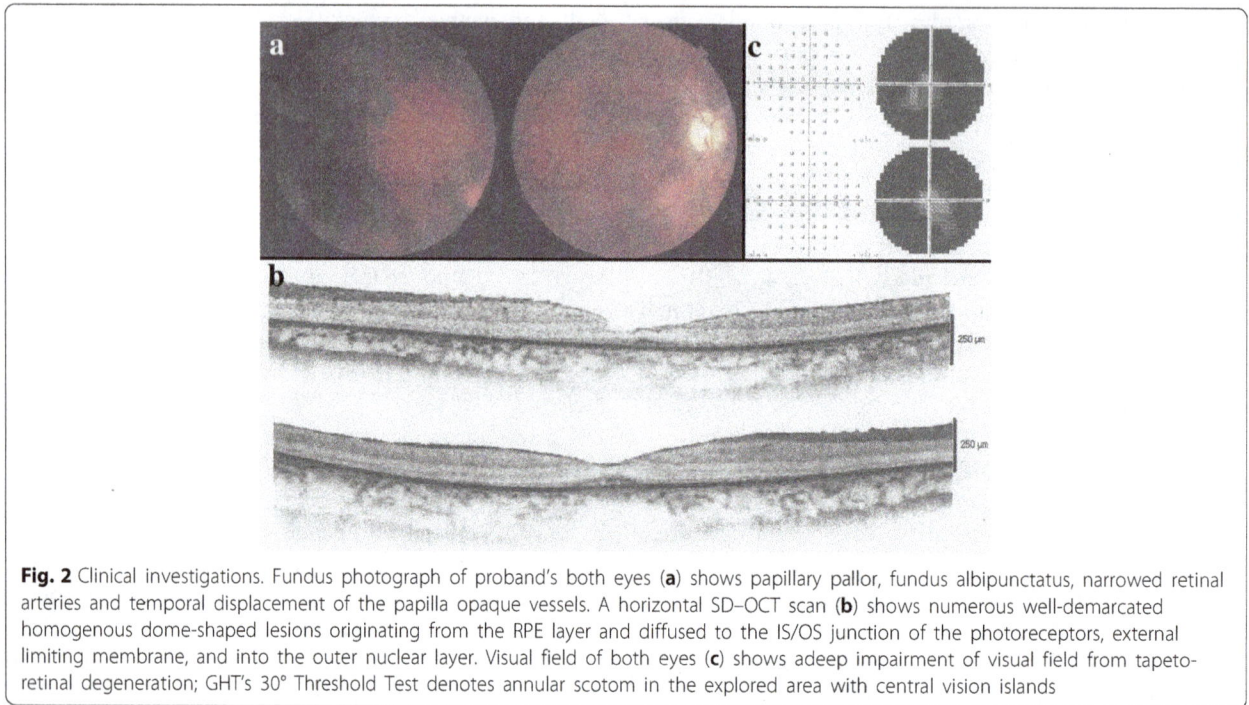

Fig. 2 Clinical investigations. Fundus photograph of proband's both eyes (**a**) shows papillary pallor, fundus albipunctatus, narrowed retinal arteries and temporal displacement of the papilla opaque vessels. A horizontal SD–OCT scan (**b**) shows numerous well-demarcated homogenous dome-shaped lesions originating from the RPE layer and diffused to the IS/OS junction of the photoreceptors, external limiting membrane, and into the outer nuclear layer. Visual field of both eyes (**c**) shows adeep impairment of visual field from tapeto-retinal degeneration; GHT's 30° Threshold Test denotes annular scotom in the explored area with central vision islands

three generations, absence of consanguinity, and absence of inherited disabling ocular diseases. The second group was collected in the Sicilian area: Ionic and Tyrrhenian municipality in province of Messina, like Santa Teresa Riva, Roccalumera, Pace del Mela, were excluded due to their geographic localization, since destinations of the inhabitants of Fiumedinisi who have left their native town. For each population, the c.398delC allele frequency was calculated as $[1 \times (h + 2H)]/2\,N$, where h represents the heterozygous genotype, H the homozygous genotype, and N the sample size for each population. Deviation from Hardy-Weinberg equilibrium (HWE) was determined using the χ^2 test with 2×3 contingency tables and 1 degree of freedom. Analysis was performed by the IBM SPSS statistical analysis software.

Molecular analysis

Buccal swabs were used for collecting saliva samples. DNA was purified by QIAamp® DNA Mini kit (Qiagen). Exon 6 of RLBP1 gene was amplified by PCR for all collected samples, then sequenced on 3500 Genetic Analyzer (Applied Biosystems), using BigDyeTermitor v3.1 chemistry.

All patients and controls involved in this study were fully informed and written consent was obtained. For underage subjects, consent was obtained from the parents. The study protocol followed the guidelines of our local ethics committee, and the investigation was conducted with the ethical requirements defined in the Helsinki Declaration.

Results
Case analysis

Direct sequencing of all known RPA causative genes *LRAT*, *RDH5*, and *RHO* showed no significant variants. Two SNPs rs390659 (c.910C > G, p.Q304E) and rs434102 (c.1013A > G, p.D338G) were detected in *PRPH2*; however, in ClinVar database, these are reported as benign (http://www.ncbi.nlm.nih.gov/clinvar/variation/138904/, http://www.ncbi.nlm.nih.gov/clinvar/variation/138906/). A novel single base-pair frameshift deletion, the c.398delC (p.P133Qfs*258), was detected in exon 6 of RLBP1 gene in a homozygous condition (Fig. 3a). It is not present in mutations and SNPs databases as HGMD, dbSNPs, ClinVar, ExAC, and Ensembl. The variant leads to substitution of proline 133 in glutamine and results in a frameshift with consequent premature termination at the 258th codon, in exon 8, causing the loss of the last 60 amino acids at the C-terminus of the protein. Figure 4 shows the results of in-silico prediction of tertiary structure alteration in mutated protein (Fig. 4b) compared to wild-type one (Fig. 4a). As evident, the c.398delC results in total disruption of functional domain as well as in an altered folding.

About other family's members, the novel mutation was observed in both parents (Fig. 1, III:5, III:6), in heterozygous condition (Fig. 3b) and was absent in the sister (Fig. 1, IV:8; Fig. 3c). Moreover, mutated allele was found both in paternal and in maternal relatives (Fig. 1, II:2, II:3, II:7, III:8).

Population study

As previously described, *RLBP1* mutations are very uncommon and founder mutations were reported. Frequency of

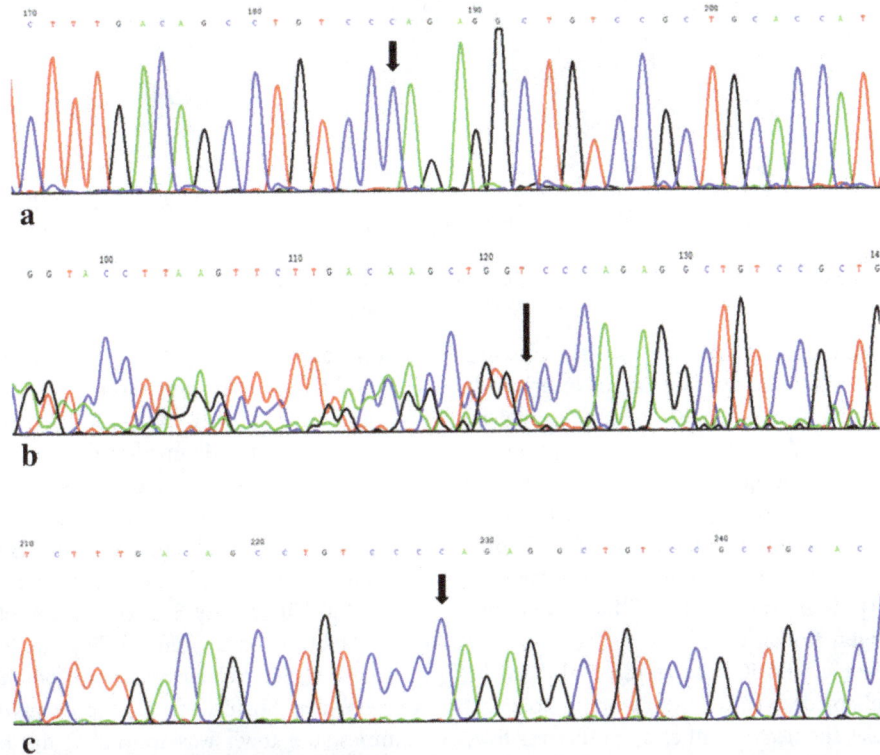

Fig. 3 Partial electropherograms of *RLBP1* exon 6. The *arrows* indicate affected nucleotide. **a** Electropherogram showing the homozygous condition for c.398delC mutation. **b** Electropherogram showing the heterozygous condition, sequence in reverse. **c** Wild-type sequence

c.398delC allele was assessed in both Fiumedinisi and Sicilian population. In the first group, the mutated allele was detected in 0.01%, while none of screened samples of general Sicilian population showed the variant. Table 1 shows the distribution of allele frequencies in Fiumedinisi population; χ^2 test results in a p value = 0.9306 showing the condition of HWE (HWE not consistent for $p < 0.05$).

Discussion

This study reports the results obtained by a molecular analysis performed on a large Sicilian family in which a case of RPA was diagnosed. Molecular screening of all known RPA causative genes showed a novel single base-pair frameshift deletion, c.398delC, in exon 6 of *RLBP1*. It leads to a truncated 258 amino acid protein. Premature

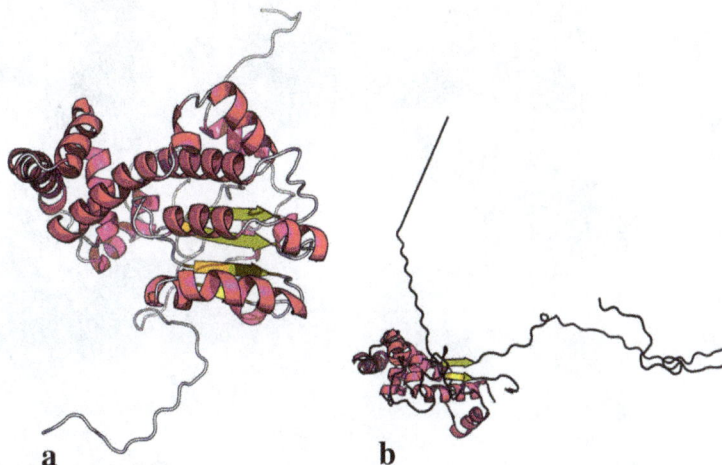

Fig. 4 CRALBP Tertiary structure alteration prediction. Structural models were generated by RaptorX tool. **a** Tertiary structure of wild-type protein. **b** Tertiary structure of p.P133Qfs*258 affected protein

Table 1 Wild-type (+) and c.398delC (−) allele frequencies in Fiumedinisi population

	Samples	Allele +	Allele −	Observed frequency	%	HW-expected frequency	%	Chi-square	p value
+/+	297	594	0	297	99.00	297.01	99.00	0.000	
+/−	3	3	3	3	1.00	2.99	1.00	0.000	
−/−	0	0	0	1	0.00	0.01	0.00	0.008	
Total	300	597	3	300	100.00	300.00	100.00	0.008	0.9306
	600	1.00	0.01	600				(p value) Chisq w 1 df	

A total of 300 samples were genotyped. Only 0.01% of screened population carries the mutated allele. Chi-square test exhibits a p value = 0.9306 suggesting the presence of the equilibrium's condition between wild-type and mutated allele in Fiumedinisi population

stop codon falls within exon 8. CRALBP protein contains one CRAL-TRIO lipid-binding domain, of 162 aminoacids (136-297). As predicted by in-silico analysis, the c.398delC affects proline 133 and causes total disruption of CRAL-TRIO domain, resulting in a loss of ability to bind its ligands. CRAL-TRIO motifs usually bind small hydrophobic molecules. In CRALBP, aminoacids 136-297 form CRAL-TRIO domain and, 12 of these, form the retinoid binding pocket [11]. Therefore, c.398delC has deleterious effects on protein's functionality.

Presence of variant c.398delC was assessed also in the other family's members; despite, they show no pathological phenotypes. Of these, the healthy father and other relatives showed this variant, in a heterozygous condition. This confirms autosomal recessive model of inheritance of RPA. The proband carries the novel c.398delC mutation in a homozygous condition. We proceeded to investigate frequency of variant in Fiumedinisi's population. Fiumedinisi, a small town in province of Messina, is located on the Ionian side, at the height of 190 above sea level (Fig. 5). It has an area of 36 km² and extends along Nisi's valley, at Mt. Belvedere's slopes, behind Valle del Mela. The city was founded in VII century B.C., by a group of Calcidesi Greek colonists, attracted by mineral deposits, who inhabited the high area of Mt. Belvedere. Later, Roman, Arab, Norman, Angevin, and Spanish dominions went on. During these centuries, the town was moved to the foot of mountain (where it remains today) and renamed as FlumenDionisyi.

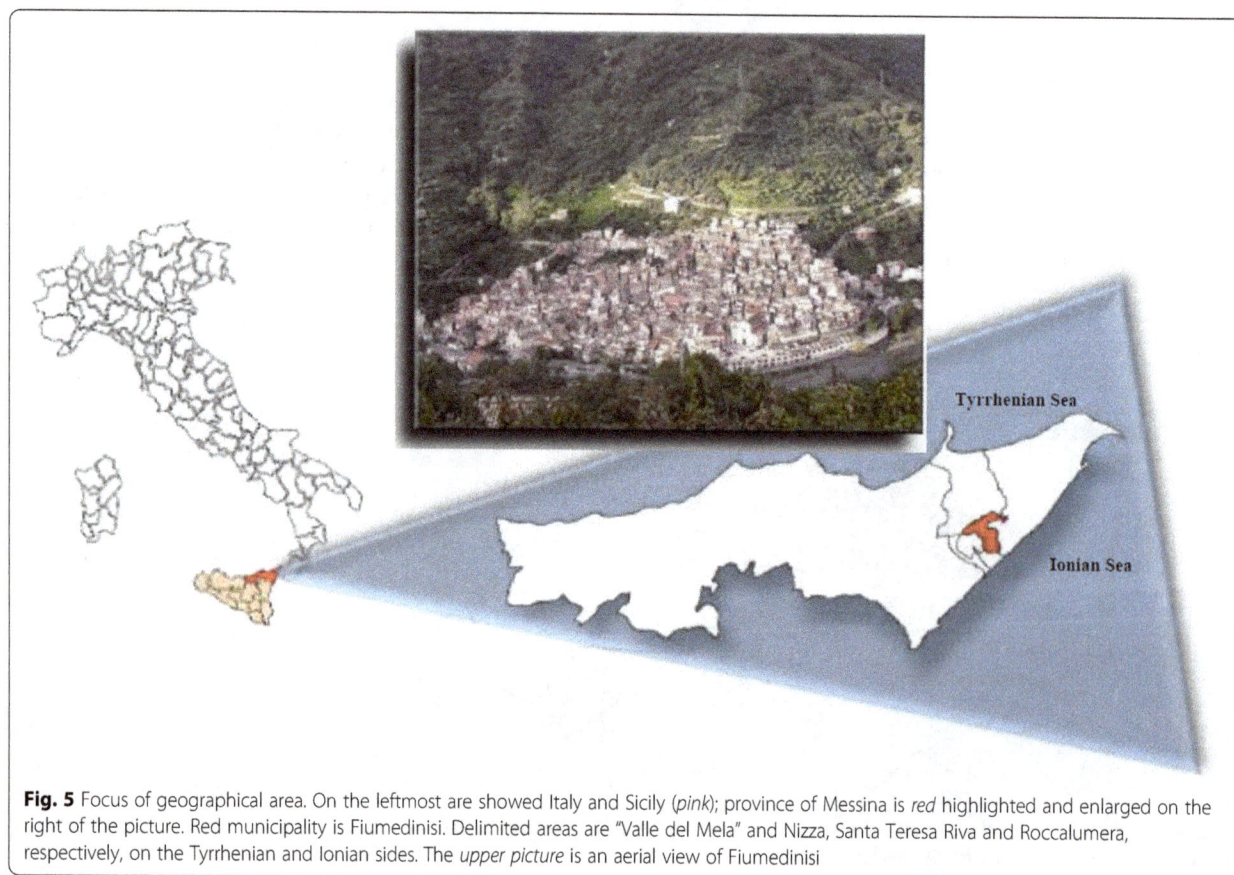

Fig. 5 Focus of geographical area. On the leftmost are showed Italy and Sicily (*pink*); province of Messina is *red* highlighted and enlarged on the right of the picture. Red municipality is Fiumedinisi. Delimited areas are "Valle del Mela" and Nizza, Santa Teresa Riva and Roccalumera, respectively, on the Tyrrhenian and Ionian sides. The *upper picture* is an aerial view of Fiumedinisi

Still today, it results in not being easy to get to. Two big disasters hit the city: an epidemic plague in 1743 and a big flood in 1855. A period of decline, then, started due to high immigration's phenomenon. To date, Fiumedinisi's population counts about 1400 inhabitants, most of which are over the age of 50 years. For our aim, we screened about 25% of population and c.398delC was found in 0.01% and it is in HWE. No other RPA cases were detected in the town. Although there is a high rate of consanguinity in Fiumedinisi's population, its low frequency may be attributed to several dominations, repeated drastic reductions in population, the probable selective disadvantage, and a recent founder effect. This last hypothesis can be demonstrated by several statistic approaches. Among these, the method proposed by Slatkin and Rannala [12, 13] based on allele frequency and coalescent process [14] is what we think to apply to estimate the age of c.398delC mutation, as next development of this paper.

Conclusions

We report a case with RPA caused by the novel mutation, the c.398delC, in RLBP1 gene in homozygous condition necessary for developing the disease. The new mutation enriches the already wide spectrum of RP causative mutations. Hypothesis of a geographic area-related mutation was induced by the detection of this allele in several non-consanguineous inhabitants and by its absence in Sicilian population. However, due to the succession of more dominations, it is very difficult to establish by which ancestral population it was introduced.

Abbreviations

CRALBP: Cellular retinaldehyde-binding protein; FA: Fundus albipunctatus; HWE: Hardy-Weinberg Equilibrium; NFRCD: Newfoundland rod-cone dystrophy; OCT: Optical coherent tomography; RLBP1: Retinaldehyde binding protein 1; RP: Retinitis pigmentosa; RPA: Retinitis punctata albescens; RPE: Retinal pigment epithelium

Acknowledgments

We thank Fiumedinisi's population for disposability, particularly Dr.Bertani Gilda for her precious collaboration in controls collection.

Funding

Authors received no financial support to perform this study.

Authors' contributions

CS wrote the manuscript; LD and TE collected samples and performed molecular analysis; CR supervised the study; RD'A designed the study; AS coordinated the research team. All authors read and approved the final manuscript.

Competing interests

The authors declare that they have no competing interests.

Author details

[1]Department of Biomedical and Dental Sciences and Morphofunctional Imaging, Division of Molecular Genetics and Preventive Medicine, University of Messina, via C. Valeria 1, I-98125 Messina, Italy. [2]Department of Cutting-Edge Medicine and Therapies, Biomolecular Strategies and Neuroscience, Section of Neuroscience-applied Molecular Genetics and Predictive Medicine, I. E. ME. S. T, via Michele Miraglia 20, I-90139 Palermo, Italy. [3]Department of Experimental Medicine, Division of Human Physiology and Integrate Biological Functions "F. Bottazzi", University of Campania Luigi Vanvitelli, ex II University of Naples, via Santa Maria di Costantinipoli 16, I-80138 Naples, Italy.

References

1. Narayan DS, Wood JP, Chidlow G, Casson RJ. A review of the mechanisms of cone degeneration in retinitis pigmentosa. Acta Ophthalmol. 2016;94:748–54.
2. Morimura H, Berson EL, Dryja TP. Recessive mutations in the RLBP1 gene encoding cellular retinaldehyde-binding protein in a form of retinitis punctata albescens. Invest Ophthalmol Vis Sci. 1999;40:1000–4.
3. Golding AM. Retinitis punctata albescens with pigmentation. Br J Ophthalmol. 1956;40:242–4.
4. Souied E, Soubrane G, Benlian P, Coscas GJ, Gerber S, Munnich A, Kaplan J. Retinitis punctata albescens associated with the Arg135Trp mutation in the rhodopsin gene. Am J Ophthalmol. 1996;121:19–25.
5. Kajiwara K, Sandberg MA, Berson EL, Dryja TP. A null mutation in the human peripherin/RDS gene in a family with autosomal dominant retinitis punctata albescens. Nat Genet. 1993;3:208–12.
6. Littink KW, Van Genderen MM, van Schooneveld MJ, Visser L, Riemslag FC, Keunen JE, et al. A homozygous frameshift mutation in LRAT causes retinitis punctata albescens. Ophthalmology. 2012;119:1899–906.
7. Hipp S, Zobor G, Glöckle N, Mohr J, Kohl S, Zrenner E, et al. Phenotype variations of retinal dystrophies caused by mutations in the RLBP1 gene. Acta Ophthalmol. 2015;93:281–6.
8. Burstedt MS, Sandgren O, Holmgren G, Forsman-Semb K. Bothnia dystrophy caused by mutations in the cellular retinaldehyde-binding protein gene (RLBP1) on chromosome 15q26. Invest Ophthalmol Vis Sci. 1999;40:995–1000.
9. Eichers ER, Green JS, Stockton DW, Jackman CS, Whelan J, McNamara JA, et al. Newfoundland rod-cone dystrophy, an early-onset retinal dystrophy, is caused by splice-junction mutations in RLBP1. Am J Hum Genet. 2002;70:955–64.
10. Kennedy BN, Li C, Ortego J, Coca-Prados M, Sarthy VP, Crabb JW. CRALBP transcriptional regulation in ciliary epithelial, retinal Müller and retinal pigment epithelial cells. Exp Eye Res. 2003;76:257–60.
11. Wu Z, Hasan A, Liu T, Teller DC, Crabb JW. Identification of CRALBP ligand interactions by photoaffinity labeling, hydrogen/deuterium exchange, and structural modeling. J Biol Chem. 2004;279:27357–64.
12. Slatkin M, Rannala B. Estimating the age of alleles by use of intraallelic variability. Am J Hum Genet. 1997;60:447–58.
13. Slatkin M, Rannala B. Estimating allele age. Annu Rev Genomics Hum Genet. 2000;01:225–49.
14. Goldstein DB, Reich DE, Bradman N, Usher S, Seligsohn U, Peretz H. Age estimates of two common mutations causing Factor XI deficiency: recent genetic drft is not necessary for elevated disease incidence among Ashkenazi Jews. Am J Hum Genet. 1999;64:1071–5.

14

Whole-exome sequencing identifies novel candidate predisposition genes for familial polycythemia vera

Elina A. M. Hirvonen[1], Esa Pitkänen[1], Kari Hemminki[2], Lauri A. Aaltonen[1,3] and Outi Kilpivaara[1*]

Abstract

Background: Polycythemia vera (PV), characterized by massive production of erythrocytes, is one of the myeloproliferative neoplasms. Most patients carry a somatic gain-of-function mutation in *JAK2*, c.1849G > T (p.Val617Phe), leading to constitutive activation of JAK-STAT signaling pathway. Familial clustering is also observed occasionally, but high-penetrance predisposition genes to PV have remained unidentified.

Results: We studied the predisposition to PV by exome sequencing (three cases) in a Finnish PV family with four patients. The 12 shared variants (maximum allowed minor allele frequency <0.001 in Finnish population in ExAC database) predicted damaging in silico and absent in an additional control set of over 500 Finns were further validated by Sanger sequencing in a fourth affected family member. Three novel predisposition candidate variants were identified: c.1254C > G (p.Phe418Leu) in *ZXDC*, c.1931C > G (p.Pro644Arg) in *ATN1*, and c.701G > A (p.Arg234Gln) in *LRRC3*. We also observed a rare, predicted benign germline variant c.2912C > G (p.Ala971Gly) in *BCORL1* in all four patients. Somatic mutations in *BCORL1* have been reported in myeloid malignancies. We further screened the variants in eight PV patients in six other Finnish families, but no other carriers were found.

Conclusions: Exome sequencing provides a powerful tool for the identification of novel variants, and understanding the familial predisposition of diseases. This is the first report on Finnish familial PV cases, and we identified three novel candidate variants that may predispose to the disease.

Keywords: Myeloproliferative neoplasm, Polycythemia vera, Genetics, Exome sequencing, Familial predisposition

Background

Myeloproliferative neoplasms (MPNs) are a group of hematological malignancies with enhanced proliferation of myeloid cells due to an acquired mutation of a single hematopoietic stem cell (HSC) resulting in clonal progeny [1, 2]. Expansion of red blood cells in the peripheral blood and bone marrow is the hallmark of polycythemia vera (PV). PV is a chronic, Philadelphia chromosome-negative myeloproliferative disorder with symptoms including fatigue, pruritus, and splenomegaly. The patients have an increased risk of thrombosis, and the disease may further progress to secondary acute myeloid leukemia (sAML) or myelofibrosis [3].

The global annual incidence rate of PV is approximately 1 per 100,000 persons [4]. Most PV patients (approximately 95%) carry a somatic mutation in exon 14 of a non-receptor tyrosine kinase-coding gene Janus kinase 2 (*JAK2*), c.1849G > T (p.Val617Phe, subsequently referred to as *JAK2V617F*) [5–8]. The major diagnostic criteria for PV according to World Health Organization (2008) are exceptionally high hemoglobin and presence of *JAK2V617F* mutation. Other criteria include consistent bone marrow morphology and low erythropoietin (Epo) levels [9, 10]. When diagnosed with PV, most patients are older than 60 years old, and survival depends on the complications and severity of the disease. In younger patients, life expectancy is reduced when compared to the general population [11].

Janus kinase 2 (JAK2) plays a crucial role in the function and maintenance of HSCs [12], as well as in myelopoiesis through binding to various cytokine receptors including

* Correspondence: outi.kilpivaara@helsinki.fi
[1]Genome-Scale Biology Research Program, Research Programs Unit and Department of Medical and Clinical Genetics, Medicum, University of Helsinki, P.O. Box 6300014 Helsinki, Finland
Full list of author information is available at the end of the article

erythropoietin receptor (Epo-R), thus, contributing to formation of red blood cells [13]. V617F mutation, which is located within the pseudokinase domain of JAK2 protein, leads to constitutive activity that promotes cytokine hypersensitivity and abnormal signaling through Janus kinase-signal transducer and activator of transcription factor (JAK-STAT) pathway [5–8]. In addition, approximately 3% of PV patients, being *JAK2V617F*-negative, harbor mutations in exon 12 of *JAK2*. The mutations in both exons 14 and 12 induce cytokine-independent proliferation of cells expressing Epo-receptors [14]. Also, certain germline mutations in *JAK2* are predicted to represent a mechanism possibly preceding the acquisition of *JAK2V617F* mutation in PV [15].

Although most PV cases appear to be sporadic, familial clustering is also observed in a subset of cases [16–18]. *JAK2V617F*-positive MPNs are strongly associated with *JAK2* 46/1, or 'GGCC' haplotype (rs10974944), which is a common, moderate penetrance predisposition allele [19–22]. Also, a single nucleotide polymorphism (SNP) in the telomerase reverse transcriptase gene (*TERT*), rs2736100, has emerged as another predisposing factor to MPNs [23]. In addition, it has been shown that germline duplication of *ATG2B* and *GSKIP* genes predisposes to familial myeloid malignancies [24], and germline *RBBP6* mutations have been associated with familial MPNs [25]. It is likely that additional inherited genetic factors contribute to PV development as well, since familial clustering of PV suggests the presence of additional susceptibility alleles. High-penetrance predisposition genes to PV have, however, remained unidentified.

Here, we report a Finnish family with four PV patients in two generations (Additional file 1: Figure S1). A family with this many cases is quite exceptional, since PV is a rare disease and usually sporadic. Also, in a familial PV case like here, the age at diagnosis is usually lower, which is an additional indication of the presence of predisposing factors. DNA from all the PV patients in this family was available. The aim of this study was to identify new predisposing gene variants by exome sequencing the DNA of three of the affected family members; the index case and two affected family members (germline) and peripheral blood DNA of the index case. Exome sequencing was not feasible in the fourth PV patient due to very low amount of archived DNA available. The observed, predicted as damaging, germline variants were analyzed in the fourth PV patient of the family, and the variants shared by all four individuals were further screened in six other families with two PV cases in each.

Methods
Patient samples
We investigated a Finnish family with four PV patients (Additional file 1: Figure S1). The index case (1.1) was

diagnosed with PV at the age of 36, and with myelofibrosis later at the age of 47. The father (1.2) of the index patient was diagnosed with PV at the age of 48, and the aunt (1.9) with PV and acute leukemia at the age of 91. The uncle (1.10) of the index patient was diagnosed with PV at the age of 83. Two individuals in the family had lymphoma; 1.19 was diagnosed with nodular lymphocyte-predominant Hodgkin lymphoma (NLPHL) at the age of 55, and with diffuse large cell non-Hodgkin lymphoma (NHL) later at the age of 68; 1.6 was diagnosed with differentiated diffuse lymphocytic lymphoma at the age of 89. The healthy daughter of the index case is currently 31 years old.

Both peripheral blood and buccal swab samples were available from the index case. Only formalin-fixed paraffin embedded (FFPE) blocks were available from three other family members diagnosed with PV: 1.2, 1.9, and 1.10. Germline DNA was also available from one of two lymphoma patients (1.19) of the family. The second sample set consisted of FFPE blocks from six other Finnish PV families with two first-degree relative cases in five, and two more distant relatives in the sixth family. The study was approved by the appropriate Ethics Review Committee. Samples were derived either after a signed informed consent or after authorization from the National Supervisory Authority for Welfare and Health. The study was conducted in accordance with the Declaration of Helsinki.

Exome capture and sequencing
DNA was extracted from FFPE blocks with a standard phenol-chloroform method, and the buccal swab sample was extracted with QIAmp DNA Mini kit (Qiagen, Hilden, Germany). DNA from the blood sample was extracted with a standard non-enzymatic TKM buffer-proteinase K method. Sample libraries of gDNA were prepared using NEBNext DNA Library Prep Reagent Set for Illumina (New England Biolabs Ltd. Catalog # E6000), and exomic regions were enriched using Agilent Sure SelectXT Human All Exon V4 + UTRs 50Mb kit (Agilent Technologies, Santa Clara, CA, USA). Paired-end short read sequencing was performed with HiSeq 2000 (Illumina Inc., San Diego, CA, USA) at Karolinska Institutet, Sweden. The DNA library for whole-genome sequencing was prepared with KAPA Hyper Prep Kit (KAPA Biosystems, Wilmington, MA, USA). Paired-end short read sequencing was performed with HiSeq 4000 (Illumina Inc.) at Karolinska Institutet.

Variant analysis
Exome and genome sequencing data was mapped against the human reference genome GRCh37 (1000 Genomes Project reference hs37d5) with Burrow-Wheeler Aligner (BWA MEM, v.0.7.12, https://arxiv.org/abs/1303.3997), and mapped reads refined following the Genome Analysis

Toolkit (GATK) Best Practices workflow including PCR duplicate removal, indel realignment, and base quality score recalibration [26]. Single-nucleotide and short-indel variants were then called using GATK HaplotypeCaller.

The SNV and indel variants in the exome sequencing data were analyzed with an in-house developed analysis and visualization tool (BasePlayer, Katainen et al., manuscript in preparation). A minimum coverage of four reads and the mutated allele present in at least 20% of the reads was required to call a variant. The variants which were present in an in-house control set of 542 Finns [93 whole genome sequenced individuals from the 1000 Genomes Project, 402 whole-genome sequenced individuals from Kuusamo, Finland (Sequencing Initiative Suomi), and 47 uterine leiomyoma patients] were excluded. To exclude common variants, we further filtered the variant set against the Exome Aggregation Consortium (ExAC v.0.3: 3,307 Finns) data [27], setting the maximum allowed minor allele frequency (MAF) in Finnish population to 0.001. Germline variants predicted benign by two independent computational methods PolyPhen-2 [28] and SIFT [29] were excluded.

Direct sequencing

The shared variants found in the exome data and *BCORL1* cDNA were validated by direct Sanger sequencing. Also, the predisposing germline variant rs10974944 in *JAK2* was checked. DNA was extracted from FFPE blocks with a standard phenol-chloroform method or with NucleoSpin® DNA FFPE XS kit (Macherey-Nagel, Düren, Germany). Primers were designed using Primer3Plus software (http://www.bioinformatics.nl/primer3plus). The DreamTaq™ DNA Polymerase (Thermo Scientific, Waltham, MA, USA) or Invitrogen™, Platinum™, SuperFi™ DNA Polymerase (Thermo Scientific) were used in PCR reactions, and PCR products were

purified with A'SAP PCR clean-up method (ArcticZymes, Tromsø, Norway). BigDye Terminator v3.1 sequencing reaction was used in the DNA sequencing, and capillary electrophoresis was performed on an ABI3730xl DNA Analyzer (Applied Biosystems, Foster City, CA, USA) at the Institute for Molecular Medicine Finland (FIMM). The results were analyzed manually using FinchTV v.1.4.0 (Geospiza Inc., Seattle, WA, USA).

For cDNA sequencing, RNA was extracted from index case's whole blood sample with NucleoSpin® RNA kit (Macherey-Nagel), and reverse-transcribed to cDNA with Promega M-MLV Reverse Transcriptase (Thermo Scientific) according to manufacturers' protocols.

Results and discussion

Novel candidate germline variants for PV predisposition

Here, we have studied a Finnish family with four PV cases with the aim of identifying novel PV-predisposing germline variants. Germline DNA exomes from three affected family members and the peripheral blood DNA exome of the index case were sequenced. The average coverage at each base was 58 reads and 88% of the captured regions had a minimum coverage of four reads. We filtered the called variants based on their predicted, damaging effect on the gene product, and their presence in an in-house control set of 542 Finns. We removed the variants that occurred in any of the 542 Finnish controls (MAF < 0.2%, 95% CI [0, 0.05%]), leaving us with 12 shared variants; 1 splice site and 11 possibly pathogenic missense variants (Table 1). We then validated the variants by Sanger sequencing in one additional family member diagnosed with PV (1.10).

From these variants predicted as damaging, 1.10 carried three rare single-nucleotide variants (SNVs): c.1254C > G (p.Phe418Leu) in *ZXDC* (ENST00000389709); c.1931C > G (p.Pro644Arg) in *ATN1* (ENST00000356654);

Table 1 A list of damaging (in silico) germline variants in PV patients detected by exome sequencing (three cases)

Gene	Ensembl gene	Ensembl transcript	Genomic location	Variation, cDNA	Variation, protein
ZXDC*	ENSG00000070476	ENST00000389709	Chr3: 126189754	c.1254C > G	p.Phe418Leu
ATN1*	ENSG00000111676	ENST00000356654	Chr12: 7046361	c.1931C > G	p.Pro644Arg
LRRC3*	ENSG00000160233	ENST00000291592	Chr21: 45877228	c.701G > A, rs148872771	p.Arg234Gln
GNL3	ENSG00000163938	ENST00000418458	Chr3: 52727477	c.1241A > G	p.Tyr414Cys
MDC1	ENSG00000137337	ENST00000376406	Chr6: 30679188	c.2221-1G > T	splice site variant
ITPR3	ENSG00000096433	ENST00000374316	Chr6: 33635026	c.1672C > T, rs780906252	p.Arg558Cys
FAM135A	ENSG00000082269	ENST00000418814	Chr6: 71190668	c.607G > A, rs143901584	p.Val203Met
SLC2A12	ENSG00000146411	ENST00000275230	Chr6: 134312391	c.1756C > T, rs200847615	p.Pro586Ser
WDR86	ENSG00000187260	ENST00000334493	Chr7: 151097265	c.226G > A, rs199824863	p.Asp76Asn
CSMD1	ENSG00000183117	ENST00000537824	Chr8: 3165238	c.3929C > T	p.Ala1310Val
SLC24A2	ENSG00000155886	ENST00000341998	Chr9: 19786283	c.582A > G, rs368590535	p.Ile194Met
ITPKC	ENSG00000086544	ENST00000263370	Chr19: 41224132	c.1092C > G, rs143757004	p.Asp364Glu

The three shared variants in all four cases are marked with an *asterisk*. Genome assembly: GRCh37

and rs148872771, c.701G > A (p.Arg234Gln) in *LRRC3* (ENST00000291592). We screened the three variants in lymphoma patient 1.19, who carried the variant in *LRRC3*. Also, we checked for the three variants in the germlines of eight PV patients from six other Finnish families, but the variants were not observed. It may still be possible, however, that some of the three variants or other variants in these genes may play a role in PV development. We identified also one rare benign (PolyPhen-2, SIFT) missense SNP, rs144332650, c.2912C > G (p.Ala971Gly), and in *BCORL1* (ENST00000540052) in all four PV patients in the family. Mutations in *BCORL1* have been associated with the leukemogenic process in AML [30–32]. PV patients in six other families did not carry the variant.

Zinc-finger X-linked duplicated family member C (ZXDC) belongs to the ZXD family of transcription factors, which has been observed to regulate transcription of major histocompatibility complex (MHC) class I and II genes in antigen presenting cells [33]. In addition to zinc fingers, ZXDC contains a transcriptional activation domain, and a specific domain used for interaction with a transcriptional co-factor class II *trans*-activator (CIITA), which leads to CIITA binding to promoter elements involved in constitutive MHC class II expression [33, 34]. By reducing the expression of ZXDC, CIITA activation of MHC class II gene transcription is significantly reduced [33]. Thus, downregulation of *ZXDC* may contribute to carcinogenesis and malignant progression of tumors by participating in the suppression of MHC class II genes. The mutated site of *ZXDC* identified in our study is the first amino acid of the ninth zinc finger repeat. Zinc fingers are necessary for full activity of cooperation with CIITA [33]. Beyond this role of acting as a co-factor in CIITA function, the *ZXDC* gene function is unknown. ZXDC is enriched in myeloid lineages and has been observed to regulate transcription of key genes during myeloid cell differentiation [35]. During hematopoiesis, it is expressed especially in stem and progenitor cells in the bone marrow, myelocytes, and leukocytes (BloodSpot http://nar.oxfordjournals.org/con tent/early/2015/10/26/nar.gkv1101.abstract, www.protei natlas.org). Solely based on gene function, *ZXDC* variant would be the most attractive predisposition candidate of the three, but further studies are warranted.

Atrophin-1 (ATN1) is a nuclear transcriptional corepressor, and aberrant form of ATN1 is associated with neurodegenerative diseases such as dentatorubral-pallidoluysian atrophy (DRPLA), and cancer in humans [36]. It is ubiquitously expressed in neurons [37] and widely in various other tissues, e.g., in hematopoietic cells in the bone marrow (www.proteinatlas.org). ATN1 contains glutamine-repeats, and two arginine-glutamic acid dipeptide-like repeats (RE-repeats) [36]. In neuronal nuclei, ATN1 has been shown to interact with a

transcriptional repressor Eight twenty-one (ETO) protein [38]. In normal hematopoiesis, it is widely expressed in differentiated blood cells, but the expression is lower in stem and progenitor cells (BloodSpot). Thus, it is likely that ATN1 interaction with ETO has no contribution to erythropoiesis or development of myeloproliferative diseases. On the other hand, in patients with AML, ATN1 is expressed more substantially (BloodSpot) compared to normal counterparts. Nevertheless, its normal function is not completely understood.

Little is known about the function of Leucine-rich repeat containing 3 (LRRC3) gene product, but it is widely expressed in different tissues, including the bone marrow. Most malignancies display moderate cytoplasmic-positive staining, and the strongest expression is observed in colorectal cancers (www.proteinatlas.org). One lymphoma patient of the family with DNA available carried the rare variant rs148872771 in *LRRC3*, too, which may indicate the particular variant not being responsible for PV predisposition exclusively.

The SNP in *JAK2*, rs10974944, was identified in all the PV patients in the family. Individuals 1.1, 1.2, and 1.10 were homozygous for the risk variant in their germline (GG genotype), whereas 1.9 was heterozygous (CG genotype). Also, all eight PV patients from the six other families carried the risk variant: two of them were heterozygous, and six were homozygous. The SNP in *TERT*, rs2736100, was also checked from the patients. All the PV patients in the studied family were homozygous for the risk variant (CC).

Germline duplication of *ATG2B* and *GSKIP* has been shown to predispose to familial myeloid malignancies [24]. A possible duplication was checked for in the whole-genome sequence data of the index case by visualizing the depth of coverage in the region. The duplication had not occurred in the index patient's genome.

Detection of somatic variants

We identified the most frequent somatic variation in PV patients, *JAK2V617F*, in index case's blood sample. Loss of heterozygosity (LOH) in the 12 damaging gene variants detected by exome sequencing was looked for in the index case's blood sample, but only the variants c.582A > G (p.Ile194Met) in *SLC24A2* and c.3929C > T (p.Ala1310Val) in *CSMD1*, in addition to *JAK2V617F*, showed clear LOH. In known MPN-associated genes, the index case carried two missense variants, c.680C > T (p.Thr227Met) in *FLT3* and c.5162 T > G (p.Leu1721Trp) in *TET2* (Illumina TruSight® Myeloid Sequencing Panel), predicted as possibly damaging by PolyPhen-2 and SIFT. In addition, we identified possibly damaging missense variants c.3263C > T (p.Ser1088Phe) and c.1235C > T (p.Ala412Val) in *FANCA*, which is one of the genes associated with other myeloid malignancies [39, 40].

BCORL1 gene is located on the X chromosome. The index case being a woman, we checked which of the alleles was expressed; the *BCORL1* variant or the wild-type. By Sanger sequencing the cDNA, we identified the expression of *BCORL1* variant.

Conclusions

Identification of predisposing genes and mutations is important for families with PV susceptibility and acknowledging family history is essential in order to unveil the genetic background. New hereditary gene defects may lead to screening and genetic counseling of family members and may improve the diagnosis and treatment thus affecting the quality of life. Also, the identification of specific gene mutations gives the possibility to screen individuals at higher risk. This is the first report on Finnish familial PV cases, and we identified three candidate predisposition variants by exome-sequencing. We would like to present these genes as candidates for PV susceptibility and for further validation by the research community.

Acknowledgements
The authors would like to thank Annukka Ruokolainen, Inga-Lill Svedberg, Iina Vuoristo, Sini Nieminen, Marjo Rajalaakso, Heikki Metsola, and Jiri Hamberg for excellent technical assistance. Institute for Molecular Medicine Finland (FIMM) is acknowledged for capillary sequencing. Minna Taipale and Jussi Taipale (Karolinska Institutet, Stockholm, Sweden) are acknowledged for providing excellent exome and genome sequencing services.

Funding
Funding for the work was supported by grants from the Academy of Finland (Finnish Centre of Excellence Program 2012-2017 (#250345), and personal grants for O.K. (#137680, #274474), the Finnish Cancer Society, and Sigrid Juselius Foundation. The funding bodies did not participate in the study design, sample collection, analysis and interpretation of data, or in the writing of the manuscript.

Author's contributions
OK, KH, and LAA designed the study. KH provided the samples. EAMH performed the laboratory experiments and data analysis. EP was responsible for the pipeline. EAMH and OK wrote the manuscript. All authors read and approved the final manuscript.

Competing interests
The authors declare that they have no competing interests.

Author details
[1]Genome-Scale Biology Research Program, Research Programs Unit and Department of Medical and Clinical Genetics, Medicum, University of Helsinki, P.O. Box 6300014 Helsinki, Finland. [2]Division of Molecular Genetic Epidemiology, German Cancer Research Center (DKFZ), Heidelberg, Germany. [3]Department of Biosciences and Nutrition, Karolinska Institutet, SE-17177 Stockholm, Sweden.

References
1. Adamson JW, Fialkow PJ, Murphy S, Prchal JF, Steinmann L. Polycythemia vera: stem-cell and probable clonal origin of the disease. N Engl J Med. 1976;295:913–6.
2. Jamieson CH, Gotlib J, Durocher JA, Chao MP, Mariappan MR, Lay M, et al. The JAK2 V617F mutation occurs in hematopoietic stem cells in polycythemia vera and predisposes toward erythroid differentiation. Proc Natl Acad Sci U S A. 2006;103:6224–9.
3. Stein BL, Oh ST, Berenzon D, Hobbs GS, Kremyanskaya M, Rampal RK, et al. Polycythemia vera: an appraisal of the biology and management 10 years after the discovery of JAK2 V617F. J Clin Oncol. 2015;33:3953–60.
4. Titmarsh GJ, Duncombe AS, Mcmullin MF, O'rorke M, Mesa R, De Vocht F, et al. How common are myeloproliferative neoplasms? A systematic review and meta-analysis. Am J Hematol. 2014;89:581–7.
5. Baxter EJ, Scott LM, Campbell PJ, East C, Fourouclas N, Swanton S, et al. Acquired mutation of the tyrosine kinase JAK2 in human myeloproliferative disorders. Lancet. 2005;365:1054–61.
6. James C, Ugo V, Le Couedic JP, Staerk J, Delhommeau F, Lacout C, et al. A unique clonal JAK2 mutation leading to constitutive signalling causes polycythaemia vera. Nature. 2005;434:1144–8.
7. Kralovics R, Passamonti F, Buser AS, Teo SS, Tiedt R, Passweg JR, et al. A gain-of-function mutation of JAK2 in myeloproliferative disorders. N Engl J Med. 2005;352:1779–90.
8. Levine RL, Wadleigh M, Cools J, Ebert BL, Wernig G, Huntly BJ, et al. Activating mutation in the tyrosine kinase JAK2 in polycythemia vera, essential thrombocythemia, and myeloid metaplasia with myelofibrosis. Cancer Cell. 2005;7:387–97.
9. Tefferi A, Thiele J, Orazi A, Kvasnicka HM, Barbui T, Hanson CA, et al. Proposals and rationale for revision of the World Health Organization diagnostic criteria for polycythemia vera, essential thrombocythemia, and primary myelofibrosis: recommendations from an ad hoc international expert panel. Blood. 2007;110:1092–7.
10. Tefferi A, Thiele J, Vardiman JW. The 2008 World Health Organization classification system for myeloproliferative neoplasms: order out of chaos. Cancer. 2009;115:3842–7.
11. Stein BL, Saraf S, Sobol U, Halpern A, Shammo J, Rondelli D, et al. Age-related differences in disease characteristics and clinical outcomes in polycythemia vera. Leuk Lymphoma. 2013;54:1989–95.
12. Akada H, Akada S, Hutchison RE, Sakamoto K, Wagner KU, Mohi G. Critical role of Jak2 in the maintenance and function of adult hematopoietic stem cells. Stem Cells. 2014;32:1878–89.
13. Witthuhn BA, Quelle FW, Silvennoinen O, Yi T, Tang B, Miura O, et al. JAK2 associates with the erythropoietin receptor and is tyrosine phosphorylated and activated following stimulation with erythropoietin. Cell. 1993;74:227–36.
14. Scott LM, Tong W, Levine RL, Scott MA, Beer PA, Stratton MR, et al. JAK2 exon 12 mutations in polycythemia vera and idiopathic erythrocytosis. N Engl J Med. 2007;356:459–68.
15. Lanikova L, Babosova O, Swierczek S, Wang L, Wheeler DA, Divoky V, et al. Coexistence of gain-of-function JAK2 germline mutations with JAK2V617F in polycythemia vera. Blood. 2016. doi:10.1182/blood-2016-04-711283.

Whole-exome sequencing identifies novel candidate predisposition genes for familial...

161

16. Hemminki K, Jiang Y. Familial polycythemia vera: results from the Swedish Family-Cancer Database. Leukemia. 2001;15:1313–5.

17. Kralovics R, Stockton DW, Prchal JT. Clonal hematopoiesis in familial polycythemia vera suggests the involvement of multiple mutational events in the early pathogenesis of the disease. Blood. 2003;102:3793–6.

18. Cario H, Goerttler PS, Steimle C, Levine RL, Pahl HL. The JAK2V617F mutation is acquired secondary to the predisposing alteration in familial polycythaemia vera. Br J Haematol. 2005;130:800–1.

19. Jones AV, Chase A, Silver RT, Oscier D, Zoi K, Wang YL, et al. JAK2 haplotype is a major risk factor for the development of myeloproliferative neoplasms. Nat Genet. 2009;41:446–9.

20. Kilpivaara O, Mukherjee S, Schram AM, Wadleigh M, Mullally A, Ebert BL, et al. A germline JAK2 SNP is associated with predisposition to the development of JAK2(V617F)-positive myeloproliferative neoplasms. Nat Genet. 2009;41:455–9.

21. Olcaydu D, Harutyunyan A, Jager R, Berg T, Gisslinger B, Pabinger I, et al. A common JAK2 haplotype confers susceptibility to myeloproliferative neoplasms. Nat Genet. 2009;41:450–4.

22. Trifa AP, Cucuianu A, Petrov L, Urian L, Militaru MS, Dima D, et al. The G allele of the JAK2 rs10974944 SNP, part of JAK2 46/1 haplotype, is strongly associated with JAK2 V617F-positive myeloproliferative neoplasms. Ann Hematol. 2010;89:979–83.

23. Oddsson A, Kristinsson SY, Helgason H, Gudbjartsson DF, Masson G, Sigurdsson A, et al. The germline sequence variant rs2736100_C in TERT associates with myeloproliferative neoplasms. Leukemia. 2014;28:1371–4.

24. Saliba J, Saint-Martin C, Di Stefano A, Lenglet G, Marty C, Keren B, et al. Germline duplication of ATG2B and GSKIP predisposes to familial myeloid malignancies. Nat Genet. 2015;47:1131–40.

25. Harutyunyan AS, Giambruno R, Krendl C, Stukalov A, Klampfl T, Berg T, et al. Germline RBBP6 mutations in familial myeloproliferative neoplasms. Blood. 2016;127:362–5.

26. Mckenna A, Hanna M, Banks E, Sivachenko A, Cibulskis K, Kernytsky A, et al. The Genome Analysis Toolkit: a MapReduce framework for analyzing next-generation DNA sequencing data. Genome Res. 2010;20:1297–303.

27. Lek M, Karczewski KJ, Minikel EV, Samocha KE, Banks E, Fennell T, et al. Analysis of protein-coding genetic variation in 60,706 humans. Nature. 2016;536:285–91.

28. Adzhubei IA, Schmidt S, Peshkin L, Ramensky VE, Gerasimova A, Bork P, et al. A method and server for predicting damaging missense mutations. Nat Methods. 2010;7:248–9.

29. Kumar P, Henikoff S, Ng PC. Predicting the effects of coding non-synonymous variants on protein function using the SIFT algorithm. Nat Protoc. 2009;4:1073–81.

30. Li M, Collins R, Jiao Y, Ouillette P, Bixby D, Erba H, et al. Somatic mutations in the transcriptional corepressor gene BCORL1 in adult acute myelogenous leukemia. Blood. 2011;118:5914–7.

31. Tiacci E, Grossmann V, Martelli MP, Kohlmann A, Haferlach T, Falini B. The corepressors BCOR and BCORL1: two novel players in acute myeloid leukemia. Haematologica. 2012;97:3–5.

32. Rotunno G, Guglielmelli P, Biamonte F, Rumi E, Cazzola M, Vannucchi AM. Mutational analysis of BCORL1 in the leukemic transformation of chronic myeloproliferative neoplasms. Ann Hematol. 2014;93:523–4.

33. Al-Kandari W, Jambunathan S, Navalgund V, Koneni R, Freer M, Parimi N, et al. ZXDC, a novel zinc finger protein that binds CIITA and activates MHC gene transcription. Mol Immunol. 2007;44:311–21.

34. Al-Kandari W, Koneni R, Navalgund V, Aleksandrova A, Jambunathan S, Fontes JD. The zinc finger proteins ZXDA and ZXDC form a complex that binds CIITA and regulates MHC II gene transcription. J Mol Biol. 2007;369:1175–87.

35. Ramsey JE, Fontes JD. The zinc finger transcription factor ZXDC activates CCL2 gene expression by opposing BCL6-mediated repression. Mol Immunol. 2013;56:768–80.

36. Wang L, Tsai CC. Atrophin proteins: an overview of a new class of nuclear receptor corepressors. Nucl Recept Signal. 2008;6:e009.

37. Yazawa I, Nukina N, Hashida H, Goto J, Yamada M, Kanazawa I. Abnormal gene product identified in hereditary dentatorubral-pallidoluysian atrophy (DRPLA) brain. Nat Genet. 1995;10:99–103.

38. Wood JD, Nucifora Jr FC, Duan K, Zhang C, Wang J, Kim Y, et al. Atrophin-1, the dentato-rubral and pallido-luysian atrophy gene product, interacts with ETO/MTG8 in the nuclear matrix and represses transcription. J Cell Biol. 2000;150:939–48.

39. Butturini A, Gale RP, Verlander PC, Adler-Brecher B, Gillio AP, Auerbach AD. Hematologic abnormalities in Fanconi anemia: an International Fanconi Anemia Registry study. Blood. 1994;84:1650–5.

40. Wijker M, Morgan NV, Herterich S, Van Berkel CG, Tipping AJ, Gross HJ, et al. Heterogeneous spectrum of mutations in the Fanconi anaemia group A gene. Eur J Hum Genet. 1999;7:52–9.

15

A hypomorphic inherited pathogenic variant in *DDX3X* causes male intellectual disability with additional neurodevelopmental and neurodegenerative features

Georgios Kellaris[1,2], Kamal Khan[1,3], Shahid M. Baig[3], I-Chun Tsai[1], Francisca Millan Zamora[6], Paul Ruggieri[4], Marvin R. Natowicz[5] and Nicholas Katsanis[1,4*] (ID)

Abstract

Background: Intellectual disability (ID) is a common condition with a population prevalence frequency of 1–3% and an enrichment for males, driven in part by the contribution of mutant alleles on the X-chromosome. Among the more than 500 genes associated with ID, *DDX3X* represents an outlier in sex specificity. Nearly all reported pathogenic variants of *DDX3X* are de novo, affect mostly females, and appear to be loss of function variants, consistent with the hypothesis that haploinsufficiency at this locus on the X-chromosome is likely to be lethal in males.

Results: We evaluated two male siblings with syndromic features characterized by mild-to-moderate ID and progressive spasticity. Quad-based whole-exome sequencing revealed a maternally inherited missense variant encoding p.R79K in *DDX3X* in both siblings and no other apparent pathogenic variants. We assessed its possible relevance to their phenotype using an established functional assay for DDX3X activity in zebrafish embryos and found that this allele causes a partial loss of DDX3X function and thus represents a hypomorphic variant.

Conclusions: Our genetic and functional data suggest that partial loss of function of *DDX3X* can cause syndromic ID. The p.R79K allele affects a region of the protein outside the critical RNA helicase domain, offering a credible explanation for the observed retention of partial function, viability in hemizygous males, and lack of pathology in females. These findings expand the gender spectrum of pathology of this locus and suggest that analysis for *DDX3X* variants should be considered relevant for both males and females.

Background

Intellectual disability (ID) is a common (estimated prevalence of 1–3% [1–3]), clinically variable phenotype, defined by impairment in both intellectual function and adaptive behavior, with onset during the developmental period [4, 5]. ID is clinically and etiologically heterogeneous, with varying disability of the two aspects of the condition [6]. In addition, ID can occur as an isolated trait but is accompanied frequently by one or more comorbidities; these can include seizures or other neurological involvement [7], microcephaly or macrocephaly [8], dysmorphic features, and structural and/or functional abnormalities in organ systems other than the brain [9].

ID is more prevalent in males than females with a ratio of 1.3–1.4:1 [10], a gender bias partially reflective of the observation that numerous genes on the X-chromosome contribute to ID under an X-linked recessive paradigm [10]. Indeed, substantial gene discovery efforts have focused on male-enriched or male-specific cohorts as a means to accelerate the discovery of ID-associated genes and mutational mechanisms [10]. Genetic and genomic

* Correspondence: natowim@ccf.org; nicholas.katsanis@duke.edu
[1]Center for Human Disease Modeling, Duke University, 300 North Duke Street, Durham, NC 27701, USA
[4]Imaging Institute, Cleveland Clinic, 9500 Euclid Avenue, Cleveland, OH 44195, USA
Full list of author information is available at the end of the article

studies of individuals, families, and populations with ID have led to the identification of more than 500 mutated genes, with some estimates predicting that number to exceed 1000, possibly reflective of the large number of transcripts expressed in and necessary for the development and maintenance of the central nervous system [10, 11]. In several instances, female carriers are protected by virtue of functional mosaicism due to random X-inactivation or by X-inactivation that favors the wild-type allele [12]. Further phenotypic analyses have also led to the appreciation of subtle phenotypic defects under a dosage model, in which males manifest the extreme range of pathology and females are partially protected [13].

The *DDX3X* locus on Xp11.4 represents an exception to the male specificity paradigm. To date, *DDX3X* pathogenic variants have been reported in 35 females with ID [3, 14], all of which were de novo. As of September 2017, 52 cases have been deposited in Decipher: 49 females, all but one of whom have de novo alleles (the 50th was inherited from a mosaic father) and three males, two harbor de novo mutations and one whose mutation is of unknown origin [15]. Consistent with the intolerance of the locus to variation [3], there are no null alleles found in control populations of either gender and a concomitant depletion of missense variants as well [16].

Herein, we report our investigation of two adult male siblings with ID, born to parents of normal intelligence. Whole-exome sequencing (WES) identified a rare, non-synonymous, maternally transmitted variant in *DDX3X* as a likely driver of their phenotype. DDX3X is necessary for canonical *Wnt* signaling [17], an observation utilized previously to develop an in vivo ventralization assay in zebrafish embryos as a means to assess the pathogenic potential of alleles [3]. Using this assay, we found that the *DDX3X* variant results in reduced DDX3X function, reinforcing the genetic hypothesis. Together, our data support the notion that partial loss of function in *DDX3X* can lead to ID in males and reinforce a gradient of severity model that is dependent on the strength of the mutation as it pertains to residual protein function.

Materials and methods

Subjects

We studied a pedigree with two affected male siblings. Diagnostic testing of subjects was done as part of their clinical evaluations with informed consent from the mother and assent of the two cases. Research-based testing protocols were approved by the Cleveland Clinic Institutional Review Board.

Whole-exome sequencing

WES was carried out at GeneDx, Inc. subsequent to informed consent of the parents and assent of the affected individuals. Using genomic DNA from the ID cases and their parents, the exonic regions and flanking splice junctions of the genome were captured using the Clinical Research Exome kit (Agilent Technologies, Santa Clara, CA). Massively parallel (NextGen) sequencing was done on an Illumina system with 100 bp paired-end reads. The percent coverage at 10X or greater in the two brothers and their two parents ranged from 97.14 to 97.49%; the younger brother had 97.18% coverage that was at least 10X and the older brother had 97.49% coverage at least at 10X. The mean coverage in the younger brother was 132X and in the older brother 197X. The mean coverage in the father and the mother was 134.29X and 222.05X, respectively.

Data analysis

Reads were aligned to human genome build GRCh37/UCSC hg19 and were analyzed for sequence variants using a custom-developed analysis tool. Additional sequencing technology and variant interpretation protocols have been described [18]. The general assertion criteria for variant classification are available on the GeneDx ClinVar submission page (http://www.ncbi.nlm.nih.gov/clinvar/submitters/26957/). Variants of possible clinical significance relative to the phenotype of interest were confirmed by Sanger sequencing. Variants were named according to the following GenBank identifiers: *DDX3X* (NM_001356) and *SPG7* (NM_003119).

In vivo complementation studies in zebrafish

We obtained a plasmid containing the wild-type (wt) human open reading frame (ORF) of *DDX3X* and *WNT3A* from Ultimate ORF Collection (LifeTechnologies; clone ID *DDX3X*: IOH13891; *WNT3A*: IOH80731). Both plasmids were sequence-confirmed and cloned into the pCS2+ vector using Gateway LR clonase II-mediated recombination (LifeTechnologies) as described [19]. For *WNT3A*, a stop codon was introduced by site-directed mutagenesis using primer (5′-ctgcaaggccgccaggcacTAG GGTGGGCGCGCCGA-3′ and its reverse complement). To generate the mutant constructs for the ID-associated variant c.236 G>A (p.R79K) along with the positive control female variant c.641T>C (p.I214T) and a negative control male variant c.898G>T (p.V300F), we conducted site-directed mutagenesis using primers (c.641T>C: 5′-CTATTCCTATTACCAAAGAGAAAAG-3′, c.898G>T: 5′CTAGAGTTCGTCCTTGCGTGTTT TATGGTGGTGCCGATATT-3′, and c.236 G>A G: 5′-TTGGATCTCGTAGTGATTCAAAAGGGAAGTCTAG CTTC-3′ and their reverse complements). We then generated capped mRNA from linearized wt-*DDX3X* and *WNT3A* pCS2+ constructs as well as for *DDX3X* variants with the mMessage mMachine SP6 kit (ThermoFisher). Injections were conducted with wt (ZDR) embryos, and resulting embryos were phenotyped at 48 hpf for eye phenotypes according to established criteria (class I: hypoplasia of the eye and class II: absence of one or both eyes; [3]. The mRNAs (wt-*WNT3A*, wt-*DDX3X*, and *DDX3X* variants) were injected in the yolk of the embryos at 1–4 cell stage as described [20]. We acquired lateral and dorsal images with an AZ100 florescent microscope (Nikon), digital sight black and white camera (Nikon), and NIS Elements software (Nikon) at ×4 magnification. We determined statistical differences between pairs of batches with an unpaired *t* test.

Results

Clinical evaluations

We evaluated two affected male siblings from a non-consanguineous family (Fig. 1; Table 1; for full clinical descriptions, see Additional file 1). The eldest affected, currently 29 years old, was diagnosed with ID, macrocephaly, dysarthria, progressive spastic paraparesis, and decreased lower extremity strength. He presented for clinical evaluation at 2 years of age; he had reduced speech output for age and was easily agitated and hyperactive. He walked at 15 months, said his first words at 1–2 years, talked in sentences at 3–4 years, and was toilet-trained at 3 years. Developmental assessment at 6.5 years showed nonverbal cognitive function and composite mental processing at 5 and 3 percentiles, respectively, and adaptive behavior functions ranging from 0.3 to 3%. At age 9.5 years, he showed verbal, performance, and full-scale IQ scores of 71, 80, and 73, respectively. Assessment of communication function showed receptive and expressive language function at about 0.5 and 0.04 percentiles, while adaptive behavior assessment showed communication, daily living, and socialization functions at 1, 2, and 10 percentiles, respectively.

At 14 years of age, he developed a stiff gait. Exam at 15 years showed an acquired macrocephaly, an asymmetric spastic gait, lower extremity hyperreflexia, and tight heel cords. He began treatment with oral baclofen for spasticity at 17 years of age. He had an adjusted curriculum during high school, graduated at 19 years, and has worked part-time afterwards in a supported workplace. His gait slowly worsened and he was last able to ambulate independently at 21 years. On neurological exam at 23 years, there was a slow, spastic gait, decreased lower extremity strength, especially with hip flexion, markedly increased the tone of the lower extremities, lower extremity hyperreflexia, and slowed fine finger and rapid alternating movements. At 29 years of age, he has progressive lower extremity and hand weakness and decreased fine motor function.

Brain MRI scan at 16 years of age (Fig. 1i) showed mildly prominent lateral ventricles and cortical sulci,

atrophy of the entire corpus callosum that was accentuated in the anterior body and genu, and mild, symmetric, confluent T2-hyperintensity in the supratentorial periventricular white matter. The follow-up study 2 years later demonstrated further interval enlargement of the lateral ventricles and periventricular white matter T2-hyperintensity, suggesting progression of central white matter volume loss. Myelination was otherwise within normal limits (Fig. 1ii). Cerebrospinal fluid analyses at 19 years showed a normal cell count, CSF glucose, and protein levels and normal CSF IgG synthesis and index. Metabolic testing included increased CSF alanine and intermittent mildly increased urinary lactate (Additional file 2: Table S1).

The younger affected brother, 25 years old, has progressive spastic paraparesis and tremor and learning disability/mixed expressive-receptive language disorder (Fig. 1; Table 1). The first concern about his neurodevelopmental status was when he was about 2 years old and had mildly delayed speech development; he spoke in sentences at 3 years and began speech therapy at that time. He developed an intentional hand tremor at about 6 years that worsened over time. Developmental assessment at 5.6 years showed normal development in all areas except for mild receptive and expressive language delay. Re-evaluation at 6 years showed receptive and expressive language skills at 39 and 16 percentiles, with weaknesses in auditory memory, interpreting directions, and categorizing words. Assessment at 7 years showed verbal, performance, and full-scale IQ scores of 84, 81, and 81, respectively. Academic achievement testing showed basic reading, reading comprehension, mathematics calculation, mathematics reasoning, and written expression at 1, 5, 16, 9, and 23 percentiles, respectively; receptive and expressive language tested at 37 and 16 percentiles. He did not have significant behavioral issues.

Examination at 15 years old, for worsening hand tremors, showed a non-dysmorphic male with lower extremity hyperreflexia and tremor; the gait and motor tone were normal. At 17 years, he was noted to have a mild spastic gait and bilateral Babinski signs. At 18 years, he was noted to have a worsening asymmetric spastic paretic gait and bilateral hip flexor weakness. Schooling involved an adjusted curriculum with training in service occupations, and he graduated from high school at 18 years of age, subsequently working part-time and requiring supports in complex daily living tasks.

His diagnostic evaluation included an abnormal brain MRI scans at 15, 16, and 17 years of age showing mild, diffuse prominence of the cortical sulci suggesting mild cortical volume loss and mild enlargement of the lateral ventricles, generalized volume loss in the corpus callosum that was more prominent in the genu and anterior body, and mild symmetric confluent periventricular T2-

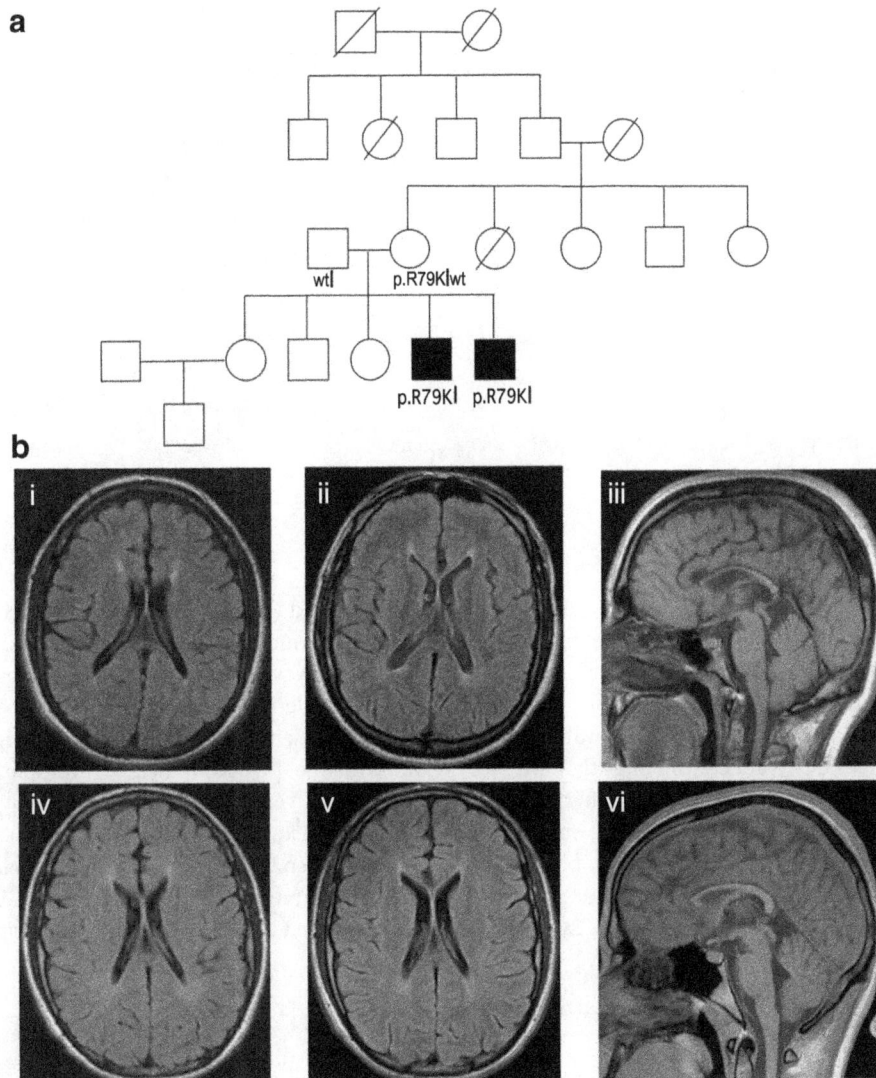

Fig. 1 Brain MRI of both affected syndromic ID cases. **a** Family pedigree showing the two affected brothers and the family pedigree. **b** (i) Axial T2 FLAIR of sibling 1 at age 16 demonstrates mild enlargement of the lateral ventricles and mild confluent hyperintensity in the adjacent white matter. (ii) Axial T2 FLAIR of sibling 1 2 years later demonstrates interval enlargement of the lateral ventricles and mild progression of the confluent hyperintensity in the adjacent white matter suggesting progressive damage to the central white matter and volume loss. (iii) Sagittal T1 demonstrates generalized volume loss in the corpus callosum that is more prominent in the genu and anterior body, further supporting central white matter volume loss that is more severe anteriorly. (iv) Axial T2 FLAIR of sibling 2 at age 15 demonstrates mild enlargement of the lateral ventricles and mild, symmetric hyperintensity in the adjacent white matter, suggesting central white matter volume loss and gliosis. (v) Axial T2 FLAIR of sibling 2 2 years later demonstrates mild interval increase in size of the lateral ventricles suggesting mild progression of central white matter volume loss, but no significant change in the periventricular hyperintensity. (vi) Sagittal T1 image is also comparable in appearance to his sibling, with prominent volume loss in the corpus callosum that is more striking anteriorly

hyperintensity within the supratentorial periventricular white matter suggesting central white matter volume loss that was more prominent in the frontal lobes (Fig. 1iv–vi). There was also slight further enlargement of the lateral ventricles without significant change in the T2-hyperintensity or the corpus callosum over the 2-year period. The MRI of the entire spinal cord was normal in caliber and signal intensity. CSF analyses showed normal cellular CSF and normal levels of CSF glucose and protein, normal CSF IgG synthesis and IgG index, normal levels of CSF lactate and pyruvate, and increased CSF alanine. Plasma amino acid analyses consistently showed mildly moderately increased levels of alanine and, sometimes, increased levels of proline and glycine (Additional file 2: Table S1).

Genomic analysis

A host of known genetic and metabolic etiologies of ID and of spasticity were ruled-out in the two cases

Table 1 Summary of clinical findings in the two subjects. Human phenotype ontology (HPO) terms and codes are shown

Phenotype	HPO code	Case 1	Case 2
Intellectual disability or related neurodevelopmental disability	HP:0001256	+	+
Macrocephaly	HP:0000256	+	+
Dysarthria	HP:0001260	+	+
Tight heel cords		+	+
Progressive spastic paraparesis	HP:0007199	+	+
Tremor	HP:0002322	–	+
Hand weakness	HP:0030237	+	–
Proximal leg weakness	HP:0007340	+	+
Brain MRI with abnormal periventricular T2 intensity	HP:0002518	+	+
Ventriculomegaly	HP:0002119	+	+
Atrophy of corpus callosum, esp. the genu and anterior body of corpus callosum	HP:0006989	+	+
Increased cerebrospinal fluid alanine level	n/a	+	+

n/a not applicable

(Additional file 2: Table S1). Consequently, given that both parents are of normal intelligence, we undertook quad-based WES analysis hypothesizing either a recessive or an X-linked paradigm of disease inheritance. Under a rare variant hypothesis, the WES data were evaluated for alleles shared among the two affected siblings that are rare (minor allele frequency < 1%) and affect coding residues or canonical splice sites. We identified several variants of potential interest (Additional file 3: Table S2), but only a single, maternally inherited variant fulfilled our stringent criteria: a c.236G>A change encoding p.R79K in *DDX3X*

was identified (Fig. 2a, b). The *DDX3X* locus has been implicated previously in ID and, sometimes, other features in females; however, nearly all published variants described to date are de novo, which has led to the hypothesis that haploinsufficiency of *DDX3X* in males might be incompatible with life [3]. Nonetheless, multiple sequence alignment across vertebrates showed the p.R79 position to be conserved (Fig. 2b). Prediction algorithms were discordant: PolyPhen2 [21] predicted the allele to be benign, whereas MutationTaster [22] predicted it to be deleterious. Overall, 11 variant prediction algorithms predict this

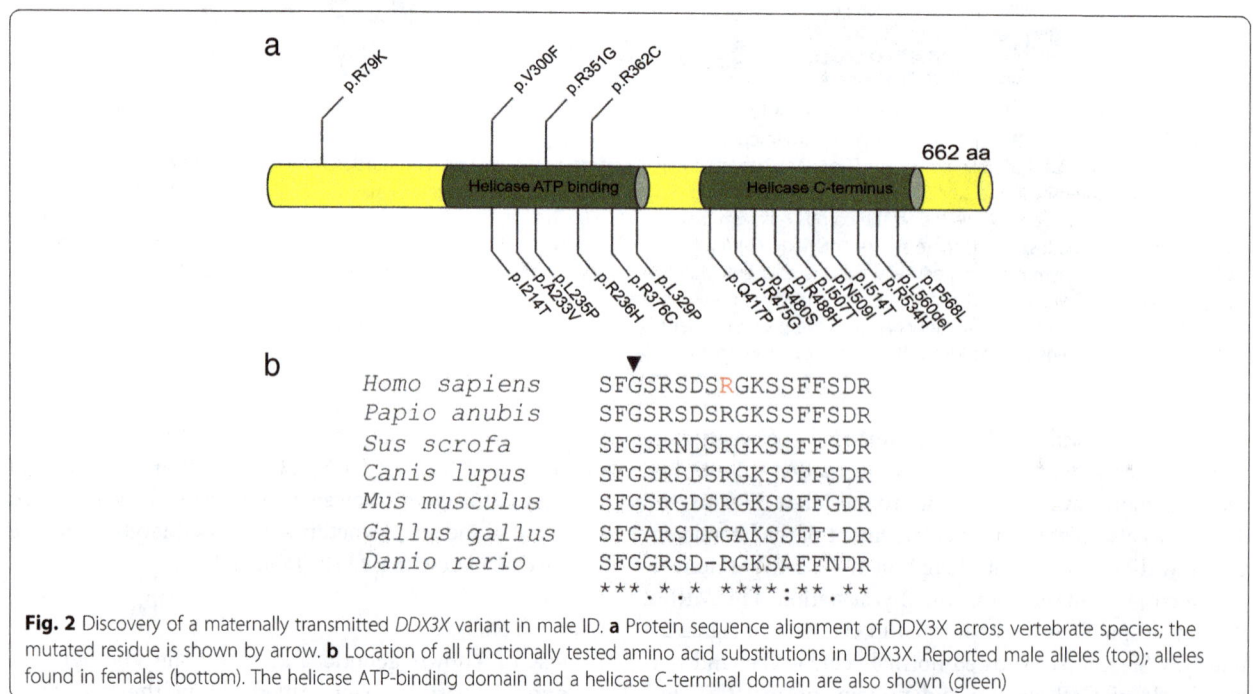

Fig. 2 Discovery of a maternally transmitted *DDX3X* variant in male ID. **a** Protein sequence alignment of DDX3X across vertebrate species; the mutated residue is shown by arrow. **b** Location of all functionally tested amino acid substitutions in DDX3X. Reported male alleles (top); alleles found in females (bottom). The helicase ATP-binding domain and a helicase C-terminal domain are also shown (green)

variant to be damaging to the structure/function of DDX3X out of a total of 21 in silico assessments [23], http://159.226.67.237/sun/varcards/welcome/index). The variant was found only once in heterozygosity, in a female, in > 170,000 control exomes [16]. We note that, in contrast to the majority of described DDX3X variants that lie in the helicase domain, the p.R79K variant maps proximal to that region (Fig. 2b). Together, these data raised the hypothesis that, in contrast to previously reported alleles in DDX3X that abrogate protein function, p.R79K might be a hypomorph, which could explain its transmission and the phenotypic outcome in this kindred.

Functional testing

We and others have shown that expression of human DDX3X mRNA exacerbates the ventralization phenotype induced by the expression of femtogram (fg) quantities of the canonical Wnt ligand WNT3A in zebrafish embryos [3]. This phenotype can be binned into two phenotypic classes (class I and class II; Fig. 3a–c) based on previously established and validated morphometric criteria [24]. Using this model system, we tested the functionality of missense DDX3X alleles discovered in ID patients and found that DNA sequence variants predicted to cause loss of function of DDX3X and which were associated with ID failed to exacerbate WNT3A-driven pathology, whereas benign alleles were indistinguishable in their activity and promoted significant Wnt-dependent pathology [3]. Here, we utilized this assay to test the activity of the p.R79K allele. First, we optimized the in vivo complementation assays to the ZDR wt genetic background by injecting progressively increasing doses of wt-WNT3A; we found that 550 fg of mRNA was sufficient to induce a modest phenotype ($\sim$ 8–15% affected embryos, n = 50–100 embryos per clutch, replicated; Fig. 3, Additional file 4: Figure S1, Additional file 5: Figure S2A). On this background sensitization with WNT3A, we titrated the amount of human DDX3X mRNA required to generate pathology. We found a dose-dependent effect that was maximal at 30 pg mRNA (Additional file 4: Figure S1). Therefore, we selected the 500 fg/30 pg mRNA doses to test the effect of the discovered allele. Next, we co-injected WNT3A-sensitized ZDR embryos with wt DDX3X, DDX3X encoding the candidate pathogenic allele p.R79K, the known benign allele p.V300F, and the known pathogenic allele p.I214T. Upon blind scoring to injection cocktail, both the positive and negative controls scored as expected: mRNA encoding p.300F was indistinguishable from wt, whereas p.214T failed to induce any significant pathology exceeding that of WNT3A alone, consistent with a null (or near null) allele. The candidate mutation of interest, p.R79K, scored intermediate, with the extent of pathology of the resulting embryos significantly different from both wt and null DDX3X (p < 0.0008 and p < 0.01 respectively; Fig. 3d). In contrast, expression of either wt or mutant DDX3X mRNA alone did not induce any appreciable pathologies, likely excluding any dominant negative mechanisms (Additional file 5: Figure S2B). Together with the human genetics and evolutionary conservation, these data suggest that the discovered allele is a likely hypomorph.

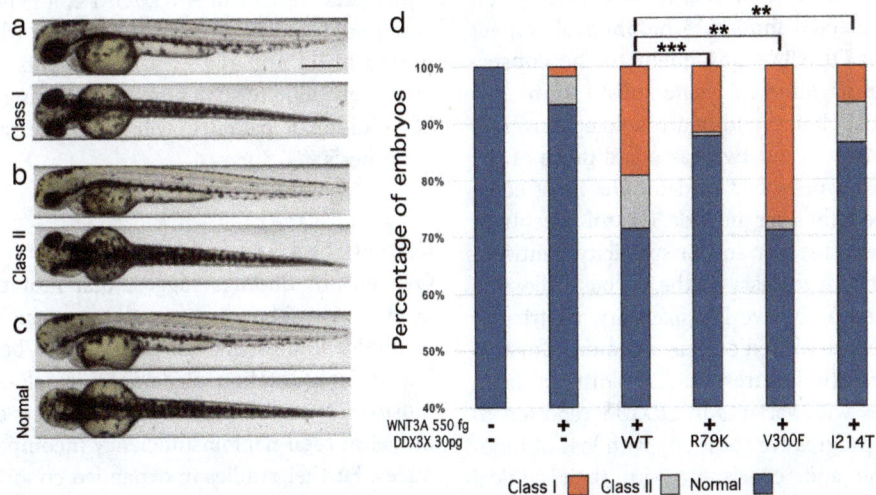

Fig. 3 Functional testing of DDX3X variants. **a–c** Representative lateral images of zebrafish embryos at 2 dpf that are either uninjected (**a**) or injected with human WNT3A without (**b**) or with (**c**) human DDX3X show a range of ventralized phenotypes. These were scored according to established criteria as normal, class I, or class II ventralization. No injection condition resulted in severe ventralization (class III or IV) [3]. **d** DDX3X variants were tested for their effect on increasing WNT3A-mediated ventralization using 550 fg of WNT3A mRNA and 30 pg of DDX3X mRNA per embryo. P values: < 0.0001 (four asterisks); 0.0001 to 0.001 (three asterisks); 0.001 to 0.01 (two asterisks); 0.01 to 0.05 (one asterisk); ≥ 0.05 not significant (ns)

Discussion

Here, we describe the clinical phenotypes of two adult males who have a rare, maternally inherited missense allele of DDX3X, a major ID locus that to date has been associated with pathology almost exclusively in females. Both genetics and functional testing support a partial loss of function disease transmission. This notion is consistent with the observation that the mother who transmitted the p.R79K is asymptomatic and that the two affected males have significant neurodevelopmental pathology but have survived. Although the formal possibility remains that the mother might exhibit sub-clinical neuroanatomical findings, careful re-examination revealed no overt neurological concerns. In addition to this notion, it would be important to identify the genotype for the maternal uncle and maternal grandfather, but DNA samples from the individuals were not available. This hypothesis is also supported by recent work in the mouse revealing essential roles of Ddx3x in placentation and embryogenesis and the differential phenotypic impacts of inheriting a paternal vs. maternal null allele [25]. Non-lethality of the p.R79K variant in our cases may be due to the maternal, as opposed to paternal, inheritance of the variant. Non-lethality of the p.R79K variant might also be because the location of the amino acid substitution is outside of the critical RNA helicase domain. The DDX3X protein has been investigated extensively [26], but the region of the protein surrounding amino acid residue 79 has only been studied sparingly, although site-directed mutagenesis of several nearby residues resulted in functional impacts [27, 28]. Finally, non-lethality of the p.R79K variant might be explained on the basis of the expected moderate biophysical impact on the structure of DDX3X consequent to the conservative nature of an arginine to lysine substitution.

There is substantial clinical and neuroradiologic overlap between the phenotype in our two cases and those of the females and few males described to date. The most common traits described thus far include ID, microcephaly, hypotonia, movement disorder and/or spasticity, ventricular enlargement, and hypoplasia of the corpus callosum; the subjects reported here have ID, spasticity, ventricular enlargement, and an attenuated corpus callosum. Our two cases also present with features that are distinct from those of other cases with variants in DDX3X reported to date; these include progressive spasticity with loss of independent ambulation and, consistent with their clinical courses, evidence of a progressive brain central white matter process including atrophy of the corpus callosum, not hypoplasia. Long-term follow-up of the previously reported cases, some of whom were young children, will be important to determine if any of the neurological findings or developmental disabilities are progressive and if there are ongoing brain white matter changes.

It is also possible that a second clinical process that is distinct from DDX3X may be present in the two subjects reported here. In this regard, both subjects have macrocephaly, as does their father and one sister although the father and the subjects' siblings have clinical phenotypes that are otherwise disparate from the clinical findings in the cases with ID. The finding of increased levels of CSF alanine in both cases and of increased plasma alanine in one case and increased urinary lactate in the other is notable and suggests a disturbance of mitochondrial bioenergetics. No evidence of a primary mitochondrial cytopathy was found, despite considerable investigation, and the relationship of these results to the variant of DDX3X is uncertain. In addition, the existence of a clinical process that is/was present in only one of the subjects is likely in view of the variability in neurodevelopmental phenotype between the subjects, although the basis of this process is unknown. Given the reported spasticity in this pedigree, we did evaluate known spastic paraplegia genes for candidate pathogenic variants. We detected a maternally inherited heterozygous variant in SPG7 in one of the subjects that has been reported to be pathogenic in patients with recessive spastic paraplegia [29]. Although this allele is by itself unable to explain the observed spasticity in our patient, it is possible that it contributes to the phenotype, possibly in epistasis with DDX3X; the same might be true for some of the other ultra-rare alleles discovered in this family (Additional file 3: Table S2). For example, it is intriguing that the older brother with the more extensive pathology is also hemizygous for candidate pathogenic variant in ARGHGAP4, a gene whose product is required for neuronal migration and which has been reported to be mutated in some patients with ID [30–32]. However, both formal functional testing and delineation of additional patients will be necessary to test this hypothesis.

Conclusions

Overall, our findings suggest that mutational analysis of DDX3X in either genetic testing panels or by whole-exome/genome sequencing should not be limited, by testing or interpretation of data, to females. The severity of most discovered DDX3X alleles remains consistent with a model of total haploinsufficiency incompatible with life in males. Further studies in expanded cohorts will illuminate this proposed phenotype-genotype correlation further.

Acknowledgements
We thank the family for the participation and encouragement of this work. We thank Erica Davis for the critical evaluation of the manuscript and data.

Funding
NK is a Brumley Distinguished Professor of Pediatrics. The study was supported by Core Funding from the Center for Human Disease Modeling at Duke University.

Authors' contributions
GK and KK performed experiments, reviewed and compiled data, and co-wrote the paper. SMB and ICT and NK reviewed and interpreted the data and provided guidance to the work. MRN assessed the family, reviewed and interpreted the WES data, and co-wrote the manuscript. FMZ reviewed and interpreted WES. PR reviewed the brain MRIs. All authors reviewed and commented on the manuscript. All authors read and approved the final manuscript.

Competing interests
NK is a paid consultant and holds founding stock in Rescindo Therapeutics.

Author details
[1]Center for Human Disease Modeling, Duke University, 300 North Duke Street, Durham, NC 27701, USA. [2]Department of Medical Genetics, University of Athens Medical School, Aghia Sophia Children's Hospital, 11527 Athens, Greece. [3]Human Molecular Genetics Laboratory, Health Biotechnology Division, National Institute for Biotechnology and Genetic Engineering (NIBGE), Faisalabad 38000, Pakistan. [4]Imaging Institute, Cleveland Clinic, 9500 Euclid Avenue, Cleveland, OH 44195, USA. [5]Pathology and Laboratory Medicine and Genomic Medicine Institutes, Cleveland Clinic, Cleveland, OH 44195, USA. [6]GeneDx, 207 Perry Parkway, Gaithersburg, MD 20877, USA.

References

1. Wolfe K, Stueber K, McQuillin A, Jichi F, Patch C, Flinter F, Strydom A, Bass N. Genetic testing in intellectual disability psychiatry: opinions and practices of UK child and intellectual disability psychiatrists. J Appl Res Intellect Disabil. 2017;31(2):273-84.
2. van Bokhoven H. Genetic and epigenetic networks in intellectual disabilities. Annu Rev Genet. 2011;45:81–104.
3. Snijders Blok L, Madsen E, Juusola J, Gilissen C, Baralle D, Reijnders MR, Venselaar H, Helsmoortel C, Cho MT, Hoischen A, et al. Mutations in DDX3X are a common cause of unexplained intellectual disability with gender-specific effects on Wnt signaling. Am J Hum Genet. 2015;97(2):343–52.
4. Harris JC. Intellectual disability: Understanding its development, causes, classification, evaluation, and treatment. New York: Oxford University Press; 2006.
5. Tasse MJ, Luckasson R, Nygren M. AAIDD proposed recommendations for ICD-11 and the condition previously known as mental retardation. Intellect Dev Disabil. 2013;51(2):127–31.
6. American Psychiatric Association. Diagnostic and statistical manual of mental disorders : DSM-5: Fifth edition. Arlington: American Psychiatric Publishing; 2013.
7. McGrother CW, Bhaumik S, Thorp CF, Hauck A, Branford D, Watson JM. Epilepsy in adults with intellectual disabilities: prevalence, associations and service implications. Seizure. 2006;15(6):376–86.
8. de Ligt J, Willemsen MH, van Bon BW, Kleefstra T, Yntema HG, Kroes T, Vulto-van Silfhout AT, Koolen DA, de Vries P, Gilissen C, et al. Diagnostic exome sequencing in persons with severe intellectual disability. N Engl J Med. 2012;367(20):1921–9.
9. Matson JL, Cervantes PE. Comorbidity among persons with intellectual disabilities. Res Autism Spectr Disord. 2013;7(11):1318–22.
10. Vissers LE, Gilissen C, Veltman JA. Genetic studies in intellectual disability and related disorders. Nat Rev Genet. 2016;17(1):9–18.
11. Kochinke K, Zweier C, Nijhof B, Fenckova M, Cizek P, Honti F, Keerthikumar S, Oortveld MA, Kleefstra T, Kramer JM, et al. Systematic phenomics analysis deconvolutes genes mutated in intellectual disability into biologically coherent modules. Am J Hum Genet. 2016;98(1):149–64.
12. Cotton AM, Price EM, Jones MJ, Balaton BP, Kobor MS, Brown CJ. Landscape of DNA methylation on the X chromosome reflects CpG density, functional chromatin state and X-chromosome inactivation. Hum Mol Genet. 2015;24(6):1528–39.
13. Fieremans N, Van Esch H, Holvoet M, Van Goethem G, Devriendt K, Rosello M, Mayo S, Martinez F, Jhangiani S, Muzny DM, et al. Identification of intellectual disability genes in female patients with a skewed X-inactivation pattern. Hum Mutat. 2016;37(8):804–11.
14. Dikow N, Granzow M, Graul-Neumann LM, Karch S, Hinderhofer K, Paramasivam N, Behl LJ, Kaufmann L, Fischer C, Evers C, et al. DDX3X mutations in two girls with a phenotype overlapping Toriello-Carey syndrome. Am J Med Genet A. 2017;173(5):1369–73.
15. Firth HV, Richards SM, Bevan AP, Clayton S, Corpas M, Rajan D, Vooren SV, Moreau Y, Pettett RM, Carter NP. DECIPHER: database of chromosomal imbalance and phenotype in humans using ensembl resources. Am J Hum Genet. 2009;84(4):524–33.
16. Lek M, Karczewski KJ, Minikel EV, Samocha KE, Banks E, Fennell T, O'Donnell-Luria AH, Ware JS, Hill AJ, Cummings BB, et al. Analysis of protein-coding genetic variation in 60,706 humans. Nature. 2016;536:285.
17. Cruciat CM, Dolde C, de Groot RE, Ohkawara B, Reinhard C, Korswagen HC, Niehrs C. RNA helicase DDX3 is a regulatory subunit of casein kinase 1 in Wnt-beta-catenin signaling. Science. 2013;339(6126):1436–41.
18. Tanaka AJ, Cho MT, Millan F, Juusola J, Retterer K, Joshi C, Niyazov D, Garnica A, Gratz E, Deardorff M, et al. Mutations in SPATA5 are associated with microcephaly, intellectual disability, seizures, and hearing loss. Am J Hum Genet. 2015;97(3):457–64.
19. Niederriter AR, Davis EE, Golzio C, Oh EC, Tsai IC, Katsanis N. In vivo modeling of the morbid human genome using Danio rerio. J Vis Exp. 2013;78:e50338.
20. Davis EE, Frangakis S, Katsanis N. Interpreting human genetic variation with in vivo zebrafish assays. Biochim Biophys Acta. 2014;1842(10):1960–70.
21. Adzhubei IA, Schmidt S, Peshkin L, Ramensky VE, Gerasimova A, Bork P, Kondrashov AS, Sunyaev SR: A method and server for predicting damaging missense mutations. In: Nat Methods. 2010;7:248–9.
22. Schwarz JM, Cooper DN, Schuelke M, Seelow D. MutationTaster2: mutation prediction for the deep-sequencing age. Nat Methods. 2014;11:361.
23. Li M, Gong L, Zhao D, Zhou J, Xiang H. The spacer size of I-B CRISPR is modulated by the terminal sequence of the protospacer. Nucleic Acids Res. 2017;45(8):4642–54.
24. Liu YP, Tsai IC, Morleo M, Oh EC, Leitch CC, Massa F, Lee BH, Parker DS, Finley D, Zaghloul NA, et al. Ciliopathy proteins regulate paracrine signaling by modulating proteasomal degradation of mediators. J Clin Invest. 2014;124(5):2059–70.
25. Chen C-Y, Chan C-H, Chen C-M, Tsai Y-S, Tsai T-Y, Wu Lee Y-H, You L-R. Targeted inactivation of murine Ddx3x: essential roles of Ddx3x in placentation and embryogenesis. Hum Mol Genet. 2016;25(14):2905–22.
26. Sharma D, Jankowsky E. The Ded1/DDX3 subfamily of DEAD-box RNA helicases. Crit Rev Biochem Mol Biol. 2014;49(4):343–60.
27. Gu L, Fullam A, Brennan R, Schroder M. Human DEAD box helicase 3 couples IkappaB kinase epsilon to interferon regulatory factor 3 activation. Mol Cell Biol. 2013;33(10):2004–15.
28. Oda S, Schroder M, Khan AR. Structural basis for targeting of human RNA helicase DDX3 by poxvirus protein K7. Structure. 2009;17(11):1528–37.
29. Elleuch N, Depienne C, Benomar A, Hernandez AM, Ferrer X, Fontaine B, Grid D, Tallaksen CM, Zemmouri R, Stevanin G, et al. Mutation analysis of the paraplegin gene (SPG7) in patients with hereditary spastic paraplegia. Neurology. 2006;66(5):654–9.
30. Vogt DL, Gray CD, Young WS 3rd, Orellana SA, Malouf AT. ARHGAP4 is anovel RhoGAP that mediates inhibiton of cell motility and axonal outgrowth. Mol Cell Neurosci. 2007;36(3):332–42.
31. Liu F, Guo H, Ou M, Hou X, Sun G, Gong W, Jing H, Tan Q, Xue W, Dai Y, Sui W. ARHGAP4 mutated in a Chinese intellectually challenged family. Gene. 2016;578(2):205–9.
32. Huang L, Poke G, Gecz J, Gibson K. A novel contiguous gene deletion of AVPR2 and ARHGAP4 genes in male dizygotic twins with nephrogenic diabetes insipidus and intellectual disability. Am J Med Genet A. 2012;158a(10):2511–8.

16

Variant effect prediction tools assessed using independent, functional assay-based datasets: implications for discovery and diagnostics

Khalid Mahmood, Chol-hee Jung, Gayle Philip, Peter Georgeson, Jessica Chung, Bernard J. Pope and Daniel J. Park*ⓘ

Abstract

Background: Genetic variant effect prediction algorithms are used extensively in clinical genomics and research to determine the likely consequences of amino acid substitutions on protein function. It is vital that we better understand their accuracies and limitations because published performance metrics are confounded by serious problems of circularity and error propagation. Here, we derive three independent, functionally determined human mutation datasets, UniFun, BRCA1-DMS and TP53-TA, and employ them, alongside previously described datasets, to assess the pre-eminent variant effect prediction tools.

Results: Apparent accuracies of variant effect prediction tools were influenced significantly by the benchmarking dataset. Benchmarking with the assay-determined datasets UniFun and BRCA1-DMS yielded areas under the receiver operating characteristic curves in the modest ranges of 0.52 to 0.63 and 0.54 to 0.75, respectively, considerably lower than observed for other, potentially more conflicted datasets.

Conclusions: These results raise concerns about how such algorithms should be employed, particularly in a clinical setting. Contemporary variant effect prediction tools are unlikely to be as accurate at the general prediction of functional impacts on proteins as reported prior. Use of functional assay-based datasets that avoid prior dependencies promises to be valuable for the ongoing development and accurate benchmarking of such tools.

Keywords: Variant effect prediction, Functional datasets, Benchmarking, Mutation assessment, Pathogenicity prediction, Protein function, Functional assays, Genomic screening

Background

Screening the entire protein-coding compartment of the human genome yields thousands of protein amino acid substitutions per individual, the majority of which are present at low frequencies (minor allele frequency (MAF) <0.1%) within the population [1]. Genetic screens typically seek to classify variants and genes of relevance to given phenotypes, including disease states. To this end, it is desirable to know whether a given variant is likely to impact protein function, with the inference being that this might influence phenotypes of interest [2–5]. However, appropriate functional assays exist for only a minority of proteins, and in those cases where functional assays do

* Correspondence: djp@unimelb.edu.au
Melbourne Bioinformatics, The University of Melbourne, Melbourne, Australia

exist, their associated resource requirements are often prohibitive to routine, large-scale application.

Widely used variant effect prediction methods include SIFT [6, 7], PolyPhen (v2) [8, 9], GERP++ [10, 11], Condel [12], CADD [13], fathmm [14], MutationTaster [15], MutationAssessor [16, 17], GESPA [18] and, more recently, REVEL [19]. These use information, variously, about local sequence phylogenetic conservation, amino acid physicochemical properties, functional domains and structural attributes (Table 1). Ensemble or consensus methods such as fathmm, Condel, CADD and REVEL integrate and weight predictions from collections of tools. Recent approaches to algorithm training have applied machine learning techniques. Training and validation (or 'benchmarking') of these algorithms

Variant effect prediction tools assessed using independent, functional assay-based...

171

Table 1 Characteristics of the protein variant effect prediction tools assessed in this study. The table indicates their scoring ranges and thresholds, training data, summary information about features and, where applicable, machine learning method

Prediction tool	Score range	Deleterious score cutoff	Training data	Features	Machine learning method
GERP++	−12.0 to 6.17	>0.047	None	Infers conserved or constrained elements from 33 mammalian genomes	–
fitCons	0 to 1	>0.4	None	Functional genomics data mainly sourced from chromatin analysis, e.g. ChIP-seq, and evolutionary conservation data	–
SIFT	1 to 0	<0.05	None	Conservation data (MSA of homologous sequences) and transformed into normalised probability matrix	–
PolyPhen	0 to 1	>0.5	HumVar, HumDiv	Conservation data (MSA of homologous sequences), protein functional domain data and protein structural features	Naïve Bayes classifier
CADD	0 to 35 +	>15	Simulated, Swissvar, HumVar	Integrates several annotations into a single score, e.g. SIFT, GERP++, PolyPhen, CPG distance, GC content	SVM
Condel	0 to 1	>0.5		Builds a unified classification by integration output from a collection of tools, e.g. SIFT, PolyPhen	Weighted average normalised scores
REVEL	0 to 1	>0.5	HGMD, EPS	HGMD and rare EPS variants used for training	Random forest
fathmm	0 to 1	>0.45	HGMD, Swiss-Prot	Combines evolutionary conservation with disease-specific protein weights for intolerance to mutation	Hidden Markov models

has been conducted using datasets that list variants with assigned classifications. Commonly used datasets include HumDiv [20], HumVar [21], Humsavar [22], EPS [23], dbSNP [24] and HGMD [25].

All of the above algorithms have reported potential merit and are widely used in practice. The original publication of REVEL, for example, reported that when this tool was tested against a set of variants from Clinvar, the resulting area under the receiver operating characteristic curve was an impressive 0.96. However, fundamental problems exist with the manner of the training and benchmarking for this and prior tools, centred primarily on the independence and truthfulness of reference sets. Indeed, the authors of REVEL acknowledged that these issues placed potential limitations on their study.

Grimm et al. [20] described the issue of data circularity and its effect on the assessment of prediction algorithms, explaining the importance of the choice and composition of variant datasets used for training and validation. Type 1 circularity results from substantial overlap between training and testing datasets, leading to artificially inflated apparent accuracy in contexts where variants or genes are well represented in training data and to deflated apparent accuracy in settings where they are poorly represented. Type 2 circularity results from all variants in featured genes having been labelled predominantly as either deleterious or benign. Grimm et al. postulated a third type of circularity. In this case, prediction tools contribute to new variant classifications, which, in turn, are used in further benchmarking. Variant classifications within training and benchmarking datasets have been guided substantially by computational predictions, resulting in imperfect 'truth sets'. Disease risk inflation has been observed in the Clinvar and HumVar

databases, whereby considerably fewer individuals in the general population are afflicted with given diseases than would be expected based on pathogenicity classifications within these clinical databases [1]. Ideally, mutation effect prediction training data for supervised machine learning methods should have good coverage of the protein landscape and mutation categorisation that is based on strong evidence from protein functional studies [26]. Miosge et al. [27] reported that of all the amino acid-substituting mutations predicted by PolyPhen to be deleterious to the mouse form of the key tumour suppressor, TP53, 42% had no assay-detectable functional consequence. Similarly, 45% of CADD-predicted deleterious mutations conferred no assay-detectable impact on protein function.

In this study, we conduct benchmarking of eight computational variant impact prediction methods. In addition to assessing their performance using commonly used benchmarking variant datasets, we have derived three independent, functional assay-determined datasets that we have called UniFun (UniProt-derived, functionally characterised, based on UniProt mutagenesis data), BRCA1-DMS (based on deep mutational scanning of BRCA1) and TP53-TA (TP53 mutational scanning via transactivation assay). Our findings have important implications with regard to our confidence in variant classifications derived from computational prediction methods and to how we should train and benchmark such methods in the future.

Results

In order to limit problems of circularity and systematic error, we derived three human protein mutation datasets that strive for independence from training data and are characterised by direct functional assays: UniFun, BRCA1-DMS and TP53-TA. UniFun represents 11,519 mutations from UniProt for which categorical assignments of protein functional consequence have been made based on direct assays ('Datasets and methods'). The UniFun variants were sourced from 2209 proteins and exhibit minimal overlap with variants featured in prior disease catalogue datasets (Fig. 1). UniFun is composed of a relatively high percentage of proteins that contribute both deleterious and benign mutations (Additional file 1: Figure S1). BRCA1-DMS (BRCA1 deep mutational scanning) was generated from measured efficiencies of BRCA1 mutants in activities required for efficient homology-directed DNA repair (HDR) and tumour suppression [28]. TP53-TA (TP53 transactivation assay) comprises variants in human TP53 classified by transactivation assay [29] ('Datasets and methods') (Table 2).

Employing the independent, 'functional' datasets UniFun, BRCA1-DMS and TP53-TA alongside four prior datasets, we conducted benchmarking of eight prominent variant effect prediction systems (Fig. 2 and Table 3). For all methods, the choice of benchmarking data influenced measured prediction accuracy markedly. When UniFun was employed across tools, the apparent prediction accuracies were consistently among the lowest two measures when compared to measures derived for all the datasets. BRCA1-DMS also tended to yield relatively low apparent prediction accuracies, although the apparent accuracies for Condel, REVEL and fathmm were somewhat elevated when benchmarked using BRCA1-DMS compared with UniFun (see Fig. 3). Compared with UniFun, the

Table 2 Composition of the variant reference datasets used in this study. This table separates mutation catalogues into those derived from clinical databases (disease mutation catalogues) and those derived directly from functional assays (functional mutation catalogues). The table provides summary information for the numbers of proteins and variants of different classifications that have contributed to each dataset. See Additional file 1: Figure S1 and Table S1 for more detailed information

	Total variants	Deleterious	Benign	Total proteins
Disease mutation catalogues				
ClinvarHC	29,752	19,461	10,291	2979
Humsavar	43,878	19,329	24,549	10,231
Swissvar	12,729	4526	8203	5036
Varibench	10,266	4309	5957	4203
Functional mutation catalogues				
TP53-TA	1886	582	1304	1
BRCA1-DMS	1683	408	1275	1
UniFun	11,519	9503	2016	2209

BRCA1-DMS and TP53-TA datasets yielded more variable apparent predictive accuracies, with apparent accuracies tending higher for TP53-TA. The apparent prediction accuracies for UniFun, BRCA1-DMS and TP53-TA were in the ranges 0.52 to 0.63, 0.54 to 0.75 and 0.53 to 0.91, respectively. To highlight the strength of influence that the benchmarking dataset choice can have, the apparent accuracy of REVEL, for example, dropped from AUC = 0.945 to AUC = 0.629 when assessment was conducted using UniFun instead of ClinvarHC. For a majority of tools, there was a general grouping of relatively high measured accuracy for the ClinvarHC, Humsavar and TP53-TA datasets. fathmm exhibited its highest apparent accuracy when benchmarked against Varibench (AUC = 0.936), consistent with the observations of [20], and appeared to perform relatively poorly when benchmarked using any of our functional datasets. Remarkably, when benchmarking was conducted using the most extensive and independent of our functional datasets, UniFun, SIFT achieved the highest measured accuracy score of any method tested, at a level comparable with recent machine learning-based methods.

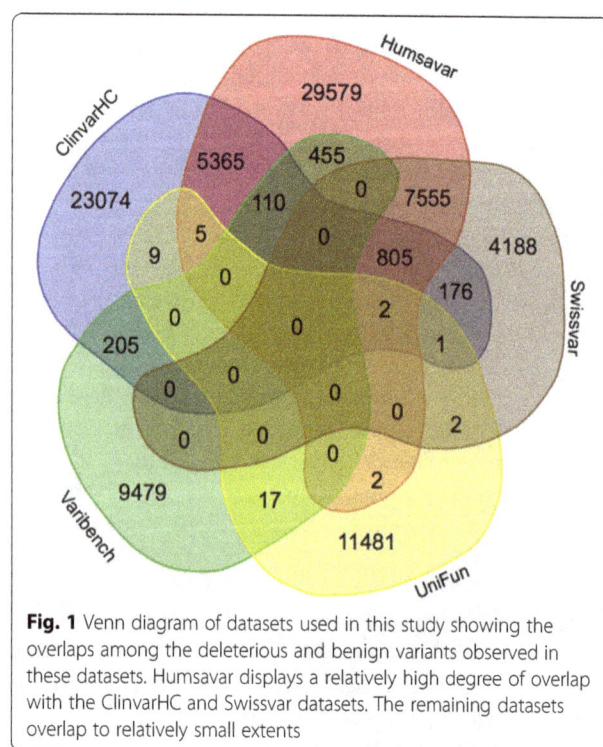

Fig. 1 Venn diagram of datasets used in this study showing the overlaps among the deleterious and benign variants observed in these datasets. Humsavar displays a relatively high degree of overlap with the ClinvarHC and Swissvar datasets. The remaining datasets overlap to relatively small extents

Discussion

We have generated three functional datasets that attempt to better represent the truth with regard to variant classifications, guided by direct in vitro functional assays. They are relatively unrelated to prior variant effect prediction tool training datasets. As such, they promise to be useful for tool benchmarking and training, along with similar, expanded datasets in the future. A potential confounder of our functional datasets (although the same applies to

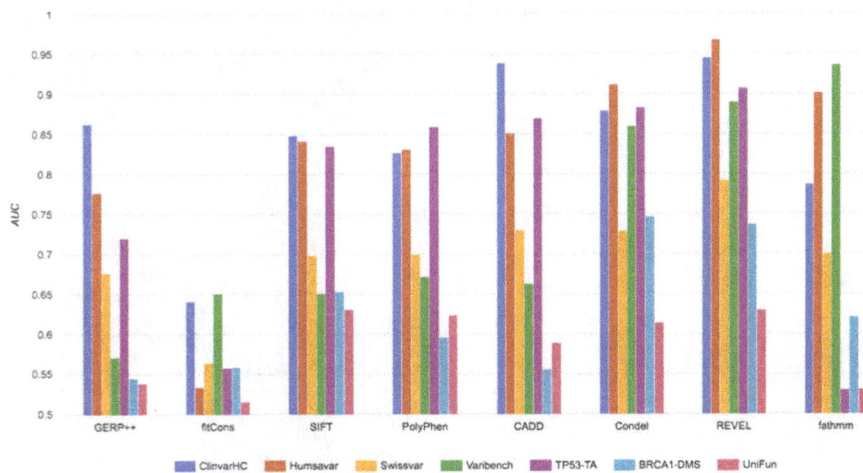

Fig. 2 Histogram depicting apparent accuracies of in silico variant effect predictors based on ROC curve AUCs for the benchmarking datasets used in this study

other datasets) is that we cannot be certain of our variant classifications—despite being guided by dedicated in vitro tests. Although our functional datasets include genetic variants that have not been observed in human populations to date, observations for established pathogenic mutations support their relevance to the disease setting. Starita et al. [28] showed that for ten known disease-causing missense mutations in BRCA1, all were found to be deleterious by functional assay. Since UniFun represents 2209 proteins, it includes a relatively broad sampling of the human protein landscape and should provide a good basis for general variant effect benchmarking, including for proteins that have not been studied in depth previously. The BRCA1-DMS and TP53-TA datasets focus on single proteins. As single-gene datasets, they do not necessarily offer good representation of the broader protein landscape. They are also likely to be confounded by type 1 circularity because BRCA1 and TP53 are relatively highly represented at the protein level, albeit

via different collections of variants, in prior training datasets.

Our observations upon benchmarking a range of in silico variant effect prediction tools against different datasets appeared to broadly reflect the properties of the datasets and how the tools had been calibrated. The high variability of observed prediction accuracies (as measured by the AUC) of the various tools depending on the benchmarking dataset casts serious doubts over the interpretation of outputs from and utility of such tools. That the 'conservation-only' tools tended to yield relatively low measured prediction accuracies across datasets is likely due to their comparative naïvety. The low measured prediction accuracies observed when UniFun was used to benchmark machine learning-derived prediction tools are likely to have been influenced by avoidance of circularity problems. This is supported by similar AUC values having been observed by Grimm et al. when they applied their VariBenchSelected and SwissVarSelected

Table 3 Measured accuracies of eight in silico predictors as benchmarked against seven different variant reference datasets. Measured accuracies are calculated as the areas under the respective ROC curves (AUCs) and Matthews correlation coefficients (MCCs). See Additional file 1: Figure S4 for the ROC curve graphs

	ClinvarHC		Humsavar		Swissvar		Varibench		TP53-TA		BRCA1-DMS		UniFun	
	AUC	MCC	AUC	MCC	AUC	MCC	AUC	MCC	AUC	MCC	AUC	MCC	AUC	MCC
GERP++	0.863	0.587	0.777	0.469	0.677	0.286	0.571	0.15	0.719	0.283	0.544	0.069	0.538	0.04
fitCons	0.641	0.3	0.533	0.033	0.564	0.008	0.651	0.024	0.557	0	0.559	0	0.515	0.033
SIFT	0.848	0.489	0.841	0.543	0.698	0.289	0.651	0.228	0.835	0.484	0.653	0.199	0.631	0.184
PolyPhen	0.827	0.447	0.831	0.541	0.699	0.301	0.672	0.256	0.859	0.469	0.596	0.088	0.623	0.168
CADD	0.939	0.731	0.851	0.57	0.73	0.331	0.663	0.25	0.869	0.418	0.556	0.032	0.589	0.119
Condel	0.879	0.51	0.911	0.664	0.728	0.333	0.86	0.57	0.883	0.074	0.747	0.172	0.614	0.098
REVEL	0.945	0.68	0.968	0.83	0.792	0.462	0.89	0.59	0.907	0.465	0.737	0.088	0.63	0.148
fathmm	0.787	0.288	0.902	0.538	0.701	0.253	0.936	0.509	0.53	0	0.621	0	0.531	0.02

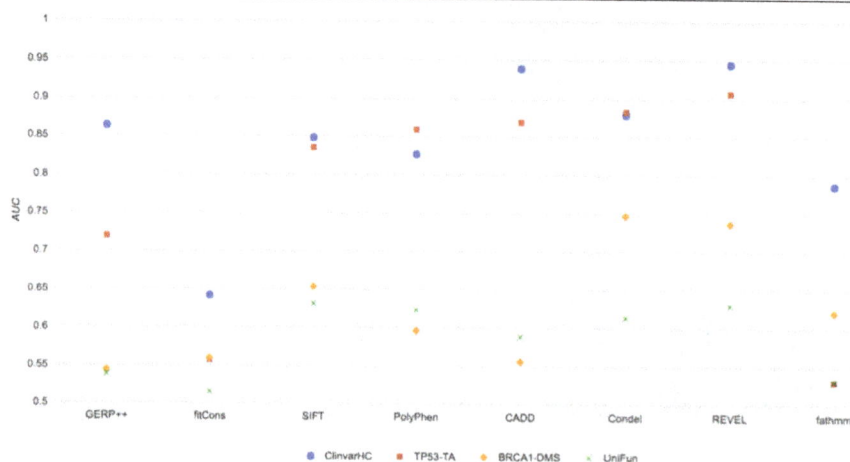

Fig. 3 Apparent prediction accuracies of variant effect prediction tools when assessed using ClinvarHC versus functional mutation derived datasets, reported as AUCs derived from ROC curves

datasets, engineered to avoid circularity, to the benchmarking of a variety of variant effect prediction tools.

The general grouping observed for the ClinvarHC, Humsavar and TP53-TA datasets with respect to apparent accuracies of variant effect prediction tools has likely been influenced by substantial protein representation overlaps between these datasets. Approximately 83% of ClinvarHC proteins overlap with Humsavar variant proteins, and TP53 mutations are represented strongly within each of these (Additional file 1: Table S2 and Figure S3). However, BRCA1 variants are even more strongly represented in ClinvarHC and Humsavar than those of TP53, without BRCA1-DMS displaying similar grouping. It is possible that TP53 behaves as a relatively highly representative protein for these datasets with respect to selected predictive features. We observe that a relatively high proportion of TP53 mutants in ClinvarHC and Humsavar are deleterious (Additional file 1: Figure S3). As inferred by Grimm et al., that fathmm's best apparent performance was observed when benchmarked using Varibench is likely due to type 2 circularity-associated inflation. Varibench contains mutations across 4203 genes, of which only 1.6% have mutations labelled as both benign and deleterious. That SIFT exhibited comparable apparent performance to more recent machine learning-based tools when tested against UniFun may be explained by their training datasets not being conducive to improved general protein effect prediction.

Important to the selection of datasets for training is the issue of whether a prediction tool aims to determine functional consequences generally or only in specific (e.g. particular disease-relevant protein set) contexts. The extent of functional damage conferred by a given variant is an important consideration, which may inform the clinical relevance and preferred classification. Future prediction tools will likely perform best when trained specifically for

particular sets of proteins and mutation/variant classes, via multiple partitioned 'sub-tools'. Regardless, in vitro assay-informed datasets similar to UniFun promise to make important contributions by enabling high-confidence protein functional consequence classifications while allowing training and benchmarking independence.

Conclusions

Our findings, consistent with those of Grimm et al. [20], indicate that the accuracies of contemporary variant effect prediction tools are likely to be considerably lower than reported in their original method publications. This has profound implications for how we use such tools in clinical diagnostic and disease-gene discovery programs. Indeed, we should treat the predictions generated by such tools with considerable caution. We offer a new paradigm for benchmarking such tools that avoids many of the prior conflicts with the ideals of machine learning. Use of these, and expansion to similar independent, functionally determined mutation datasets as training and benchmarking datasets, will be extremely valuable to the progression of this field. Investigating the properties of incorrectly classified variants and using the findings to better inform algorithm design should result in improved prediction accuracy in the future.

Datasets and methods

We have employed seven benchmarking datasets (refer to Table 1) to assess the performance of eight amino acid mutation impact prediction methods: GERP++, fitCons, SIFT, PolyPhen, CADD, Condel, REVEL and fathmm. These datasets contain variants classified as *deleterious* (likely significant effect on protein function) or *benign* (unlikely significant effect on protein function). We have used a variety of datasets that can be broadly categorised into two classes: (1) variants sourced from disease variation catalogues and (2) variants sourced from molecular functional analysis experiments. Figure 1 depicts the overlaps between parent datasets used in this study.

Disease variant catalogues

Databases such as the Swiss-Prot/UniProt-based Humsavar and others, including OMIM [30] and HGMD [25], catalogue disease-associated mutations along with relevant evidence, mainly sourced from the literature. Benign mutations are catalogued via a combination of Swiss-Prot classifications and common alleles (MAF > 1%) from population-based variant databases such as dbSNP and 1000 Genomes.

Clinvar is a database to which contributors submit variants and their classifications along with accompanying evidence. Variously, classifications are based on evidence and assertion criteria such as the Emory Genetics Laboratory Classification Definitions and the InSiGHT Variant Interpretation Committee guidelines [31]. For the present study, we have further filtered Clinvar data to include only high-confidence, expert panel-verified variants with clinical significance scores of 2 (CLNSIG = 2), in the case of benign variants, and 5 (CLNSIG = 5), in the case of deleterious mutations. We term this dataset ClinvarHC (Clinvar high confidence). Mutations classified as likely benign, likely deleterious or of uncertain significance were excluded due to insufficient evidence supporting their influence on protein function and disease.

'Functional' mutation catalogues

As indicated previously, the disease mutation catalogues in common use for in silico prediction tool training and benchmarking suffer from circularity through a lack of independence on multiple levels [20]. To address this, we have identified that data relating to biochemical assays of protein function, without significant overlap with disease mutation catalogues, should be highly valuable for variant effect prediction tool assessment (and training). These reflect validated effects on protein function while achieving independence. Since highly curated and accessible databases with these properties are not available, we have engineered three such datasets, based on (1) mining functional mutagenesis data from UniProt, (2) the deep mutational scanning (DMS) protocol applied to *BRCA1* and (3) the assessment of TP53 mutants by transactivation assay.

UniFun dataset

UniFun is derived using protein annotation data from UniProt. In particular, we employed results from human protein mutagenesis experiments in which amino acids had been mutated prior to measuring their effects on protein function. We mined the UniProt data using keywords and the SPARQL querying framework to compose two sets of variants: (1) a 'functional' set containing amino acid mutations that disrupt protein function and (2) a 'non-

functional' set of mutations that have no apparent effect on protein function. More details on how we generated this data are presented in Additional file 1: Figure S2.

BRCA1-DMS dataset

This relatively new protocol efficiently analyses the impacts of thousands of missense mutations on a protein's function [32]. Because of the relative recency of this approach, only one publicly available dataset could be sourced [28], derived from measurements of mutated BRCA1 ubiquitin ligase activity and binding to the BARD1 RING domain. Both functions are required for efficient homology-directed DNA repair (HDR) and tumour suppression. The HDR rescue score is used to measure disease risk and is derived from a functional assay to measure the ability of mutant BRCA1 to repair double-stranded DNA breaks. Starita et al. defined an HDR rescue score of 0.53 as the point of inflection between the classifications of deleterious (<0.53) and benign (≥0.53). The authors developed a support vector regression predictor based on both ubiquitin ligase activity and BARD1 RING domain binding to predict the HDR rescue scores for DMS data. In the present study, we employed the conservative approach of categorising variants as 'deleterious' if their associated HDR rescue scores were less than 0.33 (above which, no known pathogenic variant score was recorded) and 'benign' for HDR rescue scores above 0.77 (below which, the scores of no known benign variants were measured).

TP53-TA dataset

We sourced unique TP53 amino acid substitutions that had been deposited in the IARC TP53 database [33] (http://p53.iarc.fr) in accordance with the work of Kato et al. [29]. We defined the TP53-TA dataset to exclude variants exhibiting 'partial' reduction in transactivation and those variants that are present in the Clinvar and Humsavar databases.

Data processing

For consistency, Ensembl Variant Effect Predictor (VEP) [34] was employed to convert all variant datasets into variant call format (VCF), using their HGVS amino acid mutation notations as inputs. The resultant VCF files were then annotated using VEP and SnpEff [35]. Condel and fathmm scores were annotated using the VEP custom annotation tools based on precalculated scores available from FannsDB (http://bg.upf.edu/fannsdb). Similarly, GERP++ and fitCons conservation scores were annotated using custom BED files. CADD scores were annotated using CADD v1.2 (http://cadd.gs.washington.edu/download).

Assessing impact prediction

Prediction performances were evaluated using receiver operating characteristic curves (ROC curves) derived using ratios of true positive rates (TPR or sensitivity) and false positive rates (FPR or 1 – specificity), and the areas under the ROC curves (AUCs) were calculated. AUC values range between 0 and 1, inclusive, where 1 corresponds to a perfect classifier and 0.5 implies a random classification. The Matthews correlation coefficient (MCC) was calculated to measure classifier quality. A score of 1 implies perfect classification and 0 implies random classification.

Abbreviations

AUC: Area under the curve; BED: Browser extensible data; BRCA1-DMS: BRCA1 deep mutational scanning; ClinvarHC: Clinvar high confidence; FPR: False positive rate; HDR: Homology-directed DNA repair; MAF: Minor allele frequency; MCC: Matthews correlation coefficient; OMIM: Online Mendelian Inheritance in Man; ROC: Receiver operating characteristic; SPARQL: SPARQL protocol and RDF query language; TP53-TA: TP53 transactivation assay; TPR: True positive rate; UniFun: UniProt-derived, functionally characterised; VCF: Variant call format

Acknowledgements

This work was supported by Melbourne Bioinformatics through Resource Allocation VR0002.

Funding

The authors are supported by Melbourne Bioinformatics (formerly the Victorian Life Sciences Computation Initiative).

Authors' contributions

KM, DJP and BJP conceived the study and contributed to the study design, analysis and manuscript preparation. C-hJ, GP, PG and JC contributed to the analyses and manuscript preparation. All authors read and approved the final manuscript.

Competing interests

The authors declare that they have no competing interests.

References

1. Lek M, Karczewski KJ, Minikel EV, Samocha KE, Banks E, Fennell T, et al. Analysis of protein-coding genetic variation in 60,706 humans. Nature. 2016;536:285–91.
2. Spurdle AB, Healey S, Devereau A, Hogervorst FBL, Monteiro ANA, Nathanson KL, et al. ENIGMA—evidence-based network for the interpretation of germline mutant alleles: an international initiative to evaluate risk and clinical significance associated with sequence variation in BRCA1 and BRCA2 genes. Hum Mutat. 2012;33:2–7.
3. Thompson BA, Spurdle AB, Plazzer J-P, Greenblatt MS, Akagi K, Al-Mulla F, et al. Application of a 5-tiered scheme for standardized classification of 2,360 unique mismatch repair gene variants in the InSiGHT locus-specific database. Nat Genet Nature Research. 2013;46:107–15.
4. Chandler MR, Bilgili EP, Merner ND. A review of whole-exome sequencing efforts toward hereditary breast cancer susceptibility gene discovery. Hum Mutat. 2016;37:835–46.
5. Sullivan PF, Daly MJ, O'Donovan M. Genetic architectures of psychiatric disorders: the emerging picture and its implications. Nat Rev Genet. 2012;13:537–51.
6. Kumar P, Henikoff S, Ng PC. Predicting the effects of coding non-synonymous variants on protein function using the SIFT algorithm. Nat Protoc. 2009;4:1073–81.
7. Ng PC, Henikoff S. Predicting deleterious amino acid substitutions. Genome Res. 2001;11:863–74.

8. Adzhubei IA, Schmidt S, Peshkin L, Ramensky VE, Gerasimova A, Bork P, et al. A method and server for predicting damaging missense mutations. Nat Methods Nature Publishing Group. 2010;7:248–9.
9. Adzhubei I, Jordan DM, Sunyaev SR. Predicting functional effect of human missense mutations using PolyPhen-2. Curr. Protoc. Hum. Genet. 2013;Chapter 7:Unit7.20.
10. Davydov EV, Goode DL, Sirota M, Cooper GM, Sidow A, Batzoglou S. Identifying a high fraction of the human genome to be under selective constraint using GERP++. PLoS Comput Biol. 2010;6, e1001025.
11. Cooper GM, Stone EA, Asimenos G, NISC Comparative Sequencing Program, Green ED, Batzoglou S, et al. Distribution and intensity of constraint in mammalian genomic sequence. Genome Res. 2005;15:901–13.
12. González-Pérez A, López-Bigas N. Improving the assessment of the outcome of nonsynonymous SNVs with a consensus deleteriousness score. Condel Am J Hum Genet. 2011;88:440–9.
13. Kircher M, Witten DM, Jain P, O'Roak BJ, Cooper GM, Shendure J. A general framework for estimating the relative pathogenicity of human genetic variants. Nat Genet. 2014;46:310–5.
14. Shihab HA, Gough J, Cooper DN, Stenson PD, Barker GLA, Edwards KJ, et al. Predicting the functional, molecular, and phenotypic consequences of amino acid substitutions using hidden Markov models. Hum Mutat. 2013; 34:57–65.
15. Schwarz JM, Rödelsperger C, Schuelke M, Seelow D. MutationTaster evaluates disease-causing potential of sequence alterations. Nat Methods Nature Research. 2010;7:575–6.
16. Reva B, Antipin Y, Sander C. Predicting the functional impact of protein mutations: application to cancer genomics. Nucleic Acids Res. 2011;39:e118.
17. Gnad F, Baucom A, Mukhyala K, Manning G, Zhang Z. Assessment of computational methods for predicting the effects of missense mutations in human cancers. BMC Genomics bmcgenomicsbiomedcentralcom. 2013;14 Suppl 3:S7.
18. Khurana JK, Reeder JE, Shrimpton AE, Thakar J. GESPA: classifying nsSNPs to predict disease association. BMC Bioinformatics. 2015;16:228.
19. Ioannidis NM, Rothstein JH, Pejaver V, Middha S, McDonnell SK, Baheti S, et al. REVEL: an ensemble method for predicting the pathogenicity of rare missense variants. Am J Hum Genet. 2016;99:877–85.
20. Grimm DG, Azencott C-A, Aicheler F, Gieraths U, MacArthur DG, Samocha KE, et al. The evaluation of tools used to predict the impact of missense variants is hindered by two types of circularity. Hum Mutat Wiley Online Library. 2015;36:513–23.
21. Capriotti E, Calabrese R, Casadio R. Predicting the insurgence of human genetic diseases associated to single point protein mutations with support vector machines and evolutionary information. Bioinformatics. 2006;22:2729–34.
22. Wu CH, Apweiler R, Bairoch A, Natale DA, Barker WC, Boeckmann B, et al. The Universal Protein Resource (UniProt): an expanding universe of protein information. Nucleic Acids Res. 2006;34:D187–91.
23. Exome Variant Server, NHLBI GO Exome Sequencing Project (ESP) [Internet]. Seattle, WA [cited 2016 Dec 22]. Available from: http://evs.gs.washington.edu/EVS/
24. Sherry ST, Ward M-H, Kholodov M, Baker J, Phan L, Smigielski EM, et al. dbSNP: the NCBI database of genetic variation. Nucleic Acids Res. 2001;29:308–11.
25. Stenson PD, Ball EV, Mort M, Phillips AD, Shiel JA, Thomas NST, et al. Human Gene Mutation Database (HGMD®): 2003 update. Hum Mutat Wiley Subscription Services, Inc, A Wiley Company. 2003;21:577–81.
26. Ionita-Laza I, McCallum K, Xu B, Buxbaum JD. A spectral approach integrating functional genomic annotations for coding and noncoding variants. Nat Genet. 2016;48:214–20.
27. Miosge LA, Field MA, Sontani Y, Cho V, Johnson S, Palkova A, et al. Comparison of predicted and actual consequences of missense mutations. Proc Natl Acad Sci. 2015;112:E5189–98.
28. Starita LM, Young DL, Islam M, Kitzman JO, Gullingsrud J, Hause RJ, et al. Massively parallel functional analysis of BRCA1 RING domain variants. Genetics Genetics Soc America. 2015;200:413–22.
29. Kato S, Han S-Y, Liu W, Otsuka K, Shibata H, Kanamaru R, et al. Understanding the function-structure and function-mutation relationships of p53 tumor suppressor protein by high-resolution missense mutation analysis. Proc Natl Acad Sci U S A. 2003;100:8424–9.

30. Hamosh A, Scott AF, Amberger J, Bocchini C, Valle D, McKusick VA. Online Mendelian Inheritance in Man (OMIM), a knowledgebase of human genes and genetic disorders. Nucleic Acids Res Oxford Univ Press. 2002;30:52–5.

31. Richards S, Aziz N, Bale S, Bick D, Das S, Gastier-Foster J, et al. Standards and guidelines for the interpretation of sequence variants: a joint consensus recommendation of the American College of Medical Genetics and Genomics and the Association for Molecular Pathology. Genet Med. 2015;17:405–24.

32. Fowler DM, Fields S. Deep mutational scanning: a new style of protein science. Nat Methods naturecom. 2014;11:801–7.

33. Bouaoun L, Sonkin D, Ardin M, Hollstein M, Byrnes G, Zavadil J, et al. TP53 variations in human cancers: new lessons from the IARC TP53 database and genomics data. Hum Mutat. 2016;37:865–76.

34. McLaren W, Gil L, Hunt SE, Riat HS, Ritchie GRS, Thormann A, et al. The Ensembl Variant Effect Predictor. Genome Biol. 2016;17:122.

35. Cingolani P, Platts A, Wang LL, Coon M, Nguyen T, Wang L, et al. A program for annotating and predicting the effects of single nucleotide polymorphisms, SnpEff: SNPs in the genome of Drosophila melanogaster strain w1118; iso-2; iso-3. Fly. 2012;6:80–92.

17

Secondary findings in 421 whole exome-sequenced Chinese children

Wen Chen[1,2], Wenke Li[2], Yi Ma[1,2], Yujing Zhang[2], Bianmei Han[1], Xuewen Liu[1], Kun Zhao[1], Meixian Zhang[3], Jie Mi[3], Yuanyuan Fu[2*] and Zhou Zhou[1,2*]

Abstract

Background: Variants with known or possible pathogenicity located in genes that are unrelated to primary disease conditions are defined as secondary findings. Secondary findings are not the primary targets of whole exome and genome sequencing (WES/WGS) assay but can be of great practical value in early disease prevention and intervention. The driving force for this study was to investigate the impact of racial difference and disease background on secondary findings. Here, we analyzed secondary findings frequencies in 421 whole exome-sequenced Chinese children who are phenotypically normal or bear congenital heart diseases/juvenile obesity. In total, 421 WES datasets were processed for potential deleterious variant screening. A reference gene list was defined according to the American College of Medical Genetics and Genomics (ACMG) recommendations for reporting secondary findings v2.0 (ACMG SF v2.0). The variant classification was performed according to the evidence-based guidelines recommended by the joint consensus of the ACMG and the Association for Molecular Pathology (AMP).

Results: Among the 421 WES datasets, we identified 11 known/expected pathogenic variants in 12 individuals, accounting for 2.85% of our samples, which is much higher than the reported frequency in a Caucasian population. In conclusion, secondary findings are not so rare in Chinese children, which means that we should pay more attention to the clinical interpretation of sequencing results.

Keywords: Secondary findings, Chinese children, Whole exome sequencing, Variant classification, ACMG recommendation

Introduction

During whole exome and whole genome sequencing (WES/WGS) data interpretation, variants with known or possible pathogenicity located in genes that are unrelated to primary disease conditions are defined as incidental findings or secondary findings. These mutated genes are not first-tier targets of the test but indicate a high risk of certain medically actionable diseases. Hence, the early awareness of risk could be of great importance for disease prevention and intervention.

Since the American College of Medical Genetics and Genomics first published recommendations for reporting clinical exome and genome sequencing secondary findings [1], close attention has been paid to the incidence and clinical significance of secondary findings [2–7]. Considering the genetic variation of different populations and the insufficiencies in the genotype-phenotype database, technical and ethical issues regarding these findings and reports have also concerned practitioners. On the one hand, the early awareness of secondary findings provides clues for patients and clinicians to prevent diseases at a relatively early stage. On the other hand, reporting the genetic variants related to certain severe diseases before the occurrence of any phenotype may bring about an unnecessary psychological burden on individuals and even hurt the trust between patients and clinicians. The debates have never been settled, especially about the ethical issues in child patients [8].

* Correspondence: wistaria97@126.com; zhouzhou@fuwaihospital.org
[2]State Key Laboratory of Cardiovascular Disease, Beijing Key Laboratory for Molecular Diagnostics of Cardiovascular Diseases, Diagnostic Laboratory Service, Fuwai Hospital, National Center for Cardiovascular Diseases, Peking Union Medical College, Chinese Academy of Medical Sciences, Beijing, China
[1]State Key Laboratory of Cardiovascular Disease, Fuwai Hospital, National Center for Cardiovascular Diseases, Peking Union Medical College, Chinese Academy of Medical Sciences, Beijing, China
Full list of author information is available at the end of the article

To contribute to database accumulation and put some of those concerns to rest, we analyzed whole exome sequencing data from 421 Chinese children who were divided into phenotypically normal (96 of 421), juvenile obesity (96 of 421), and congenital heart disease (CHD) (229 of 421) groups and calculated the frequency of the secondary findings. The entire process was performed by following the ACMG recommendations for reporting secondary findings (ACMG SF v2.0) and the pathogenic classification criteria recommended by the 2015 ACMG/AMP Standards and Guidelines [9, 10]. This work is an extensive analysis of the secondary findings in Chinese children, which will provide a general view of secondary findings incidence in the Chinese population and help us to better understand the relationship between secondary findings and preexisting disease conditions. Moreover, our data analysis and interpretation could be used as a reference by other medical researchers and clinical genetic testing practitioners.

Materials and methods

Subject and consent

Phenotypically normal cohort and juvenile obesity cohort were recruited from the Capital Institute of Paediatrics. The CHD cohort was recruited from Fuwai Hospital. All structural heart phenotypes were confirmed by echocardiography. The WHO Child Growth Standards and International Obesity Task Force criteria were used for recruiting patients younger or older than 2 years old, respectively.

All experimental protocols were approved by the ethics committee of Fuwai Hospital and Capital Institute of Paediatrics. The guardians of the children participating in this study signed the provided written informed consent forms approved by the ethics committee of Fuwai Hospital and Capital Institute of Pediatrics and were free to quit at any stage of this study. All 421 subjects were under 18 years old at the time of sample collection. The average and median ages were 6.69 and 9 years, respectively, see Additional file 1 for the participants' age and gender distributions.

Whole exome sequencing

Briefly, genomic DNA was extracted from ethylenediaminetetraacetic acid (EDTA) anti-coagulated whole blood using the Wizard® Genomic DNA Purification Kit (Promega Corporation, Madison, WI, US). The quantity and quality of DNA from each sample were measured using a NanoDrop2000 (Thermo Scientific, Waltham, MA, USA). Genomic DNA was captured with NimbleGen's SeqCap EZ Human Exome Library v3.0 kit (Roche, Pleasanton, CA, USA). Whole exome sequencing was performed on an Illumina HiSeq2500 platform (Illumina Inc., San Diego, CA, USA) using the TruSeq Rapid PE Cluster kit V2 or TruSeq Rapid SBS kit V2 - HS (Illumina Inc., San Diego, CA, USA).

Alignment and variant calling

The Burrows-Wheeler Aligner (BWA) tool [11] was used to align the sequence reads to NCBI Build 37 (hg19). Picard tools (https://github.com/broadinstitute/picard) were used to mark the duplicate reads. The aligned sequences were then stored in BAM format and underwent variant calling using the GATK HaplotypeCaller.

Automatic filtering

Variants of the 59 genes recommended by ACMG SF v2.0 were extracted. Particularly, we only kept the homozygous variants in MUTYH and ATP7B, which showed autosomal recessive inheritance. We initially extracted all rare variants defined as variants with the highest minor allele frequencies (MAFs) ≤ 0.005 in any gnomAD population (gnomAD_popmax) [12] and added the homozygote variants with the highest MAFs ≤ 0.02 in any gnomAD population for MUTYH and ATP7B. Then, the variants reported as disease-causing mutations ("DM") or "DM?" in the Human Gene Mutation Database (HGMD), pathogenic/likely pathogenic in the ClinVar database, or protein-truncating mutations ("PTMs"), including frame-shift, stop-gain, start-loss, and splicing mutations, were kept for manual assessment. The process workflow is shown in Fig. 1.

Manual assessment

The in silico filtered variants required evaluation for their pathogenicity according to the recommendations in the 2015 ACMG/AMP Standards and Guidelines. We also adopted the MYH7-associated inherited cardiomyopathy recommendations from ClinGen's working group [13]. Each variant was considered to be known pathogenic ("KP"), expected pathogenic ("EP"), or "others." The pathogenicity of each variant was evaluated according to the 2015 ACMG/AMP Standards and Guidelines. The previously reported variants that met the criteria for "pathogenic/likely pathogenic" were classified as KP. When analyzing a novel PTM, we only took the variants in genes recommended as "EP" in ACMG SF v2.0 into consideration. A category of EP would be given to a variant that met the pathogenic criteria; otherwise, it was defined as "others." We only analyzed the pathogenicity of the reported non-PTMs; novel missense variants of these 59 genes were not considered as secondary findings according to the ACMG SF v2.0 [10], see Fig. 1 for an overview of the assessment process.

To prevent interpersonal bias, two experts specialized in data analysis and annotation simultaneously performed the assessment. When inconsistencies were present, supporting evidence was provided for further

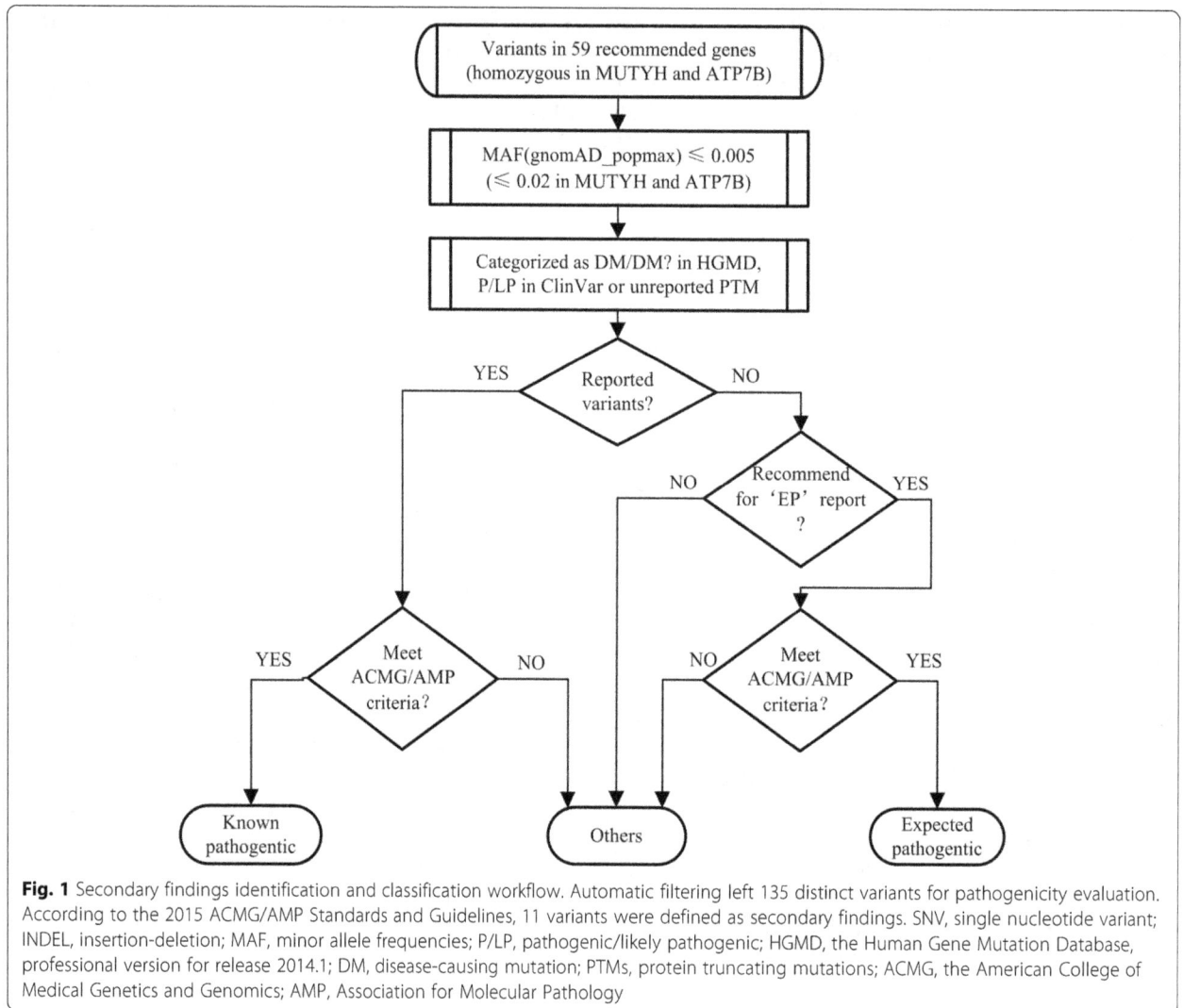

Fig. 1 Secondary findings identification and classification workflow. Automatic filtering left 135 distinct variants for pathogenicity evaluation. According to the 2015 ACMG/AMP Standards and Guidelines, 11 variants were defined as secondary findings. SNV, single nucleotide variant; INDEL, insertion-deletion; MAF, minor allele frequencies; P/LP, pathogenic/likely pathogenic; HGMD, the Human Gene Mutation Database, professional version for release 2014.1; DM, disease-causing mutation; PTMs, protein truncating mutations; ACMG, the American College of Medical Genetics and Genomics; AMP, Association for Molecular Pathology

discussion and decision-making. As a final step, the lab director checked all the variant classifications along with the supporting evidence for the final reported list. All reported variants were confirmed by Sanger sequencing.

Results

The average target region coverage was 99.54%, and 92.60% of the target regions with more than 20-fold coverage were successfully detected. The average coverage for the 59 genes was 99.74%, and 94.13% of target regions with more than 20-fold coverage were successfully detected. Specifically, the average sequencing depth of the 59 target genes was 69-fold, which contributed a reliable resource for analyzing the secondary findings. More detailed information is shown in Additional file 2.

In 421 individuals, we identified 251 rare (MAFs ≤ 0.005) variants using the 59-gene list (0.60 variants per individual). The criteria we used to classify the variants were in complete agreement with the 2015 ACMG/AMP

Standards and Guidelines [9, 10]. After the automated variant filtering process, 135 unique variants remained for manual annotation, 11 of which were reportable secondary findings. Overall, we identified 5 reportable variants classified as KP or EP in the *DSP, MYH7*, and *FBN1* genes, which have been reported to cause different types of cardiovascular diseases. Four variants classified as KP or EP in the *BRCA2, PMS2*, and *SDHB* genes have been recognized to cause different types of hereditary cancer. We also identified 2 reportable variants in the *LDLR* and *APOB* genes (Table 1). Detailed evidence-based information is shown in Additional file 3. The genetic mode for all these genes is autosomal dominant inheritance with high penetrance, suggesting that the carriers are at high risk of these diseases.

According to our protocol, 135 potentially pathogenic variants were defined in 198 of 421 individuals (47.03%), and 42 of the 59 genes were affected. Among the 135 variants that required manual annotation, 34 of them

Table 1 Variants defined as secondary findings according to the ACMG recommendations for the reportable gene list

Category	Gene	Variants	Evidence	Associated condition	Group	RCFs
Pathogenic variants:						
KP	APOB	NM_000384: exon26:c.10579C>T p.Arg3527Trp	PS3, PS4, PP3	Familial hypercholesterolemia	Normal/ CHD	LDL-c 7.16 mmol/ L 2.46 mmol/ L
KP	BRCA2	NM_000059: exon11: c.2806-2809del p.Lys936fs	PVS1, PS4, PM2	Hereditary breast and ovarian cancer	Obesity	None
KP	DSP	NM_004415: exon2: c.268C>T p.Gln90Term	PVS1, PM2, PP3	Arrhythmogenic right ventricular cardiomyopathy	Obesity	None
KP	MYH7	NM_000257: exon18: c.1988G>A p.Arg663His	PS4, PP1_Strong, PM1, PM2, PP3	Hypertrophic cardiomyopathy, dilated cardiomyopathy	Normal	None
KP	MYH7	NM_000257: exon13: c.1207C>T p.Arg403Trp	PS4, PP1_Strong, PM1, PM2, PM5, PP3	Hypertrophic cardiomyopathy, dilated cardiomyopathy	Normal	None
KP	PMS2	NM001322010: exon8: c.498+2T>C	PVS1, PS3, PM2, PP3	Lynch syndrome	CHD	None
KP	SDHB	NM_003000: exon7: c.724C>T p.Arg242Cys	PS4, PM2, PM5, PP3, PS3_Supporting	Hereditary paraganglioma-pheochromocytoma syndrome	CHD	None
Likely pathogenic variants:						
KP	LDLR	NM_000527: exon4:c.459delC p.Phe153fs	PVS1, PM2	Familial hypercholesterolemia	Normal	LDL-c 5.13 mmol/ L
KP	MYH7	NM_000257: exon22: c.2608C>T p.Arg870Cys	PM1, PM2, PM5, PP3, PS4_Supporting	Hypertrophic cardiomyopathy, dilated cardiomyopathy	Obesity	None
EP	BRCA2	NM_000059: exon11: c.2944_2945del p.Ile982fs	PVS1, PM2	Hereditary breast and ovarian cancer	Normal	None
EP	FBN1	NM_000138: exon25: c.3042dupT p.Ala1015fs	PVS1, PM2	Marfan syndrome, Loeys-Dietz syndromes, familial thoracic aortic aneurysms and dissections	Normal	None

RCFs related clinical features, *EP* expected pathogenic, *KP* known pathogenic, *ACMG* American College of Medical Genetics and Genomics, *HGMD* Human Gene Mutation Database, professional version for release 2014.1, *dbSNP* single-nucleotide polymorphism database, *CHD* congenital heart diseases, *PVS* very strong evidence of pathogenicity, *PS* strong evidence of pathogenicity, *PM* moderate evidence of pathogenicity, *PP* supporting evidence of pathogenicity, *NA* not available

were shared in two or more individuals; the remaining 101 variants were observed only once. Most of the variants were missense mutations (98/135 or 72.59%); the others included 7 synonymous variants (5.19%), 18 insertion/deletions (13.42%), 8 stop-gain/start-loss variants (5.92%), and 4 splicing region variants (2.96%). Among the affected genes, *ATP7B*, *BRCA1/2*, *MYBPC3*, and *SCN5A* bore the largest number of variations among the total variants (52/135 or 38.52%). These results may be caused by gene size and evolutionary conservation and were in accordance with Petrovski's findings [14].

As shown in Table 1, different groups have different reportable findings, with six individuals from the

phenotypically normal group, three individuals from the obesity group, and three individuals from the CHD group showing secondary findings. The reportable rates were 6.25%, 3.13%, and 1.31%, respectively. Because the patients in our cohort have not shown any of the phenotypes mentioned in the ACMG SF v2.0, all these P/LP variants were defined as secondary findings. Hence, we found 12 individuals bearing secondary findings, which accounted for 2.85% of our sample.

Discussion

Eleven of the 135 distinct variants were reported as secondary findings after annotation and classification.

Among these distinct variants, although 115 distinct variants have been reported as "potentially pathogenic" in at least one of the two most popular variation reference databases (HGMD and ClinVar), only 9 variants in 10 different individuals were finally defined as secondary findings. These results indicate that the pathogenicity of other distinct non-PTM variants in our sample might be overrated by these databases, which suggests the need to be particularly cautious when using these databases to perform clinical data interpretation. Additionally, a careful curation of these databases might be of great urgency and importance.

During the manual interpretation of these variants, in addition to the 28 criteria for classifying pathogenicity recommended by the ACMG/AMP, we also applied the latest recommendations for MYH7-associated inherited cardiomyopathies given by ClinGen's inherited cardiomyopathy expert panel [13]. Additionally, when reporting familial hypercholesterolemia (FH)-related secondary findings, much more attention should be paid to the carriers' conditions. Two FH-related pathogenic gene mutation carriers in our cohort had elevated LDL-c levels—7.16 and 5.13 mmol/L at the time of sample collection. The third pathogenic mutation carrier has not shown a related phenotype (LDL-c level 2.46 mmol/L). Considering the age of testing, it is understandable for such a finding.

During the past few years, many groups have focused on secondary findings reporting based on different candidate gene lists and analytical criteria. As a result, the positive rates were also different. Following the automatic filtering process and the mutation classification rules embedded in the next generation sequencing analysis workflow routines, the additional workload would be controlled at an acceptable level in actual clinical practice. Our automatic filter system called 135 distinct variants from 421 individuals, which means an average of 0.32 variants per individual during manual annotation. In comparison, the post-filtration variants per person in other studies were higher, ranging from 0.39 to 1.1 [3–5]. In our study, we tried to be more accurate and clinically practical, as shown in the following aspects: first, we adopted an authoritative and updated 59-gene list recommended by the ACMG; second, we combined the most prevalent quality control strategy, which made the remaining variants more confirmable and reliable; third, we set a stringent filter condition, which significantly reduced the workload of subsequent manual analysis; and lastly, we simplified the classification of variants into three categories (KP, EP, or "others"); thus, all we needed to consider was the ACMG pathogenicity criteria and the related published literature. The variants in the "others" category did not need to be distinguished as "variants with uncertain significance" or "(likely) benign," which lightened the burden for laboratories.

We found a similar rate of reportable secondary findings within a family cohort [3], the Korean population [15] and East Asians [16], which is much higher than the rates in adults of European and African ancestry as reported by different groups [2, 3, 5, 17]. Several of the following reasons could explain this discrepancy: [1] the analysis was performed within different population contexts; [2] differences in the candidate gene list, variant evaluation criteria, and analytical process existed in these studies; and [3] the participants in our cohort were all relatively young (< 18 years), suggesting that some phenotypes may not show up at this age, which then led us to believe that the EP and KP variants were unrelated to primary disease and should be defined as secondary findings. Based on these assumptions, we suggest that special attention should be paid to secondary findings reporting in children and young patients.

There were also some limitations in our study. First, the samples in our cohort were from sporadic patients or phenotypically normal person and lacked family member information/samples, which made it hard for us to evaluate the pathogenicity of a de novo mutation or identify compound heterozygous/hemizygous mutations. Second, our study only included children and juvenile participants, which may have some age-related bias. Further study of random samples will be meaningful to confirm or validate our results. However, considering the unavailability of open-access Chinese population WES data, our work could reflect, to a certain degree, the secondary findings incidence in this largest population in the world.

There are always ethical issues accompanied by the interpretation of the secondary findings. Performing secondary findings on children has been a controversial topic invariably. Some groups hold the opinion that predictive testing should not be performed on children considering the consequent unrealistic burden and ethical concerns [8, 18]. However, the ACMG workgroup recommends that seeking and reporting secondary findings should not be restricted to the age of the person being sequenced [1]. The aim of secondary findings reporting is to notify the medically actionable disease-causing genetic mutation and allow the doctors and potential patients to take action in advance. From this point of view, the participants could receive additional benefit from their genomic data. To pull the two ends together, it might be more appropriate for us to respect the test receivers' wishes, only report the portion of data they would like to know and keep the rest in the black box.

Conclusions

In summary, by sequencing the whole exome of CHD/obesity patients and normal children, we evaluated the secondary findings incidence in Chinese minors.

Secondary findings are not so rare in Chinese children, and much more attention should be paid to the clinical interpretation of genome sequencing results. Our work demonstrates some feasible interpretation criteria as well as a simplified analytical workflow for clinical practice.

Abbreviations
ACMG: American College of Medical Genetics and Genomics; BWA: Burrows-Wheeler Aligner; DM: Disease-causing mutation; EDTA: Ethylenediaminetetraacetic acid; EP: Expected pathogenic; FH: Familial hypercholesterolemia; KP: Known pathogenic; MAF: Minor allele frequencies; PTMs: Protein truncating mutations; WES/WGS: Whole exome and whole genome sequencing

Acknowledgements
The authors gratefully acknowledge the support of the patients in this study.

Funding
This work was supported by the CAMS Initiative for Innovative Medicine (CAMS-I2M, 2016-I2M-1-016).

Authors' contributions
ZZ and YF conceived the project. WC and WL designed the experiments. WC, MZ, and JM collected the samples and clinical information. BH, XL, and KZ performed the experimental process. WL and YZ performed the in silico analysis and data interpretation. WC, YM, and YF analyzed the data and interpreted all the variants. WC drafted the manuscript, and YF refined the final approved version of the paper. ZZ supervised the project. All authors have discussed the data and provided some advice. All authors read and approved the final manuscript.

Competing interests
The authors declare that they have no competing interests.

Author details
[1]State Key Laboratory of Cardiovascular Disease, Fuwai Hospital, National Center for Cardiovascular Diseases, Peking Union Medical College, Chinese Academy of Medical Sciences, Beijing, China. [2]State Key Laboratory of Cardiovascular Disease, Beijing Key Laboratory for Molecular Diagnostics of Cardiovascular Diseases, Diagnostic Laboratory Service, Fuwai Hospital, National Center for Cardiovascular Diseases, Peking Union Medical College, Chinese Academy of Medical Sciences, Beijing, China. [3]Department of Epidemiology, Capital Institute of Paediatrics, Beijing, China.

References
1. Green RC, Berg JS, Grody WW, et al. ACMG recommendations for reporting of incidental findings in clinical exome and genome sequencing. Genet Med. 2013;15:565–74.
2. Dorschner MO, Amendola LM, Turner EH, et al. Actionable, pathogenic incidental findings in 1,000 participants' exomes. Am J Hum Genet. 2013;93:631–40.
3. Lawrence L, Sincan M, Markello T, et al. The implications of familial incidental findings from exome sequencing: the NIH Undiagnosed Diseases Program experience. Genet Med. 2014;16:741–50.
4. Jang MA, Lee SH, Kim N, et al. Frequency and spectrum of actionable pathogenic secondary findings in 196 Korean exomes. Genet Med. 2015;17:1007–11.
5. Jurgens J, Ling H, Hetrick K, et al. Assessment of incidental findings in 232 whole-exome sequences from the Baylor-Hopkins Center for Mendelian Genomics. Genet Med. 2015;17:782–8.
6. Dewey FE, Murray MF, Overton JD, et al. Distribution and clinical impact of functional variants in 50,726 whole-exome sequences from the DiscovEHR study. Scie. 2016;354(6319).
7. Amendola LM, Dorschner MO, Robertson PD, et al. Actionable exomic incidental findings in 6503 participants: challenges of variant classification. Genome Res. 2015;25:305–15.
8. Committee on Bioethics, Committee on Genetics, American College of Medical Genetics, Genomics Social, Ethical, Legal Issues Committee. Ethical and policy issues in genetic testing and screening of children. Pediatrics. 2013;131:620–2.
9. Richards S, Aziz N, Bale S, et al. Standards and guidelines for the interpretation of sequence variants: a joint consensus recommendation of the American College of Medical Genetics and Genomics and the Association for Molecular Pathology. Genet Med. 2015;17:405–24.
10. Kalia SS, Adelman K, Bale SJ, et al. Recommendations for reporting of secondary findings in clinical exome and genome sequencing, 2016 update (ACMG SF v2.0): a policy statement of the American College of Medical Genetics and Genomics. Genet Med. 2017;19:249-55.
11. Li H, Durbin R. Fast and accurate short read alignment with Burrows-Wheeler transform. Bioinformatics. 2009;25:1754–60.
12. Lek M, Karczewski KJ, Minikel EV, et al. Analysis of protein-coding genetic variation in 60,706 humans. Nature. 2016;536:285–91.
13. Kelly MA, Caleshu C, Morales A, et al. Adaptation and validation of the ACMG/AMP variant classification framework for MYH7-associated inherited cardiomyopathies: recommendations by ClinGen's inherited cardiomyopathy expert panel. Genet Med. 2018;20:351–9.
14. Petrovski S, Wang Q, Heinzen EL, et al. Genic intolerance to functional variation and the interpretation of personal genomes. PLoS Genet. 2013;9:e1003709.
15. Kwak SH, Chae J, Choi S, et al. Findings of a 1303 Korean whole-exome sequencing study. Exp Mol Med. 2017;49:e356.
16. Tang CS, Dattani S, So MT, et al. Actionable secondary findings from whole-genome sequencing of 954 East Asians. Hum Genet. 2018;137:31–7.
17. Johnston JJ, Rubinstein WS, Facio FM, et al. Secondary variants in individuals undergoing exome sequencing: screening of 572 individuals identifies high-penetrance mutations in cancer-susceptibility genes. Am J Hum Genet. 2012;91:97–108.
18. Ross LF, Saal HM, David KL, et al. Technical report: ethical and policy issues in genetic testing and screening of children. Genet Med. 2013;15:234–45.

18

Trans-activation-based risk assessment of *BRCA1* BRCT variants with unknown clinical significance

Jonas Langerud[1], Elisabeth Jarhelle[2], Marijke Van Ghelue[2], Sarah Louise Ariansen[1] and Nina Iversen[1*]

Abstract

Background: Deleterious variants in the tumour suppressor *BRCA1* are known to cause hereditary breast and ovarian cancer syndrome (HBOC). Missense variants in *BRCA1* pose a challenge in clinical care, as their effect on protein functionality often remains unknown. Many of the pathogenic missense variants found in *BRCA1* are located in the *BRCA1* C-terminal (BRCT) domains, domains that are known to be vital for key functions such as homologous recombination repair, protein-protein interactions and trans-activation (TA). We investigated the TA activity of 12 *BRCA1* variants of unknown clinical significance (VUSs) located in the BRCT domains to aid in the classification of these variants.

Results: Twelve *BRCA1* VUSs were investigated using a modified version of the dual luciferase TA activity assay (TA assay) that yielded increased sensitivity and sample throughput. Variants were classified according to American College of Medical Genetics and Genomics (ACMG) criteria using TA assay results and available data. In combining our TA-assay results and available data, in accordance with the ACMG guidelines for variant classification, we proposed the following variant classifications: c.5100A>G, c.5326C>T, c.5348T>C and c.5477A>T as likely benign (class 2) variants. c.5075A>C, c.5116G>A and c.5513T>G were likely pathogenic (class 4), whereas c.5096G>A likely represents a likely pathogenic variant with moderate penetrance. Variants c.5123C>T, c.5125G>A, c.5131A>C and c.5504G>A remained classified as VUSs (class 3).

Conclusions: The modified TA assay provides efficient risk assessment of rare missense variants found in the BRCA1 BRCT-domains. We also report that increased post-transfection incubation time yielded a significant increase in TA assay sensitivity.

Keywords: *BRCA1*, HBOC, BRCT, Trans-activation, Functional assay, VUS

Background

Breast cancer is the most prevalent cancer in women worldwide, representing 25.1% of all new cancer cases and 14.7% of cancer-related deaths [1]. Roughly, 10% of breast cancer incidents can be attributed to pathogenic germline variants. These germline variants are inherited in an autosomal dominant manner and result in what is known as hereditary breast and ovarian cancer syndrome (HBOC) [2]. HBOC confers a 45–65% lifetime risk of developing breast cancer and a 11–44% risk of ovarian cancer in addition to the association with an increased

risk of tumour development in other tissues exposed to elevated hormone levels, such as the fallopian tubes, pancreas and prostate [3, 4]. Monoallelic variants in the high penetrance genes *BRCA1* and *BRCA2* are estimated to account for 30% of HBOC cases [2, 5].

The *BRCA1, DNA repair associated (BRCA1)* gene encodes a 220 kDa nuclear phosphoprotein, consisting of 1863 amino acids (aa). N-terminally, the protein contains a Really Interesting New Gene (RING) domain (aa 8–96) with E3-ubiquitin ligase activity [6]. BRCA1 also includes a nuclear export signal (aa 81–99), a non-canonical NLS (aa 252–257), two canonical nuclear localisation signals (NLS; aa 503–508 and aa 607–617), a coiled-coil domain (aa 1364–1437) and various binding sites and phosphorylation targets for a variety of protein

* Correspondence: ninaiversenous@gmail.com
[1]Department of Medical Genetics, Oslo University Hospital, Oslo, Norway
Full list of author information is available at the end of the article

interaction partners [7–10]. C-terminally, BRCA1 contains a domain consisting of two BRCA1 C-terminal (BRCT) domains with trans-activation activity [11, 12]. The BRCT domains are located at aa 1646–1736 and aa 1760–1855 [6].

BRCA1 is directly involved in homologous recombination repair (HRR), and as such is vital for maintaining genomic stability [13]. Deleterious variants in the BRCA1 BRCT domains may halt the interactions between BRCA1 and important facilitators of HRR such as Abraxas, BRCA1 interacting protein C-terminal helicase 1 (BRIP1) or RB-binding protein 8, endonuclease (RBBP8; alias: CtIP) [14]. BRCA1 also regulates the progression of the cell cycle through the S-phase [15, 16] and is associated with the G2/M checkpoint control [17–20]. Additionally, BRCA1 interact with oestrogen receptor-α (ER-α) and is important for the regulation of transcription factors involved in epithelial mesenchymal transition [21–23]. Furthermore, BRCA1 has been implicated in enhancing nucleotide excision repair and transcription-coupled repair via its connection to the RNA polymerase II holoenzyme complex [24]. In addition to the abovementioned roles, BRCA1 has been shown to possess trans-activation (TA) activity, and pathogenic variants in the BRCT domains can abrogate this ability, indicating the importance of TA as a mechanism of tumour suppression [12].

With the rising number of patients undergoing predictive BRCA1/2 screening, the incidence of variants of unknown clinical significance (VUS) increases. The correct classification of these rare variants is paramount for the right clinical assessment of the patient. Accordingly, in order to classify the 12 BRCA1 BRCT VUSs found in our patients, we optimised the sensitivity and efficiency of a TA assay (Fig. 1).

Methods

Variants included in this study

Twelve missense variants in the BRCA1 BRCT domains were found in patients during routine diagnostics at the Oslo University Hospital, Department of Medical Genetics. These variants were chosen for functional trans-activation studies (Table 1). Additionally, we tested two variant combinations in cis (c.5075A>C/c.5411T>A and c.5252G>A/c.5477A>T) to investigate possible additive or synergistic effects. Variant annotation follows HGVS nomenclature. The reference sequence used was BRCA1 NM_007294.3 (custom exon numbering). The classifications of the included variants at the beginning of this study were performed at the Oslo University Hospital, Department of Medical Genetics prior to implementation of the ACMG criteria.

In silico assessment of BRCA1 variants

All variants included in this study were analysed in silico using Alamut Visual 2.9.0. Table 1 displays entries in databases dbSNP, ClinVar, and HGMD, allele frequencies reported by gnomAD and ESP, where available, as well as the predicted effects of the variants based on reports from SIFT, AlignGVGD and Mutation taster. The maximal pathogenic allele frequency (MPAF) for BRCA1 is estimated at 0.1%, variant allele frequencies above the MPAF (> 0.1) were considered evidence for the variant to be benign [25]. Splice predictions were based on SpliceSiteFinder-like, MaxEntScan, NNSPLICE and GeneSplicer, alterations of ≥ 10% and agreement between three or more programs were used as criteria for a variant to likely result in aberrant splicing. Variant effects on splicing regulatory elements (SREs) were not included in the predictions.

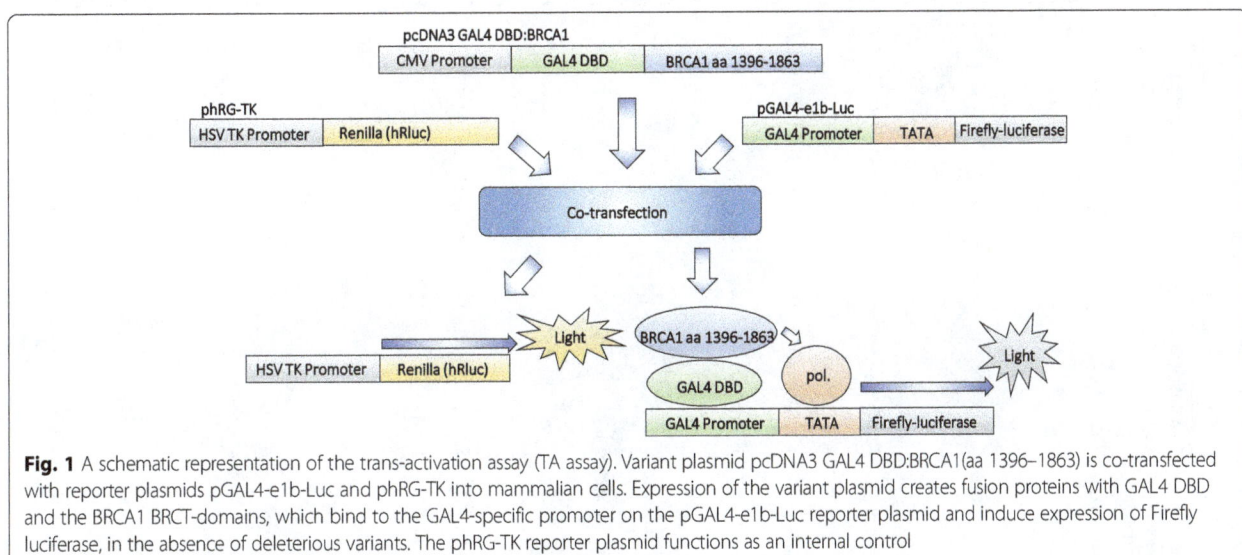

Fig. 1 A schematic representation of the trans-activation assay (TA assay). Variant plasmid pcDNA3 GAL4 DBD:BRCA1(aa 1396–1863) is co-transfected with reporter plasmids pGAL4-e1b-Luc and phRG-TK into mammalian cells. Expression of the variant plasmid creates fusion proteins with GAL4 DBD and the BRCA1 BRCT-domains, which bind to the GAL4-specific promoter on the pGAL4-e1b-Luc reporter plasmid and induce expression of Firefly luciferase, in the absence of deleterious variants. The phRG-TK reporter plasmid functions as an internal control

Table 1 Variant entries in databases dbSNP, ClinVar and HGMD, as well as allele frequencies reported by gnomAD and ESP (ALL: All, AFR: African/African American, NFE: Non-Finnish European, AMR: Latino, EAS: East Asian, SAS: South Asian, OTH: Other)

HGVS nucleotide variant	HGVS protein variant	Exon	Type	dbSNP	ClinVar	gnomAD	ESP	HGMD	SIFT	Align GVGD	Mutation taster	Splice prediction	Class
c.4956G>A	p.(Met1652Ile)	16	Missense	rs1799967	RCV000112434.6: Benign (ENIGMA) RCV000048709.9: Benign/Likely benign RCV000034756.3: Benign RCV000476093.1: Benign RCV000128916.4: Benign/VUS RCV000120261.7: Benign	ALL: 1.82% AFR: 0.18% AMR: 0.40% EAS: 0.012% SAS: 3.78% NFE: 1.53% FIN: 5.08% OTH: 1.66%	EA: 1.5%AA: 0.2%	CM014325(Disease-causing?)	Tolerated	C0	Polymorphism (p = 0.964)	None	1[a]
c.4964C>T	p.(Ser1665Phe)	16	Missense	rs80357390	RCV000112436.1: VUS RCV000223580.1: Likely pathogenic			CM041700(Disease-causing)	Deleterious	C25	Disease-causing (p = 1)	None	4[b]
c.5075A>C	p.(Asp1692Ala)	18	Missense	rs397509222	RCV000500821.1: VUS RCV000241473.1: VUS			CM169296(Disease-causing)	Deleterious	C65	Disease-causing (p = 1)	None	4
c.5095C>T	p.(Arg1699Trp)	18	Missense	rs55770810	RCV000048789.10: Pathogenic RCV000159999.4: Pathogenic RCV000077595.6: Pathogenic (ENIGMA) RCV000191041.1: Pathogenic RCV000457515.1: Pathogenic RCV000239322.2: Pathogenic RCV000131821.4: PathogenicRCV000148390.1: Pathogenic	ALL: 0.0024%EAS: 0.0058% NFE: 0.0018%FIN: 0.0090%OTH: T = 0.11%	EA: 0.01%	CM041706(Disease-causing)	Deleterious	C65	Disease-causing (p = 1)	None	5[b]
c.5096G>A	p.(Arg1699Gln)	18	Missense	rs41293459	RCV000031217.14: Likely pathogenic RCV000048790.6: Pathogenic/Likely pathogenic RCV000195350.6: Pathogenic/Likely pathogenicRCV000131564.6: Pathogenic/Likely pathogenic	ALL: 0.0024%NFE: 0.0054%		CM034007(Disease-causing)	Deleterious	C35	Disease-causing (p = 1)	None	4
c.5100A>G	p.(Thr1700Thr)	18	Synonymous	rs45519437	RCV000199783.5: Likely benign RCV000428938.2: Benign/Likely benign RCV000494789.2: Likely benign (ENIGMA) RCV000163399.2: Likely benign	ALL: 0.0028%AMR: 0.0060%SAS: 0.0032%NFE: 0.0036%	EA: 0.01%					None	2

Table 1 Variant entries in databases dbSNP, ClinVar and HGMD, as well as allele frequencies reported by gnomAD and ESP (ALL: All, AFR: African/African American, NFE: Non-Finnish European, AMR: Latino, EAS: East Asian, SAS: South Asian, OTH: Other) (Continued)

HGVS nucleotide variant	HGVS protein variant	Exon	Type	dbSNP	ClinVar	gnomAD	ESP	HGMD	SIFT	Align GVGD	Mutation taster	Splice prediction	Class
c.5116G>A	p.(Gly1706Arg)	18	Missense	rs886040864	RCV000494689.1: Pathogenic RCV000257990.3: Likely pathogenic/VUS			CM1612904(Disease-causing?)	Deleterious	C65	Disease-causing ($p=1$)	None	4
c.5123C>T	p.(Ala1708Val)	18	Missense	rs28897696	RCV000212194.4: VUS RCV000148393.1: VUS RCV000031221.5: VUS RCV000131166.5: VUS RCV000048803.10: VUS	ALL: 0.0024% AFR: 0.039%	EA: 0.01%AA: 0.05%	CM065004(Disease-causing)	Deleterious	C65	Disease-causing ($p=1$)	None	3
c.5125G>A	p.(Gly1709Arg)	18	Missense	rs886038197	RCV000546570.2: VUS RCV000241163.1: VUS RCV000571176.2: VUS				Deleterious	C15	Disease-causing ($p=1$)	None	3
c.5131A>C	p.(Lys1711Gln)	18	Missense		RCV000463327.1: VUS				Tolerated	C0	Disease-causing ($p=0.974$)	None	3
c.5252G>A	p.(Arg1751Gln)	20	Missense	rs80357442	RCV000112579.2: Benign (ENIGMA) RCV000257892.6: Benign RCV000162992.3: Benign/Likely benign RCV000168520.7: Benign/Likely benign/VUS RCV000148392.1: VUS	ALL: 0.00041% AMR: 0.00060% NFE: 0.00072%	EA: 0.01%	CM022328(Disease-causing?)	Deleterious	C0	Disease-causing ($p=0.999$)	None	1[a]
c.5309G>T	p.(Gly1770Val)	21	Missense		RCV000502156.1: Likely pathogenic RCV000477771.1: Likely pathogenic			CM133533(Disease-causing)	Deleterious	C0	Disease-causing ($p=1$)	None	4[b]
c.5326C>T	p.(Pro1776Ser)	21	Missense	rs1800757	RCV000480229.1: VUS RCV000477350.2: VUS		EA: 0.01%		Tolerated	C0	Polymorphism ($p=0.741$)	None	2
c.5348T>C	p.(Met1783Thr)	22	Missense	rs55808233	RCV000048954.7: Likely benign RCV000414204.1: VUS RCV000129758.4: Benign/Likely benign RCV000167822.8: Benign/Likely benign/VUS RCV000031240.7: Likely benign	ALL: 0.012%AFR: 0.18%AMR: 0.0060% OTH: 0.018%	AA: 0.18%	CM041721(Disease-causing?)	Deleterious	C45	Disease-causing ($p=0.999$)	None	2
c.5411T>A	p.(Val1804Asp)	23	Missense	rs80356920	RCV000167770.7: Benign RCV000162993.3: Benign/Likely benign RCV000120302.4: Likely benign RCV000148405.1: VUS	ALL: 0.010% AMR: 0.048%NFE: 0.0027%	EA: 0.02%	CM044859(Disease-causing?)	Tolerated	C0	Polymorphism ($p=1$)	None	2[a]

Table 1 Variant entries in databases dbSNP, ClinVar and HGMD, as well as allele frequencies reported by gnomAD and ESP (ALL: All, AFR: African/African American, NFE: Non-Finnish European, AMR: Latino, EAS: East Asian, SAS: South Asian, OTH: Other) (Continued)

HGVS nucleotide variant	HGVS protein variant	Exon	Type	dbSNP	ClinVar	gnomAD	ESP	HGMD	SIFT	Align GVGD	Mutation taster	Splice prediction	Class
					RCV001112647.4: Benign (ENIGMA)								
c.5477A>T	p.(Glu1826Leu)	24	Missense	rs730881499	RCV000160011.1: VUS	ALL: 0.0033% NFE: 0.00018% FIN: 0.0027%			Tolerated	C0	Polymorphism (p = 0.763)	None	2
c.5504G>A	p.(Arg1835Gln)	24	Missense	rs273902776	RCV000049023.6: VUS RCV000240743.1: VUS RCV000130437.5: VUS RCV000112685.1: VUS RCV000120265.3: VUS	ALL: 0.0028% AFR: 0.013% EAS: 0.0058% NFE: 0.00090%			Tolerated	C0	Disease-causing (p = 0.965)	None	3
c.5513T>G	p.(Val1838Gly)	24	Missense	rs80357107	RCV000241502.1: Likely pathogenic			CM169297(Disease-causing)	Deleterious	C35	Disease-causing (p = 1)	None	4

Variant predictions by SIFT, AlignGVGD and Mutation taster, as well as splicing effects predicted by SpliceSiteFinder-like, MaxEntScan, NNSPLICE and GeneSplicer. Alterations of ≥ 10% and agreement between three or more splice software were used as criteria for a variant to likely result in aberrant splicing. Class is the final classification following the ACMG 5-tier scheme, combining TA assay results and available data. Class with indications for benign (b) and pathogenic (p) were used as controls and were classified according to the ACMG criteria prior to this study

Plasmid preparation and mutagenesis

The *BRCA1* BRCT variants were introduced into the pcDNA3 GAL4 DBD:BRCA1(aa 1396–1863) plasmid (kindly provided by Alvaro N. A. Monteiro) with the QuikChange II XL Site-Directed Mutagenesis Kit procedure (Agilent Technologies, Santa Clara, CA, USA), as per manufacturer's instructions. Primers used for mutagenesis are summarised in Additional file 1: Table S1. Purification of plasmids was performed using the ZymoPURE™ Plasmid Maxiprep Kit and Zyppy™ Plasmid Miniprep Kit (Zymo Research, Irvine, CA, USA). Miniprep and the subsequent Maxiprep was performed once for each plasmid and used for all downstream applications. Plasmid quantification was performed using the Nanodrop® ND1000, and a 260/280 ratio between 1.7 and 1.9 was deemed satisfactory for plasmid purity. The quality of the plasmids was checked on an agarose gel. Correct incorporation of variants into pcDNA3 GAL4 DBD:BRCA1(aa 1396–1863) plasmid was verified using Sanger sequencing and the Big-Dye® Terminator v3.1. Cycle Sequencing Kit (Thermo Fisher, Waltham, MA, USA).

Transfection and cell cultivation

HEK293T (ATCC® CRL-3216™) and MDA-MB-231 (ATCC® HTB-26™) cells were cultured in Dulbecco's modified Eagle medium (DMEM) supplemented with 10% foetal bovine serum (FBS) and kept below 90% confluency prior to transfection experiments. The Lipofectamine® 3000 Transfection Reagent Kit (Invitrogen, Thermo Fisher, Waltham, MA, USA) was used for reverse-co-transfection of 0.2 µg reporter plasmid pGAL4-e1b-Luc (Firefly luciferase), 0.2 µg of pcDNA3 GAL4 DBD:BRCA1(aa 1396–1863) plasmid and 20 ng of reporter plasmid phRG-TK (Renilla luciferase). Ratios of Lipofectamine 3000 to P3000 were 1.75:1 for HEK293T and 1.2:1 for the MDA-MB-231. Cell suspensions of 4.0×10^4 HEK293T or MDA-MB-231 cells were added to the transfection mix in 96-well plates. Cells transfected exclusively with reporter plasmids pGAL4-e1b-Luc and phRG-TK were used to measure background. Cells transfected with pcDNA3 GAL4 DBD:BRCA1(aa 1396–1863) containing *BRCA1*(aa 1396–1863) wild type (wt) sequence, benign/likely benign variants c.4956G>A, c.5252G>A and c.5411T>A or pathogenic/likely pathogenic variants c.4964C>T, c.5095C>T and c.5309G>T, were used as controls. Cells were harvested 24 and 48 h post-transfection. All experiments were performed in sextuplicates and repeated at least three times.

Luciferase measurement

Luciferase measurements were conducted using the Dual Luciferase® Reporter Assay System Kit (Promega, Madison, Wi, USA) according to manufacturer's instructions. Using a BioTek® Synergy H1 luminometer (BioTek, Winooski, VT, USA); 50 µL of Luciferase Assay Reagent II (LARII) was injected into 5 µL cell lysate in a white half area µclear® 96-well plate (Greiner bio-one, Monroe, NC, USA) followed by light emission measurement and subsequent injection of 50 µL Stop&Glo reagent and final measurement. The Firefly/Renilla ratio was used to mitigate possible differences in transfection efficiencies and cell numbers. The mean of each sextuplicate was calculated and presented as the percentage of wt pcDNA3 GAL4 DBD:BRCA1(aa 1396–1863) activity. Student T test was used for statistical analysis, and p values < 0.05 was considered significant.

Western blot

The transfection experiments described under *Transfection and cell cultivation* were scaled to a 12-well plate setup for expression analysis of the GAL4 DBD:BRCA1(aa 1396–1863) fusion protein constructs by western blot analysis. Ten microgramme of sample protein was run on a 10% Mini-PROTEAN® TGX™ gel (Bio-Rad Laboratories, Hercules, CA, USA) and blotted onto 0.2 µm Nitrocellulose Membranes (Bio-Rad Laboratories, Hercules, CA, USA). The membranes were blocked with 5% BSA. Primary immunoblot staining was done using BRCA1 (D-9):sc-6954 (Santa Cruz Biotechnology, Dallas, TX, USA) in a 1:1000 dilution, overnight at 4 °C, and followed by staining with secondary antibody m-IgGκ BP-HRP: sc-516102 (Santa Cruz Biotechnology, Dallas, TX, USA) (1:1000) for 1 h at room temperature, before exposure using the ECL™ Prime Western Blotting Detection Reagent (GE Healthcare, Buckinghamshire, UK) with ImageQuant™ LAS 4000 and ImageQuant™ TL 1D v8.1 (GE Healthcare, Buckinghamshire, UK).

cDNA synthesis and mRNA expression

The cDNA synthesis was performed on equal amounts of RNA isolated from a 12-well transfection experiment, using the High Capacity cDNA Reverse Transcription kit (Applied Biosystems®, Thermo Fisher, Waltham, MA, USA) in accordance with manufacturer's instructions. Relative expression was measured with Applied Biosystems™ QuantStudio™ 12K Flex Real-Time System using SYBR™ green (Thermo Fisher, Waltham, MA, USA), and with *GAPDH* as reference gene. Relative expression (RQ) of pcDNA3 GAL4 DBD:BRCA1(aa 1396–1863) was calculated utilising the comparative ΔCt method with *GAPDH* as reference gene. Since amplification of pcDNA3 GAL4 DBD:BRCA1(aa 1396–1863) using SYBR™ green and *BRCA*-specific primers (Additional file 1: Table S2) also targets expression of endogenous *BRCA1*, non-transfected cells were used as reference to account for this.

Results

Trans-activation activity

Studying the effect of the *BRCA1* BRCT variants on the TA activity was performed in HEK293T and MDA-MB-231 cells after 48-h post-transfection incubation, for all variants included. The results (Fig. 2) revealed a high degree of TA activity similarity between the two cell lines. Variants with prior classification as likely benign/benign or likely pathogenic/pathogenic were used to estimate the range of TA activity in benign and deleterious variants, respectively. The 12 variants investigated in this study were divided into three groups based on a strict interpretation of the TA assay controls; no or low risk (TA ≥ 44%), high risk (TA ≤ 14%) and intermediate (14% < TA < 44%) (Fig. 2). Variants c.5096G>A and c.5123C>T displayed TA activities slightly above the estimated 14% threshold for pathogenicity (16.1–19.9% and 15.7–16.0% in MDA-MB-231 and HEK293T, respectively), but were not significantly different from the pathogenic control in the MDA-MB-231 cell line (p values 0.12 and 0.18 for c.5096G>A and c.5123C>T, respectively).

The effect of prolonged post-transfection incubation time on the sensitivity of the TA assay yielded a significant increase for variants with TA activities < 50% after 48-h incubation, compared to 24-h in both HEK293T and MDA-MB-231 cells (p values < 0.001, Fig. 3a, b). The

difference in TA activity between variants c.5131A>C and c.5348T>C (Fig. 3b) illustrated the increased sensitivity after 48 h by displaying a variation in TA activities that were not as clearly evident after 24 h.

Additive effects of variants

The TA activity of the plasmids containing the *in cis* variant combinations c.5075A>C/c.5411T>A and c.5252G>A/c.5477A>T were significantly different compared to the activity of plasmids containing each of these variants separately (Fig. 4, p values < 0.0001). The TA activity of c.5075A>C was low to begin with (0.86% in HEK293T and 0.91% in MDA-MB-231), inclusion of c.5411T>A reduced the TA activities additionally to 0.48% in HEK293T and 0.61% in MDA-MB-231. Variant c.5252G>A had TA activities of 52 and 44% of wt activity in cell lines HEK293T and MDA-MB-231, respectively, while variant c.5477A>T displayed increased TA activities in both cell lines; 136% in HEK293T and 150% in MDA-MB-231. The plasmid containing both variants had a TA activity of 76% in

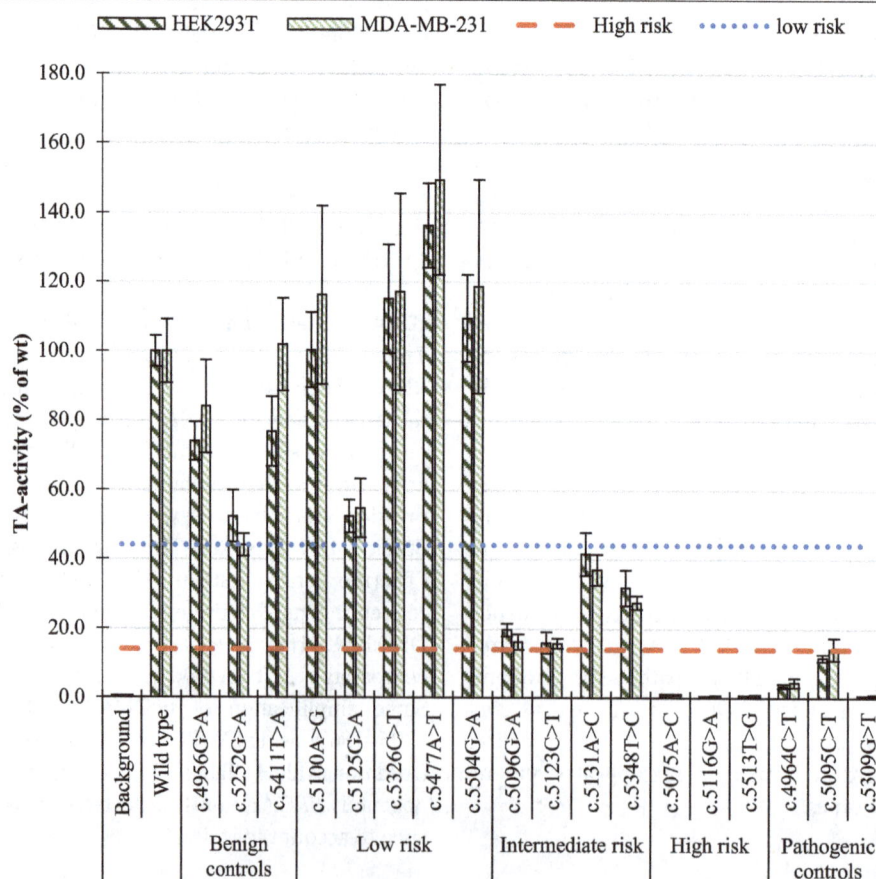

Fig. 2 TA activity of *BRCA1* BRCT variants in HEK293T (dark green), MDA-MB-231 (light green) cells. Activities were measured after 48-h post-transfection incubation. The area below the lower (red) line indicates high risk, the area above the upper (blue) line indicates low risk. The area between these lines identifies variants of intermediate risk. TA activity is displayed as mean percentage of wt for three to four experiments conducted in sextuplicates, with error bars representing the standard deviation ($n \geq 18$). The background is measured in cells transfected exclusively with reporter plasmids pGAL4-e1b-Luc (Firefly) and phRG-TK (Renilla)

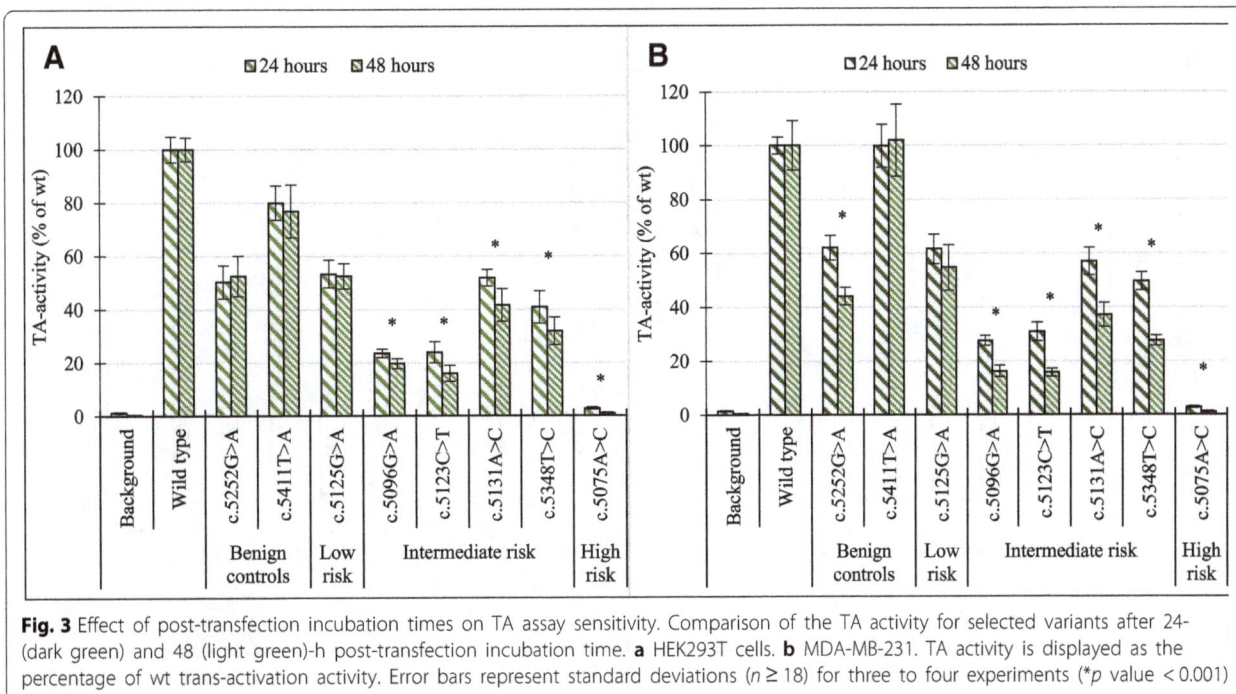

Fig. 3 Effect of post-transfection incubation times on TA assay sensitivity. Comparison of the TA activity for selected variants after 24- (dark green) and 48 (light green)-h post-transfection incubation time. **a** HEK293T cells. **b** MDA-MB-231. TA activity is displayed as the percentage of wt trans-activation activity. Error bars represent standard deviations ($n \geq 18$) for three to four experiments (*p value < 0.001)

HEK293T and 78% in MDA-MB-231, and c.5477A>T seemed to rescue some of the loss in TA activity caused by c.5252G>A.

Expression of the GAL4 DBD:BRCA1(aa 1396–1863) fusion protein

To confirm that the lack of TA activity was a result of the variant in question and not an inability to express the variant fusion protein, western blot analysis was performed on RIPA lysates from transfected HEK293T and MDA-MB-231 cells 48 h post-transfection (Additional file 1: Figure S1A and B, and Table S3). Cells transfected exclusively with the reporter plasmids and non-transfected cells were used as controls. Bands specific for the GAL4 DBD:BRCA1(aa 1396–1863) fusion protein were detected for all tested variants. Variants lacking TA activity (c.5075A>C and c.5309G>T) displayed weaker bands compared to the wt in HEK293T, but intensities comparable to the

wt in MDA-MB-231. Whereas variant c.5326C>T (TA activity > 100% in both cell lines) displayed weaker band intensity in MDA-MB-231 lysates than wt. Variant c.4964C>T, a positive control, with TA activity of 3.5% displayed band intensity comparable to the wt in HEK293T, and was stronger than the band observed for c.5348T>C with 32% TA activity, indicating a lack of correlation between TA activity and band intensity.

mRNA expression of the pcDNA3 GAL4 DBD:BRCA1(aa 1396–1863) fusion protein

The pcDNA3 GAL4 DBD:BRCA1(aa 1396–1863) mRNA expression results provided a control of the TA assay in addition to the western blots. The variability observed in pcDNA3 GAL4 DBD:BRCA1(aa 1396–1863) mRNA expression between wt, variants and cell lines (Fig. 5a, b) does not translate to the TA activities. Measured TA activity remains highly similar between cell lines despite

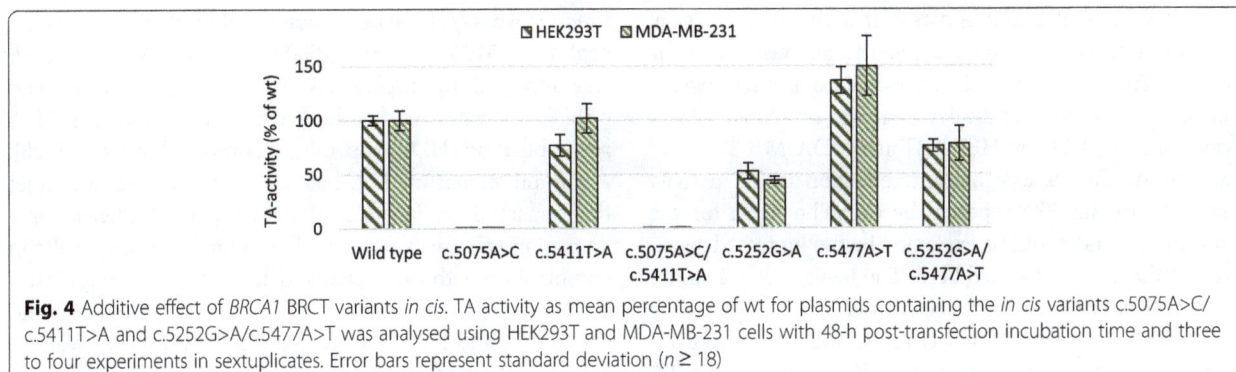

Fig. 4 Additive effect of *BRCA1* BRCT variants *in cis*. TA activity as mean percentage of wt for plasmids containing the *in cis* variants c.5075A>C/ c.5411T>A and c.5252G>A/c.5477A>T was analysed using HEK293T and MDA-MB-231 cells with 48-h post-transfection incubation time and three to four experiments in sextuplicates. Error bars represent standard deviation ($n \geq 18$)

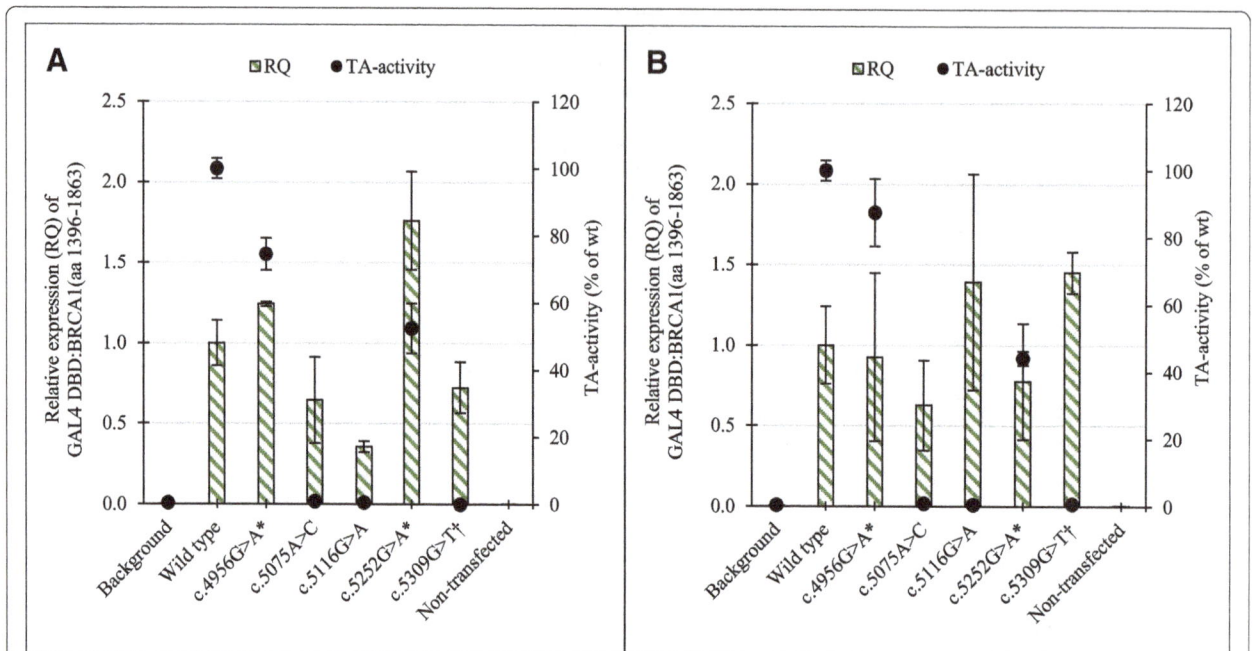

Fig. 5 Mean relative expression (RQ) of variant GAL4 DBD:BRCA1(aa 1396–1863) fusion protein in transfected cell lines. **a** HEK293T and **b** MDA-MB-231 (green bars) with corresponding TA activities (black dots). RQ is displayed as the relative expression between pcDNA3 GAL4 DBD:BRCA1(aa 1396–1863) and GAPDH. Error bars represent standard deviations ($n_{RQ} = 6$, $n_{TA} \leq 18$). The graph illustrates the independence between RQ and TA activity and is based on three qPCR experiments and three to four TA assay experiments

variations in the observed mRNA levels. There seem, however, to be a correlation between the western blot band intensities and the mRNA expression levels. Our results suggest that the measured TA activities were independent of mRNA levels and that they represent functional variant effects on the protein level.

Discussion
Risk thresholds
In order to use the TA assay for dividing variants into high- or low-risk categories, it was useful to define thresholds for measured TA activities representing a high- or low-risk variant. In a study by Carvalho et al., TA activity thresholds of $\leq 45\%$ and $\geq 50\%$ were proposed for categorising a variant as *high risk* or *low risk*, respectively [26]. While these thresholds likely remain true for the Carvalho et al.'s version of the TA assay, it is not apparent that this is a universal threshold that can be readily applied to all versions of the assay. Variant c.5095C>T (class 5) was used as a pathogenic control in our version of the TA assay and presented TA activities of 12 and 14% in HEK293T and MDA-MB-231 cells, respectively. This is a significant reduction in TA activity compared to the 45% reported by Carvalho et al. for the same variant and could be explained by the increased sensitivity of the assay presented here. The benign class 1 and 2 controls (c.4956G>A, c.5252G>A and c.5411T>A) were used to define the wt TA activity range, with the lowest observed TA activity in variant c.5252G>A, displaying TA

activities of 52 and 44% in HEK293T and MDA-MB-231 cells, respectively. The threshold for what ought to be regarded as high risk in this version of the TA assay was set at $\leq 14\%$, and the low-risk threshold at $\geq 44\%$. As no gain-of-function regarding TA activity has been reported to confer with pathogenicity, no upper wt boundary was set.

Risk assessment of *BRCA1* variants
The variants c.5100A>G, c.5125G>A, c.5326C>T, c.5477A>T and c.5504G>A presented with TA activities in the likely no/low-risk range defined by the TA assay controls and were therefore placed in the low-risk category. Four of these variants (c.5100A>G, c.5326C>T, c.5477A>T and c.5504G>A) presented TA activities higher than wt, whereas variant c.5125G>A displayed TA activity at the lower end of the low-risk range. To our knowledge, no functional assays have been performed on these variants except for c.5125G>A and c.5504G>A. Variant c.5125G>A was reported to display TA activity similar to wt, and c.5504G>A was found to have reduced homologous DNA recombination (HDR) capabilities compared to wt. [27, 28]. A computational method has also been utilised to predict the impact of variant c.5504G>A, but no evidence for a damaging effect was reported [29]. Our TA assay results in combination with the available data support a benign interpretation of variants c.5100A>G, c.5326C>T and c.5477A>T and that they are likely benign (class 2). Variant c.5125G>A could be considered a benign variant based on

the TA assay results. However, due to in silico predictions of a deleterious nature and the lack of alleles in a control population, the classification of this variant should be further investigated to rule out any uncertainty and therefore retains its status as a VUS (class 3). Variant c.5504G>A remains classified as a VUS despite wt-like results on the TA assay due to conflicting reports of a possibly deleterious impact on HDR functionality.

Variants c.5075A>C, c.5116G>A and c.5513T>G displayed a complete lack of TA activity on our TA assay, consistent with pathogenic variant behaviour and previously reported TA results for c.5075A>C and c.5513T>G [27]. The three variants were predicted to have a deleterious nature by all applied software, and none were reported in control populations, further supporting a deleterious interpretation. The variants were known to ClinVar where variants c.5075A>C and c.5513T>G were reported as VUSs, while c.5116G>A was reported as disease-causing. Variants c.5075A>C and c.5513T>G have been reported previously to abolish TA activity [27], and to our knowledge, no other functional assays have been performed on these variants prior to this study. Based on these data, it seems likely that all three variants represent likely pathogenic (class 4) BRCA1 variants.

Variants c.5096G>A, c.5123C>T, c.5131A>C and c.5348T>C presented TA activities in the intermediate range on the TA assay, and therefore, any risk related to these variants could not be ascertained based on the TA assay alone. However, variants c.5096G>A and c.5123C>T failed to present a significant difference in TA activity compared to pathogenic control c.5095C>T in the MDA-MB-231 cell line. Variant c.5096G>A has been reported to possess a deleterious effect on BRCA1 in multiple functional assays [30–33], with in silico analysis predicting a deleterious effect. However, the variant has been shown to result in a lower risk of cancer development than what is typically observed for BRCA1 variants [33, 34]. Variant c.5123C>T has been reported to be functionally compromised in multiple functional assays [30] and was suggested to be a moderately penetrant variant in a study using a multifactorial likelihood analysis and multiple functional assays [35]. The status of variant c.5096G>A as a likely pathogenic variant with moderate penetrance is rather well documented, and while c.5123C>T may prove to be of a similar nature, we believe it should retain its status as a VUS until more data can be acquired.

Unlike the aforementioned intermediate variants, c.5131A>C displayed TA activities closer to the low-risk threshold. Analysis using in silico prediction software failed to agree on the nature of the variant, and it was absent in control populations, supporting a deleterious interpretation. Until a better assessment of c.5131A>C can be performed, it should likely remain classified as a VUS (class 3).

Variant c.5348T>C presented TA activities in the middle of the intermediate range established by the TA assay controls. In silico analysis of the variant predicted a deleterious effect on the BRCA1 protein, in all applied software. The influence of the variant on the function of the protein has been illustrated in some functional assays, whereas others have shown the variant to be either wt or inconclusive [30, 36–38]. The variant is known to ClinVar, with three reports of a benign nature, three reports of a likely benign nature and one report of unknown significance. The allele frequencies reported for the c.5348T>C variant were higher than what was expected of a pathogenic variant (Table 1) and has largely been found in an African and Afro-American population [39]. It is uncertain if the variant represents a benign variant with a lower TA activity than defined in this study or a potential risk factor. However, given the amount of evidence indicating a benign nature, c.5348T>C could be regarded as a likely benign, class 2, variant.

Recent advances in functional studies of BRCA1 variants allow for a high throughput assessment of virtually any single nucleotide variant in the gene, or in functional domains of particular interest [40–42]. These methods have the distinct advantage of providing functional data on variants prior to their discovery in patients, thereby providing efficient classification relevant to clinical treatment. Comparing our results with those of Findlay et al. [40], we observe a high concordance between the TA assay and the saturation genome editing (SGE) data, particularly in the TA assay groups of high and low risk, including the pathogenic and benign controls. The only variant in the high-/low-risk groups that was classified differently between the two studies was c.5504G>A, that presented with a low-risk TA result but scored as an intermediate risk variant in the SGE dataset. The highest variability between the studies was found in variants placed in the intermediate risk category on the TA assay; variants c.5123C>T, c.5131A>C and c.5348T>C scored as functional on the SGE assay (c.5096G>A was not evaluated in the SGE assay).

Additive variant effects

To our knowledge, no publications have investigated the effects of BRCA1 variants in cis prior to our work, except for an investigation into the possible effects of including a polymorphism in combination with deleterious variants and VUSs that were unable to find any significant impact on TA activities [26]. We found that both in cis variant combinations tested revealed a significant effect. The combined variants c.5075A>C/c.5411T>A displayed an additional reduction in the TA activities compared to c.5075A>C alone; this could indicate that neutral variants can affect the performance of deleterious variants on the TA assay. Interestingly, the combination of c.5252G>A/c.5477A>T displayed TA activities in-between c.5252G>A and c.5477A>T alone, implying that the elevated TA activity of c.5477A>T was able to rescue some of the loss in the TA activity displayed by c.5252G>A. Considering the rarity of these particular variants, it seems unlikely that they will co-occur in any significant number of patients. However, it is an interesting observation that the co-occurrence of variants seemingly influences the performance of the TA assay in a synergistic manner and can potentially act as risk modifiers.

Increased post-transfection incubation time

The effect of increased post-transfection incubation time on the sensitivity of the TA assay revealed a significant benefit using 48-h incubation instead of 24 h on variants with TA activity < 50%. Other attempts at investigating BRCA1 variants utilising TA assays have usually been conducted with a post-transfection incubation period of 24 h [27, 30, 31, 43–45]. The improved sensitivity of the assay should enable a more precise distinction of intermediate variants that could be of clinical importance.

Reproducibility of TA activities in different cell lines

The data obtained from the TA assays revealed little variability between cell lines, especially at low TA activities. The MDA-MB-231 cells generally displayed larger variability in the data than the HEK293T cells, especially in variants with TA activity > 70%. We conclude that the reproducibility of the TA assay results was high and that variant risk assessment did not differ between the cell lines.

Limitations

There are several limitations to the TA assay, mainly that investigations of BRCA1 variants utilising the TA assay are limited to variants in or near the BRCT domains. Second, the assay is performed only on a subsection of the protein, and how well the TA assay reflects variant effect on full-length BRCA1 is largely unknown. Additionally, a wt-like result on the TA assay cannot be regarded as conclusive evidence towards harmlessness, as the biological effect of the missense variant can escape detection on this assay (e.g. variants resulting in aberrant splicing). Despite this, the TA assay provides a reliable assessment of the BRCT-domain integrity, and the reported correlation between cancer predisposing variants and TA results is high [46]. The ability of the TA assay to assess the integrity of the BRCT domains makes it well suited for efficiently dividing BRCA1 BRCT variants into risk groups but provides little or no explanation to the biological mechanism of how the variant contributes to tumorigenesis.

Conclusion

In conclusion, the modified TA assay presented here provides efficient risk assessment of rare missense variants found in the BRCA1 BRCT domains. The increased post-transfection incubation time yielded a significant increase in TA assay sensitivity which may enable a better characterisation of BRCA1 BRCT variants with intermediate TA activity. The results presented here may aid in a better classification of the 12 included VUSs, a classification that is vital for the proper clinical care of affected patients.

Additional file

Additional file 1: Table S1. Mutagenic primers used for introducing the variants into plasmid pcDNA3 GAL4 DBD:BRCA1(aa 1396–1863) by in vitro mutagenesis. The introduced variants are displayed in bold capital letters. Primers were designed according to the QuikChange II XL Site-Directed Mutagenesis Kit procedure (Agilent Technologies, Santa Clara, CA, USA) and provided by Eurofins (MWG Synthesis, GmbH). Table S2. Primers used for real-time quantification of endogenous BRCA1 and plasmid pcDNA3 GAL4 DBD:BRCA1(aa 1396–1863). Figure S1. Western blot illustrating the presence of GAL4 DBD:BRCA1(aa 1396–1863) fusion protein in transfected cell lines A) HEK293T and B) MDA-MB-231 protein lysates from TA assay. Figure legends are shown in Additional file 1: Table S2. Variant c.5513T>G was only analysed on western blot in MDA-MB-231 cells. Band specific for GAL4 DBD:BRCA1(aa 1396–1863) (~ 80 kDa) and loading control β-actin (42 kDa) are indicated by black arrows. Ladder sizes 50 and 75 kDa are indicated. Blots represent one representative gel for each transfected cell line. Table S3. Western blot legend displaying the well number for each variant/sample and its corresponding TA activity for blots A and B (Figure S1a, b). Variants with indications were benign (*) and pathogenic (†

Abbreviations

aa: Amino acid; BRCT: BRCA1 C-terminal; DBD: DNA-binding domain; HBOC: Hereditary Breast and Ovarian Cancer; HRR: Homologous recombination repair; MPAF: Maximal pathogenic allele frequency; RQ: Relative quantification; SRE: Splicing regulatory element; TA: Transactivation; wt: Wild type

Acknowledgements

We would like to thank Alvaro N. Monteiro for kindly providing the plasmid, Marit Sletten for helpful assistance with the transfection procedures and Deeqa Ahmed and Magnhild Fjeldvær for valuable help regarding variant interpretation.

Funding

This work was funded by the Oslo University Hospital, Ullevål, Oslo.

Authors' contributions

JL designed experiments, analysed results and wrote the paper. EJ and MVG provided and interpreted western blot analyses and edited the paper. SA and NI planned the project, interpreted results and edited the paper. NI designed the research. All authors have read and approved the final manuscript.

Competing interests

The authors declare that they have no competing interests.

Author details

[1]Department of Medical Genetics, Oslo University Hospital, Oslo, Norway. [2]Department of Medical Genetics, Division of Child and Adolescent Health, University Hospital of North Norway, Tromsø, Norway.

References

1. IARC. GLOBOCAN 2012: estimated cancer incidence, mortality and prevalence worldwide in 2012 http://globocan.iarc.fr/Pages/fact_sheets_population.aspx?country=900 Available from: http://globocan.iarc.fr/Pages/fact_sheets_population.aspx?country=900.
2. van Marcke C, De Leener A, Berliere M, Vikkula M, Duhoux FP. Routine use of gene panel testing in hereditary breast cancer should be performed with caution. Crit Rev Oncol Hematol. 2016;108:33–9.
3. Roy R, Chun J, Powell SN. BRCA1 and BRCA2: different roles in a common pathway of genome protection. Nat Rev Cancer. 2011;12(1):68–78.
4. Nielsen FC, van Overeem HT, Sorensen CS. Hereditary breast and ovarian cancer: new genes in confined pathways. Nat Rev Cancer. 2016;16(9):599–612.
5. Katsuki Y, Takata M. Defects in homologous recombination repair behind the human diseases: FA and HBOC. Endocr Relat Cancer. 2016;23(10):T19–37.
6. Millot GA, Carvalho MA, Caputo SM, Vreeswijk MP, Brown MA, Webb M, et al. A guide for functional analysis of BRCA1 variants of uncertain significance. Hum Mutat. 2012;33(11):1526–37.
7. Korlimarla A, Bhandary L, Prabhu JS, Shankar H, Sankaranarayanan H, Kumar P, et al. Identification of a non-canonical nuclear localization signal (NLS) in BRCA1 that could mediate nuclear localization of splice variants lacking the classical NLS. Cell Mol Biol Lett. 2013;18(2):284–96.
8. Chen CF, Li S, Chen Y, Chen PL, Sharp ZD, Lee WH. The nuclear localization sequences of the BRCA1 protein interact with the importin-alpha subunit of the nuclear transport signal receptor. J Biol Chem. 1996;271(51):32863–8.
9. Thakur S, Zhang HB, Peng Y, Le H, Carroll B, Ward T, et al. Localization of BRCA1 and a splice variant identifies the nuclear localization signal. Mol Cell Biol. 1997;17(1):444–52.
10. Clark SL, Rodriguez AM, Snyder RR, Hankins GD, Boehning D. Structure-function of the tumor suppressor BRCA1. Comput Struct Biotechnol J. 2012; 1(1). https://doi.org/10.5936/csbj.201204005.
11. Miki Y, Swensen J, Shattuck-Eidens D, Futreal PA, Harshman K, Tavtigian S, et al. A strong candidate for the breast and ovarian cancer susceptibility gene BRCA1. Science. 1994;266(5182):66–71.
12. Monteiro AN, August A, Hanafusa H. Evidence for a transcriptional activation function of BRCA1 C-terminal region. Proc Natl Acad Sci U S A. 1996;93(24): 13595–9.
13. Prakash R, Zhang Y, Feng W, Jasin M. Homologous recombination and human health: the roles of BRCA1, BRCA2, and associated proteins. Cold Spring Harb Perspect Biol. 2015;7(4):a016600.
14. Shakya R, Reid LJ, Reczek CR, Cole F, Egli D, Lin CS, et al. BRCA1 tumor suppression depends on BRCT phosphoprotein binding, but not its E3 ligase activity. Science. 2011;334(6055):525–8.
15. Gartel AL, Radhakrishnan SK. Lost in transcription: p21 repression, mechanisms, and consequences. Cancer Res. 2005;65(10):3980–5.
16. Somasundaram K, Zhang H, Zeng YX, Houvras Y, Peng Y, Zhang H, et al. Arrest of the cell cycle by the tumour-suppressor BRCA1 requires the CDK-inhibitor p21WAF1/CiP1. Nature. 1997;389(6647):187–90.
17. MacLachlan TK, Somasundaram K, Sgagias M, Shifman Y, Muschel RJ, Cowan KH, et al. BRCA1 effects on the cell cycle and the DNA damage response are linked to altered gene expression. J Biol Chem. 2000;275(4):2777–85.
18. Yarden RI, Pardo-Reoyo S, Sgagias M, Cowan KH, Brody LC. BRCA1 regulates the G2/M checkpoint by activating Chk1 kinase upon DNA damage. Nat Genet. 2002;30(3):285–9.
19. Mullan PB, Quinn JE, Harkin DP. The role of BRCA1 in transcriptional regulation and cell cycle control. Oncogene. 2006;25(43):5854–63.
20. Wang XW, Zhan Q, Coursen JD, Khan MA, Kontny HU, Yu L, et al. GADD45 induction of a G2/M cell cycle checkpoint. Proc Natl Acad Sci U S A. 1999; 96(7):3706–11.
21. Fan S, Ma YX, Wang C, Yuan RQ, Meng Q, Wang JA, et al. Role of direct interaction in BRCA1 inhibition of estrogen receptor activity. Oncogene. 2001;20(1):77–87.
22. Wang L, Di LJ. BRCA1 and estrogen/estrogen receptor in breast cancer: where they interact? Int J Biol Sci. 2014;10(5):566–75.
23. Simoes BM, Piva M, Iriondo O, Comaills V, Lopez-Ruiz JA, Zabalza I, et al. Effects of estrogen on the proportion of stem cells in the breast. Breast Cancer Res Treat. 2011;129(1):23–35.
24. Moisan A, Larochelle C, Guillemette B, Gaudreau L. BRCA1 can modulate RNA polymerase II carboxy-terminal domain phosphorylation levels. Mol Cell Biol. 2004;24(16):6947–56.
25. Song W, Gardner SA, Hovhannisyan H, Natalizio A, Weymouth KS, Chen W, et al. Exploring the landscape of pathogenic genetic variation in the ExAC population database: insights of relevance to variant classification. Genet Med. 2016;18(8):850–4.
26. Carvalho MA, Marsillac SM, Karchin R, Manoukian S, Grist S, Swaby RF, et al. Determination of cancer risk associated with germ line BRCA1 missense variants by functional analysis. Cancer Res. 2007;67(4):1494–501.
27. Jarhelle E, Riise Stensland HMF, Mæhle L, et al. Familial Cancer. 2017;16:1. https://doi.org/10.1007/s10689-016-9916-2.
28. Lu C, Xie M, Wendl MC, Wang J, McLellan MD, Leiserson MD, et al. Patterns and functional implications of rare germline variants across 12 cancer types. Nat Commun. 2015;6:10086.
29. Iversen ES Jr, Couch FJ, Goldgar DE, Tavtigian SV, Monteiro AN. A computational method to classify variants of uncertain significance using functional assay data with application to BRCA1. Cancer Epidemiol Biomark Prev. 2011;20(6):1078–88.
30. Lee MS, Green R, Marsillac SM, Coquelle N, Williams RS, Yeung T, et al. Comprehensive analysis of missense variations in the BRCT domain of BRCA1 by structural and functional assays. Cancer Res. 2010;70(12):4880–90.
31. Vallon-Christersson J, Cayanan C, Haraldsson K, Loman N, Bergthorsson JT, Brondum-Nielsen K, et al. Functional analysis of BRCA1 C-terminal missense mutations identified in breast and ovarian cancer families. Hum Mol Genet. 2001;10(4):353–60.
32. Bouwman P, van der Gulden H, van der Heijden I, Drost R, Klijn CN, Prasetyanti P, et al. A high-throughput functional complementation assay for classification of BRCA1 missense variants. Cancer Discov. 2013;3(10):1142–55.
33. Spurdle AB, Whiley PJ, Thompson B, Feng B, Healey S, Brown MA, et al. BRCA1 R1699Q variant displaying ambiguous functional abrogation confers intermediate breast and ovarian cancer risk. J Med Genet. 2012;49(8):525–32.
34. Moghadasi S, Meeks HD, Vreeswijk MP, Janssen LA, Borg A, Ehrencrona H, et al. The BRCA1 c. 5096G>A p.Arg1699Gln (R1699Q) intermediate risk variant: breast and ovarian cancer risk estimation and recommendations for clinical management from the ENIGMA consortium. J Med Genet. 2018;55(1):15–20.
35. Lovelock PK, Spurdle AB, Mok MT, Farrugia DJ, Lakhani SR, Healey S, et al. Identification of BRCA1 missense substitutions that confer partial functional activity: potential moderate risk variants? Breast Cancer Res. 2007;9(6):R82.
36. Coyne RS, McDonald HB, Edgemon K, Brody LC. Functional characterization of BRCA1 sequence variants using a yeast small colony phenotype assay. Cancer Biol Ther. 2004;3(5):453–7.
37. Gaboriau DC, Rowling PJ, Morrison CG, Itzhaki LS. Protein stability versus function: effects of destabilizing missense mutations on BRCA1 DNA repair activity. Biochem J. 2015;466(3):613–24.
38. Drikos I, Nounesis G, Vorgias CE. Characterization of cancer-linked BRCA1-BRCT missense variants and their interaction with phosphoprotein targets. Proteins. 2009;77(2):464–76.
39. McKean-Cowdin R, Spencer Feigelson H, Xia LY, Pearce CL, Thomas DC, Stram DO, et al. BRCA1 variants in a family study of African-American and Latina women. Hum Genet. 2005;116(6):497–506.
40. Findlay GM, Daza RM, Martin B, Zhang MD, Leith AP, Gasperini M, et al. Accurate classification of BRCA1 variants with saturation genome editing. Nature. 2018;562(7726):217–22.
41. Starita LM, Islam MM, Banerjee T, Adamovich AI, Gullingsrud J, Fields S, et al. A multiplex homology-directed DNA repair assay reveals the impact of more than 1,000 BRCA1 missense substitution variants on protein function. Am J Hum Genet. 2018;103(4):498–508.
42. Starita LM, Young DL, Islam M, Kitzman JO, Gullingsrud J, Hause RJ, et al. Massively parallel functional analysis of BRCA1 RING domain variants. Genetics. 2015;200(2):413–22.

19

Multiple genotype–phenotype association study reveals intronic variant pair on *SIDT2* associated with metabolic syndrome in a Korean population

Sanghoon Moon[1†], Young Lee[1,2†], Sungho Won[3] and Juyoung Lee[1*]

Abstract

Background: Metabolic syndrome is a risk factor for type 2 diabetes and cardiovascular disease. We identified common genetic variants that alter the risk for metabolic syndrome in the Korean population. To isolate these variants, we conducted a multiple-genotype and multiple-phenotype genome-wide association analysis using the family-based quasi-likelihood score (MFQLS) test. For this analysis, we used 7211 and 2838 genotyped study subjects for discovery and replication, respectively. We also performed a multiple-genotype and multiple-phenotype analysis of a gene-based single-nucleotide polymorphism (SNP) set.

Results: We found an association between metabolic syndrome and an intronic SNP pair, rs7107152 and rs1242229, in *SIDT2* gene at 11q23.3. Both SNPs correlate with the expression of *SIDT2* and *TAGLN*, whose products promote insulin secretion and lipid metabolism, respectively. This SNP pair showed statistical significance at the replication stage.

Conclusions: Our findings provide insight into an underlying mechanism that contributes to metabolic syndrome.

Keywords: Multiple variants, Multiple traits, Metabolic syndrome, 11q23.3, *SIDT2*

Introduction

Metabolic syndrome is a cluster of metabolic risk factors for cardiovascular disease and type 2 diabetes that are attributable to both genetic and environmental factors [1–3]. The National Cholesterol Education Program's Adult Treatment Panel III report (2001) defined metabolic syndrome as a combination of components such as high blood pressure, elevated fasting plasma glucose, high serum triglycerides, and abnormal low-density lipoprotein (LDL) and high-density lipoprotein (HDL) cholesterol levels [4]. Because of the fast-growing economy and rapid industrialization of Korea, metabolic syndrome is likely to become a major public health problem [5].

Many genetic variants that are associated with metabolic syndrome have been identified by genome-wide association studies (GWASs). However, because these known genetic variants account for only a fraction of the heritability of metabolic syndrome, the genetic determinants of this condition remain undefined [6, 7]. Many common variants with very small effect sizes that are widely distributed across the genome cannot be identified by the use of traditional GWAS cutoffs [8]. Experimental sample sizes must be large because the statistical power to detect associations between DNA variants and a trait depends on the sample size [9]. However, the cost and difficulties of sample collection inhibit the ability to continuously increase the sample size of GWASs [10]. Joint analysis approaches that analyze multiple genotypes and phenotypes have shown improved ability to detect variants relative to single-variant association analyses of the same-size sample [11–13]. A statistical approach called the MFQLS (http://healthstat.snu.ac.kr/software/mfqls/) test enables the estimation of the genetic relation matrix from population-based samples [14]. From the results of a single test for association with a set of traits, multiple genotype–multiple phenotype analysis reduces the number of

* Correspondence: jylee@cdc.go.kr
†Sanghoon Moon and Young Lee contributed equally to this work.
[1]Division of Genome Research, Center for Genome Science, Korea National Institute of Health, Cheongju, Chungcheongbuk-do 28159, South Korea
Full list of author information is available at the end of the article

tests and mitigates the multiple testing issues, resulting in increased statistical power [13, 14]. This approach identifies genetic variants that have pleiotropic effects for metabolic syndrome and other diseases.

We conducted a multiple single nucleotide polymorphism (SNP)–multiple trait analysis to identify genetic variants associated with metabolic syndrome by utilizing 10,049 samples from Korean subjects. After the multiple-genotype and multiple-phenotype analysis (multi-SNP–multi-trait analysis), 27 SNP pairs were associated with metabolic syndrome in the discovery stage and successfully replicated. Of those pairs, from the joint analysis of a single genotype and multiple phenotypes (single-SNP–multi-trait analysis), we found that three SNP pairs in the respective genes *SIDT2*, *UBASH3B*, and *CUX2* were significant in the multi-SNP–multi-trait analysis but not significant in the single-SNP–multi-trait analysis. *SIDT2* was not previously reported in the NHGRI-EBI GWAS Catalog (https://www.ebi.ac.uk/gwas/) [15] and was significant in the gene-based SNP set and multi-trait analysis. The Genotype-Tissue Expression (GTEx) database shows rs7107152 and rs1242229 on *SIDT2* correlates with *SIDT2* and *TAGLN* expression (https://www.gtexportal.org/home/) [16]. Our findings support the effectiveness of the multi-SNP–multi-trait analysis to identify new susceptible loci in complex diseases.

Results
Multi-SNP-multi-trait analysis
We conducted the multi-SNP–multi-trait genome-wide analysis of metabolic syndrome using 10,049 samples from Korean subjects. We considered six quantitative components of metabolic syndrome: systolic blood pressure (SBP), diastolic blood pressure (DBP), high-density lipoprotein (HDL), fasting plasma glucose (FPG), triglyceride, and waist circumference. Through the multi-SNP–multi-trait genome-wide analysis, adjusted for age and sex, 27 SNP pairs satisfied a Bonferroni-adjusted P value threshold of $P < 0.05$ ($P = 1.45 \times 10^{-7}$) and were successfully replicated (Tables 1 and 2). All but four of the mapped genes (*SIK3*, *SIDT2*, *UBASH3B*, and *CUX2*) had been previously reported to be associated with metabolic syndrome, as indicated by a keyword search of "metabolic syndrome" in the GWAS catalog (Tables 1 and 2).

Single SNP set-multi-trait analysis
The relation of the individual SNPs, including those on *SIK3*, *SIDT2*, *UBASH3B*, and *CUX2*, to metabolic syndrome was further examined by single-SNP–multi-trait analysis, adjusted for age and sex. Intronic SNPs on *SIK3* showed genome-wide significance in single-SNP–multi-trait analysis (Table 1), but SNPs on *SIDT2*, *UBASH3B*, and *CUX2* not identified by this approach (Table 2).

Gene-based SNP set-multi-trait analysis
We conducted gene-based SNP set–multi-trait analysis on 14,475 SNP sets. The mean and median numbers of SNPs in a set were 6.895 and 3, respectively (Additional file 1: Table S1). Table 3 shows the gene-based test results. Three genes reached a Bonferroni-adjusted P value threshold ($P < 3.45 \times 10^{-6}$). All three genes satisfied statistical significance in the meta-analysis. The number of SNPs in three genes ranges from 3 to 14. SNP sets in two genes (*PAFAH1B2* and *SIDT2*) showed significant P values of $< 3.45 \times 10^{-6}$ in the gene-based test and reached a nominal P value threshold of < 0.05 in the replication stage. Although the results of tests in which 14 SNPs were utilized in *CUX2* were significant in the discovery stage, there was only a suggested P value of 0.06 in the replication analysis (Table 3). Table 3 also shows the SNPs used in each SNP set.

Expression QTL pattern of identified SNP pair
To examine the correlation between two SNPs (rs7107152 and rs1242229) on the *SIDT2* gene and gene expression, we utilized three online resources: the Genotype-Tissue Expression (GTEx) project (https://www.gtexportal.org/home/) [16], the NESDA NTR Conditional Expression Quantitative Trait Loci (eQTL) catalog (https://eqtl.onderzoek.io/), and RegulomeDB (http://www.regulomedb.org/) [17]. All three databases showed that the two SNPs correlated with *SIDT2* and *TAGLN* expressions. The GTEx project showed that for rs7107152, the statistical significance of *SIDT2* and *TAGLN* expression in whole blood was $P = 3.89 \times 10^{-14}$ and $P = 3.59 \times 10^{-47}$, respectively (Additional file 1: Figure S1A), and for rs1242229, the P values were 3.64×10^{-13} and 4.78×10^{-12}, respectively (Additional file 1: Figure S1B) [16]. Additional file 1: Figure S1C–F show gene expression patterns by genotype for the two SNPs. The eQTL catalog showed similar gene expression patterns for the two SNPs (Additional file 1: Figure S2). The SNP rs1242229 was mainly expressed in *SIDT2* and *TAGLN*, whereas the SNP rs7107152 showed gene expression patterns not only in *SIDT2* and *TAGLN* but also in *PCSK7* and *PAFAH1B2* (Additional file 1: Figure S2). Additional file 1: Figure S3 shows the gene expression pattern for rs1242229 in RegulomeDB [17].

Correlation test with previously reported SNPs
To calculate the correlation of the identified SNPs (rs7107152 and rs1242229) in the current study and nearby SNPs reported in the GWAS catalog (intronic variant rs530885291, associated with HDL cholesterol level, and intergenic variant rs508487, associated with triglyceride level), we conducted a pairwise linkage disequilibrium (LD) analysis utilizing the SNP Annotation and Proxy Search (SNAP) server (https://www.broadinstitute.org/snap/snap) [18]. The pairwise LD analysis showed that

Table 1 Twenty-four SNP pairs that were significant in both single- and multi-SNP–multi-trait analyses

SNP pair	Gene	Publication of mapped gene in GWAS catalog	P value from a single SNP–multi trait analysis			P value from multi SNP–multi trait analysis (A Bonferroni-adjusted P value = 1.45×10^{-7})		
			Discovery	Replication	Meta P value	Discovery	Replication	Meta P value
rs2293571, **rs780094**	GCKR	[6, 19, 20, 36]	2.39E-03, 2.55E-12	9.46E-02, 1.85E-06	2.12E-03, 1.93E-16	4.98E-14	6.21E-05	1.28E-16
rs780094, rs780092	GCKR	[6, 19, 20, 36]	2.55E-12, 2.08E-11	1.85E-06, 1.36E-02	1.93E-16, 8.46E-12	2.02E-14	5.62E-05	4.80E-17
rs780092, rs8179252	GCKR	[6, 19, 20, 36]	2.08E-11, 1.93E-03	1.36E-02, 1.26E-02	8.46E-12, 2.83E-04	1.02E-13	4.17E-05	1.74E-16
rs263, rs271	LPL	[6, 19, 37]	2.09E-10, 6.96E-11	1.40E-05, 1.57E-05	1.01E-13, 3.87E-14	2.30E-09	2.43E-05	1.76E-12
rs12545984, **rs10503669**	LPL-SLC18A1	[6, 19, 37]	2.43E-01, 1.74E-15	2.24E-01, 9.06E-11	2.13E-01,9.16E-24	1.81E-14	9.20E-10	8.90E-22
rs10503669, rs17410962	LPL-SLC18A1	[6, 19, 37]	1.74E-15, 1.85E-16	9.06E-11, 4.76E-11	9.16E-24, 5.37E-25	3.35E-14	5.28E-09	9.04E-21
rs17489282, rs4922117	LPL-SLC18A1	[6, 19, 37]	4.80E-12, 1.09E-12	2.82E-07, 1.82E-07	5.70E-17, 8.74E-18	3.35E-11	6.59E-06	8.18E-15
rs765547, rs11986942	LPL-SLC18A1	[6, 19, 37]	7.30E-13, 1.54E-12	3.55E-07, 1.46E-07	1.13E-17, 9.88E-18	1.79E-11	2.43E-07	1.78E-16
rs11986942, rs1837842	LPL-SLC18A1	[6, 19, 37]	1.54E-12, 2.16E-12	1.46E-07, 3.57E-07	9.88E-18, 3.29E-17	1.21E-10	1.24E-06	5.62E-15
rs1837842, rs1919484	LPL-SLC18A1	[6, 19, 37]	2.16E-12, 1.57E-12	3.57E-07, 4.14E-07	3.29E-17, 2.79E-17	4.43E-10	3.19E-05	4.65E-13
rs1919484, rs7461115	LPL-SLC18A1	[6, 19, 37]	1.57E-12, 1.77E-12	4.14E-07, 2.61E-07	2.79E-17, 2.00E-17	8.62E-11	1.68E-05	5.09E-14
rs7013777, rs4442164	LPL-SLC18A1	[6, 19, 37]	7.61E-13, 1.08E-01	2.12E-07, 3.63E-01	7.14E-18, 1.66E-01	1.40E-16	1.09E-07	8.17E-22
rs4442164, **rs4244457**	LPL-SLC18A1	[6, 19, 37]	1.08E-01, 3.42E-14	3.63E-01, 4.04E-06	1.66E-01, 6.14E-18	1.39E-15	1.50E-05	9.66E-19
rs4244457, rs4449813	LPL-SLC18A1	[6, 19, 37]	3.42E-14, 3.20E-01	4.04E-06, 2.28E-01	6.14E-18, 2.64E-01	3.54E-14	1.69E-05	2.57E-17
rs12686004, rs3905000	ABCA1	[6]	1.25E-09, 6.74E-02	1.13E-02, 7.66E-01	3.67E-10, 2.05E-01	3.08E-10	4.22E-02	3.39E-10
rs481843, rs486394	LOC101929011	[38]	2.40E-06, 4.03E-08	6.85E-03, 1.79E-03	3.11E-07, 1.76E-09	3.33E-08	1.85E-02	1.37E-08
rs180344, **rs11216126**	LOC101929011-BUD13	[19, 38]	9.22E-02, 3.70E-20	9.04E-01, 3.25E-08	2.90E-01, 7.57E-26	5.54E-20	5.66E-07	1.87E-24
rs6589566, rs603446	ZPR1	[6]	8.27E-26, 9.02E-14	2.69E-12, 1.15E-05	1.90E-35, 4.40E-17	1.03E-28	3.51E-12	3.32E-38
rs6589566, rs6589567	APOA5-APOA4	[38]	8.27E-06, 1.14E-06	2.95E-02, 1.82E-05	3.96E-06, 5.31E-10	6.60E-09	2.32E-05	4.67E-12
rs12279433, rs11827828	SIK3	--	2.29E-07, 3.35E-05	2.85E-05, 6.27E-01	1.75E-10, 2.47E-04	1.35E-09	6.84E-04	2.65E-11
rs11827828, rs2044426	SIK3	--	3.35E-05, 2.23E-07	6.27E-01, 9.96E-06	2.47E-04, 6.18E-11	1.30E-09	2.84E-04	1.09E-11
rs10892044, rs11216186	SIK3	--	7.85E-05, 1.14E-06	6.58E-01, 5.91E-05	5.62E-04, 1.65E-09	1.64E-08	1.40E-03	5.85E-10
rs2074356, rs11066194	HECTD4	[21]	8.85E-24, 4.83E-02	9.27E-07, 4.76E-01	5.58E-28, 1.10E-01	1.19E-20	2.49E-05	1.70E-23
rs11631342, **rs6494005**	LIPC	[6, 19]	6.22E-08, 1.41E-10	3.16E-01, 1.51E-02	3.68E-07, 5.93E-11	1.63E-14	1.24E-02	7.51E-15

SNPs that are listed in GWAS catalog are shown in boldface

Table 2 Three SNP pairs that were significant only in the multi-SNP–multi-trait analysis

SNP pair	CHR	Position (hg19)	Gene	Annotation	Single-multi P value			Multi-multi P value (A Bonferroni-adjusted P value of discovery stage = 1.45×10^{-7})		
					Discovery	Replication	Meta P value	Discovery	Replication	Meta P value
rs7107152	11	117,056,080	SIDT2	Intronic	2.59E-01	8.43E-01	5.51E-01	1.40E-08	2.32E-03	8.17E-10
rs1242229	11	117,062,370	SIDT2	Intronic	5.39E-03	7.68E-02	3.64E-03			
rs10892876	11	122,540,281	UBASH3B	Intronic	2.93E-01	1.27E-01	1.60E-01	3.34E-12	3.82E-03	4.21E-13
rs12290043	11	122,540,528	UBASH3B	Intronic	1.62E-01	1.46E-01	1.12E-01			
rs886126	12	111,679,214	CUX2	Intronic	3.51E-01	1.79E-01	2.37E-01	5.09E-13	3.35E-03	5.97E-14
rs2078851	12	111,690,579	CUX2	Intronic	7.31E-05	6.63E-02	6.42E-05			

Single-multi P value P value from a single-SNP–multi-trait association analysis, *multi-multi P value* P value from a multi-SNP–multi-trait association analysis, *CHR* chromosome, *Meta P value* P value from meta-analysis

rs1242229 had a squared correlation of $r^2 = 0.167$ with rs508487 (Fig. 1). The correlation score between rs7107152 and rs530885291, however, was lower than the cutoff score.

SNP pair-single trait analysis

A radar chart shows the results of the rs7107152 and rs1242229 SNP metabolic syndrome-component trait association pair analysis (Additional file 1: Figure S4). The SNP pair correlated with HDL ($P = 5.87 \times 10^{-5}$) and triglycerides ($P = 1.67 \times 10^{-9}$). Moreover, it showed a suggestive association with diastolic blood pressure ($P = 0.07$). But it did not correlate with waist circumference ($P = 0.75$), fasting plasma glucose ($P = 0.55$), systolic blood pressure ($P = 0.29$).

Discussion

Utilizing the MFQLS test, we found 27 SNP pairs associated with metabolic syndrome based on multi-SNP–multiple continuous phenotypes. Our keyword search

Table 3 Results from a gene-based SNP set and multi-trait analysis

Gene	The number of SNP	Chromosome	Position (hg19)	Maximum r^2	P value (a Bonferroni-adjusted P value of discovery stage P = 3.45×10^{-6})		
					Discovery	Replication	Meta P value
PAFAH1B2	rs12420127	11	117,035,319	0.466	4.00E-07	3.99E-03	3.39E-08
	rs10790175		117,034,729				
	rs10892082		117,039,325				
SIDT2	rs2269399	11	117,066,353	0.456	2.31E-07	3.83E-03	1.93E-08
	rs1242229		117,062,370				
	rs1784042		117,065,476				
	rs7107152		117,056,080				
CUX2	rs7952972	12	111,646,519	0.561	3.28E-10	6.34E-02	5.32E-10
	rs886126		111,679,214				
	rs7300082		111,737,115				
	rs4766553		111,634,281				
	rs1265566		111,716,376				
	rs9783423		111,639,456				
	rs7398833		111,786,892				
	rs16941414		111,779,792				
	rs6489979		111,614,736				
	rs16941284		111,610,723				
	rs16941319		111,646,853				
	rs11065851		111,723,739				
	rs756825		111,598,202				
	rs7300860		111,754,597				

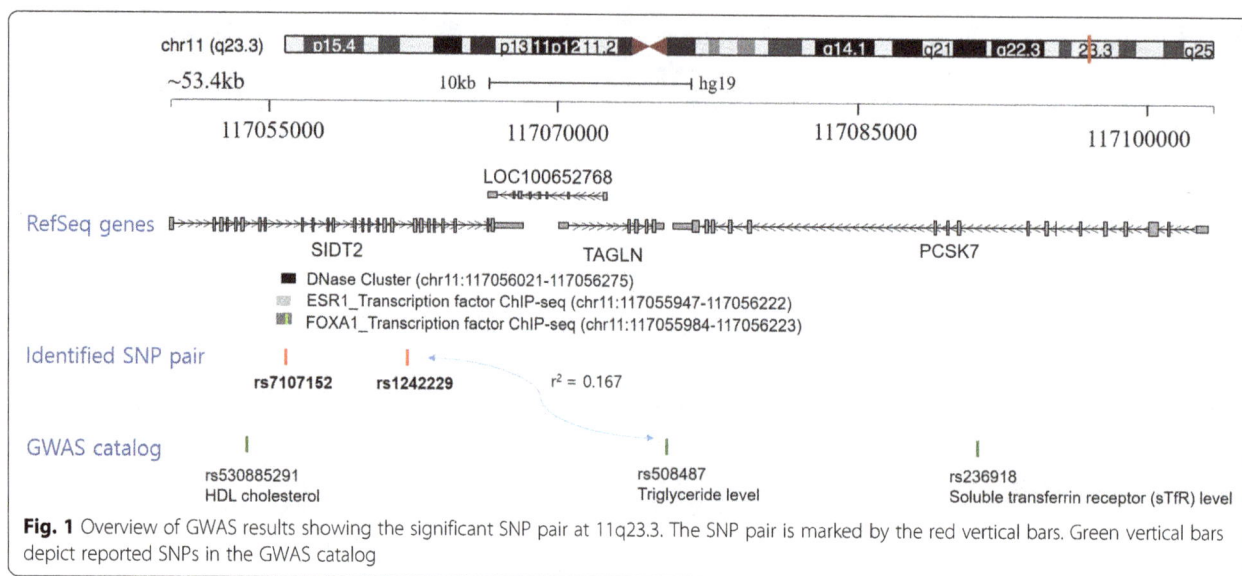

Fig. 1 Overview of GWAS results showing the significant SNP pair at 11q23.3. The SNP pair is marked by the red vertical bars. Green vertical bars depict reported SNPs in the GWAS catalog

for the term "metabolic syndrome" found single-variant association results in the GWAS catalog. The association of metabolic syndrome or metabolic syndrome-component traits with 21 SNP pairs was found in the GWAS catalog [15], whereas the association of 6 SNP pairs on the genes SIK3, SIDT2, UBASH3B, and CUX2 was not found (Table 1). Not only lipid loci but also insulin-associated loci associated with metabolic syndrome. However, most of the variants identified were present in known lipid loci. In contrast, a relatively small number of variants were in other metabolic syndrome-component traits. For example, genetic variants such as rs780092 and rs780094 mapped on the GCKR gene were susceptible variants relative to total cholesterol, fasting glucose level, and lipid metabolism phenotypes [6, 19, 20]. An SNP from the pairs identified here, rs2074356, which mapped on the HECTD4 gene, was previously associated with the glycemic trait [21]. Six of the SNP pairs identified have shown an association with the lipid trait–associated LD region spanning BUD13-ZNF259, APOA5-A4-C3-A1, and SIK3 [6, 13, 19, 22]. Povel et al. [22] reported a systematic review of genetic variants and metabolic syndrome. They suggested that although disturbances in metabolic syndrome-component traits have been proposed to activate metabolic syndrome, most SNPs associated with metabolic syndrome are in genes involved in lipid metabolism [23]. Moreover, Kristiansson et al. [6] showed that genes from the lipid metabolism pathway are factors in metabolic syndrome. However, these investigators found little evidence associated with other metabolic syndrome-component traits such as hypertension and glucose intolerance [6]. Our results were consistent with previous studies.

Through the single-SNP–multi-trait analysis, we identified four SNP pairs that were associated with metabolic

syndrome but were not in the GWAS catalog. Intronic SNPs on the SIK3 gene showed genome-wide significance in the single-SNP–multi-trait analysis (Table 1). SNPs on the UBASH3B and CUX2 genes could not be identified by single-SNP–multi-trait analysis (Table 2), whereas the association of UBASH3B and CUX2 with metabolic syndrome-component traits was reported in the GWAS catalog. For example, two variants, rs7128198 on the 5'-untranslated region and rs7941030 upstream of UBASH3B, were associated with total cholesterol and HDL level, respectively [24, 25]. The intergenic variant rs12229654 between MYL2 and CUX2 showed a pleiotropic effect associated with metabolic syndrome, HDL, and glycemic traits [21, 26]. An association between cardiovascular disease and rs886126, which also identified in our study, was previously reported [27].

Utilizing multi-SNP–multi-trait analysis, we found an association between the SIDT2 gene and metabolic syndrome or metabolic syndrome-component traits based on an association between metabolic syndrome and rs7107152 and rs1242229. The SNP rs7107152 is within the DNase cluster in the region of transcription factors such as ESR1 and FOXA1 (Fig. 1). The SNPs rs530885291 and rs508487 showed in the GWAS catalog as proximal to rs7107152 and rs1242229, respectively [15]. However, the pairwise LD score between rs1242229 and rs508487 was low ($r^2 = 0.167$), indicating little correlation between these two SNPs.

We performed another multi-SNP–multi-trait analysis based on the SNP set test (gene-based test). SNP sets on the PAFAH1B2, SIDT2, and CUX2 genes showed significant P values in the gene-based test (a Bonferroni-adjusted P value threshold is $P = 3.45 \times 10^{-6}$). PAFAH1B2 and SIDT2 reached a replication P value of < 0.05. The SNP set on CUX2 suggested a P value of 0.06 in the replication stage (Table 3); a larger sample size might have resulted in a significant P value. The SNP set rs7107152 and rs1242229 on *SIDT2* was also significant, supporting the association of *SIDT2* with metabolic syndrome.

We found evidence from the three online databases that rs7107152 and rs1242229, which are in an intron of *SIDT2*, correlated with the expression of *SIDT2* and *TAGLN* (Additional file 1: Figure S1). Two recent eQTL studies provide further evidence that these two SNPs alter gene expression that is relevant to metabolic syndrome-component traits [28, 29]. From the eQTL analysis between SNP and whole-blood gene expression in 5,257 Framingham Heart Study participants, rs1242229 was reported as a proxy SNP for altered *SIDT2* and *TAGLN* expression in triglyceride [28]. Huan et al. [29] investigated *cis* and *trans* eQTL by utilization of the human whole-blood transcriptome data from Framingham Heart Study pedigrees. The SNP rs7107152 also altered *SIDT2* expression in triglyceride [8]. The radar chart shows that these variants increase HDL and triglyceride levels among metabolic syndrome-component traits, supporting the hypothesis that genes are a key factor in the link between lipid metabolism and metabolic syndrome (Additional file 1: Figure S4) [6, 22]. We conferred that lipid traits such as HDL and TG have the greatest impact on metabolic syndrome, but weak associations such as DBP may also have an impact. However, due to the limitations of current research, the potential weak association must interpret carefully. The eQTL SNPs correlated with *SIDT2* and *TAGLN* expression enriched in the 100-kb region (117000–117,100 kb) around *SIDT2* and *TAGLN* (Additional file 1: Figure S5).

SID1 transmembrane family member 2 (SIDT2) is a lysosomal integral membrane protein that promotes insulin secretion [30]. Recently, Gao et al. [31] described its activity in insulin secretion. $Sidt2^{-/-}$ mice exhibit weight loss and increased fasting glucose levels and impaired glucose tolerance. These investigators identified mouse SIDT2 function in lipid metabolism. SIDT2-deficient mice have increased serum triglyceride [32]. TAGLN (Transgelin, sm22α) is an actin-binding protein expressed in smooth muscle cells [33]. Yang et al. [34] revealed that the most enriched pathways caused by SM22α knockout in mice were lipid metabolism, inflammation, and hematopoiesis. We hypothesize that the SNP pair associated with metabolic syndrome activate expression of the genes *SIDT2* and *TAGLN*. A difference in gene expression might inhibit insulin secretion, lipid metabolism, and adipogenesis, resulting in metabolic syndrome (Additional file 1: Figure S6). Although evidence supports the association between the identified SNPs and metabolic syndrome, functional investigations of the SNPs are needed. However, functional investigation using identified 27 SNP pairs in non-coding regions is limited. Given additional information such as imputed SNPs, a metabolic syndrome-associated genetic variant in coding regions may be detected by the statistical test used in the present study.

Conclusions

Our results show that a multi-SNP–multi-trait analysis is an efficient approach for finding variants that have not previously been isolated from single-variant–multi-trait analysis. The advantage of this approach is an increase in statistical power that results from considering the combined effects of two variants. Because P values of identified variants such as rs7107152 and rs1242229 did not reach statistical significance, these variants cannot be identified by single-variant analysis of the same sample size. Although previously identified variants are in lipid loci, these variants and their mapped genes are not reported in metabolic syndrome. Our findings provide insight into the genetic variant contribution to metabolic syndrome.

Methods

Study design and participants

To identify susceptible variant sets associated with metabolic syndrome, we conducted a multi-SNP–multi-trait analysis through the two stages: discovery and replication analysis (Fig. 2). For the discovery stage, we used genome data from the Ansan/Ansung cohort in the Korean Genome Epidemiology Study, which is known as the Korea Association REsource (KARE) project [35]. In the subsequent replication stage, we used the Health Examinees (HEXA) study cohort, data from which were also used in the GWASs [26, 27]. All participants were between 40 and 69 years of age. Informed consent was obtained from all participants. This study was approved by the ethical committee of the Korea Centers for Disease Control and Prevention Institutional Review Board. Detailed demographic information of participants is shown in Table 4.

Quality control in GWAS

The KARE data consisted of 10,004 samples genotyped with Affymetrix Genome-Wide Human SNP array 5.0 [26, 35]. We selected 8,842 individuals genotyped with 352,228 SNPs from the quality control process. The quality control criteria and process have been described [21, 26, 35]. We used 351,983 SNPs for the multi-SNP–multi-trait analysis after exclusion of 245 SNPs with ambiguous chromosome numbers and positions. We selected 7,211 of 8,842 participants who did not take lipid-lowering or anti-diabetes medication. For the replication analysis, we selected 2,838 of 3,701 participants from the HEXA study after those taking medication were excluded.

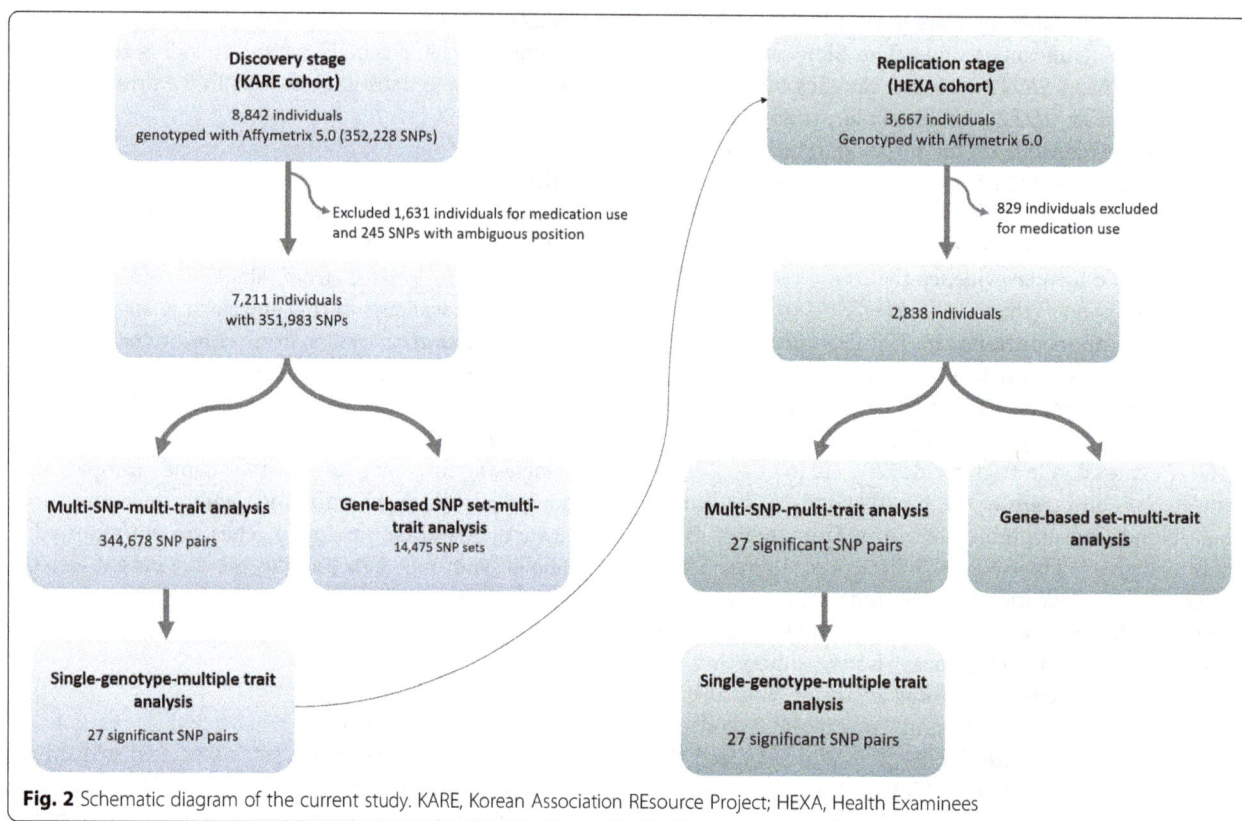

Fig. 2 Schematic diagram of the current study. KARE, Korean Association REsource Project; HEXA, Health Examinees

Phenotyping

We considered six quantitative traits as components of metabolic syndrome. We used the National Cholesterol Education Program Expert Panel on Detection, Evaluation, and Treatment of High Blood Cholesterol in Adults (Adult Treatment Panel III) final report guideline as metabolic syndrome definition [4]. For waist circumference, we used modified Asian guidelines, which reduce the limit from > 102 cm to > 90 cm for men and from > 88 cm to > 80 cm for women. Thus, a participant was considered to have

metabolic syndrome if he or she had three of the five following features: (1) triglyceride > 150 mg/dL, (2) HDL < 40 mg/dL for men and < 50 mg/dL for women, (3) waist circumference > 90 cm for men and > 80 cm for women, (4) fasting plasma glucose > 110 mg/dL, and (5) blood pressure threshold > 130 mmHg (SBP) and > 85 mmHg (DBP).

Multiple SNP set–multiple trait association analysis

Previously, Won et al. [14] proposed a statistical method for the joint analysis of multiple phenotypes and

Table 4 Characteristics of the study participants

	KARE			HEXA	
	Case (n = 1328)	Control (n = 5870)	Not determined (n = 13)	Case (n = 309)	Control (n = 2529)
Age	53.9 (8.65)	50.52 (8.62)	61.31 (8.02)	54 (7.92)	51.48 (7.88)
Sex (m/f)	561/767	3000/2870	4/9	184/125	1039/1490
SBP	128.15 (18.13)	112.36 (15.52)	128.36 (16.07)	132.19 (13.77)	118.68 (13.47)
DBP	81.97 (11.46)	72.32 (10.49)	74.92 (6.43)	83.54 (9.12)	75.39 (9.47)
FPG	94 (29.82)	84.31 (14.79)	80.67 (1.53)	101.49 (25.38)	90.15 (22.3)
Triglyceride	241.35 (134.62)	138.94 (83.58)	180.92 (122.1)	224.38 (134.91)	106.35 (74.49)
log triglyceride	5.38 (0.44)	4.82 (0.44)	5.04 (0.55)	5.28 (0.5)	4.52 (0.52)
HDL	38.35 (6.78)	46.54 (10.06)	42.58 (8.39)	43.5 (8.88)	57 (13.16)
WC	90.33 (7.01)	79.98 (7.82)	87.27 (7.97)	90.69 (6.86)	80.44 (8.13)

n sample size; *SBP* systolic blood pressure, *DBP* diastolic blood pressure, *FPG* fasting plasma glucose, *HDL* high-density lipoprotein, *WC* waist circumference
KARE Korean Association Resource Project, *HEXA* Health Examinee cohort
Data are shown as the mean (SD)

genotypes. This method, the MFQLS (http://health-stat.snu.ac.kr/software/mfqls/), can be utilized for both quantitative and dichotomous phenotypes. It can be applied to large-scale, genome-wide association analysis as well as family-based samples. The empirical power test showed that it is statistically more efficient than existing methods. In addition, the genome-wide association analysis of 1,801 individuals with obesity showed that P values from the MFQLS were markedly less than those from other methods [14]. In our study, two types of multiple SNP sets, such as paired SNPs and gene-based SNPs having more than three variants, were considered to be multiple genotypes. For the multi-SNP–multi-trait analysis, the MFQLS incorporates both multiple traits and SNPs into a single test statistic. For example, given two traits and two SNPs, the MFQLS tests H_0: $\beta_{11} = \beta_{12} = \beta_{21} = \beta_{22} = 0$, where β_{ij} denotes the effect of association between the ith SNP and the jth trait. The effect of these genotypes and the statistical significance of this effect are greater when multiple genotypes and phenotypes are correlated. Of 351,983 SNPs, 344,677 SNP pairs with MAF > 0.01 were selected (a Bonferroni-adjusted P value threshold, $P = 1.45 \times 10^{-7}$). Additional file 1: Table S2 shows MAF of identified SNPs. We extended the gene-based genome-wide association analysis with multiple traits. To select an SNP set for gene-based analysis, we included common SNPs in the first set on the platform used in the discovery and replication stages. We selected gene-based tag SNPs captured with $r^2 \geq 0.8$ by the use of Tagger (http://www.broad.mit.edu/mpg/tagger/) for the second set. Consequently, 14,475 SNP sets were selected for gene-based analysis (a Bonferroni-adjusted P value threshold, $P = 3.45 \times 10^{-6}$). Table 3 and Additional file 1: Table S1 show information about the SNP sets used for the gene-based test.

Two-stage analyses such as estimation of correlation between each SNP and calculation of statistics are used to run the MFQLS.

The Fisher's combined probability test was used to calculate the meta-analysis from discovery and replication results by application of MADAM in the R package.

Single-SNP–multi-trait association analysis

To determine whether a significant SNP pair identified in the multi-SNP–multi-trait analysis was still significant if a different approach was used, we performed a joint analysis between single genotype and multiple phenotypes. An SNP and multiple traits were incorporated into the statistics of a single test and three traits were given, H_0: $\beta_1 = \beta_2 = \beta_3 = 0$ and H_1: not H_0, where β_i denotes the effect of association between a SNP and the ith trait. Covariates such as age and sex were adjusted in the analysis.

SNP pair–metabolic syndrome-component trait association analysis

To determine which metabolic syndrome-component traits are related to the SNP pair rs7107152 and rs1242229, we performed an association analysis between the SNP pair and each metabolic syndrome-component trait.

Additional analyses from online data resources

To examine the expression pattern of each SNP of an identified SNP pair, we utilized three online data resources that provide eQTL information: the portal for GTEx [16], RegulomeDB [17], and the NESDA NTR Conditional eQTL Catalog. SNAP was applied to calculate the correlation between identified SNPs and previously known GWAS SNPs [18].

Abbreviations
DBP: Diastolic blood pressure; eQTL: Expression quantitative trait loci; FPG: Fasting plasma glucose; GTEx: Genotype-tissue expression; GWAS: Genome-wide association study; HDL: High-density lipoprotein cholesterol; HEXA: Health Examinees; KARE: Korean Association REsource Project; LDL: Low-density lipoprotein cholesterol; MFQLS: The family-based quasi-likelihood score test; SBP: Systolic blood pressure; SIDT2: SID1 transmembrane family member 2; TAGLN: Transgelin; TC: Total cholesterol; TG: Triglyceride

Funding
This work was funded by intramural grants from the Korean National Institute of Health (2013-NG73002-00, 2016-NI73005-00) and supported by the Basic Science Research Program through the National Research Foundation of Korea Grant funded by the Korean Government (NRF-2014S1A2A2028559). Data were also provided by the Korean Genome Analysis Project (4845-301) and the National Biobank of Korea, which were supported by the Korea Center for Disease Control and Prevention, Republic of Korea.

Author's contributions
SM contributed to the analysis and interpretation of data and to the drafting of the manuscript. YL contributed to the design of the study, analysis of the data, and drafting of the manuscript. SW contributed to the revision of the manuscript. JL contributed to the concept and design of the study and to the revision of the manuscript. All authors approved submission of the final version of the article for publication.

Competing interests
The authors declare that they have no competing interests.

Author details
[1]Division of Genome Research, Center for Genome Science, Korea National Institute of Health, Cheongju, Chungcheongbuk-do 28159, South Korea. [2]Veterans Medical Research Institute, Veterans Health Service Medical Center, Seoul 05368, South Korea. [3]Department of Public Health Science, Seoul National University, Seoul 08826, South Korea.

References

1. Ordovas JM, Shen J. Gene-environment interactions and susceptibility to metabolic syndrome and other chronic diseases. J Periodontol. 2008;79: 1508–13.

2. Brown AE, Walker M. Genetics of insulin resistance and the metabolic syndrome. Curr Cardiol Rep. 2016;18:75.

3. Dragsbaek K, Neergaard JS, Laursen JM, Hansen HB, Christiansen C, Beck-Nielsen H, Karsdal MA, Brix S, Henriksen K. Metabolic syndrome and subsequent risk of type 2 diabetes and cardiovascular disease in elderly women: challenging the current definition. Medicine (Baltimore). 2016;95:e4806.

4. Third Report of the National Cholesterol Education Program (NCEP). Expert panel on detection, evaluation, and treatment of high blood cholesterol in adults (adult treatment panel III) final report. Circulation. 2002;106:3143–421.

5. Hong AR, Lim S. Clinical characteristics of metabolic syndrome in Korea, and its comparison with other Asian countries. J Diabetes Investig. 2015;6:508–15.

6. Kristiansson K, Perola M, Tikkanen E, Kettunen J, Surakka I, Havulinna AS, Stancakova A, Barnes C, Widen E, Kajantie E, Eriksson JG, Viikari J, Kahonen M, et al. Genome-wide screen for metabolic syndrome susceptibility Loci reveals strong lipid gene contribution but no evidence for common genetic basis for clustering of metabolic syndrome traits. Circ Cardiovasc GenetCirc Cardiovasc Genet. 2012;5:242–9.

7. Abou Ziki MD, Mani A. Metabolic syndrome: genetic insights into disease pathogenesis. Curr Opin Lipidol. 2016;27:162–71.

8. Pare G, Asma S, Deng WQ. Contribution of large region joint associations to complex traits genetics. PLoS Genet. 2015;11:e1005103.

9. Klein RJ. Power analysis for genome-wide association studies. BMC Genet. 2007;8:58.

10. Spencer CC, Su Z, Donnelly P, Marchini J. Designing genome-wide association studies: sample size, power, imputation, and the choice of genotyping chip. PLoS Genet. 2009;5:e1000477.

11. Klei L, Luca D, Devlin B, Roeder K. Pleiotropy and principal components of heritability combine to increase power for association analysis. Genet Epidemiol. 2008;32:9–19.

12. Stephens M. A unified framework for association analysis with multiple related phenotypes. PLoS One. 2013;8:e65245.

13. Zhou X, Stephens M. Efficient multivariate linear mixed model algorithms for genome-wide association studies. Nat Methods. 2014;11:407–9.

14. Won S, Kim W, Lee S, Lee Y, Sung J, Park T. Family-based association analysis: a fast and efficient method of multivariate association analysis with multiple variants. BMC Bioinformatics. 2015;16:46.

15. MacArthur J, Bowler E, Cerezo M, Gil L, Hall P, Hastings E, Junkins H, McMahon A, Milano A, Morales J, Pendlington ZM, Welter D, Burdett T, et al. The new NHGRI-EBI catalog of published genome-wide association studies (GWAS catalog). Nucleic Acids Res. 2017;45:D896–901.

16. GTEx consortium. Genetic effects on gene expression across human tissues. Nature. 2017;550:204–13.

17. Boyle AP, Hong EL, Hariharan M, Cheng Y, Schaub MA, Kasowski M, Karczewski KJ, Park J, Hitz BC, Weng S, Cherry JM, Snyder M. Annotation of functional variation in personal genomes using RegulomeDB. Genome Res. 2012;22:1790–7.

18. Johnson AD, Handsaker RE, Pulit SL, Nizzari MM, O'Donnell CJ, de Bakker PI. SNAP: a web-based tool for identification and annotation of proxy SNPs using HapMap. Bioinformatics. 2008;24:2938–9.

19. Kraja AT, Vaidya D, Pankow JS, Goodarzi MO, Assimes TL, Kullo IJ, Sovio U, Mathias RA, Sun YV, Franceschini N, Absher D, Li G, Zhang Q, et al. A bivariate genome-wide approach to metabolic syndrome: STAMPEED consortium. Diabetes. 2011;60:1329–39.

20. Setoh K, Terao C, Muro S, Kawaguchi T, Tabara Y, Takahashi M, Nakayama T, Kosugi S, Sekine A, Yamada R, Mishima M, Matsuda F. Three missense variants of metabolic syndrome-related genes are associated with alpha-1 antitrypsin levels. Nat Commun. 2015;6:7754.

21. Go MJ, Hwang JY, Kim YJ, Hee OJ, Heon Kwak S, Soo Park K, Lee J, Kim BJ, Han BG, Cho MC, Cho YS, Lee JY. New susceptibility loci in MYL2, C12orf51 and OAS1 associated with 1-h plasma glucose as predisposing risk factors for type 2 diabetes in the Korean population. J Hum Genet. 2013;58:362–5.

22. Povel CM, Boer JMA, Reiling E, Feskens EJM. Genetic variants and the metabolic syndrome: a systemic review. Obes Rev. 2011;12:952–67.

23. Braun TR, Been LF, Singhal A, Worsham J, Ralhan S, Wander GS, Chambers JC, Kooner JS, Aston CE, Sanghera DK. A replication study of GWAS-derived lipid genes in Asian Indians: the chromosomal region 11q23.3 harbors loci contributing to triglycerides. PLoS One. 2012;7:e37056.

24. Willer CJ, Schmidt EM, Sengupta S, Peloso GM, Gustafsson S, Kanoni S, Ganna A, Chen J, Buchkovich ML, Mora S, Beckmann JS, Bragg-Gresham JL, Chang HY, et al. Discovery and refinement of loci associated with lipid levels. Nat Genet. 2013;45:1274–83.

25. Teslovich TM, Musunuru K, Smith AV, Edmondson AC, Stylianou IM, Koseki M, Pirruccello JP, Ripatti S, Chasman DI, Willer CJ, Johansen CT, Fouchier SW, Isaacs A, et al. Biological, clinical and population relevance of 95 loci for blood lipids. Nature. 2010;466:707–13.

26. Kim YJ, Go MJ, Hu C, Hong CB, Kim YK, Lee JY, Hwang JY, Oh JH, Kim DJ, Kim NH, Kim S, Hong EJ, Kim JH, et al. Large-scale genome-wide association studies in East Asians identify new genetic loci influencing metabolic traits. Nat Genet. 2011;43:990–5.

27. Lee JY, Lee BS, Shin DJ, Woo Park K, Shin YA, Joong Kim K, Heo L, Young Lee J, Kyoung Kim Y, Jin Kim Y, Bum Hong C, Lee SH, Yoon D, et al. A genome-wide association study of a coronary artery disease risk variant. J Hum Genet. 2013;58:120–6.

28. Yao C, Chen BH, Joehanes R, Otlu B, Zhang X, Liu C, Huan T, Tastan O, Cupples LA, Meigs JB, Fox CS, Freedman JE, Courchesne P, et al. Integromic analysis of genetic variation and gene expression identifies networks for cardiovascular disease phenotypes. Circulation. 2015;131:536–49.

29. Huan T, Liu C, Joehanes R, Zhang X, Chen BH, Johnson AD, Yao C, Courchesne P, O'Donnell CJ, Munson PJ, Levy D. A systematic heritability analysis of the human whole blood transcriptome. Hum Genet. 2015;134: 343–58.

30. Jialin G, Xuefan G, Huiwen Z. SID1 transmembrane family, member 2 (Sidt2): a novel lysosomal membrane protein. Biochem Biophys Res Commun. 2010; 402:588–94.

31. Gao J, Yu C, Xiong Q, Zhang Y, Wang L. Lysosomal integral membrane protein Sidt2 plays a vital role in insulin secretion. Int J Clin Exp Pathol. 2015;8:15622–31.

32. Gao J, Zhang Y, Yu C, Tan F, Wang L. Spontaneous nonalcoholic fatty liver disease and ER stress in Sidt2 deficiency mice. Biochem Biophys Res Commun. 2016;476:326–32.

33. Sayar N, Karahan G, Konu O, Bozkurt B, Bozdogan O, Yulug IG. Transgelin gene is frequently downregulated by promoter DNA hypermethylation in breast cancer. Clin Epigenetics. 2015;7:104.

34. Yang M, Jiang H, Li L. Sm22alpha transcription occurs at the early onset of the cardiovascular system and the intron 1 is dispensable for its transcription in smooth muscle cells during mouse development. Int J Physiol Pathophysiol Pharmacol. 2010;2:12–9.

35. Cho YS, Go MJ, Kim YJ, Heo JY, Oh JH, Ban HJ, Yoon D, Lee MH, Kim DJ, Park M, Cha SH, Kim JW, Han BG, et al. A large-scale genome-wide association study of Asian populations uncovers genetic factors influencing eight quantitative traits. Nat Genet. 2009;41:527–34.

36. Ridker PM, Pare G, Parker A, Zee RY, Danik JS, Buring JE, Kwiatkowski D, Cook NR, Miletich JP, Chasman DI. Loci related to metabolic-syndrome pathways including LEPR, HNF1A, IL6R, and GCKR associate with plasma C-reactive protein: the Women's Genome Health Study. Am J Hum Genet. 2008;82:1185–92.

37. Zabaneh D, Balding DJ. A genome-wide association study of the metabolic syndrome in Indian Asian men. PLoS One. 2010;5:e11961.

38. Zhu Y, Zhang D, Zhou D, Li Z, Fang L, Yang M, Shan Z, Li H, Chen J, Zhou X, Ye W, Yu S, Cai L, et al. Susceptibility loci for metabolic syndrome and metabolic components identified in Han Chinese: a multi-stage genome-wide association study. J Cell Mol Med. 2017;21:1106–16.

20

Link between short tandem repeats and translation initiation site selection

Masoud Arabfard[1,2], Kaveh Kavousi[2*], Ahmad Delbari[3] and Mina Ohadi[3*] ⓘ

Abstract

Background: Despite their vast biological implication, the relevance of short tandem repeats (STRs)/microsatellites to the protein-coding gene translation initiation sites (TISs) remains largely unknown.

Methods: We performed an Ensembl-based comparative genomics study of all annotated orthologous TIS-flanking sequences in human and 46 other species across vertebrates, on the genomic DNA and cDNA platforms (755,956 TISs), aimed at identifying human-specific STRs in this interval. The collected data were used to examine the hypothesis of a link between STRs and TISs. BLAST was used to compare the initial five amino acids (excluding the initial methionine), codons of which were flanked by STRs in human, with the initial five amino acids of all annotated proteins for the orthologous genes in other vertebrates (total of 5,314,979 pair-wise TIS comparisons on the genomic DNA and cDNA platforms) in order to compare the number of events in which human-specific and non-specific STRs occurred with homologous and non-homologous TISs (i.e., ≥ 50% and < 50% similarity of the five amino acids).

Results: We detected differential distribution of the human-specific STRs in comparison to the overall distribution of STRs on the genomic DNA and cDNA platforms (Mann Whitney U test $p = 1.4 \times 10^{-11}$ and $p < 7.9 \times 10^{-11}$, respectively). We also found excess occurrence of non-homologous TISs with human-specific STRs and excess occurrence of homologous TISs with non-specific STRs on both platforms ($p < 0.00001$).

Conclusion: We propose a link between STRs and TIS selection, based on the differential co-occurrence rate of human-specific STRs with non-homologous TISs and non-specific STRs with homologous TISs.

Keywords: Translation initiation site, Short tandem repeat, Genome-scale, Human-specific, Selection

Introduction

An increasing number of human protein-coding genes are unraveled to consist of alternative translation initiation sites (TISs), which are selected based on complex and yet not fully known scanning mechanisms [1, 2]. The alternative TISs result in various protein structures and functions [3, 4]. Selection of TISs and the level of translation and protein synthesis depend partially on the *cis*-regulatory elements in the mRNA sequence and its secondary structure such as the formation of hair-pins and thermal stability [5–7]. Genomic DNA *cis*-elements

can also affect translation and TISs through various mechanisms (for a review see [8]).

One of the important and understudied *cis*-regulatory elements affecting translation is short tandem repeats (STRs)/microsatellites. In physiological terms, STRs can dramatically influence TIS and the amount of protein synthesis. Poly(A) tracts in the 5′-untranslated region (UTR) are important sites for translation regulation in yeast. These poly(A) tracts can interact with translation initiation factors or poly(A) binding proteins (PABP) to either increase or decrease translation efficiency. Pre-AUG A_N can enhance internal ribosomal entry both in the presence of PABP and eIF-4G in *Saccharomyces cerevisiae* [9], and in the complete absence of PABP and eIF-4G [10]. Biased distribution of dinucleotide repeats is a known phenomenon in the region immediately upstream of the TISs in *Escherichia coli* [11]. In pathological instances,

* Correspondence: kkavousi@ut.ac.ir; mi.ohadi@uswr.ac.ir; ohadi.mina@yahoo.com
[2]Laboratory of Complex Biological Systems and Bioinformatics (CBB), Department of Bioinformatics, Institute of Biochemistry and Biophysics (IBB), University of Tehran, Tehran, Iran
[3]Iranian Research Center on Aging, University of Social Welfare and Rehabilitation Sciences, Tehran, Iran
Full list of author information is available at the end of the article

expansion of STRs in the RNA structure results in toxic RNAs and non-AUG translation and the development of several human-specific neurological [12–14].

Genomic DNA STRs can affect TISs through their effect on alternative splicing and shuffling of novel ATG translation sites in novel exons [15]. Genome-scale findings of the evolutionary trend of a number of STRs have begun to unfold their implication in respect to speciation and species-specific characteristics/phenotypes [16–27]. The hypermutable nature of STRs and their large unascertained reservoir of functionality make them an ideal source of evolutionary adaptation, speciation, and disease [28–35]. In line with the above, recent reports indicate a role of repetitive sequences in the creation of new transcription start sites (TSSs) in human [36–39].

This research aimed to examine a possible link between STRs and TIS selection through studying the occurrence rate of TIS-flanking human-specific and non-specific STRs with homologous and non-homologous proteins.

Methods
Data collection
Forty-seven species encompassing major classes of vertebrates were selected, and in each species, the 120 bp upstream genomic DNA and cDNA sequences flanking all annotated protein-coding TISs ($n = 755,956$) were downloaded based on the Ensembl database version 90 (https://asia.ensembl.org). The species studied are alphabetically listed as follows: anole lizard, armadillo, bush baby, cat, chicken, chimpanzee, cow, dog, dolphin, duck, ferret, fugu, gibbon, golden hamster, gorilla, guinea pig, hedgehog, human, horse, kangaroo rat, lamprey, lesser hedgehog tenrec, macaque, marmoset, megabat, microbat, mouse, mouse lemur, olive baboon, opossum, orangutan, pig, platypus, prairie vole, rabbit, rat, sheep, shrew, shrew mouse, squirrel, tarsier, Tasmanian devil, tree shrew, turkey, vervet-AGM, Xenopus, and zebrafish.

For each gene in each species, its Ensembl ID, all the annotated transcript IDs, the genomic DNA sequence, the cDNA, and the coding DNA sequence (CDS) were retrieved (the list of genes is available upon request). The genomic DNA, CDS, and the annotated cDNAs were downloaded using REST API from the Ensembl database. The first start codon for each transcript was determined using BLAST between the CDS and cDNA. The 120 bp genomic DNA and cDNA interval upstream of the start codon (ATG) were investigated for the presence of STRs of ≥ 3-repeats (Additional file 1).

Retrieval of gene IDs across species
Using the Enhanced REST API tools, a set of functions were developed to analyze genes and their transcripts information, including *func_get_ensemblID* and *func_get_TranscriptsID*. The genomic DNA, cDNA, and CDS

sequences of genes and their respective transcripts were obtained using *func_get_GenomicSequence, func_get_cDNASequence*, and *func_get_CDSSequence* functions.

Identification of STRs in the human TIS-flanking genomic and cDNA intervals
A general method of finding human-specific and non-specific STRs (≥ 3-repeats in all classes of STRs, except the mononucleotide repeats, in which STRs of ≥ 6-repeats were studied) for each individual gene was developed and applied as follows: the 120 bp genomic DNA and cDNA sequence upstream of the TISs of all annotated protein-coding gene transcripts was screened in human and 46 other species across vertebrates for the presence of STRs. A list of all STRs and their abundance was prepared for each gene in every species. The data obtained on the human STRs was compared to those of other species, and the term "human-specific" was applied to STRs that were not detected at ≥ 3-repeats in any other species. Exceptionally, in the mononucleotide category, the threshold of repeats for "human-specificity" was set at > 6-repeats. The relevant pseudo-code for the identification of repeated substrings was used for STR identification (Additional file 2).

Mann-Whitney U test was used to compare the distribution of human-specific vs. the overall (specific and non-specific) STR distribution in human.

TIS homology threshold estimation
Weighted homology scoring was performed, in which the initial five amino acids (excluding the initial methionine) of the human protein-coding TISs, codons of which were flanked by STRs, were BLASTed (compared using BLAST) against all initial protein-coding five amino acids annotated for the orthologous genes in 46 species across vertebrates [(3,872,779 pair-wise TIS comparisons on the genomic DNA platform (Ensembl 91) and 1,442,200 pair-wise TIS comparisons on the cDNA platform (Ensembl 92)]. The above was aimed at comparing the number of events in which human-specific and non-specific STRs occurred with homologous and non-homologous TISs.

The following equation was developed for the weighted scoring of homology (Eq. 1), where A refers to the five amino acid sequence (excluding the initial methionine M), codons of which were flanked by a STR at the genomic DNA or cDNA sequence, j refers to the gene, and B refers to all the transcripts of the same gene that contain the STR in other species.

If M is the first methionine amino acid of two sequences, for all five successive positions represented by i in the equation, we defined five weight coefficients W_1 to W_5 based on the importance of the amino acid position, i.e., proximity to the methionine starting codon, observed in the W vector. The degree of homology between the two sequences A and B was calculated using function ϕ for all five positions with the operations $\sum_{i=1}^{L=5} W_i \phi(A_{jik}, B_{jik'})$. We repeated this operation for k transcripts, where k stands for the number of transcripts in human. k' refers to all transcripts of the gene j in other species.

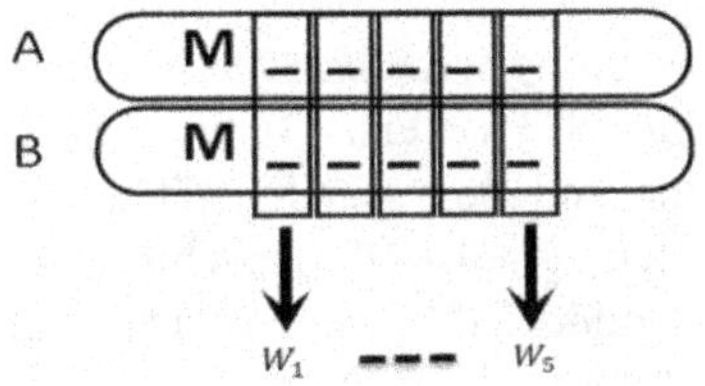

$$H_k^j = \sum_{i=1}^{L=5} W_i \phi\left(A_{jik}, B_{jik'}\right); \text{for all } k \text{ and } k' \quad (1)$$

$$\phi(x, y) = \begin{cases} 1; \text{if } x \neq y \\ 0; \text{otherwise} \end{cases}$$

$$W = \{25, 25, 25, 12.5, 12.5\}$$

Homology of the five amino acids, and therefore the TISs, was inferred based on the %similarity scoring. We validated the homology threshold by measuring the %similarity of 3000 random pairs of human proteins (the first five amino acids excluding the initial methionine),

where similarity of $\geq 50\%$ was virtually non-existent in that sample (6 in 3000, false positive rate = 0.001) (Additional file 3).

Finally, the two by two table and Fisher exact statistics were used to examine the link between STRs and TISs.

Results

Genome-scale distribution of human STRs in the 120 bp upstream sequence of TISs

Genomic DNA platform

Mono- and dinucleotide STRs dominated STRs of > 1000 counts, and the (T)6 mononucleotide repeat was the most abundant STR in this interval, succeeded by the (CT)3 and (TC)3 dinucleotide STRs (Fig. 1). Trinucleotide STRs were less abundant, observed at counts between 100 and 1000, and predominated by GC-rich composition such as (GGC)3, (GCC)3, (CCG)3, and (GCG)3. In the non-GC composition, (CTC)3 and (CCT)3 were the most common trinucleotide STRs. Tetra-, penta-, and hexanucleotide STRs were at lesser abundance than the above categories and observed at < 100 counts, where (CCTC)3 and (CCGC)3 were the most abundant tetranucleotide STRs. Only three pentanucleotide STR classes, (GGGGC)3, (TTTTG)3, and (GTTTT)3, were observed at counts > 10 in the screened interval.

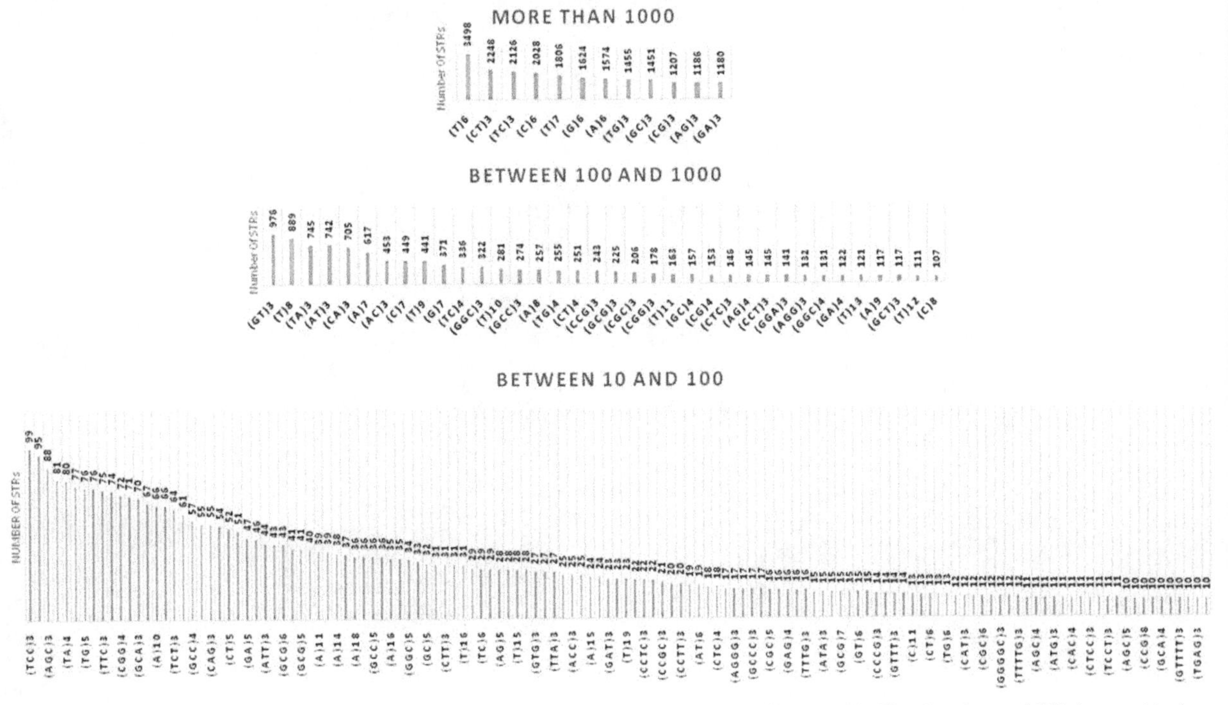

Fig. 1 Genome-scale landscape of STRs in the 120 bp genomic DNA sequence upstream of human TISs. The abundance of STRs is sorted in the ascending order

cDNA platform

The overall distribution of STRs in the 120 bp TIS-flanking cDNA sequences was significantly different in comparison to the genomic DNA STRs (Fig. 2). In comparison to the genomic DNA platform on which T(6) was the most abundant STR, GC-rich dinucleotide repeats were the most abundant on the cDNA platform. Numerous other instances at high, medium, and low abundance differentiated the genomic DNA vs. cDNA platforms (e.g., differential abundance of (T)8, (GT)3, (TA)3, and (CA)3 between the two platforms).

Human-specific STR fingerprints on the TIS-flanking genomic DNA and cDNA platforms and differential distribution of these compartments in comparison to the overall STR distribution

Genomic DNA platform

The flanking sequence of 755,956 TISs was screened in human and 46 other species in order to identify human-specific STRs. One thousand eight hundred eighty-seven genes contained human-specific TIS-flanking STRs on the genomic DNA platform, which were of a wide range of nucleotide compositions of mono-, di-, tri-, tetra-, penta-, and hexanucleotide repeats, of which poly(A) and poly(T) STRs were the longest (the 1st percentile, based on STR length, is listed in Table 1, and the list of all genes is provided as Additional file 4).

As an extreme example, the TIS of the *NVL* gene was flanked by a human-specific (T)22 STR, which was the longest STR detected in a human protein-coding gene TIS-flanking sequence. The TIS of the gene, *SULT1A3*, was flanked by the longest poly(A) at (A)18. Short- and medium-length STRs were also detected in the human-specific compartment (Additional file 4).

Significant skewing was observed in the distribution of human-specific STRs (Fig. 3) vs. the overall (i.e., human-specific and non-specific) STRs (Fig. 1) (Mann Whitney U test, $p = 1 \times 10^{-5}$). While the (GC)3 and (CG)3 dinucleotide STRs were enriched in the overall STR compartment, their abundance was significantly lower in the human-specific compartment. Instead, (CA)3 and (AC)3 were significantly more abundant in the human-specific compartment. Differences in the distribution of tri- and tetranucleotide STRs were also observed between the two compartments. While trinucleotide and tetranucleotide STRs of GC composition were more abundant in the overall compartment, non-GC STR compositions (e.g., GGA, TTC, GCA, and ATAA) were more abundant in the human-specific compartment.

cDNA platform

Two thousand six hundred genes contained human-specific STRs in their TIS cDNA flanking sequence (the 1st percentile based on length is represented in Table 2 and

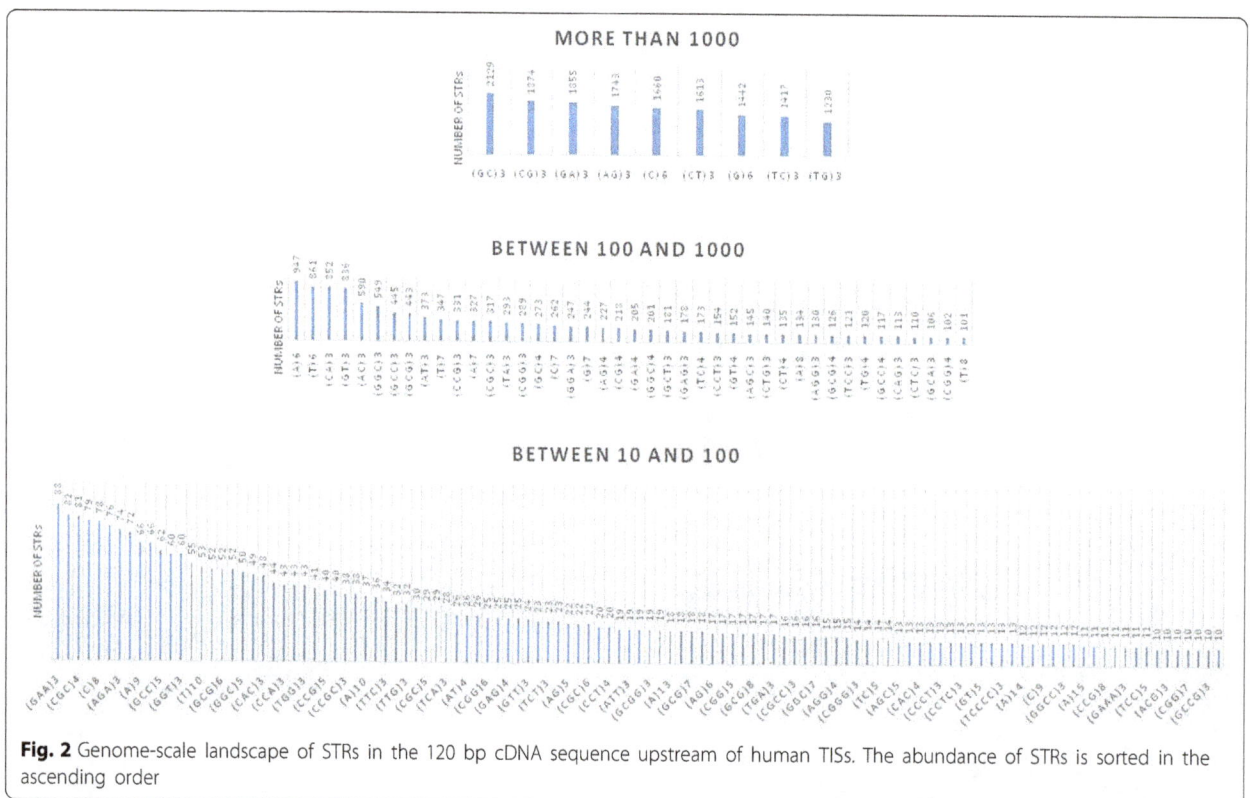

Fig. 2 Genome-scale landscape of STRs in the 120 bp cDNA sequence upstream of human TISs. The abundance of STRs is sorted in the ascending order

Table 1 The 1st percentile of human protein-coding genes which contain human-specific STRs (length-wise) in their TIS-flanking genomic DNA sequence

Gene symbol	Gene Ensembl ID	Transcript ID	STR	GO term
NVL	ENSG00000143748	ENST00000436927	(T)22	ATP binding
OR4K2	ENSG00000165762	ENST00000641885	(T)20	Olfactory receptor activity
MGRN1	ENSG00000102858	ENST00000591895	(A)18	–
SULT1A3	ENSG00000261052	ENST00000338971		Sulfotransferase activity
		ENST00000395138		
GDI2	ENSG00000057608	ENST00000380127	(T)17	GTPase activator activity
		ENST00000609712		
SULT1A4	ENSG00000213648	ENST00000360423	(A)17	Sulfotransferase activity
ZNF283	ENSG00000167637	ENST00000618787	(T)17	Regulation of transcription
		ENST00000593268		
ADAP2	ENSG00000184060	ENST00000581548	(A)16	GTPase activator activity
DDX20	ENSG00000064703	ENST00000475700		Nucleic acid binding
SGIP1	ENSG00000118473	ENST00000435165	(A)16	Clathrin-dependent endocytosis
LCA5L	ENSG00000157578	ENST00000288350		Intraciliary transport
		ENST00000485895		
		ENST00000418018		
		ENST00000448288		
		ENST00000434281		
		ENST00000438404		
		ENST00000411566		
		ENST00000415863		
		ENST00000426783		
		ENST00000456017		
		ENST00000451131		
LRRC36	ENSG00000159708	ENST00000569499	(T)14	–
		ENST00000568804		
OR7A10	ENSG00000127515	ENST00000641129	(CT)14	G protein-coupled receptor activity
POLR2F	ENSG00000100142	ENST00000492213	(T)14	Transcription, DNA templated
SNX19	ENSG00000120451	ENST00000528555	(T)14	Integral component of membrane
		ENST00000530356		
TEX11	ENSG00000120498	ENST00000395889	(TTCC)14	Meiotic cell cycle
ACAT1	ENSG00000075239	ENST00000527942	(T)13	Transferring acyl groups
CHRFAM7A	ENSG00000166664	ENST00000299847	(T)13	Ion transmembrane transport
		ENST00000562729		
GALK2	ENSG00000156958	ENST00000560654	(TG)13	Phosphotransferase activity
		ENST00000396509		
		ENST00000558145		
		ENST00000544523		
		ENST00000560138		

the complete list as Additional file 5). Similar to the genomic DNA platform, poly(A) and Poly(T) STRs were the longest STRs identified in the interval. The longest STR in this interval was (A)20 and belonged to *KCTD19*.

The distribution of human-specific STRs on the cDNA platform (Fig. 4) was unique to this platform and different from the overall STR distribution on the cDNA platform (Fig. 2) (Mann-Whitney U test $p = 1 \times 10^{-5}$). While

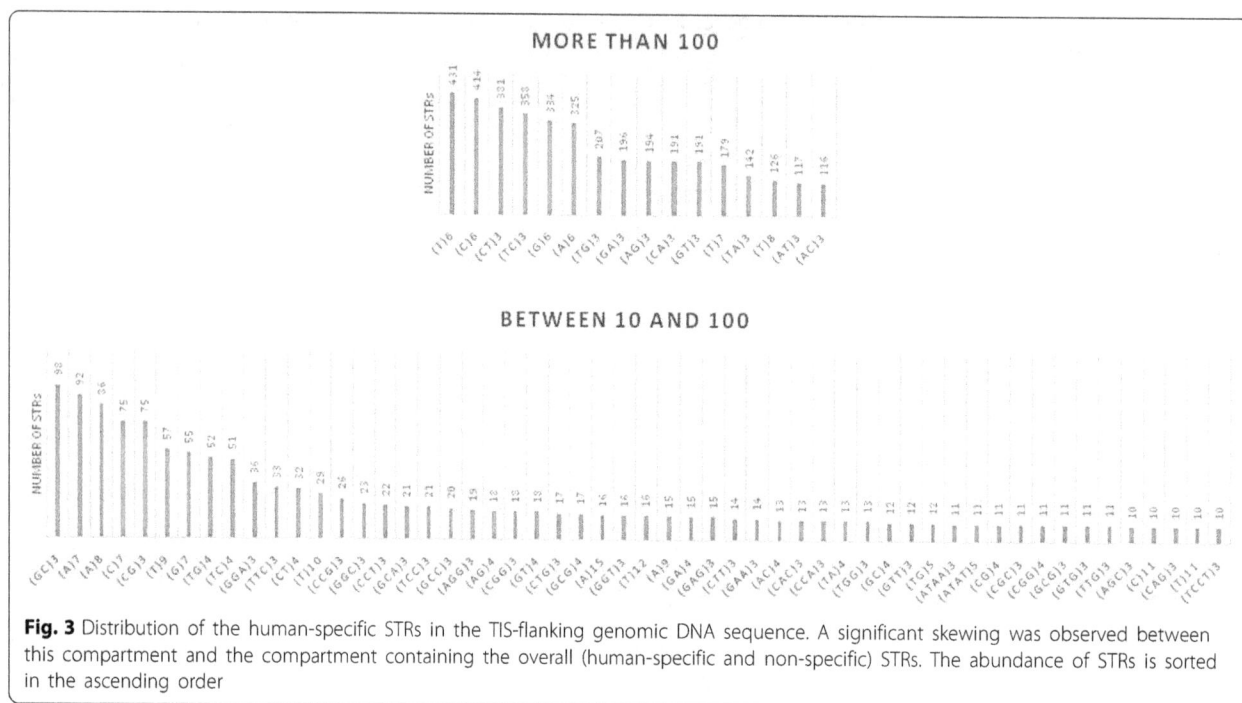

Fig. 3 Distribution of the human-specific STRs in the TIS-flanking genomic DNA sequence. A significant skewing was observed between this compartment and the compartment containing the overall (human-specific and non-specific) STRs. The abundance of STRs is sorted in the ascending order

the CG and CG dinucleotide STRs were more abundant in the overall distribution, CT, CA, and TG repeats were more abundant in the human-specific compartment. Various other differences were detected in other classes of STRs (e.g., more abundance of non-GC compositions in the trinucleotide STRs such as GGA, GCT, and CTG).

STRs link to TIS selection on both genomic DNA and cDNA platforms

We examined the hypothesis that there may be a link between STRs and TIS selection. The initial five amino acids (excluding the initial methionine) of the human protein sequences, codons of which were flanked by STRs at the genomic DNA and cDNA, were BLASTed (compared using BLAST) against the initial five amino acids of all the proteins annotated for the orthologous genes in 46 species across vertebrates in order to compare the number of events in which human-specific and non-specific STRs occurred with homologous and non-homologous TISs (≥ 50% and < 50% similarity of the five amino acids). Total of 5,314,979 pair-wise TIS comparisons were performed, and significant correlation was observed between STRs and TIS selection both on the genomic DNA (Fig. 5a) and cDNA platforms (Fig. 5b) ($p < 0.00001$), where there was excess occurrence of non-homologous TISs with human-specific STRs, and vice versa (i.e., excess occurrence of homologous TISs with non-specific STRs).

Discussion

In this study, we characterized the genome-scale STR landscape of the immediate 120 bp upstream sequence

of human TISs on the genomic DNA and cDNA platforms, cataloged the human-specific compartment of these STRs, and investigated a possible link between STRs and TIS selection. Our findings provide the first evidence of a link between STRs and TIS selection on both platforms. This link is primarily deduced based on the differential co-occurrence rate of human-specific STRs with non-homologous TISs and non-specific STRs with homologous TISs.

Sequence similarity searches can reliably identify "homologous" proteins or genes by detecting excess similarity [40]. The TIS homology threshold of ≥ 50% was validated based on 3000 random similarity scorings of the initial protein-coding five amino acids (excluding the initiating methionine) of human proteins, in which that threshold was non-existent in effect (false-positive rate = 0.001). This scoring methodology was consistently applied to the TISs linked to human-specific and non-specific STRs.

We also observed differential distribution of the human-specific STRs vs. the overall distribution of STRs on both genomic and cDNA platforms. Importantly, each platform had a unique pattern of STR distribution, indicating differential selection of STRs based on their location and evolutionary course. Genome-scale skewing of STRs, albeit at a lesser scale of STR classes, was reported by our group in a preliminary study of the gene core promoter interval [36].

It is imperative to envision that human-specific *cis* elements at the mRNA and DNA may result in the production of proteins that are specific to humans. The RNA structure influences recruitment of various RNA binding

Table 2 The 1st percentile of human protein-coding genes which contain human-specific STRs (length-wise) in their TIS-flanking cDNA sequence

Gene symbol	Gene Ensembl ID	Transcript ID	STR	GO term
KCTD19	ENSG00000168676	ENST00000566295	(A)20	Protein homooligomerization
ATP8B1	ENSG00000081923	ENST00000585322	(A)17	Magnesium ion binding
C1QTNF1	ENSG00000173918	ENST00000583904		Collagen trimer
SEC11A	ENSG00000140612	ENST00000558196		Peptidase activity
SHQ1	ENSG00000144736	ENST00000463369		–
SPRY1	ENSG00000164056	ENST00000505319		Multicellular organism development
		ENST00000610581		
DDX20	ENSG00000064703	ENST00000475700	(A)16	ATP binding
NAB1	ENSG00000138386	ENST00000409641	(T)16	Negative regulation of transcription
SGIP1	ENSG00000118473	ENST00000435165	(A)16	–
SOX6	ENSG00000110693	ENST00000528252	(A)14	Multicellular organism development
DPP6	ENSG00000130226	ENST00000406326	(T)13	Proteolysis
		ENST00000377770		
MLF1	ENSG00000178053	ENST00000482628	(G)13	–
SHC4	ENSG00000185634	ENST00000558220	(T)13	Stem cell differentiation
ITGB1BP2	ENSG00000147166	ENST00000538820	(T)12	Calcium ion binding
NELL2	ENSG00000184613	ENST00000548531		Calcium ion binding
GIPC1	ENSG00000123159	ENST00000393028	(GCG)11	–
		ENST00000345425		
		ENST00000587210		
HBS1L	ENSG00000112339	ENST00000527578	(T)11	GTPase activity
HOPX	ENSG00000171476	ENST00000556376	(A)11	Cell differentiation
OR7D2	ENSG00000188000	ENST00000642043	(T)11	G protein-coupled receptor activity
RNF145	ENSG00000145860	ENST00000520638		Integral component of membrane
TXNL4A	ENSG00000141759	ENST00000592837		mRNA splicing, via spliceosome
ABCF1	ENSG00000204574	ENST00000468958	(A)10	ATP binding
ARHGEF18	ENSG00000104880	ENST00000359920	(T)10	Rho guanyl-nucleotide exchange factor activity
ARL14	ENSG00000179674	ENST00000320767	(A)10	GTP binding
ASNS	ENSG00000070669	ENST00000448127	(T)10	Asparagine biosynthetic process
EIF2S1	ENSG00000134001	ENST00000466499		Translation initiation factor activity

proteins and determines alternative TISs [41]. Indeed, the ribosomal machinery has the potential to scan and use several open reading frames (ORFs) at a particular mRNA species [42]. When located at the 5′ or 3′ UTR, STRs can modulate translation, the effect of which has biological and pathological implications [13, 43, 44]. The disorders linked to the 5′ UTR STRs encompass a number of human-specific neurological disorders.

On the genomic DNA platform, proximity to the splice sites may increase the biological/pathological implication of repeats [45]. Similar to the cDNA STRs, we observed significant enrichment of non-homologous TISs co-occurring with human-specific genomic STRs, which were substantially near the exons (within 120 bp upstream of the TISs).

Gene Ontology (GO) search yielded a variety of terms across the identified genes, including neuron cell fate specification, multicellular organism development, translation initiation factor activity, and cell differentiation (https://www.ebi.ac.uk/QuickGO/), examples of which are presented in Tables 1 and 2.

EMBOSS Needle (https://www.ebi.ac.uk/Tools/psa/emboss_needle) pair-wise comparison was performed between human and three other species (chimpanzee, macaque, and mouse), of the proteins encoded by the transcripts in Table 1 (Fig. 6a), Table 2 (Fig. 6b), and several randomly selected proteins, codons of which were

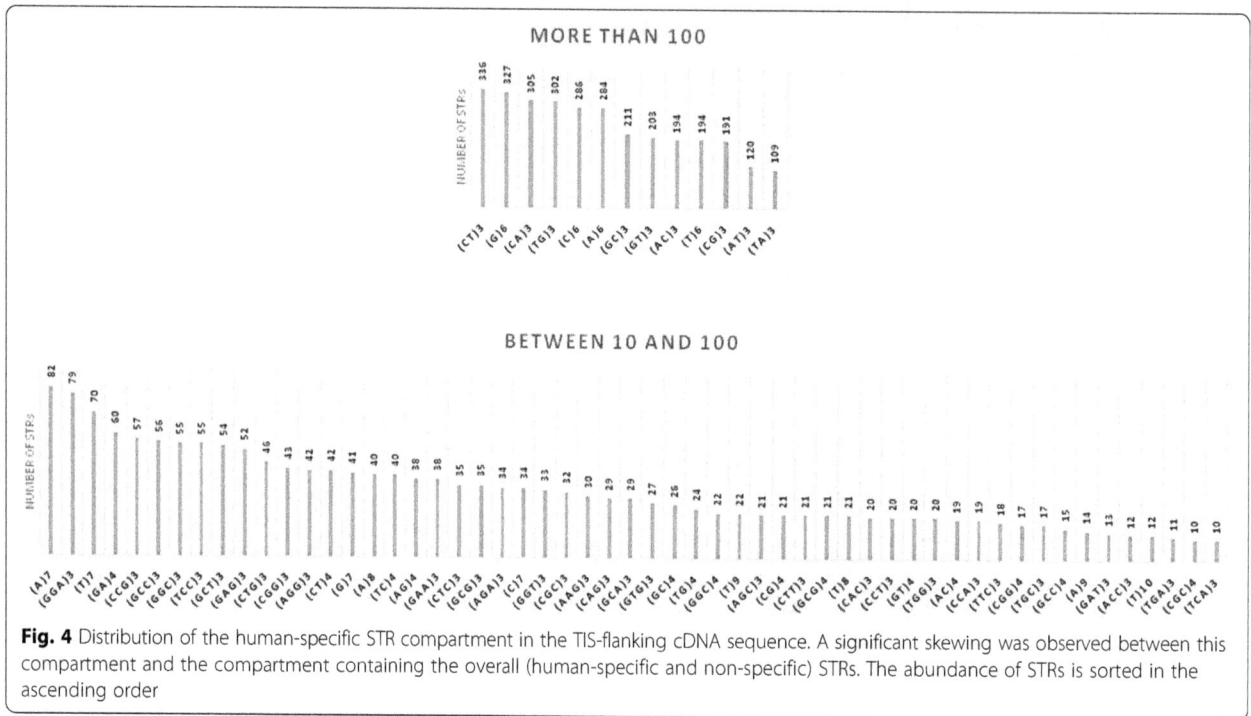

Fig. 4 Distribution of the human-specific STR compartment in the TIS-flanking cDNA sequence. A significant skewing was observed between this compartment and the compartment containing the overall (human-specific and non-specific) STRs. The abundance of STRs is sorted in the ascending order

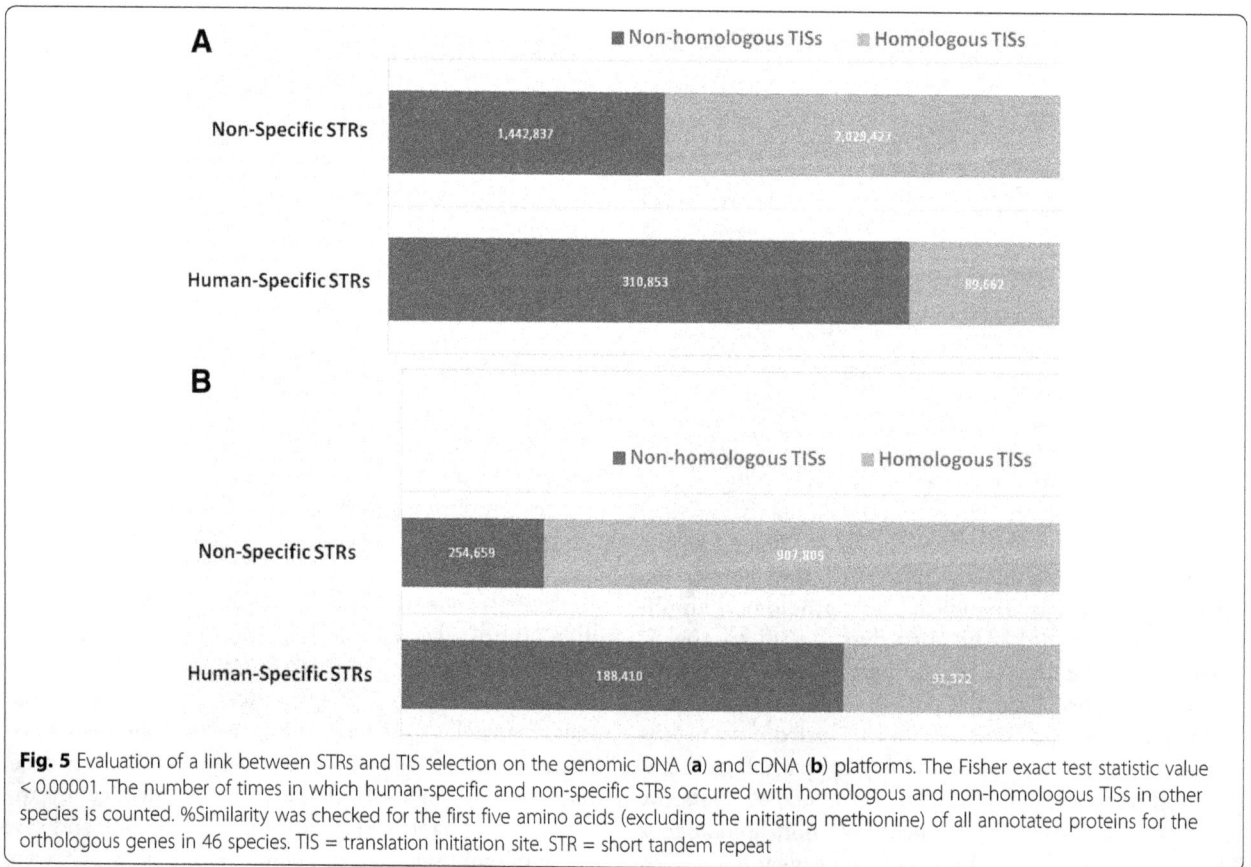

Fig. 5 Evaluation of a link between STRs and TIS selection on the genomic DNA (**a**) and cDNA (**b**) platforms. The Fisher exact test statistic value < 0.00001. The number of times in which human-specific and non-specific STRs occurred with homologous and non-homologous TISs in other species is counted. %Similarity was checked for the first five amino acids (excluding the initiating methionine) of all annotated proteins for the orthologous genes in 46 species. TIS = translation initiation site. STR = short tandem repeat

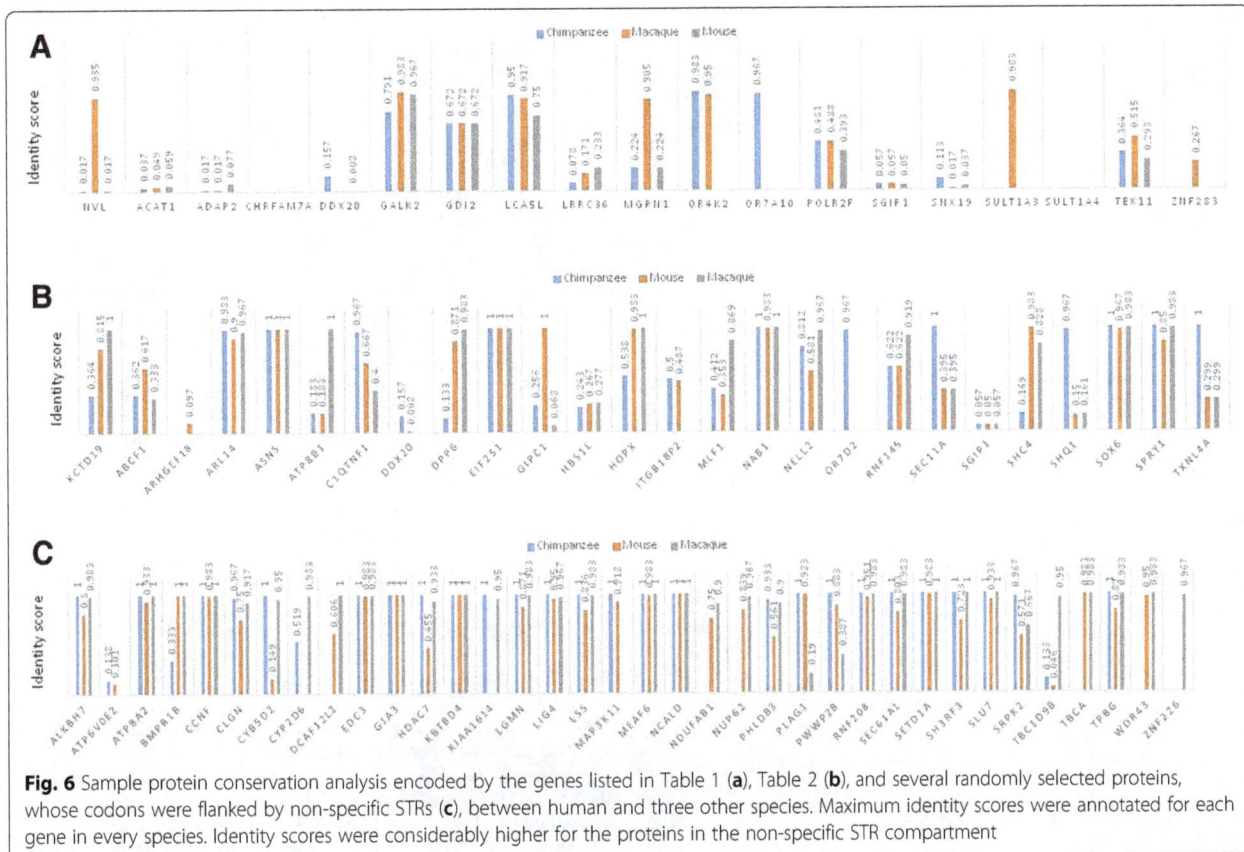

Fig. 6 Sample protein conservation analysis encoded by the genes listed in Table 1 (**a**), Table 2 (**b**), and several randomly selected proteins, whose codons were flanked by non-specific STRs (**c**), between human and three other species. Maximum identity scores were annotated for each gene in every species. Identity scores were considerably higher for the proteins in the non-specific STR compartment

flanked by non-specific STRs (Fig. 6c). Identity scores were considerably lower across the three species for the genes in Tables 1 and 2, compared to the identity scores for the genes in the non-specific STR compartment.

A number of the identified genes such as *ACAT1* (Table 1) and *SGIP1* (Table 2) confer risk for diseases or endophenotypes that are predominantly specific to the human species, such as complex psychiatric disorders [46, 47]. *SULT1A4* (Table 1) plays a critical role in neurotransmitter metabolism in the human brain and is also linked to neurodegeneration [48]. *APOA2* (Additional file 4) along with several other lipoproteins is linked to cognitive health [49]. In another remarkable example, *TBR1* (Additional file 5) is involved in *FOXP2* gene expression, which has pivotal role in speech and language in human [50]. *SRGAP2* (Additional file 5) family proteins may have increased the density of dendritic spines and promoted neoteny of the human brain during crucial periods of human evolution [51].

GO terms, protein conservation comparisons, and phenotypes stated above are only a few examples of the identified genes, in which human-specific STRs and the linked TISs may contribute to human evolution and disease. Future studies are warranted to examine the implication of the identified STRs and genes at the inter- and intra-species levels.

Conclusion

We characterized the landscape of STRs at the immediate upstream genomic DNA and cDNA sequences flanking the human protein-coding gene TISs and found differential distribution of the human-specific STRs in comparison to the overall distribution of STRs on both platforms. Further, we propose a link between STRs and TIS selection, based on the differential co-occurrence rate of human-specific STRs with non-homologous TISs and non-specific STRs with homologous TISs. The data presented here have implications at the inter- and intraspecies levels, which warrant further functional and evolutionary studies.

Additional files

Additional file 1: Workflow of STR identification in the TIS-flanking

Additional file 2:

Additional file 3: Homology threshold validation. Three thousand random pair-wise similarity checks were performed on the five initial amino acids (excluding methionine) of human protein sequences. A similarity threshold of ≥ 50% was considered "homology." (JPG 24 kb)

Additional file 4: List of all human protein-coding genes which contain human-specific STRs in their TIS-flanking genomic DNA

Additional file 5: List of all human protein-coding genes which contain

Abbreviations
cDNA: Complementary DNA; CDS: Coding DNA sequence; GO: Gene
Ontology; mRNA: Messenger RNA; STR: Short tandem repeat; TIS: Translation
initiation site; TSS: Transcription start site

Acknowledgements
Not applicable

Funding
This research was funded jointly by the University of Social Welfare and
Rehabilitation Sciences, Tehran, Iran, and University of Tehran, Iran.

Authors' contributions
MA carried out the bioinformatics studies. KK participated in project supervision,
data analysis, and co-ordination. AD helped in coordination. MO conceived the
study, designed the project, supervised the analysis, and wrote the manuscript.
All authors read and approved the final manuscript.

Competing interests
The authors declare that they have no competing interests.

Author details
[1]Department of Bioinformatics, Kish International Campus University of
Tehran, Kish, Iran. [2]Laboratory of Complex Biological Systems and
Bioinformatics (CBB), Department of Bioinformatics, Institute of Biochemistry
and Biophysics (IBB), University of Tehran, Tehran, Iran. [3]Iranian Research
Center on Aging, University of Social Welfare and Rehabilitation Sciences,
Tehran, Iran.

References
1. Andreev DE, O'Connor PBF, Loughran G, Dmitriev SE, Baranov PV, Shatsky IN. Insights into the mechanisms of eukaryotic translation gained with ribosome profiling. Nucleic Acids Res. 2017;45(2):513–26. https://doi.org/10.1093/nar/gkw1190.
2. Lee S, Liu B, Lee S, Huang S-X, Shen B, Qian S-B. Global mapping of translation initiation sites in mammalian cells at single-nucleotide resolution. Proc Natl Acad Sci U S A. 2012;109(37):E2424–32. https://doi.org/10.1073/pnas.1207846109.
3. Fukushima M, Tomita T, Janoshazi A, Putney JW. Alternative translation initiation gives rise to two isoforms of Orai1 with distinct plasma membrane mobilities. J Cell Sci. 2012;125(18):4354–61. https://doi.org/10.1242/jcs.104919.
4. Bazykin GA, Kochetov AV. Alternative translation start sites are conserved in eukaryotic genomes. Nucleic Acids Res. 2011;39(2):567–77. https://doi.org/10.1093/nar/gkq806.
5. Cenik C, Cenik ES, Byeon GW, Grubert F, Candille SI, Spacek D, Snyder MP. Integrative analysis of RNA, translation, and protein levels reveals distinct regulatory variation across humans. Genome Res. 2015;25(11):1610–21. https://doi.org/10.1101/gr.193342.115.
6. Babendure JR, Babendure JL, Ding J-H, Tsien RY. Control of mammalian translation by mRNA structure near caps. RNA. 2006;12(5):851–61. https://doi.org/10.1261/rna.2309906.
7. Master A, Wójcicka A, Giżewska K, Popławski P, Williams GR, Nauman A. A novel method for gene-specific enhancement of protein translation by

8. Park E, Pan Z, Zhang Z, Lin L, Xing Y. The expanding landscape of alternative splicing variation in human populations. Am J Hum Genet. 2018;102(1):11–26. https://doi.org/10.1016/j.ajhg.2017.11.002.
9. Gilbert WV, Zhou K, Butler TK, Doudna JA. Cap-independent translation is required for starvation-induced differentiation in yeast. Science. 2007;317:1224–7. https://doi.org/10.1126/science.1144467.
10. Shirokikh NE, Spirin AS. Poly(A) leader of eukaryotic mRNA bypasses the dependence of translation on initiation factors. Proc Natl Acad Sci U S A. 2008;105(31):10738–43. https://doi.org/10.1073/pnas.0804940105.
11. Yamagishi K, Oshima T, Masuda Y, Ara T, Kanaya S, Mori H. Conservation of translation initiation sites based on dinucleotide frequency and codon usage in *Escherichia coli* K-12 (W3110): non-random distribution of A/T-rich sequences immediately upstream of the translation initiation codon. DNA Res. 2002;9(1):19–24. https://doi.org/10.1093/dnares/9.1.19.
12. Glineburg MR, Todd PK, Charlet-Berguerand N, Sellier C. Repeat-associated non-AUG (RAN) translation and other molecular mechanisms in Fragile X Tremor Ataxia Syndrome. Brain Res. 2018. https://doi.org/10.1016/j.brainres.2018.02.006.
13. Rovozzo R, Korza G, Baker MW, Li M, Bhattacharyya A, Barbarese E, Carson JH. CGG repeats in the 5'UTR of FMR1 RNA regulate translation of other RNAs localized in the same RNA granules. PLoS One. 2016;11(12):e0168204. https://doi.org/10.1371/journal.pone.0168204.
14. Krauss S, Griesche N, Jastrzebska E, Chen C, Rutschow D, Achmüller C, Dorn S, Boesch SM, Lalowski M, Wanker E, Schneider R, Schweiger S. Translation of HTT mRNA with expanded CAG repeats is regulated by the MID1-PP2A protein complex. Nat Commun. 2013;4:1511. https://doi.org/10.1038/ncomms2514.
15. Gymrek M, Willems T, Guilmatre A, Zeng H, Markus B, Georgiev S, Erlich Y. Abundant contribution of short tandem repeats to gene expression variation in humans. Nat Genet. 2016;48(1):22–9. https://doi.org/10.1038/ng.3461.
16. Yuan Z, Liu S, Zhou T, Tian C, Bao L, Dunham R, Liu Z. Comparative genome analysis of 52 fish species suggests differential associations of repetitive elements with their living aquatic environments. BMC Genomics. 2018;19:141. https://doi.org/10.1186/s12864-018-4516-1.
17. Emamalizadeh B, Movafagh A, Darvish H, Kazeminasab S, Andarva M, Namdar-Aligoodarzi P, Ohadi M. The human RIT2 core promoter short tandem repeat predominant allele is species-specific in length: a selective advantage for human evolution? Mol Genet Genomics. 2017;292(3):611–7. https://doi.org/10.1007/s00438-017-1294-4.
18. Abe H, Gemmell NJ. Evolutionary footprints of short tandem repeats in avian promoters. Sci Rep. 2016;6:19421. https://doi.org/10.1038/srep19421.
19. Bushehri A, Barez MR, Mansouri SK, Biglarian A, Ohadi M. Genome-wide identification of human- and primate-specific core promoter short tandem repeats. Gene. 2016;587:83–90. https://doi.org/10.1016/j.gene.2016.04.041.
20. Namdar-Aligoodarzi P, Mohammadparast S, Zaker-Kandjani B, Talebi Kakroodi S, Jafari Vesiehsari M, Ohadi M. Exceptionally long 5' UTR short tandem repeats specifically linked to primates. Gene. 2015;569:88–94. https://doi.org/10.1016/j.gene.2015.05.053.
21. Nikkhah M, et al. An exceptionally long CA-repeat in the core promoter of SCGB2B2 links with the evolution of apes and Old World monkeys. Gene. 2016;576(1 Pt 1):109–14. https://doi.org/10.1016/j.gene.2015.09.070.
22. Bilgin Sonay T, Carvalho T, Robinson MD, Greminger MP, Krützen M, Comas D, Wagner A. Tandem repeat variation in human and great ape populations and its impact on gene expression divergence. Genome Res. 2015;25(11):1591–9. https://doi.org/10.1101/gr.190868.115.
23. Rezazadeh M, Gharesouran J, Mirabzadeh A, Khorram Khorshid HR, Biglarian A, Ohadi M. A primate-specific functional GTTT-repeat in the core promoter of CYTH4 is linked to bipolar disorder in human. Prog Neuro-Psychopharmacol Biol Psychiatry. 2015;56:161–7. https://doi.org/10.1016/j.pnpbp.2014.09.001.
24. Khademi E, Alehabib E, Shandiz EE, Ahmadifard A, Andarva M, Jamshidi J, Rahimi-Aliabadi S, Pouriran R, Nejad FR, Mansoori N, Shahmohammadibeni N, Taghavi S, Shokraeian P, Akhavan-Niaki H, Paisán-Ruiz C, Darvish H, Ohadi M. Support for "disease-only" genotypes and excess of homozygosity at the CYTH4 primate-specific GTTT-repeat in schizophrenia. Genet Test Mol Biomarkers. 2017;21:485–90. https://doi.org/10.1089/gtmb.2016.0422.
25. Mohammadparast S, et al. Exceptional expansion and conservation of a CT-repeat complex in the core promoter of PAXBP1 in primates. Am J Primatol. 2014;76:747–56. https://doi.org/10.1002/ajp.22266.

26. Ohadi M, Mohammadparast S, Darvish H. Evolutionary trend of exceptionally long human core promoter short tandem repeats. Gene. 2012; 507(1):61–7. https://doi.org/10.1016/j.gene.2012.07.001.

27. King DG. Evolution of simple sequence repeats as mutable sites. Adv Exp Med Biol. 2012;769:10–25.

28. Hannan AJ. Tandem repeats mediating genetic plasticity in health and disease. Nat Rev Genet. 2018;19:286–98.

29. Bagshaw ATM. Functional mechanisms of microsatellite DNA in eukaryotic genomes. Genome Biol Evol. 2017;9(9):2428–43. https://doi.org/10.1093/gbe/evx164.

30. Press MO, McCoy RC, Hall AN, Akey JM, Queitsch C. Massive variation of short tandem repeats with functional consequences across strains of Arabidopsis thaliana. Genome Res. 2018;28:1169–78. https://doi.org/10.1101/gr.231753.117.

31. Press MO, Carlson KD, Queitsch C. The overdue promise of short tandem repeat variation for heritability. Trends Genet. 2014;30(11):504–12. https://doi.org/10.1016/j.tig.2014.07.008.

32. Ohadi M, Valipour E, Ghadimi-Haddadan S, Namdar-Aligoodarzi P, Bagheri A, Kowsari A, Rezazadeh M, Darvish H, Kazeminasab S. Core promoter short tandem repeats as evolutionary switch codes for primate speciation. Am J Primatol. 2015;77(1):34–43. https://doi.org/10.1002/ajp.22308.

33. Valipour E, et al. Polymorphic core promoter GA-repeats alter gene expression of the early embryonic developmental genes. Gene. 2013;531(2):175–9. https://doi.org/10.1016/j.gene.2013.09.032.

34. Darvish H, Heidari A, Hosseinkhani S, Movafagh A, Khaligh A, Jamshidi J, Noorollahi-Moghaddam H, Heidari-Rostami HR, Karkheiran S, Shahidi GA, Togha M, Paknejad SM, Ashrafian H, Abdi S, Firouzabadi SG, Jamaldini SH, Ohadi M. Biased homozygous haplotypes across the human caveolin 1 upstream purine complex in Parkinson's disease. J Mol Neurosci. 2013;51(2):389–93. https://doi.org/10.1007/s12031-013-0021-9.

35. Heidari A, Nariman Saleh Fam Z, Esmaeilzadeh-Gharehdaghi E, Banan M, Hosseinkhani S, Mohammadparast S, Oladnabi M, Ebrahimpour MR, Soosanabadi M, Farokhashtiani T, Darvish H, Firouzabadi SG, Farashi S, Najmabadi H, Ohadi M. Core promoter STRs: novel mechanism for inter-individual variation in gene expression in humans. Gene. 2012;492:195–8. https://doi.org/10.1016/j.gene.2011.10.028.

36. Nazaripanah N, Adelirad F, Delbari A, Sahaf R, Abbasi-Asl T, Ohadi M. Genome-scale portrait and evolutionary significance of human-specific core promoter tri- and tetranucleotide short tandem repeats. Hum Genomics. 2018;12:17 https://doi.org/10.1186/s40246-018-0149-3.

37. Alizadeh F, Bozorgmehr A, Tavakkoly-Bazzaz J, Ohadi M. Skewing of the genetic architecture at the ZMYM3 human-specific 5′ UTR short tandem repeat in schizophrenia. Mol Gen Genomics. 2018;293:747–52. https://doi.org/10.1007/s00438-018-1415-8.

38. Li C, Lenhard B, Luscombe NM. Integrated analysis sheds light on evolutionary trajectories of young transcription start sites in the human genome. Genome Res. 2018. https://doi.org/10.1101/gr.231449.117.

39. Kramer M, Sponholz C, Slaba M, Wissuwa B, Claus RA, Menzel U, Bauer M. Alternative 5′ untranslated regions are involved in expression regulation of human heme oxygenase-1. PLoS One. 2013;8(10):e77224. https://doi.org/10.1371/journal.pone.0077224.

40. Pearson, W. R. (2013). An introduction to sequence similarity ("homology") searching. Current protocols in bioinformatics/editoral board, Andreas D. Baxevanis. [et al.]. doi: https://doi.org/10.1002/0471250953.bi0301s42

41. Martínez-Salas E, Lozano G, Fernandez-Chamorro J, Francisco-Velilla R, Galan A, Diaz R. RNA-binding proteins impacting on internal initiation of translation. Int J Mol Sci. 2013;14(11):21705–26. https://doi.org/10.3390/ijms141121705.

42. Kochetov AV, Allmer J, Klimenko AI, Zuraev BS, Matushkin YG, Lashin SA. AltORFev facilitates the prediction of alternative open reading frames in eukaryotic mRNAs. Bioinformatics. 2017;33:923–5. https://doi.org/10.1093/bioinformatics/btw736.

43. Usdin K. The biological effects of simple tandem repeats: lessons from the repeat expansion diseases. Genome Res. 2008;18(7):1011–9. https://doi.org/10.1101/gr.070409.107.

44. Kumari S, Bugaut A, Huppert JL, Balasubramanian S. An RNA G-quadruplex in the 5′ UTR of the NRAS proto-oncogene modulates translation. Nat Chem Biol. 2007;3(4):218–21. https://doi.org/10.1038/nchembio864.

45. Zhang X, Lin H, Zhao H, Hao Y, Mort M, Cooper DN, Liu Y. Impact of human pathogenic micro-insertions and micro-deletions on post-transcriptional regulation. Hum Mol Genet. 2014;23(11):3024–34. https://doi.org/10.1093/hmg/ddu019.

46. Shibuya Y, Niu Z, Bryleva EY, Harris BT, Murphy SR, Kheirollah A, Bowen ZD, Chang CCY, Chang TY. Acyl-coenzyme A: cholesterol acyltransferase 1 blockage enhances autophagy in the neurons of triple transgenic Alzheimer's disease mouse and reduces human P301L-tau content at the presymptomatic stage. Neurobiol Aging. 2015;36(7):2248–59. https://doi.org/10.1016/j.neurobiolaging.2015.04.002.

47. Hodgkinson CA, Enoch MA, Srivastava V, Cummins-Oman JS, Ferrier C, Iarikova P, Sankararaman S, Yamini G, Yuan Q, Zhou Z, Albaugh B, White KV, Shen PH, Goldman D. Genome-wide association identifies candidate genes that influence the human electroencephalogram. Proc Natl Acad Sci U S A. 2010;107(19):8695–700. https://doi.org/10.1073/pnas.0908134107.

48. Butcher NJ, Horne MK, Mellick GD, Fowler CJ, Masters CL, AIBL research group, Minchin RF. Sulfotransferase 1A3/4 copy number variation is associated with neurodegenerative disease. Pharmacogenomics J. 2017. https://doi.org/10.1038/tpj.2017.4.

49. Muenchhoff J, Song F, Poljak A, Crawford JD, Mather KA, Kochan NA, Yang Z, Trollor JN, Reppermund S, Maston K, Theobald A, Kirchner-Adelhardt S, Kwok JB, Richmond RL, McEvoy M, Attia J, Schofield PW, Brodaty H, Sachdev PS. Plasma apolipoproteins and physical and cognitive health in very old individuals. Neurobiol Aging. 2017;55:49–60. https://doi.org/10.1016/j.neurobiolaging.2017.02.017.

50. Becker M, Devanna P, Fisher SE, Vernes SC. Mapping of human FOXP2 enhancers reveals complex regulation. Front Mol Neurosci. 2018;11:47. https://doi.org/10.3389/fnmol.2018.00047.

51. Lucas B, Hardin J. Mind the (sr)GAP - roles of Slit-Robo GAPs in neurons, brains and beyond. J Cell Sci. 2017;130:3965–74. https://doi.org/10.1242/jcs.207456.

21

Perceptions of students in health and molecular life sciences regarding pharmacogenomics and personalized medicine

Lejla Mahmutovic[1], Betul Akcesme[1,2], Camil Durakovic[1], Faruk Berat Akcesme[1,3], Aida Maric[1], Muhamed Adilovic[1], Nour Hamad[1], Matthias Wjst[4], Oliver Feeney[5] and Sabina Semiz[1]* 🄳

Abstract

Background: Increasing evidence is demonstrating that a patient's unique genetic profile can be used to detect the disease's onset, prevent its progression, and optimize its treatment. This led to the increased global efforts to implement personalized medicine (PM) and pharmacogenomics (PG) in clinical practice. Here we investigated the perceptions of students from different universities in Bosnia and Herzegovina (BH) towards PG/PM as well as related ethical, legal, and social implications (ELSI). This descriptive, cross-sectional study is based on the survey of 559 students from the Faculties of Medicine, Pharmacy, Health Studies, Genetics, and Bioengineering and other study programs.

Results: Our results showed that 50% of students heard about personal genome testing companies and 69% consider having a genetic test done. A majority of students (57%) agreed that PM represents a promising healthcare model, and 40% of students agreed that their study program is well designed for understanding PG/PM. This latter opinion seems to be particularly influenced by the field of study (7.23, CI 1.99–26.2, $p = 0.003$). Students with this opinion are also more willing to continue their postgraduate education in the PM (OR = 4.68, CI 2.59–8.47, $p < 0.001$). Furthermore, 45% of students are aware of different ethical aspects of genetic testing, with most of them (46%) being concerned about the patient's privacy.

Conclusions: Our results indicate a positive attitude of biomedical students in Bosnia and Herzegovina towards genetic testing and personalized medicine. Importantly, our results emphasize the key importance of pharmacogenomic education for more efficient translation of precision medicine into clinical practice.

Keywords: Precision medicine, Pharmacogenomics, Education, Ethical, legal, and social issues, Survey

Background

Personalized or precision medicine (PM) refers to an innovative approach to the disease diagnosis and treatment by considering differences in people's genetic background, lifestyle, and environment [1–3]. Importantly, it has the potential to shape many if not all aspects of clinical care from prevention and early diagnosis to treatment of disease [4, 5]. Pharmacogenomics (PG) studies individuals' genetic material in order to determine whether that person would benefit from a drug, require a different dose, or experience side effects, and as such is considered as an essential tool in personalized medicine [1, 6]. The successful completion of the Human Genome Project in 2003 was a first crucial step towards personalized medicine [7] and that eventually led to the Precision Medicine Initiative in the USA in 2015 to advance biomedical research in PM and facilitate its transition to clinical care [8–10]. In order to ensure the benefits of personalized diagnosis and treatment, the Food and Drug Administration (FDA) has

* Correspondence: ssemiz@ius.edu.ba
[1]Faculty of Engineering and Natural Sciences, International University of Sarajevo, Hrasnicka cesta 15, 71210 Ilidza, Sarajevo, Bosnia and Herzegovina
Full list of author information is available at the end of the article

listed about 140 drugs with pharmacogenetic/pharmaco-genomic (PG) information included in their labeling [9, 11]. Importantly, the identification of genetic variants by PG tests increases the prediction regarding drug efficacy and adverse reactions [10, 12, 13]. The guidelines provided by the Pharmacogenomics Knowledgebase (PharmGKB at https://www.pharmgkb.org/) and the Clinical Pharmaco-genomics Implementation Consortium (CPIC at https://cpicpgx.org/) are important educational and clinical resources for the healthcare professionals interested in introducing PG tests in their patient care.

Previous studies have shown that many physicians and pharmacists have positive attitudes towards the clinical application(s) of PG/PM [14, 15]. However, it appears that an inadequate knowledge and experience among some physicians and other healthcare professionals are the key drawbacks in more efficient clinical application of pharmacogenomics [14, 16–18], suggesting that it would be pertinent to introduce more PG topics in their professional education.

There are also many additional challenges that have to be addressed in order to facilitate its broader clinical implementation [19–21]. For example, the ethical, legal, and social implications (ELSI) of personalized medicine, such as informed consent, patient privacy, confidentiality, safety monitoring, reporting of adverse events, patient-centered practices, and other potential conflicting interests, have been addressed in existing bioethical analyses [20, 22–24]. However, further ethical implications associated with personalized medicine are emerging, for example, where it can be observed that different ethnicities may have different response to drugs [25–27]. Furthermore, some bioethicists are also concerned about the increased trend of human genome sequencing, processing, and storing of databases, private genetic bio/databanks, as well as about the increasingly popular direct-to-consumer (DTC) genetic tests, incidental (unsolicited) non-PG findings, potential health disparities, and other socioeconomic barriers in a broad PG application [28–32].

It is also important to mention here an issue which is often overlooked and that is of the fairness (or lack thereof) related to how the benefits of pharmacogenetic research, such as an increasing number of genomic advances relevant to disease prevention, diagnosis, and treatment [3] together with the decreasing costs of genetic testing [33], are currently being shared at the global level. A recent study performed by Manolio et al. [34] identified the major barriers to global implementation of genomic medicine, including high costs and/or lack of reimbursement and limited access to reliable standardized genotyping or sequencing platforms. Previous studies concluded that countries with limited research sources should have a chance to also express their opinions in making global decisions regarding public access

and benefits from the commercialized products, such as (pharmaco) genetic tests [35]. Transnational collaboration through the large research consortia and sharing information in the areas of health information technology, pharmacogenomics, education, professional development, and policy and regulatory issues seems to be pertinent for the future efficient clinical implementation of personalized medicine at the global level [34]. Increasing evidence is demonstrating different views and attitudes regarding PG testing, including patients' concerns about privacy, discrimination, quality of care, and value of the relationship between patient and physician [32]. Recently, several survey-based studies have been performed in order to assess the knowledge and awareness of health science students in the area of pharmacogenomics, personalized medicine, and bioethics [36–39]. Results of these studies demonstrated that health science students' knowledge and appreciation of PG is very important for optimal patient care. They should have the necessary skills and knowledge to make more rational therapy decisions based on patients' genetic information [38].Thus, education and raising awareness of biomedical students are of key importance for the future practice of precision medicine.

More than a decade ago, the International Society of Pharmacogenomics proposed recommendations regarding PG education standards to the medical, pharmacy, and health schools globally [40]. Consequently, many medical and pharmacy schools around Europe adopted these recommendations and included PG topics in their curricula [41–45], while only a few programs have been evaluated.

This is the first study of students' perception of pharmacogenomics in Bosnia and Herzegovina (BH). Although there are a few pharmacogenetic studies that have been performed in BH [46–50], an inadequate understanding of pharmacogenomics, expertise, and limited resources of the healthcare system in this middle-income country appears to represent the major challenges in clinical application of PG. Since the views of BH students have not been investigated yet on this topic, it is pertinent to understand the current status and needs for pharmacogenomic education in order to develop appropriate educational and training programs among professionals and students in health and molecular life sciences. Here we investigate the awareness and attitudes of health science (medical, pharmacy, health studies) and molecular life science (genetics and bioengineering) students in BH towards genetic testing, pharmacogenomics, and personalized medicine. As a second outcome, different ethical, legal, and social issues (ELSI) of personalized treatment have been also investigated. While health and molecular life science university students are not representative of the population as a whole, given their roles as the future medical doctors, nurses, pharmacists, and other health care professionals in BH society, it is important to capture their views.

Methods

This descriptive, cross-sectional study was done using online and hard copy questionnaires (survey is accessible as Additional file 1) between the second and eighth week of the spring semester in February and March 2016. Surveys were distributed by the teachers during a class or they were accessed online. Eligible participants included current students from several universities in Bosnia and Herzegovina (BH) located in four different cities, including Sarajevo, Tuzla, Mostar, and Bihac. The total number of 559 students participating in the survey involved students from the Faculty of Pharmacy, Faculty of Medicine, Faculty of Health Studies (FHS), Genetics and Bioengineering (GBE), as well as students from other non-health science (HS) and non-molecular life science (MLS)-related faculties.

The survey consisted of four clusters from a total of 33 questions on the following: (i) demographic and professional characteristics of the participants, (ii) participants' diseases and treatment, (iii) awareness and attitudes towards genetic testing and personalized medicine approach, and (iv) challenges towards genetic tests, PG, and its clinical application. Key definitions of genetic testing, personalized medicine, and pharmacogenomic/pharmacogenetic test were provided to the participants in the instruction section of the survey. All survey questions were consistent across all participating faculties. The survey included yes/no/I do not know (not sure) questions. In addition, the survey asked for levels of agreement with various statements using a Likert scale (i.e., agree, disagree, no opinion, neutral) and also offered multiple choice questions. Before being sent to students for the study, this questionnaire was reviewed by three experts from various backgrounds (clinical genetics, genomics, genetic counseling, genetic education, ethics, and social sciences). Along with the survey, an introductory cover page was attached describing the purpose and objectives of the study and inviting the students to participate in the study. Participants were assured their identity and all data are confidential. Participation was voluntary, and the study was approved by the Ethical Committee of the International University of Sarajevo.

Statistical analysis

All categorical variables including participants' demographics, professional information, and answers to questions regarding the perceptions about PG and PM were expressed as frequencies and percentages. Descriptive analysis was performed by using chi-square test and ANOVA for categorical variables. In addition, the binary logistic regression was performed in order to assess association between question of interest and hypothetically related covariates, while adjusting for age, gender, and level of education. In model I, we present this association prior to adjustment; in model II, we analyzed this association adjusted for age and gender, while model III additionally included an adjustment for the level of education. Odds ratio (OR) and corresponding 95% confidence intervals (CI) were computed, using a significance level of 5% for all statistical tests. Statistical analysis was performed by using IBM Statistical Package for Social Sciences (IBM SPSS®23).

Results

Participants' characteristics

Table 1 summarizes the students' demographics characteristics and professional information. The response rate was calculated for all students who completed the survey ($N = 559$, 10% response rate), including students from the Faculty of Pharmacy ($N = 183$), students from the Faculty of Medicine ($N = 158$), students from the Faculty of Health Studies ($N = 64$), students from the Genetics and Bioengineering ($N = 66$), and 88 students from other non-HS- and non-MLS-related study programs (architecture; psychology; industrial, mechanical, and electrical engineering; computer sciences; law; political sciences; and visual arts) ($N = 88$). The majority of participants were female (71%) and undergraduate students ($N = 398$, 84%), while 12% ($N = 60$) were attending Master and 3% ($N = 13$) PhD programs, with age ranging from 19 to 26 years old (86%).

Students' attitudes towards pharmacogenetic testing and personalized medicine

Participants' responses to almost all survey questions regarding their awareness and attitudes towards genetic testing, pharmacogenomics, personalized medicine, and corresponding ELSI are shown in the tables, with selected ones that are further elaborated in the discussion. As shown in Table 2, about 30–40% of participants from medicine, pharmacy, health studies, and genetics and bioengineering experienced that a particular drug did not work for them, while about 15–25% of these students had an adverse drug reaction. When asked about personal genome testing companies, about half of the participants from all HS and MLS faculties responded that they have heard about these companies and the majority of students (69%) showed an interest in having a genetic test done. About 40% of students would also consider contacting a personal genome testing company and ordering a PG test. The majority of students (70%) believe that genes moderately influence their health, with 13% of them thinking that genes completely affect it. When asked would they take the drug if a PG test revealed that prescribed drug would either be ineffective

Table 1 Students' demographic characteristics and professional information

	Total	Faculty of Pharmacy	Faculty of Medicine	Genetics and Bioengineering	Faculty of Health Studies	Non-ML&HS faculties	p^*
Gender							
Male	153 (29)[a]	25 (15)	46 (29)	16 (26)	19 (29)	47 (54)	< 0.01
Female	382 (71)	140 (85)	110 (71)	46 (74)	46 (71)	40 (46)	
Total	535	165	156	62	65	87	
Age							
< 19	37 (6.8)	–	–	19 (30)	10 (15)	8 (9)	< 0.01
19–26	465 (86)	141 (85)	154 (97)	44 (70)	54 (82)	72 (82)	
26–40	37 (6.8)	24 (14)	4 (2)	–	2 (3)	7 (8)	
41–50	1 (0.2)	–	–	–	–	1 (1)	
51–60	1 (0.2)	1 (1)	–	–	–	–	
> 60	1 (0.2)	–	1 (1)	–	–	–	
Total	542	166	159	63	66	88	
Level of education							
Less than high school	3 (1)	–	1 (1)	–	–	2 (2)	< 0.01
BSc	398 (84)	89 (63)	129 (95)	56 (97)	60 (97)	64 (82)	
MSc	60 (12)	46 (33)	4 (3)	2 (3)	2 (3)	6 (8)	
PhD	13 (3)	6 (4)	1 (1)	–	–	6 (8)	
Total	474	141	135	58	62	78	

ML&HS, Molecular Life and Health Science;
*Chi-square test, Bonferroni-adjusted *p* values
[a]Percentage (%)

or cause severe side effects, about 40% of all students responded that they would accept the test result and take the drug only if the disease might be life-threatening (Table 2). Furthermore, more than half of all students (57%) agreed that personalized medicine represents a promising healthcare model.

The level of awareness about companies offering PG tests appears to be similar between medicine and pharmacy students (not significantly different; see Additional file 2). Students from the Faculty of Health Studies are less aware of genome testing companies than their colleagues from the medicine and pharmacy ($p = 0.010$ and $p = 0.025$, respectively). A significantly lower number of these students agreed that PM represents the new and promising healthcare model as compared to the pharmacy and genetics students ($p < 0.01$ and $p = 0.01$, respectively; Additional file 3).

As shown in Table 2, respondents from the other non-health and non-molecular life sciences-related studies are generally aware that genes affect their health, and about half of them agree that personalized medicine represents a new and promising healthcare model. Furthermore, the majority of these students (60%) from non-HS and non-MLS faculties would consider having genetic test done to find out what illnesses they might develop in the future. However, their awareness of personal genome testing companies is significantly lower as

compared to their peers from medicine, pharmacy, and genetics ($p < 0.01$, $p < 0.01$, and $p = 0.02$, respectively; Additional file 2). In addition, as shown in Table 2, a lower number of these students (23%) from the non-health and non-molecular life science studies would consider contacting a personal genome testing company to order a PG test, as compared to the number of students from pharmacy (52%), health sciences (44%), and GBE (45%).

Our results of logistic regression analysis, performed to determine which independent variables were the strongest predictors of the specific students' responses, demonstrated belief that genes influence health in moderate to complete extent. Students with this belief would consider having a genetic test done to find out which illnesses they might develop in the future (OR = 3.02, CI 1.16–7.85, $p = 0.024$) (Table 3). This association does not appear to be affected by age, gender, and/or levels of education. Furthermore, our results demonstrated that those students who agreed that personalized medicine represents a new and promising healthcare model were also willing to do a genetic test, as compared to those who think the opposite (OR = 3.11, CI 1.60–6.06, $p = 0.001$). In addition, students who are ready to make necessary changes in their lifestyle to reduce disease risk would also consider having a genetic test done to know their genetic tendency to develop a disease (OR = 0.198, CI 0.114–0.283, $p = 0.001$). Our results also indicated that students'

Table 2 Students' attitudes towards pharmacogenetic testing and personalized medicine

	Total	Faculty of Pharmacy	Faculty of Medicine	Genetics and Bioeng.	Faculty of Health Studies	Non- ML&HS faculties	p*
Have you heard about personal genome testing companies?							
Yes	271 (50)[a]	95 (57)	101 (64)	29 (44)	23 (37)	23 (27)	< 0.01
No	136 (26)	39 (23)	26 (16)	25 (38)	22 (36)	24 (18)	
Do not know	131 (24)	32 (20)	31 (20)	12 (18)	17 (27)	39 (31)	
Total	538	166	158	66	62	86	
To what extent do you think genes influence your health?							
Completely	74 (13)	30 (18)	18 (11)	8 (13)	7 (11)	11 (13)	< 0.01
Moderately	375 (69)	129 (78)	132 (80)	43 (68)	36 (56)	35 (41)	
Not at all	37 (7)	1 (1)	10 (6)	4 (6)	1 (2)	21 (24)	
Do not know	58 (11)	6 (3)	5 (3)	8 (13%)	20 (31)	19 (22)	
Total	544	166	165	63	64	86	
Would you consider having a genetic test done to find out what illnesses you might develop in the future?							
Yes	374 (69)	138 (83)	101 (64)	45 (68)	38 (59)	52 (60)	< 0.01
No	110 (21)	20 (12)	36 (23)	15 (23)	20 (31)	19 (22)	
Not sure	56 (10)	8 (5)	20 (13)	6 (9)	6 (10)	16 (18)	
Total	540	166	157	66	64	87	
Do you agree that personalized medicine represents a new and promising healthcare model?							
Agree	295 (57)	116 (70)	83 (52)	31 (74)	24 (37)	41 (48)	< 0.01
Disagree	62 (12)	14 (8)	17 (11)	1 (2)	10 (16)	20 (23)	
Not sure	160 (31)	37 (22)	58 (37)	10 (24)	30 (47)	25 (29)	
Total	517	167	158	42	64	86	
Have you ever had an adverse drug reaction?							
Yes	91 (17)	41 (25)	22 (14)	8 (13)	10 (16)	10 (11)	< 0.01
No	328 (61)	82 (51)	112 (71)	45 (69)	42 (67)	47 (54)	
Do not know	89 (16)	38 (23)	20 (13)	10 (15)	8 (13)	13 (15)	
I have never taken any medication	29 (6)	2 (1)	4 (2)	2 (3)	3 (5)	18 (20)	
Total	537	163	158	65	63	88	
Have you ever found that a particular drug did not work for you?							
Yes	184 (34)	67 (41)	47 (30)	26 (39)	25 (39)	19 (22)	
No	226 (42)	69 (42)	76 (49)	25 (38)	25 (39)	31 (35)	
Do not know	90 (17)	27 (16)	26 (18)	11 (17)	7 (11)	19 (22)	
I have never taken any medication	37 (6)	2 (1)	5 (3)	4 (6)	7 (11)	19 (22)	
Total	537	165	154	66	64	88	
If a PG test revealed that prescribed drug would either be ineffective or cause severe side effects, would you take the drug anyway?							
Take the drug anyway	62 (12)	17 (10)	38 (23)	6 (10)	9 (14)	2 (2)	< 0.01
Accept the test result and not take the drug	117 (22)	34 (20)	27 (16)	20 (30)	20 (32)	16 (19)	
Accept the test result and take the drug only if the disease might be life-threatening	207 (39)	79 (48)	61(37)	24 (36)	15 (24)	28 (33)	
Not sure	150 (28)	36 (22)	39 (24)	16 (24)	19 (30)	40 (46)	
Total	536	166	165	66	63	66	

Perceptions of students in health and molecular life sciences regarding pharmacogenomics...

221

Table 2 Students' attitudes towards pharmacogenetic testing and personalized medicine *(Continued)*

	Total	Faculty of Pharmacy	Faculty of Medicine	Genetics and Bioeng.	Faculty of Health Studies	Non- ML&HS faculties	p*
Would you consider contacting a personal genome testing company and ordering a PG test for yourself?							
Yes	211 (39)	85 (52)	54 (33)	30 (45)	28 (44)	20 (23)	0.01
No	117 (22)	24 (14)	39 (24)	14 (21)	17 (27)	21 (24)	
Do not know	210	57 (34)	69(43)	22 (34)	18 (29)	45 (53)	
Total	538	166	162	66	63	86	

ML&HS Molecular Life and Health Science
*Chi-square test, Bonferroni-adjusted *p* values
[a]Percentage (%)

response on how much money they would be willing to spend to examine the effectiveness of a specific drug by using PG test was associated with their family monthly income (OR = 0.229, CI 0.065–0.392, p = 0.006), regardless of the field of their study (OR = 0.033, CI – 0.075–0.141, p = 0.543). This association does not seem to be affected by age, gender, and/or levels of education.

Importance of pharmacogenomics education
Results presented in Table 4 demonstrated similar opinion between medical, pharmacy, and health studies students regarding their study curriculum and future plans related to PG. When asked about their study curriculum, 44% of pharmacy students, 51% of medical students, and 61% of health studies students agreed that their study

Table 3 Students' attitudes towards pharmacogenomics and personalized medicine

Would you consider having a genetic test done to find out what illnesses you might develop in the future?

	Model I OR (CI)	Model II OR (CI)	Model III OR (CI)
Q1			
To what extent do you think that genes influence your health?	3.02 (1.16–7.85) p = 0.024	3.04 (1.17–7.92) p = 0.023	2.81 (1.07–7.36) p = 0.035
Q2			
Do you agree that PM represents a new and promising healthcare model?	3.11 (1.60–6.06) p = 0.001	3.11 (1.60–6.06) p = 0.001	3.14 (1.61–6.15) p = 0.001
Q3			
If you know your genetic tendency to develop a disease, would you be ready to make necessary changes in your lifestyle, to reduce disease risk?	0.198 (0.114–0.283) p = 0.001	0.195 (0.109–0.281) p = 0.001	0.191 (0.102–0.210) p = 0.001

Model I: without adjustment; model II: adjusted to age and gender; model III: adjusted to age, gender, and level of education
Answer as a reference for Q1: completely; answer as a reference for Q2 and Q3: yes

program is well designed for understanding PG. However, we found that only 20% of GBE students share this opinion, while 71% of them believe that PG should be an important part of their study curriculum (p < 0.01, see Additional file 4). About 30% of respondents are mostly interested to learn about pharmacogenomics in general, its clinical examples and benefits, while about 20% of students would like to learn more about its corresponding ethical, legal, and social issues. More than half of GBE students (55%) would like to continue their postgraduate education in the field of personalized medicine. Similarly, 74% of health studies students, 65% of pharmacy students, and 48% of medical students are also interested to continue their education in personalized medicine, which was significantly different as compared to the students from non-ML and non-HS study programs (p < 0.01; see Additional file 5). A similar finding was observed related to the students' opinion of PG position in their study curriculum, where significantly more medical, pharmacy, and genetics students agreed about an importance of PG as compared to their peers from other study programs (p < 0.01).

Our findings presented in Table 5 showed that students who believe that their study curriculum is well designed agreed that PG should be an important part of their study curriculum (OR = 0.54, CI 0.33–0.87, p = 0.01). They also believe that in their future practice they should be able to identify patients that could benefit from genetic testing (OR = 0.48, CI 0.31–0.75, p = 0.001) as well as to be able to answer patients' questions regarding PG and PM (OR = 1.70, CI 1.01–2.82, p = 0.047).

As shown in Table 6, our results suggest that the field of study significantly affects students' attitudes related to their study curriculum (OR = 3.94, CI 1.37–11.33, p = 0.011) as well as influences students' wish to continue their postgraduate education in the area of personalized medicine. As compared to other respondents, it appears that the highest number of GBE students would like to continue their postgraduate education in this field (OR = 14.7 CI 4.31–49.9, p < 0.001, upon adjustment to students' gender, age, and level of education).

Table 4 Students' opinion regarding the study curriculum and their future plans in pharmacogenomics

	Total	Faculty of Pharmacy	Faculty of Medicine	Genetics and Bioengineering	Faculty of Health Studies	Non- ML&HS faculties	p*
Do you think that the curriculum of your study program is well designed for understanding pharmacogenomics?							
Agree	219 (40)[a]	74 (44)	78 (51)	15 (20)	37 (61)	15 (18)	< 0.01
Disagree	185 (34)	71 (43)	40 (26)	25 (32)	17 (28)	32 (37)	
Not sure	139 (26)	21 (13)	36 (23)	37 (48)	7 (11)	38 (45)	
Total	543	166	154	77	61	85	
Pharmacogenomics should be an important part of my study curriculum.							
Agree	204 (38)	65 (39)	61 (39)	46 (71)	7 (11)	25 (29)	< 0.01
Disagree	112 (21)	86 (52)	8 (5)	1 (1)	–	17 (20)	
Not sure	318 (41)	15 (9)	86 (56)	18 (28)	55 (89)	44 (51)	
Total	534	166	155	65	62	86	
Would you like to continue your postgraduate education in the field of personalized medicine?							
Yes	275 (53)	107 (65)	74 (48)	36 (55)	45 (74)	13 (16)	< 0.01
No	97 (18)	17 (10)	41 (27)	6 (9)	10 (16)	32 (39)	
Do not know	146 (29)	40 (25)	39 (25)	24 (36)	6 (10)	37 (45)	
Total	527	164	154	66	61	82	

ML&HS, Molecular Life and Health Science
*Chi-square test, Bonferroni-adjusted p values
[a]Percentage (%)

Furthermore, our results suggest that students who believe that their study program is well designed to provide them with an adequate understanding of PG are also more willing to continue their postgraduate education in the area of personalized medicine (OR = 4.68, CI 2.59–8.47,*p* < 0.001). Similarly, it appears that these students also believe that PG should be an important part of their study curriculum (OR = 1.79 CI 1.01–3.19, *p* = 0.045), and this opinion is particularly affected by the level of education (OR = 2.40 CI 1.28–4.48, *p* = 0.006).

Furthermore, as shown in Table 7, our results demonstrated an interesting difference in attitude between pharmacy students from Sarajevo and Tuzla. A significantly higher number of pharmacy students at the University of Sarajevo, who have an elective course "Pharmacogenomics and Personalized Therapy" included in their study curriculum, believe that genes influence their health (*p* = 0.011), consider having genetic test done (*p* < 0.05), and agree that PM represents a new and promising healthcare model (*p* < 0.001), as compared to their colleagues from the Faculty of Pharmacy in Tuzla whose curriculum seems to cover PG education only as a few topics built into other coursework. In addition, the higher number of pharmacy students from Sarajevo agree that PG should be an important part of their study curriculum (*p* < 0.001). All surveyed pharmacy students from the University of Tuzla disagree that PG should be an important part of their study curriculum as opposed to only 6% of pharmacy students from the University of Sarajevo who believe that PG is not essential for their education.

Students' awareness about the ethical, legal, and social implications (ELSI)

Our results showed that about 45% of all students participating in our survey are aware of different ethical aspects of genetic testing, ranging from 27% of students at the Faculty of Health Studies to 54% of pharmacy students (*p* < 0.01, Table 8 and Additional file 6). The highest percentage (46%) of all respondents believed that patient privacy is the most related ethical issue to pharmacogenetic testing, while 18% believed that the key issue is data confidentiality (*p* < 0.01). Other ethical issues, such as incidental findings, racial issues, and stigma, were selected by 9%, 5%, and 4% of students, respectively. Our results revealed that 44% of students are worried about the possibility that PG test results may be passed to the unauthorized persons, and this opinion was shared similarly across different faculties (no significant difference). When asked which of the healthcare professionals should have an access to their PG information, 75% of students believe that a physician, 50% of students selected a genetic counselor, while 35% of them believe that a pharmacist should have this information. Furthermore, approximately one third of the respondents believe that they would be disadvantaged at work or job seeking in a case of unfavorable results of genetic test. Our analysis of questions related to the social issues showed that about half of participating students would not feel "helpless" or "pessimistic" (49%) nor they would feel "different" or "inadequate" (50%) in case of the unfavorable test results. Students' answers regarding all

Perceptions of students in health and molecular life sciences regarding pharmacogenomics...

223

Table 5 Students' attitudes towards continued education in pharmacogenomics

Do you think that the curriculum of your study program is well designed for understanding PG?

	Model I OR (CI)	Model II OR (CI)	Model III OR (CI)
Q1			
PG should be an important part of my study curriculum.	0.54 (0.33–0.87) $p = 0.012$	0.54 (0.33–0.88) $p = 0.014$	0.75 (0.43–1.30) $p = 0.307$
Q2			
In my future practice, I should be able to identify patients that could benefit from genetic testing.	0.48 (0.31–0.75) $p = 0.001$	0.48 (0.31–0.70) $p = 0.002$	0.57 (0.35–0.91) $p = 0.020$
Q3			
In my future practice, I should be able to answer patients' questions regarding PG and personalized medicine.	1.70 (1.01–2.82) $p = 0.047$	1.71 (1.02–2.87) $p = 0.044$	1.51 (0.87–2.62) $p = 0.146$
Q4			
In my future practice, I should be able to identify drugs that would require PG testing prior to their administration to the patient.	0.043 (0.011–0.098) $p = 0.121$	0.050 (0.006–0.107) $p = 0.079$	0.049 (0.007–0.106) $p = 0.086$
Q5			
What is your field of study?	3.94 (1.37–11.33) $p = 0.011$	7.23 (1.99–26.2) $p = 0.003$	7.23 (1.99–26.2) $p = 0.003$

Model I: without adjustment; model II: adjusted to age and gender; model III: adjusted to age, gender, and level of education
Answer as a reference for Q1: agree; answer as a reference for Q2: agree; answer as a reference for Q3: agree; answer as a reference for Q4: agree; answer as a reference for Q5: Genetics and Bioengineering

Table 6 Students' attitudes towards continued education in pharmacogenomics

Would you like to continue your postgraduate education (master, PhD, specialization) in the field of personalized medicine?

	Model I OR (CI)	Model II OR (CI)	Model III OR (CI)
Q1			
PG should be an important part of my study curriculum.	1.73 (0.99–3.02) $p = 0.056$	1.79 (1.01–3.19) $p = 0.045$	2.40 (1.28–4.48) $p = 0.006$
Q2			
Do you think that the curriculum of your study program is well designed for understanding PG?	4.68 (2.59–8.47) $p < 0.001$	4.71 (2.59–8.57) $p < 0.001$	4.27 (2.28–7.99) $p < 0.001$
Q3			
What is your field of study?	14.7 (4.31–49.9) $p < 0.001$	14.1 (3.94–50.6) $p < 0.001$	16.05 (4.05–63.6) $p < 0.001$

Model I: without adjustment; model II: adjusted to age and gender; model III: adjusted to age, gender, and level of education
Answer as a reference for Q1: agree; answer as a reference for Q2: agree; answer as a reference for Q3: Genetics and Bioengineering

above ELSI were similar across all participating disciplines (no significant difference). Our results presented in Table 9 showed that students who are worried about the possibility that PG test may reveal that they have additional risk factors for other diseases would also feel "different" and "inadequate" (OR = 2.48, CI 1.34–4.60, $p = 0.004$). A similar finding was demonstrated upon adjustment to students' age, gender, and level of education (OR = 2.15, CI 1.13–4.10, $p = 0.020$).

Discussion

This is the first study that analyzed the level of awareness and attitude towards genetic tests, pharmacogenomics, and personalized medicine among students from several different universities in Bosnia and Herzegovina (BH). Our results showed that health and molecular life science students are generally aware of PG, and the level of awareness about personal genome testing companies appears to be similar between medicine and pharmacy students. However, students from the Faculty of Health Studies (FHS) seem to be less aware of these companies and less interested to employ PM as the novel healthcare model as compared to pharmacy, medicine, or genetics students. Although the respondents from the other non-health- and molecular life science-related studies are also generally aware of genes influence on their health, our results suggest that the level of their awareness about personal genome testing companies is significantly lower than that of their peers from medicine, pharmacy, and genetics.

Importantly, here we also demonstrated that about 40% of pharmacy students believe that PG should be an important part of their study curriculum and more than 60% of these students would like to continue their postgraduate education in the field of personalized medicine. This is in line with the recent study, which showed that the majority of students from the eight pharmacy schools in California were aware of pharmacogenomics, agreed that PG is important for the future pharmacist, and would be interested in a residency, fellowship, and/ or career specializing PG [51]. However, Latif [8] reported that in the USA by 2005, PG was only being taught at a cursory level and highlighted the need to incorporate PG into the pharmacy curriculum. A recent survey of pharmacy students in California concluded that the presence of a stand-alone PG course did not impact student-perceived preparedness for a career in pharmacogenomics [51]. These findings are in accordance with the other studies including students from the medical schools in the UK [41] and USA [52], which also

Table 7 Pharmacy students' awareness and opinion regarding genetic tests and pharmacogenomics

	Total	Faculty of Pharmacy, University of Sarajevo	Faculty of Pharmacy, University of Tuzla	p^*
Have you heard about personal genome testing companies?				
Yes	95 (57)[a]	53 (62)	42 (52)	0.261
No	39 (24)	17 (20)	22 (27)	
Do not know	32 (19)	15 (18)	17 (21)	
Total	166	85	81	
To what extent do you think genes influence your health?				
Completely	30 (18)	20 (24)	10 (12)	0.011
Moderately	129 (78)	64 (75)	65 (80)	
Not at all	1 (1)	–	1 (1)	
Do not know	6 (4)	1 (1)	5 (6)	
Total	166	85	81	
Would you consider having a genetic test?				
Yes	85 (51)	51 (60)	34 (42)	0.047
No	24 (14)	9 (11)	15 (18)	
Not sure	57 (34)	25 (29)	32 (40)	
Total				
Do you agree that personalized medicine represents a new and promising healthcare model?				
Agree	116 (70)	78 (92)	38 (46)	$p < 0.001$
Disagree	14 (8)	2 (2)	12 (15)	
Not sure	37 (22)	5 (5.9)	32 (39)	
Total	167	85	82	
Pharmacogenomics should be an important part of my study curriculum.				
Agree	65 (39)	65 (76)		$p < 0.001$
Disagree	86 (52)	5 (5.9)	81 (100)	
Not sure	15 (9)	15 (18)		
Total	166	85	81	
Would you like to continue your postgraduate education in the field of personalized medicine?				
Yes	107 (64)	31 (36)	76 (94)	$p < 0.001$
No	19 (11)	16 (19)	3 (4)	
Do not know	40 (24)	38 (45)	2 (2)	
Total	166	85	81	

*Chi-square test, Bonferroni-adjusted p values
[a]Percentage (%)

clearly indicated that inadequate education at undergraduate and postgraduate medical programs is an important obstacle to more broad use of PG. A recent study performed at the Stanford School of Medicine showed that almost all students taking a course in personalized medicine believed that physicians are not trained to interpret results of PG tests and thus are not able to effectively practice PM [52]. In line with this study, more than a third of the total number of students participating in our survey disagree that the curriculum of their study program is well designed to understand PG, suggesting that the majority of faculties do not have PG-related courses implemented in their curricula.

Similar to our finding that 52% of pharmacy students disagree that their study program is well designed for understanding PG, half of the pharmacy students at the University of Minnesota also argued that their curriculum is not well designed to grasp pharmacogenomics [38]. Interestingly, in contrast to the pharmacy students from the University of Tuzla whose curriculum covers PG topics cursorily, usually not more than a week in a semester as a part of other coursework based on their current curriculum (http://frmf.untz.ba/web/bs/integri sani-i-i-ii-ciklus/), pharmacy students from the University of Sarajevo think that their curriculum is well designed to understand PG and PM. The Faculty of

Perceptions of students in health and molecular life sciences regarding pharmacogenomics...

225

Table 8 Students' awareness and opinion regarding the ethical, legal, and social implications (ELSI)

	Total	Faculty of Pharmacy	Faculty of Medicine	Genetics and Bioengineering	Faculty of Health Studies	Non- ML&HS	p^*
Ethical							
Are you aware of the different ethical aspects of genetic testing?							
Yes	244 (45)[a]	90 (54)	50 (36)	28 (43)	17 (27)	26 (30)	< 0.01
No	155 (29)	32 (19)	60 (43)	22 (34)	32 (50)	33 (38)	
Not sure	139 (26)	44 (27)	30 (21)	15 (23)	15 (23)	27 (32)	
Total	538	166	140	65	64	86	
What ethical issues do you believe might be related to genetic or PG testing?							
Patient privacy	237 (46)	88 (40)	63 (34)	29 (38)	30 (41)	27 (29)	< 0.01
Data confidentiality	91 (18)	82 (37)	56 (30)	14 (18)	13 (18)	8 (8)	
Racial issues	27 (5)	10 (5)	4 (3)	2 (3)	12 (17)	9 (10)	
Stigma	20 (4)	7(3)	17 (9)	–	–	3 (3)	
Incidental findings	47 (9)	21 (9)	21 (11)	9 (12)	9 (12)	8 (8)	
Other	93 (18)	14 (6)	24 (13)	21 (28)	9 (12)	39 (42)	
Total	515	222	185	75	73	94	
Legal							
Are you worried about the possibility that the results of a PG test may be passed to unauthorized persons?							
Worried	238 (44)	71 (43)	69 (44)	30 (46)	24 (37)	44 (51)	1.0
Not worried	190 (35)	65 (39)	60 (38)	24 (36)	21 (33)	20 (23)	
No opinion	112 (21)	30 (18)	29 (18)	12 (18)	19 (30)	22 (26)	
Total	540	166	158	66	64	86	
In case unfavorable test results should be disclosed, do you believe that you would be disadvantaged at work or job seeking?							
Yes	165 (31)	45 (27)	49 (31)	26 (39)	21 (35)	24 (28)	0.400
No	219 (41)	86 (51)	71 (45)	17 (26)	15 (25)	30 (35)	
Not sure	152 (28)	38 (22)	38 (24)	23 (35)	24 (40)	32 (37)	
Total	536	169	158	66	60	86	
Social							
In case of an unfavorable test result, do you believe you would feel "helpless" or "pessimistic"?							
Yes	174 (33)	63 (38)	40 (25)	26 (39)	18 (29)	27 (32)	0.170
No	265 (49)	69 (42)	93 (58)	35 (53)	32 (52)	36 (42)	
Not sure	98 (18)	34 (20)	25 (16)	5 (8)	12 (19)	22 (26)	
Total	537	166	158	66	62	85	
In case of an unfavorable test result, do you believe you would feel "different" or "inadequate"?							
Yes	152 (28)	51 (31)	32 (20)	25 (38)	19 (31)	25 (30)	0.100
No	268 (50)	84 (50)	95 (60)	32 (48)	27 (44)	30 (36)	
Not sure	115 (22)	31 (19)	31 (20)	9 (14)	15 (25)	29 (34)	
Total	535	166	158	66	61	84	

ML&HS, Molecular Life and Health Science
*Chi-square test, Bonferroni-adjusted *p* values
[a]Percentage (%)

Pharmacy in Sarajevo implemented changes in their curriculum in 2012. Based on our knowledge and information available at the Faculty's website (http://ffsa.unsa.ba/wp-content/uploads/2014/03/ECTS-katalog-2015.pdf), so far in BH only this Faculty included an elective course Pharmacogenomics and Personalized Therapy in the biomedical study course. In addition, pharmacy students from Sarajevo have a lot of subject education built into their other coursework. This is may be the reason why student pharmacists from Sarajevo had more positive attitude and future plans towards PG, while the majority of the pharmacy

Table 9 Students' opinion regarding the confidentiality and data privacy in pharmacogenomic testing

	Model I OR (CI)	Model II OR (CI)	Model III OR (CI)
In case of an unfavorable test result, do you believe that you would feel "different" or "inadequate"?			
Q1			
Are you worried about the possibility that a pharmacogenomics test may reveal that you have additional risk factors for other diseases?	2.48 (1.34–4.60) $p = 0.004$	2.17 (1.15–4.09) $p = 0.017$	2.15 (1.13–4.10) $p = 0.020$

Model I: without adjustment; model II: adjusted to age and gender; model III: adjusted to age, gender, and level of education
Answer as a reference for Q1: yes

students from Tuzla disagree that PG should be an important part of their study curriculum.

Students of the Genetics and Bioengineering program at the International University of Sarajevo have special PG topics included in the syllabus of several undergraduate and graduate courses, including courses Pharmaceutical Biotechnology and Omics Technologies. Interestingly, more than 70% of GBE students agree that PG should be an important part of their study curriculum and more than half of them would like to continue their postgraduate education in the field of personalized medicine. Furthermore, as expected, in contrast to students from HS and MLS studies, half of students from other non-related study programs are not interested to continue their education in the field of pharmacogenomics and personalized medicine. Thus, in line with previous studies [38, 51], our results confirmed that if students do not gain enough PG knowledge during their studies, that would affect their attitudes towards PG as well as their future interest for this area of research or professional practice. Specifically, McCullough et al. [16] showed that pharmacists included in their study lacked the knowledge and self-confidence to act properly based on the results of PG testing. However, an education emphasizing medical applications of PG can significantly increase students' knowledge and comfort in their PG practice. Recently, Pisanu et al. [53] investigated the discrepancy in PG education in Southeast Europe and recommended that PG should be thought as a stand-alone course or at least as a part of existing genetics courses. The lack of education and clinical guidelines appear to be among the major barriers perceived by participants towards the clinical application of PG [51].

It is expected that PG will continue to evolve over time and become one of the most relevant aspects of patient care. For this reason, it is of key importance to increase the number of professional practitioners in this new and expanding area of PG and to modify the current curricula to increase students' knowledge and interests. The survey performed in the UK in 2008 found that typically 2–8 h of PG teaching were included in the pharmacology curricula of UK medical schools [41]. Previous studies have shown that incorporating active learning experiences in PG would increase student interests [54]. Additional innovative learning methods in PG have been recently adopted, such as Pharmacogenomics Education Program 3 (PharmGenEd™) open online courses [9] and personal genotyping [52, 55, 56]. When teaching PG through practical applications, students learn to use genetic information in the framework of medication management, allowing them to understand the significance of PG applications in clinical practice [51].

As our results indicate, BH students are interested to continue their education in PG. They would like to learn more about pharmacogenomics, its clinical examples and benefits, as well as about ELSI and future developments in this field. Students consider performing genetic tests in their future practice to optimize therapy for their patients as well as answering patients' questions regarding PG and personalized medicine. Interestingly, our results suggest that the field of study significantly influences students' wish to continue their education in this area. This is in line with the previous studies which indicated that healthcare students believe that PG is important for patient care [16, 40] and that they should have the knowledge to employ genetic tests results to optimize therapy and educate their patients [38].

Students participating in our survey have shown to be aware of different ethical aspects of genetic testing. Interestingly, our results demonstrated that the majority of students appear to be concerned about the patient's privacy and data confidentiality, followed by other ethical issues, such as autonomy, trust, beneficence relating to incidental findings, racial issues, and stigma. The majority of participants in our survey believe that the physician, pharmacist, and genetic counselor should have an access to their PG information. If genetic information is inappropriately disclosed, individuals may suffer from embarrassment, stigma, and discrimination, and these issues are recently considered as the key aspects of respecting confidentiality [25]. This is increasingly a salient point with developments and prevalence of information and communication technology, especially in the context of health, with emerging EU regulations in context of data sharing. Information and tools that were previously accessible to physicians only under controlled clinical setting within the last decade have been made freely available through the increasing variety of the direct-to-consumer (DTC) genetic tests on the Internet and social networks, often without the public's ability to understand the health risk information that are sold without genetic counseling [57, 58]. This issue is particularly important in the low- and middle-income countries, where the use of commercial genomics and DTC tests might not be adequately regulated yet.

Our results suggest that students from non-HS- and non-MLS-related faculties, including architecture, psychology, industrial, mechanical, electrical engineering, and others, are also generally aware of genes influence on their own health as well as about benefits of PM-based healthcare model. About half of these students agree that personalized medicine represents a new and promising healthcare model, and the majority of them would consider having a genetic test done to find out what illnesses they might develop in the future. However, their awareness of personal genome testing companies is lower as well as their readiness to contact a personal genome testing company and order a PG test, as compared to their peers from medicine, pharmacy, and genetics. Furthermore, these students from non-HS- and non-MLS-related faculties appear to be less aware regarding the potential ethical implications of PG testing, as compared to the students from medicine and pharmacy. These findings may indicate the significance of educating the public about genomics and its relevant bioethical implications. As recently suggested by Dressler et al. [59], roundtable discussions, a body of experts' discussions, workshops, and symposia are needed to bring together key interdisciplinary stakeholders in academia, government, profit, and nonprofit organizations to create programs of genomic education for the public. Such efforts can lead to enhanced knowledge and widespread acceptance of PG.

Interestingly, our findings revealed that almost half of all respondents are worried about the possibility that PG test results may be passed to the unauthorized persons, and this opinion was shared similarly across different study programs. Students who are worried about the possibility that PG test may reveal that they have additional risk factors for other diseases would also feel "different" and "inadequate" in case of the unfavorable test results. Otherwise, about half of respondents would not feel "helpless" or "pessimistic," nor they would not feel "different" or "inadequate." This is in line with the previous study, which indicated that every individual would respond in a different way to the genetic test results, and it is considered essential for patients to have a proper counseling to help them understand the meaning and significance of the test results related to their own health [60, 61]. This also emphasizes the importance of sociological disciplines in public perceptions of pharmacogenomics and personalized medicine in order to examine and understand better the society's needs, concerns, and attitudes towards the utilization of PG testing and its wider clinical implementation as well as to be an asset in instituting policies and regulating the use of genetic information. This is in line with the findings of the recent survey of the general public in Belgium on genetics and genetic testing [62], which indicated that recognizing the attitudes and concerns of the general public is the key in ensuring ethically reliable and socially acceptable application of new genetic technologies. Sociology students should be also approached to expand such studies of people's reactions to genetics and PM/PG, where it would be pertinent to compare expected attitudes with actual attitudes upon receiving results of genetic tests [22].

An important strength of our study was that we recruited a variety of health science students across the nation within three different settings (medicine, pharmacy, health studies), genetics students, and students from other non-molecular life and non-health science programs. Another key aspect of our study was that, for the first time in BH, we have investigated students' perceptions regarding their knowledge, skills, and attitudes towards pharmacogenomics and personalized medicine as well as their ethical, legal, and social implications. In addition, we compared opinions and attitudes of students who were exposed vs. students who were non-exposed to the PG course that further strengthens our results. Although our survey explored students' interest in learning more about PG, we did not investigate which teaching tools students would favor in order to determine the most effective way to educate students in PG. Another limitation is that the survey which we designed assessed perceived (or self-reported) understanding and skills in pharmacogenomics and personalized medicine, with the limited possibility to evaluate actual students' knowledge and capabilities. Lastly, survey tools that employ Likert scale are prone to central tendency bias due to selection of neutral answers. However, the potential impact of this type of bias on our results is probably small due to low percentage of neutral answers in the majority of our questions. Notwithstanding these limitations, our study will offer an important reference point for future comparative studies between different regions and countries as well as between different disciplines.

Conclusions

Here we investigated for the first time students' perceptions about pharmacogenomics and personalized medicine across the nation and various study programs that was, based on our knowledge, never studied before in Bosnia and Herzegovina. Our results show that most of the students participating in our survey, other than pharmacy students from Sarajevo, believe that they do not have well-designed curricula for understanding and practicing PG. The large number of students enrolled in molecular life and health sciences clearly expressed their wish to be more educated in this field. This implies the need for the development of study programs in the area of PG in order to equip future providers with the knowledge, skills, and attitude required to practice personalized medicine. This could also further highlight the need for increased genetic literacy education throughout high school levels throughout Europe and beyond. In order to accomplish this important goal, it would be pertinent to enhance collaboration between universities, healthcare institution, and governing bodies to incorporate more training and continued education topics related to pharmacogenomics and genetic testing. There could also be a potential here for increasing the number of interdisciplinary events or training between different disciplines, such as those highlighted in this study, both for students and for educators and researchers in order to discuss various forms of curriculum development. Thus, expanding the pharmacogenomic path of biomedical education represents an essential step for ensuring the widespread clinical implementation of personalized medicine.

Additional files

Additional file 1: The survey questionnaire—the file describes the

Additional file 2: Students' awareness about pharmacogenomics—the table represents p values calculated with chi-square test between each faculty, based on the first question from Table 2

Additional file 3: Levels of students' awareness about genetic tests and pharmacogenomics—the table represents p values calculated with chi-square test between each faculty, based on the fourth question from Table 2

Additional file 4: Students' opinion regarding the study curriculum and their future plans in pharmacogenomics—the table represents p values calculated with chi-square test between each faculty, based on the first question from Table 4

Additional file 5: Students' opinion regarding the study curriculum and their future plans in pharmacogenomics—the table represents p values calculated with chi-square test between each faculty, based on the third question from Table 4

Additional file 6: Students' awareness and opinion regarding the ethical, legal, and social issues—the table represents p values calculated with chi-square test between each faculty, based on the first question from Table 8

Abbreviations

BH: Bosnia and Herzegovina; CI: Confidence intervals; DTC: Direct-to-consumer; ELSI: Ethical, legal, and social implications; FDA: Food and Drug Administration; FHS: Faculty of Health Studies; GBE: Genetics and Bioengineering; HS: Health Studies; IBM SPSS®23: IBM Statistical Package for Social Science, Version 23; MLS: Molecular and life sciences; OR: Odds ratio; PG: Pharmacogenomics; PharmGenEd™: Pharmacogenomics Education Program; PharmGKB: Pharmacogenomics Knowledgebase; PM: Personalized medicine

Acknowledgements

The authors would like to thank all students participating in this survey, as well as all managerial and administrative staff for the survey distribution in participating institutions. We thank Dr. Emin Tahirovic for his kind help with the statistical analysis. This article is based upon work from COST Action IS1303 "Citizen's Health through public-private Initiatives: Public health, Market and Ethical perspectives," supported by COST (European Cooperation in Science and Technology) (http://www.cost.eu).

Funding

This study was partially funded by the grants received from the Council of Ministers of BH/Ministry of Civil Affairs BH, awarded to SS.

Authors' contributions

MW, SS, and CD participated in the development of the questionnaire. LM, CD, AM, and NH were involved in the survey distribution and data acquisition. LM was responsible for the statistical analysis and has made substantial contribution to the data interpretation. MA was involved in the statistical analysis. LM and BA were engaged in the writing of the initial draft of the manuscript. FBA helped in the data collection process. MW and OF revised the manuscript critically for its important intellectual content. SS conceived and designed the study, coordinated and supervised the study, provided its financial support, interpreted data, and revised the manuscript critically for its important intellectual content. All authors read and approved the final manuscript.

Authors' information

Sabina Semiz, PhD, is a Professor in Genetics and Bioengineering at the International University of Sarajevo (IUS). She is the Head of the Bosnia and Herzegovina Unit of the UNESCO Chair in Bioethics, Chair of the Cambridge Bioethics Education Network Working Group, and a member of the Management Committee of the CHIP ME COST Action IS1303 "Citizen's Health through public-private Initiatives: Public health, Market and Ethical perspectives." Matthias Wjst, PhD, and Oliver Feeney, PhD, (Researcher in Political Theory and Bioethics at the Centre of Bioethical Research and Analysis) are members of the Management Committee and Working Group 2 and Working Group 3 of the CHIP ME COST Action IS1303. Faruk Berat Akcesme, PhD, and Betul Akcesme, PhD, were Assistant Professors at the Genetics and Bioengineering Program at FENS, and they recently joined the Faculty of Medicine, University of Health Sciences, Istanbul, Turkey. Lejla Mahmutovic and Muhamed Adilovic are PhD students, while Camil Durakovic, Aida Maric, and Nour Hamad were master students at the IUS. Aida Maric recently started her PhD program at the Plant Biotechnology Department, Faculty of Pharmacy and Food Sciences, at the University of Barcelona, Spain.

Competing interests

The authors declare that they have no competing interests.

Author details

¹Faculty of Engineering and Natural Sciences, International University of Sarajevo, Hrasnicka cesta 15, 71210 Ilidza, Sarajevo, Bosnia and Herzegovina. ²Department of Medical Biology, Faculty of Medicine, University of Health Sciences, Istanbul, Turkey. ³Department of Biostatistics and Medical Informatics, Faculty of Medicine, University of Health Sciences, Istanbul, Turkey. ⁴Helmholtz Zentrum Muenchen, German Research Center for Environmental Health (GmbH), Ingolstaedter Landstraße 1, D-85764 Munich, Neuherberg, Germany. ⁵Centre of Bioethical Research and Analysis, National University of Ireland (Galway), Galway, Republic of Ireland.

References

1. Abul-Husn NS, et al. Implementation and utilization of genetic testing in personalized medicine. Pharmgenomics Pers Med. 2014;7:227–40.
2. Manolio TA, et al. Implementing genomic medicine in the clinic: the future is here. Genet Med. 2013;15(4):258–67.
3. McCarthy JJ, et al. Genomic medicine: a decade of successes, challenges, and opportunities. Sci Transl Med. 2013;5(189):189sr4.
4. Shuldiner AR, et al. The pharmacogenomics research network translational pharmacogenetics program: overcoming challenges of real-world implementation. Clin Pharmacol Ther. 2013;94(2):207–10.

5. Phillips E, Mallal S. Successful translation of pharmacogenetics into the clinic: the abacavir example. Mol Diagn Ther. 2009;13(1):1–9.

6. Goldspiel BR, et al. Integrating pharmacogenetic information and clinical decision support into the electronic health record. J Am Med Inform Assoc. 2014;21(3):522–8.

7. Collins FS, Morgan M, Patrinos A. The Human Genome Project: lessons from large-scale biology. Science. 2003;300(5617):286–90.

8. Latif DA. Pharmacogenetics and pharmacogenomics instruction in schools of pharmacy in the USA: is it adequate? Pharmacogenomics. 2005;6(4):317–9.

9. Ma JD, Lee KC, Kuo GM. A massive open online course on pharmacogenomics: not just disruptive innovation but a possible solution. Pharmacogenomics. 2013;14(10):1125–7.

10. Collins FS, Varmus H. A new initiative on precision medicine. N Engl J Med. 2015;372(9):793–5.

11. Wang B, Canestaro WJ, Choudhry NK. Clinical evidence supporting pharmacogenomic biomarker testing provided in US Food and Drug Administration drug labels. JAMA Intern Med. 2014;174(12):1938–44.

12. Johnson JA. Pharmacogenetics in clinical practice: how far have we come and where are we going? Pharmacogenomics. 2013;14(7):835–43.

13. Olivier C, Williams-Jones B. Global pharmacogenomics: where is the research taking us? Glob Public Health. 2014;9(3):312–24.

14. Elewa H, et al. A survey on the awareness and attitude of pharmacists and doctors towards the application of pharmacogenomics and its challenges in Qatar. J Eval Clin Pract. 2015;21(4):703–9.

15. Obara T, et al. Awareness regarding clinical application of pharmacogenetics among Japanese pharmacists. Pharmgenomics Pers Med. 2015;8:35–41.

16. McCullough KB, et al. Assessment of the pharmacogenomics educational needs of pharmacists. Am J Pharm Educ. 2011;75(3):51.

17. Carlberg C. The need for education in personalized medicine. Personalized Med. 2012;9(2):147–50.

18. Dickinson BD. Pharmacogenomic knowledge gaps and educational resource needs among physicians in selected specialties. Pharmacogenomics Personalized Med. 2014;7:145–62.

19. Frueh FW, Gurwitz D. From pharmacogenetics to personalized medicine: a vital need for educating health professionals and the community. Pharmacogenomics. 2004;5(5):571–9.

20. Salari P, Larijani B. Ethical issues surrounding personalized medicine: a literature review. Acta Med Iran. 2017;55(3):209–17.

21. Javitt GH. Policy implications of genetic testing: not just for geneticists anymore. Adv Chronic Kidney Dis. 2006;13(2):178–82.

22. Corrigan OP. Pharmacogenetics, ethical issues: review of the Nuffield Council on Bioethics Report. J Med Ethics. 2005;31(3):144–8.

23. Rothstein MA, Epps PG. Ethical and legal implications of pharmacogenomics. Nat Rev Genet. 2001;2(3):228–31.

24. Motulsky AG. Bioethical problems in pharmacogenetics and ecogenetics. Hum Genet Suppl. 1978;1:185–92.

25. Brothers KB, Rothstein MA. Ethical, legal and social implications of incorporating personalized medicine into healthcare. Per Med. 2015;12(1):43–51.

26. Lala M, et al. Genetics-based pediatric warfarin dosage regimen derived using pharmacometric bridging. J Pediatr Pharmacol Ther. 2013;18(3):209–19.

27. Egalite N, Ozdemir V, Godard B. Pharmacogenomics research involving racial classification: qualitative research findings on researchers' views, perceptions and attitudes towards socioethical responsibilities. Pharmacogenomics. 2007;8(9):1115–26.

28. Vogenberg FR, Barash CI, Pursel M. Personalized medicine: part 2: ethical, legal, and regulatory issues. P T. 2010;35(11):624–42.

29. Netzer C, Biller-Andorno N. Pharmacogenetic testing, informed consent and the problem of secondary information. Bioethics. 2004;18(4):344–60.

30. Spector-Bagdady K. "The Google of healthcare": enabling the privatization of genetic bio/databanking. Ann Epidemiol. 2016;26(7):515–9.

31. Niemiec E, Howard HC. Ethical issues in consumer genome sequencing: use of consumers' samples and data. Appl Transl Genom. 2016;8:23–30.

32. Trinidad SB, et al. "Getting off the bus closer to your destination": patients' views about pharmacogenetic testing. Perm J. 2015;19(3):21–7.

33. Mardis ER. A decade's perspective on DNA sequencing technology. Nature. 2011;470(7333):198–203.

34. Manolio TA, et al. Global implementation of genomic medicine: we are not alone. Sci Transl Med. 2015;7(290):290ps13.

35. Ndebele P, Musesengwa R. Will developing countries benefit from their participation in genetics research? Malawi Med J. 2008;20(2):67–9.

36. Murphy JE, et al. Pharmacogenomics in the curricula of colleges and schools of pharmacy in the United States. Am J Pharm Educ. 2010;74(1):7.

37. Ormond KE, et al. Medical and graduate students' attitudes toward personal genomics. Genet Med. 2011;13(5):400–8.

38. Moen M, Lamba J. Assessment of healthcare students' views on pharmacogenomics at the University of Minnesota. Pharmacogenomics. 2012;13(13):1537–45.

39. Jr JP, et al. Pre-graduate and post-graduate education in personalized medicine in the Czech Republic: statistics, analysis and recommendations. EPMA J. 2014;5(1):22.

40. Gurwitz D, et al. Pharmacogenomics education: International Society of Pharmacogenomics recommendations for medical, pharmaceutical, and health schools deans of education. Pharmacogenomics J. 2005;5(4):221–5.

41. Higgs JE, et al. Pharmacogenetics education in British medical schools. Genomic Med. 2008;2(3–4):101–5.

42. Cavallari LH, et al. Institutional profile: University of Florida Health Personalized Medicine Program. Pharmacogenomics. 2017;18(5):421–6.

43. Patrinos GP, Katsila T. Pharmacogenomics education and research at the Department of Pharmacy, University of Patras, Greece. Pharmacogenomics. 2016;17(17):1865–72.

44. Eden C, et al. Medical student preparedness for an era of personalized medicine: findings from one US medical school. Per Med. 2016;13(2):129–41.

45. Krynetskiy E. Institutional profile: Jayne Haines Center for Pharmacogenomics and Drug Safety: educating future generations of healthcare professionals. Pharmacogenomics. 2013;14(5):465–8.

46. Ceric T, et al. Investigation of IVS14 + 1G > A polymorphism of DPYD gene in a group of Bosnian patients treated with 5-fluorouracil and capecitabine. Bosn J Basic Med Sci. 2010;10(2):133–9.

47. Hadzagic-Catibusic F, et al. Effects of carbamazepine and valproate on serum aspartate aminotransferase, alanine aminotransferase and gamma - glutamyltransferase in children. Med Arch. 2017;71(4):239–42.

48. Dujic T, et al. Organic cation transporter 1 variants and gastrointestinal side effects of metformin in patients with type 2 diabetes. Diabet Med. 2016; 33(4):511–4.

49. Zhou K, et al. Variation in the glucose transporter gene SLC2A2 is associated with glycemic response to metformin. Nat Genet. 2016;48(9):1055–9.

50. Semiz S, et al. Analysis of CYP2C9*2, CYP2C19*2, and CYP2D6*4 polymorphisms in patients with type 2 diabetes mellitus. Bosn J Basic Med Sci. 2010;10(4):287–91.

51. Vaksman N, et al. The impact of incorporating of pharmacogenomics into the pharmacy curriculum on student interest. Pharm Educ. 2012;12.

52. Salari K, et al. Evidence that personal genome testing enhances student learning in a course on genomics and personalized medicine. PLoS One. 2013;8(7):e68853.

53. Pisanu C, et al. Assessment of the pharmacogenomics educational environment in Southeast Europe. Public Health Genomics. 2014;17(5–6):272–9.

54. Knoell DL, et al. A genotyping exercise for pharmacogenetics in pharmacy practice. Am J Pharm Educ. 2009;73(3):43.

55. Adams SM, et al. Advancing pharmacogenomics education in the Core PharmD curriculum through student personal genomic testing. Am J Pharm Educ. 2016;80(1):3.

56. Frick A, et al. Transitioning pharmacogenomics into the clinical setting: training future pharmacists. Front Pharmacol. 2016;7:241.

57. Borry P, Cornel MC, Howard HC. Where are you going, where have you been: a recent history of the direct-to-consumer genetic testing market. J Community Genet. 2010;1(3):101–6.

58. Collins RE, Wright AJ, Marteau TM. Impact of communicating personalized genetic risk information on perceived control over the risk: a systematic review. Genet Med. 2011;13(4):273–7.

59. Dressler LG, et al. Genomics education for the public: perspectives of genomic researchers and ELSI advisors. Genet Test Mol Biomarkers. 2014; 18(3):131–40.

60. Winkler EC, Wiemann S. Findings made in gene panel to whole genome sequencing: data, knowledge, ethics–and consequences? Expert Rev Mol Diagn. 2016;16(12):1259–70.

61. Howard HC, Borry P. Survey of European clinical geneticists on awareness, experiences and attitudes towards direct-to-consumer genetic testing. Genome Med. 2013;5(5):45.

62. Chokoshvili D, et al. Public views on genetics and genetic testing: a survey of the general public in Belgium. Genet Test Mol Biomarkers. 2017;21(3): 195–201.

22

Identification of gross deletions in *FBN1* gene by MLPA

Hang Yang[1†], Yanyun Ma[1†], Mingyao Luo[2], Kun Zhao[1], Yinhui Zhang[1], Guoyan Zhu[1], Xiaogang Sun[2], Fanyan Luo[3], Lin Wang[3*], Chang Shu[2*] and Zhou Zhou[1*] (iD)

Abstract

Background: Marfan syndrome (MFS) is an autosomal dominant connective tissue disorder caused by mutations in the *FBN1* gene. Approximately 90% of classic MFS patients have a *FBN1* mutation that can be identified by single-gene sequencing or gene-panel sequencing targeting *FBN1*. However, a small proportion of MFS patients carry a large genomic deletion in *FBN1*, which cannot be detected by routine sequencing. Here, we performed an MLPA (multiplex ligation-dependent probe amplification) test to detect large deletions and/or duplications in *FBN1* and *TGFBR2* in 115 unrelated Chinese patients with suspected MFS or early-onset aneurysm/dissection.

Results: Five novel large deletions encompassing a single exon or multiple exons in the *FBN1* gene were characterized in five unrelated patients, of which four were proven by Sanger sequencing, and the breakpoints were identified. Three of them met the revised Ghent criteria when genetic results were not available, and the other two patients were highly suspected and diagnosed with MFS until the *FBN1* deletions were identified.

Conclusions: Our finding expands the mutation spectrum of large *FBN1* deletions and emphasizes the importance of screening for large *FBN1* deletions in clinical genetic testing, especially for those with classic Marfan phenotype.

Keywords: Marfan syndrome, MLPA, *FBN1* gene, Deletion

Background

Marfan syndrome (MFS) is a connective tissue disorder with high clinical heterogeneity, mainly involving ocular, skeletal, and cardiovascular systems, with an estimated prevalence of 1:3000–1:5000 [1]. A large proportion of patients have visible signs, such as tall and slender stature, arachnodactyly, chest deformity, and scoliosis. Most patients have rapidly progressive myopia, and approximately 60% of affected individuals have ectopia lentis. However, cardiovascular abnormality might be the only defect in some MFS patients that is insidious and fatal.

MFS is caused by mutations in the *FBN1* gene, which is located on chromosome 15q21.1 and encodes a 320-kDa extracellular matrix glycoprotein fibrillin-1 [2, 3], a major component of microfibrils. So far, more than 2500 mutations (HGMD Professional 2018.1 total) have been identified throughout *FBN1*, while missense mutations are the most common type [4, 5]. Sanger sequencing of *FBN1* and panel sequencing including *FBN1* as well as a number of other genes associated with inherited aortopathies are commonly used to identify mutations [6]; however, both of these methods have a limitation for detecting *FBN1* large deletions (del) or duplications (dup), which have been reported in up to 7% of MFS patients [7].

Additionally, Loeys-Dietz syndrome (LDS), another inherited connective tissue disorder, which is caused mostly by *TGFBR1* and *TGFBR2* mutations, is often clinically indistinguishable from MFS [8]. However, up to now, no large genomic rearrangements in *TGFBR1*

---

* Correspondence: wanglin79922@csu.edu.cn;
changshu01@fuwaihospital.org; zhouzhou@fuwaihospital.org
†Hang Yang and Yanyun Ma contributed equally to this work.
[3]Department of Cardiovascular Surgery, Xiangya Hospital Central South University, Changsha 410008, Hunan, China
[2]State Key Laboratory of Cardiovascular Disease, Center of Vascular Surgery, Fuwai Hospital, National Center for Cardiovascular Diseases, Chinese Academy of Medical Sciences and Peking Union Medical College, Beijing 100037, China
[1]State Key Laboratory of Cardiovascular Disease, Beijing Key Laboratory for Molecular Diagnostics of Cardiovascular Diseases, Diagnostic Laboratory Service, Fuwai Hospital, National Center for Cardiovascular Diseases, Chinese Academy of Medical Sciences and Peking Union Medical College, Beijing 100037, China

Table 1 The baseline clinical characteristics of the 115 unrelated patients

Characteristics	Statistics ($n = 115$)
Age (years)	29.4 ± 14.9
Male gender	87 (75.7%)
Primary diagnosis	
Marfan syndrome	19 (16.5%)
Suspected Marfan syndrome	43 (37.4%)
Thoracic aortic aneurysm and dissection	53 (46.1%)

Values are presented as mean ± SD or n (%)

or *TGFBR2* have been reported in patients with aortic aneurysm/dissection and LDS features.

In this study, we performed a multiplex ligation-dependent probe amplification (MLPA) testing of *FBN1* and *TGFBR2* in 115 unrelated Marfan or early-onset aortopathy patients that were previously proven to be negative in a panel testing involving 15 genes associated with inherited aortopathy.

Results

A total of 115 patients with suspected MFS or early-onset aortic aneurysm/dissection, who had a negative result in a 15-gene panel testing, were included in this study and evaluated for gross deletions and

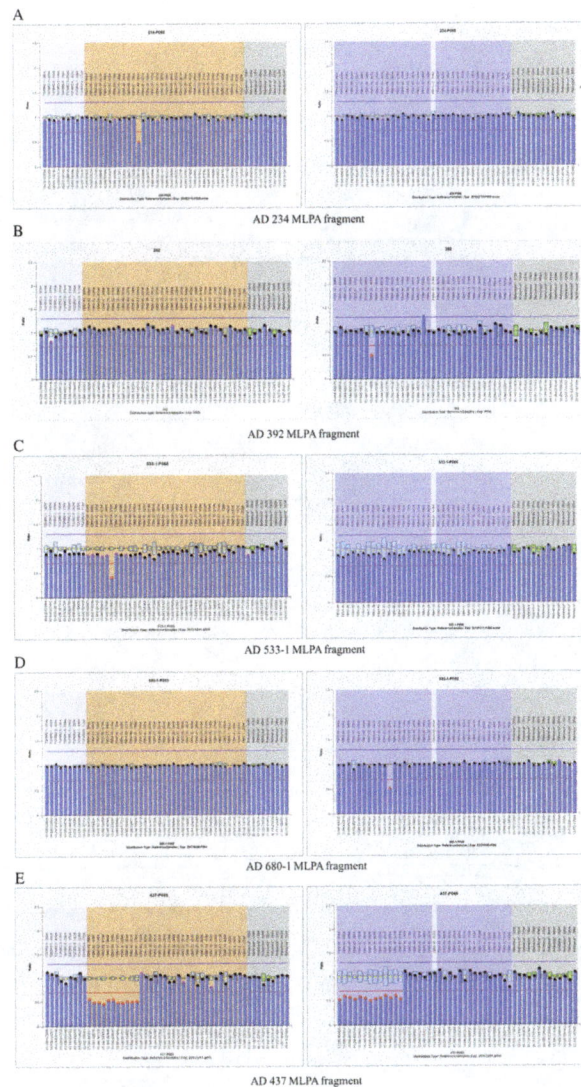

Fig. 1 Results of semiquantitative MLPA. The results of MLPA for five patients. **a** Reduced relative peak areas of *FBN1* exon 43 for patient AD234. **b** Reduced relative peak areas of *FBN1* exon 56 for patient AD392. **c** Reduced relative peak areas of *FBN1* exon 54 for patient AD533-1. **d** Reduced relative peak areas of *FBN1* exon 50 for patient AD680-1. **e** Reduced relative peak areas of *FBN1* exon 44–66 for patient AD437

Table 2 Overview of cases with large deletions in *FBN1* gene

Patient No.	Age (y)	Deletion breakpoints	Deletion (*FBN1* exon affected)	Phenotype
AD234	24	g.48749026-48753819	*FBN1*: exon 43	Classic MFS
AD392	38	g.48724560-48722281	*FBN1*: exon 56	Classic MFS
AD533-1	5	g.48727672-48726338	*FBN1*: exon 54	Suspected MFS
AD680-1	14	g.48734801-48730690	*FBN1*: exon 50	Suspected MFS
AD437	37	NA	*FBN1*: exon 44–66	Classic MFS

All nucleotide positions are represented in relation to the human genome reference sequence (GRCh37/hg19), and position + 1 corresponds to the first nucleotide of the *FBN1* reference sequence (GenBank NC_000015.9) at the genomic DNA (g) level
NA not available

duplications in *FBN1* and *TGFBR2* gene by MLPA assay. The baseline clinical characteristics are summarized in Table 1. Of all patients, 19 were classic MFS, which referred to those who met the Ghent criteria independent of genetic results, and 43 were suspected MFS, which referred to those with some positive signs (either aortic dilation or positive family history AND systemic score ≥ 3) but not meeting the criteria yet. Almost half of the patients had no other systemic abnormality except for aortic events. Five novel large deletions encompassing a single exon or multiple exons in the *FBN1* gene were identified in five unrelated patients (Fig. 1, Table 2). Patients AD234, AD392, AD533-1, and AD680-1 harbored *FBN1* deletions of exon 43, exon 56, exon 54, and exon 50, respectively, while patient AD437

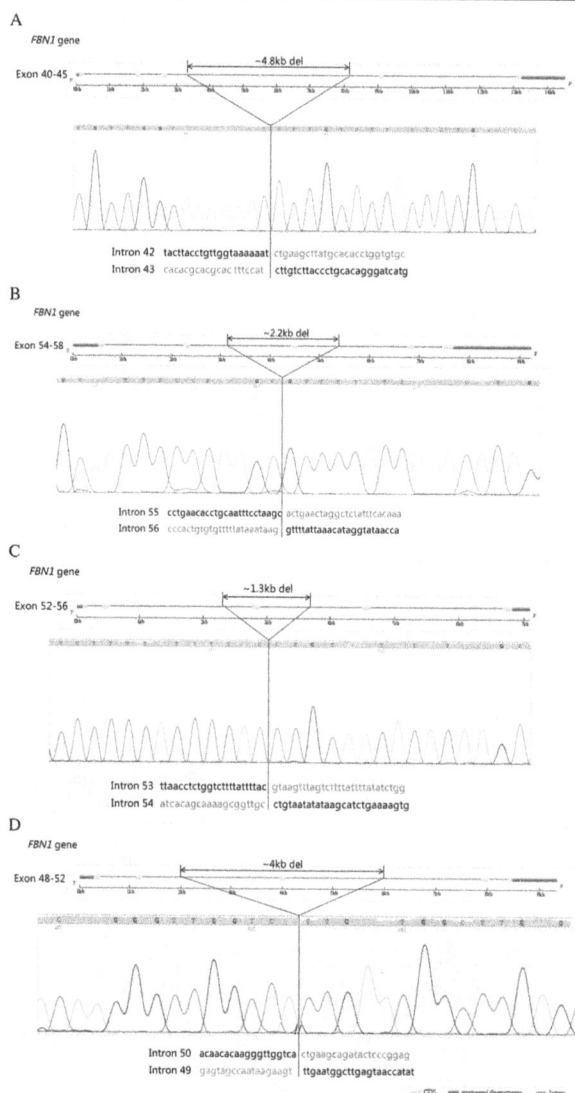

Fig. 2 Sequences of PCR products spanning the breakpoint junctions of the four single exon deletions. **a** ~ 4.8 kb deletion encompassing exon 43 in patient AD234. **b** ~ 2.2 kb deletion encompassing exon 56 in patient AD392. **c** ~ 1.3 kb deletion encompassing exon 54 in patient AD533-1. **d** ~ 4.0 kb deletion encompassing exon 50 in patient AD680-1

had a large deletion encompassing exons 44–66 in *FBN1*. These data had been submitted to ClinVar (ClinVar accessions SCV000804313-000804317).

To detect the breakpoints of deletions, we performed a long-range PCR followed by Sanger sequencing. Finally, the four single-exon deletions were all confirmed, and the breakpoints were found (Fig. 2). Regrettably, the deletion in AD437 could not be verified by the same method, since the mutated allele did not amplify well. Hence, we performed a quantitative PCR instead. Figure 3 shows that the quantity of genomic DNA from the proband amplified by primer pairs targeting exon 55 and exon 66 was half of that in the control samples, suggesting the true presence of a heterozygous deletion in this region.

All five *FBN1* large deletion carriers had multiple system deformities. Information on the clinical manifestation of the disease and family history is summarized in Table 3. Three patients (AD234, AD392, and AD437) were classic MFS, while the other two (AD533-1 and AD680-1) both had a systemic score of 6 but did not meet the criteria yet when genetic results were not available, probably due to their young ages. Combined with genetic results, these two patients were eventually diagnosed with MFS. Notably, patient AD437 had a gross deletion involving the last 23 exons, but there was no significant difference in the severity of clinical phenotypes when compared with the other four single-exon deletion carriers.

Table 3 The information of patients' clinical manifestation and family history

	Patients				
	AD234	AD392	AD533-1	AD680-1	AD437
Age (y)	24	38	5	14	37
Gender	Male	Female	Male	Male	Female
Height (cm)	178	167	120	180	177
Weight (kg)	70	58	23	52	71
Cardiovascular system					
Aortic diameter (cm)	5.6	3.5	3.3	3.2	4.7
Z-score	8.8	2.0	6.8	2.1	6.2
Aortic dissection	Y	N	N	N	Y
Skeletal system					
Pectus carinatum deformity	Y	NA	Y	N	Y
Wrist and thumb signs	Y	Y	Y	Y	Y
Scoliosis or thoracolumbar kyphosis	N	N	N	Y	N
Joint hypermobility	NA	Y	N	N	N
Reduced upper segment/lower segment ratio AND increased arm/height	N	N	NA	Y	N
Hindfoot deformity	NA	Y	N	N	NA
Ocular					
Ectopia lentis	N	Y	N	N	NA
Myopia/strabismus	Y	Y	Y	Y	N
Other features					
Skin striae	N	Y	N	N	Y
Family history	Y	NA	N	N	Y

Y presence of criterion, *N* absence of criterion, *NA* not available

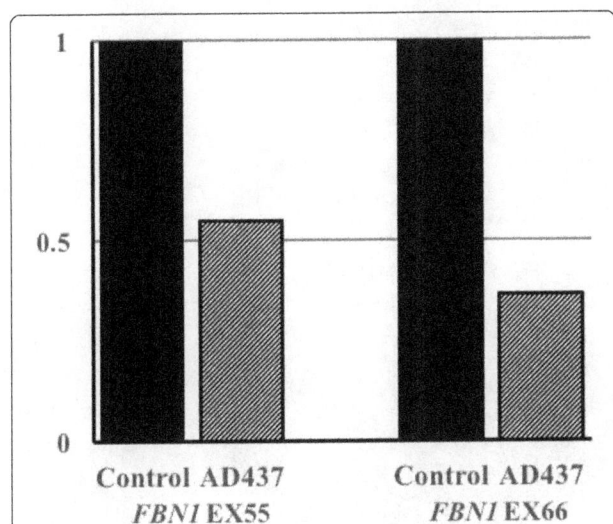

Fig. 3 Verification of gross deletions in AD437 by quantitative PCR. The bar graph shows the relative ratio of DNA from AD437, indicating the presence of a heterozygous deletion in the region

Discussion

Marfan syndrome has a highly variable manifestation, from a mild phenotype to early-onset and rapidly progressive MFS. Cardiovascular abnormality could be the only defect in some affected individuals. According to the 2010 revised Ghent criteria, in the absence of family history, the combination of aortic root dilation ($Z \geq 2$)/dissection and identification of a causal *FBN1* mutation was sufficient to establish a diagnosis of MFS [9]. Accordingly, we performed an MLPA assay to screen for *FBN1* and *TGFBR2* large genomic rearrangements not only in the diagnosed/suspected MFS patients but also in those early-onset aneurysm/dissection patients with minor skeletal and ocular involvement, who had a negative result in a 15-gene panel testing associated with heritable aortopathy.

Finally, five patients with large *FBN1* deletions were identified in our cohort. All five patients had multiple systemic deformities, and three of them met the 2010

Table 4 Overview of MFS cases with gross deletions in *FBN1* gene

Variation		Patient		Reference PMID (year)
Deletion (*FBN1* exon affected)	Affected domains	Age (y)	Phenotype in papers	
Single-exon deletion				
FBN1:g.46,701,985_46,728,871 (Ex1)	–	25	Classic MFS	17492313 (2002)
FBN1:Ex1	–	NA	Classic MFS	24501682 (2013)
FBN1:Ex1	–	NA	Classic MFS	24793577 (2014)
FBN1:Ex2	–	52	Classic MFS	11700157 (2001)
FBN1:Ex3	1st EGF-like	NA	MFS	21907952 (2011)
FBN1:Ex6	3rd EGF-like	49	Potential MFS	28842177 (2017)
FBN1:c.3603_3668 del (Ex29)	18th cbEGF-like	After birth	Neonatal MFS	10441700 (1999)
FBN1:Ex30	19–20th cbEGF-like	< 1	Suspected Beals-Hecht syndrome	25944730 (2015)
FBN1:Ex32	21–22th cbEGF-like	1	Neonatal MFS	18412115 (2008)
FBN1:Ex36	25–26th cbEGF-like	NA	Classic MFS	19839986 (2009)
FBN1:g.48,749,026_48,753,819 del (Ex43)	7th TB, 29th cbEGF-like	24	Classic MFS	In this study
FBN1:g.48,734,801-48,730,690 del (Ex50)	35th cbEGF-like	14	MFS	In this study
FBN1:Ex52	8th TB, 36th cbEGF-like	40	Classic MFS	11700157 (2001)
FBN1:g.48,727,672-48,726,338 del (Ex54)	37–38th cbEGF-like	5	MFS	In this study
FBN1:g.48,724,560_48,722,281 del (Ex56)	39–40th cbEGF-like	38	Classic MFS	In this study
Multi-exon deletion				
FBN1:Ex1–5	1–3rd EGF-like	27	Classic MFS	21936929 (2011)
FBN1:g.46,580,456_46,883,035 (Ex1-16)	1–3rd EGF-like, 1st TB, 4–10th cbEGF-like	40	Classic MFS	17492313 (2002)
FBN1:Ex1–36	1–3rd EGF-like, 4–26th cbEGF-like, 1–5th TB	15	Classic MFS	28842177 (2017)
FBN1:g.48,890,962_48,922,918 (Ex2-4)	1–2nd EGF-like	32	Classic MFS	29850152 (2018)
FBN1:Ex6–65	3rd EGF-like, 4–47th cbEGF-like, 1–9th TB	NA	Classic MFS	24793577 (2014)
FBN1:Ex13–49	7–34th cbEGF-like, 3–7th TB	5	MFS	18412115 (2008)
FBN1:Ex24–26	14–16th cbEGF-like	After birth	Neonatal MFS	20455198 (2010)
FBN1:Ex33–38	21–26th cbEGF-like, 6th TB	1	Neonatal MFS	24199744 (2014)
FBN1:Ex34–43	23–29th cbEGF-like, 6–7th TB	22	Classic MFS	19863550 (2010)
FBN1:Ex37–65	26–47th cbEGF-like, 3–9th TB	NA	Classic MFS	24793577 (2014)
FBN1:Ex42–43	7th TB, 29th cbEGF-like	> 46	Classic MFS	11710961 (2001)
FBN1:Ex44–46	29–31th cbEGF-like	> 6	Childhood onset MFS	11710961 (2001)
FBN1:Ex44–66	29–47th cbEGF-like, 8–9th TB	37	Classic MFS	In this study
FBN1:Ex48–53	33–37th cbEGF-like, 8th TB	15	Neonatal MFS	28842177 (2017)
FBN1:Ex49–50	34–35th cbEGF-like	3	Neonatal MFS	28842177 (2017)
FBN1:Ex50–63	35–46th cbEGF-like, 8–9th TB	65	MFS	19659760 (2009)
FBN1:Ex58–63	41–46th cbEGF-like	17	Juvenile onset classic MFS	17189636 (2007)
FBN1:c.7456_7821 del* (Ex61–64)	43–46th cbEGF-like	48	Classic MFS	1631074 (1994)
Whole gene deletion				
FBN1:Ex1–66	Full gene	16	Incomplete MFS	20478419 (2010)
FBN1:Ex1–66	Full gene	42	Classic MFS	21936929 (2011)
FBN1:Ex1–66	Full gene	15	Classic MFS	21936929 (2011)
FBN1:Ex1–66	Full gene	12	Classic MFS	21936929 (2011)
FBN1:Ex1–66	Full gene	41	MFS	21063442 (2011)
FBN1:Ex1–66	Full gene	39	MFS	21063442 (2011)
FBN1:Ex1–66	Full gene	16	MFS	21063442 (2011)
FBN1:Ex1–66	Full gene	13	MFS	21063442 (2011)
FBN1:Ex1–66	Full gene	27	MFS	21063442 (2011)
FBN1:Ex1–66	Full gene	21	MFS	21063442 (2011)
FBN1:Ex1–66	Full gene	34	MFS	21063442 (2011)

Table 4 Overview of MFS cases with gross deletions in *FBN1* gene (*Continued*)

Variation		Patient		Reference PMID (year)
Deletion (*FBN1* exon affected)	Affected domains	Age (y)	Phenotype in papers	
FBN1:Ex1–66	Full gene	5	Potential MFS	21063442 (2011)
FBN1:Ex1–66	Full gene	13	Potential MFS	21063442 (2011)
FBN1:Ex1–66	Full gene	8	Potential MFS	21063442 (2011)
FBN1:Ex1–66	Full gene	13	Classic MFS	22260333 (2012)
FBN1:g.48,931,968_51,102,375 (Ex1–66)	Full gene	14	MFS	27615407 (2016)

NA not available

*The deletion was represented as nt. 4762_5127 in partial cloned sequence of *FBN1* (PMID:1852207), and it was converted into its standardized nomenclature in accordance with HGVS (Human Genome Variation Society), in which the position + 1 corresponds to the A of the ATG start codon of the mRNA reference sequence (GenBank NM_000138) at the cDNA (c) level. Except for this, all of the other nucleotide positions and patient phenotypes were shown as it was reported in the reference article

Ghent criteria when genetic results were not available, while the other two met the diagnostic criteria until *FBN1* gross deletions were detected, probably due to their young ages. Meanwhile, no gross deletions/duplications were identified in patients with only aortic aneurysm/dissection but without other systemic involvement. This result supported the hypothesis that *FBN1* gross deletions usually lead to classic MFS [10–12].

Although gross genomic rearrangement within the *FBN1* gene only contributed to a small proportion of MFS genetic causes (1.8–2.9%) (UMD, http://www.umd.be/FBN1/; HGMD, http://www.hgmd.cf.ac.uk/ac/gene.php?gene=FBN1), it was important to identify the pathogenic mutation to afford the patient an opportunity for prenatal testing and preimplantation genetic diagnosis (PGD). *FBN1* mutations could be identified by sequencing in most Marfan patients (up to 93% in classic Marfan patients) [13]. However, Sanger sequencing and next-generation sequencing are commonly used in clinical genetic testing and are limited in their ability to detect large deletions and duplications. MLPA is a commonly used method to screen large del/dup, commercially, easily, and rapidly. In our cohort, 5 out of 62 patients (8.1%) with diagnosed or suspected MFS but with negative results in panel sequencing had large *FBN1* deletions, which proved it to be efficacious and cost-effective to screen for *FBN1* large genomic rearrangement in those MFS patients with multiple systemic involvements and a negative *FBN1* sequencing result.

Since MLPA and SNP (single-nucleotide polymorphism) arrays are more applicable in clinical genetic testing, increasing gross *FBN1* genomic deletions/duplications has been reported (summarized in Table 4), but until now, there has been no definite and conclusive genotype-phenotype correlation. Current studies reveal that the whole gene deletion of *FBN1* did not lead to a more severe phenotype [12], and in-frame deletion involving exon 24–53 seemed to result in a high risk of early-onset and rapidly progressive form of MFS [11, 14–16].

Conclusions

In summary, our data expand the number of large *FBN1* deletions and emphasize that screening for gross deletions in *FBN1* genes is necessary for clinically suspected MFS patients, especially in those who have a negative result in conventional sequencing methods.

Methods

Participants

Patients with MFS or early-onset aortopathy were referred for a genetic test from the Center of Vascular Surgery in Fuwai Hospital and Department of Cardiovascular Surgery in Xiangya Hospital Central South University. Of these, 115 patients in whom no causal mutation was identified in a 15-gene panel associated with heritable aortopathy, including *ACTA2*, *CLO3A1*, *FBN1*, *FBN2*, *MYH11*, *MYLK*, *NOTCH1*, *PRKG1*, *SKI*, *SLC2A10*, *SMAD3*, *SMAD4*, *TGFB2*, *TGFBR1*, and *TGFBR2*, were enrolled in this study to screen for *FBN1* and *TGFBR2* large del/dup.

Multiplex ligation-dependent probe amplification (MLPA)

MLPA assays were performed to detect *FBN1* and *TGFBR2* large deletions or duplications using the commercially available SALSA MLPA kits P065 and P066 (MRC-Holland, Amsterdam, The Netherlands), which contained probes for all exons of *FBN1* and *TGFBR2*. According to the manufacturer's instructions, a total of 100–200 ng of genomic DNA of each patient was used for hybridization, and amplification products from each MLPA assay were separated by capillary electrophoresis on an ABI 3500XL Dx Genetic Analyzer (Life Technologies, USA). The results were analyzed using Coffalyser software. Deletions and duplications with deviations more than 30% were suspected as significant alterations.

Sanger sequencing

To verify the results of MLPA and identify the breakpoints of the deletions, we performed a long-range PCR and subsequent Sanger sequencing. Primers flanking the predicted deletions were designed and LA Taq Hot Start Version kit (Takara, Japan) was used in the PCR system with the following cycling process: 5-min initial denaturation at 96 °C, 30 cycles of 10 s at 98 °C, and 15 min at 68 °C, finished by a 10-min final extension step at 72 °C. Then, the products were detected through agarose gel electrophoresis and sequenced by the inner primers on the ABI 3730XL Genetic Analyzer.

Quantitative PCR

Quantitative PCR (qPCR) with the SYBR green reporter dye was performed to quantify relative target gene regions copy number in genomic DNA, and housekeeping gene *GAPDH* (glyceraldehyde 3-phosphate dehydrogenase) was used as the reference gene. The primer pairs were designed by Primer3 Input (http://bioinfo.ut.ee/primer3-0.4.0/) (see Additional file 1). All qPCRs were performed using 2 × SYBR FAST qPCR Kit Master Mix (KAPA Biosystems, America) with the QuantStudio 6 Flex Real-Time PCR System.

Abbreviations

del: Deletion; dup: Duplication; *FBN1*: Fibrillin-1; *GAPDH*: Glyceraldehyde 3-phosphate dehydrogenase; HGMD: Human Gene Mutation Database; HGVS: Human Genome Variation Society; LDS: Loeys-Dietz syndrome; MFS: Marfan syndrome; MLPA: Multiplex ligation-dependent probe amplification; NA: Not available; qPCR: Quantitative PCR; SNP: Single-nucleotide polymorphism; UMD: Universal Mutation Database

Acknowledgements

We thanked all the subjects who participated in this study.

Funding

This work was supported by the grant of CAMS Initiative for Innovative Medicine (2016-I2M-1-016) and the grant from the Youth Foundation of Fuwai Hospital, National Center for Cardiovascular Disease, China (NO. 2016-F05).

Authors' contributions

HY coordinated the project and wrote the manuscript. YM and KZ performed MLPA and quantitative PCR. ML, XS, and FL recruited patients and collected clinical information. YZ and GZ were in charge of sample handling and quality control. LW and CS were in charge of the clinical evaluation and sample management. ZZ designed the project and revised the manuscript. All authors had read and approved the final manuscript.

Competing interests

The authors declare that they have no competing interests.

References

1. Judge DP, Dietz HC. Marfan's syndrome. Lancet (London). 2005;366(9501):1965–76.
2. Keane MG, Pyeritz RE. Medical management of Marfan syndrome. Circulation. 2008;117(21):2802–13.
3. Maddox BK, Sakai LY, Keene DR, Glanville RW. Connective tissue microfibrils. Isolation and characterization of three large pepsin-resistant domains of fibrillin. J Biol Chem. 1989;264(35):21381–5.
4. Groth KA, Von Kodolitsch Y, Kutsche K, Gaustadnes M, Thorsen K, Andersen NH, Gravholt CH. Evaluating the quality of Marfan genotype-phenotype correlations in existing FBN1 databases. Genet Med. 2017;19(7):772–7.
5. Dordoni C, Ciaccio C, Santoro G, Venturini M, Cavallari U, Ritelli M, Colombi M. Marfan syndrome: report of a complex phenotype due to a 15q21.1 contiguos gene deletion encompassing FBN1, and literature review. Am J Med Genet A. 2017;173(1):200–6.
6. Yang H, Luo M, Fu Y, Cao Y, Yin K, Li W, Meng C, Ma Y, Zhang J, Fan Y, et al. Genetic testing of 248 Chinese aortopathy patients using a panel assay. Sci Rep. 2016;6:33002.
7. Lerner-Ellis JP, Aldubayan SH, Hernandez AL, Kelly MA, Stuenkel AJ, Walsh J, Joshi VA. The spectrum of FBN1, TGFbetaR1, TGFbetaR2 and ACTA2 variants in 594 individuals with suspected Marfan syndrome, Loeys-Dietz syndrome or thoracic aortic aneurysms and dissections (TAAD). Mol Genet Metab. 2014;112(2):171–6.
8. Loeys BL, Chen J, Neptune ER, Judge DP, Podowski M, Holm T, Meyers J, Leitch CC, Katsanis N, Sharifi N, et al. A syndrome of altered cardiovascular, craniofacial, neurocognitive and skeletal development caused by mutations in TGFBR1 or TGFBR2. Nat Genet. 2005;37(3):275–81.
9. Loeys BL, Dietz HC, Braverman AC, Callewaert BL, De Backer J, Devereux RB, Hilhorst-Hofstee Y, Jondeau G, Faivre L, Milewicz DM, et al. The revised Ghent nosology for the Marfan syndrome. J Med Genet. 2010;47(7):476–85.
10. Furtado LV, Wooderchak-Donahue W, Rope AF, Yetman AT, Lewis T, Plant P, Bayrak-Toydemir P. Characterization of large genomic deletions in the FBN1 gene using multiplex ligation-dependent probe amplification. BMC Med Genet. 2011;12:119.
11. Li J, Wu W, Lu C, Liu Y, Wang R, Si N, Liu F, Zhou J, Zhang S, Zhang X. Gross deletions in FBN1 results in variable phenotypes of Marfan syndrome. Clin Chimica Acta. 2017;474:54–9.
12. Hilhorst-Hofstee Y, Hamel BC, Verheij JB, Rijlaarsdam ME, Mancini GM, Cobben JM, Giroth C, Ruivenkamp CA, Hansson KB, Timmermans J, et al. The clinical spectrum of complete FBN1 allele deletions. Eur J Human Genet. 2011;19(3):247–52.
13. Radonic T, de Witte P, Groenink M, de Bruin-Bon RA, Timmermans J, Scholte AJ, van den Berg MP, Baars MJ, van Tintelen JP, Kempers M, et al. Critical appraisal of the revised Ghent criteria for diagnosis of Marfan syndrome. Clin Genet. 2011;80(4):346–53.
14. Singh KK, Elligsen D, Liersch R, Schubert S, Pabst B, Arslan-Kirchner M, Schmidtke J. Multi-exon out of frame deletion of the FBN1 gene leading to a severe juvenile onset cardiovascular phenotype in Marfan syndrome. J Mol Cell Cardiol. 2007;42(2):352–6.
15. Liu W, Schrijver I, Brenn T, Furthmayr H, Francke U. Multi-exon deletions of the FBN1 gene in Marfan syndrome. BMC Med Genet. 2001;2:11.
16. Apitz C, Mackensen-Haen S, Girisch M, Kerst G, Wiegand G, Stuhrmann M, Niethammer K, Behrwind G, Hofbeck M. Neonatal Marfan syndrome: unusually large deletion of exons 24–26 of FBN1 associated with poor prognosis. Klinische Padiatrie. 2010;222(4):261–3.

Permissions

The contributors of this book come from diverse backgrounds, making this book a truly international effort. This book will bring forth new frontiers with its revolutionizing research information and detailed analysis of the nascent developments around the world.

We would like to thank all the contributing authors for lending their expertise to make the book truly unique. They have played a crucial role in the development of this book. Without their invaluable contributions this book wouldn't have been possible. They have made vital efforts to compile up to date information on the varied aspects of this subject to make this book a valuable addition to the collection of many professionals and students.

This book was conceptualized with the vision of imparting up-to-date information and advanced data in this field. To ensure the same, a matchless editorial board was set up. Every individual on the board went through rigorous rounds of assessment to prove their worth. After which they invested a large part of their time researching and compiling the most relevant data for our readers.

The editorial board has been involved in producing this book since its inception. They have spent rigorous hours researching and exploring the diverse topics which have resulted in the successful publishing of this book. They have passed on their knowledge of decades through this book. To expedite this challenging task, the publisher supported the team at every step. A small team of assistant editors was also appointed to further simplify the editing procedure and attain best results for the readers.

Apart from the editorial board, the designing team has also invested a significant amount of their time in understanding the subject and creating the most relevant covers. They scrutinized every image to scout for the most suitable representation of the subject and create an appropriate cover for the book.

The publishing team has been an ardent support to the editorial, designing and production team. Their endless efforts to recruit the best for this project, has resulted in the accomplishment of this book. They are a veteran in the field of academics and their pool of knowledge is as vast as their experience in printing. Their expertise and guidance has proved useful at every step. Their uncompromising quality standards have made this book an exceptional effort. Their encouragement from time to time has been an inspiration for everyone.

The publisher and the editorial board hope that this book will prove to be a valuable piece of knowledge for researchers, students, practitioners and scholars across the globe.

List of Contributors

Garima Kushwaha
Christopher S. Bond Life Sciences Center, University of Missouri, Columbia, MO 65211, USA
Informatics Institute, University of Missouri, Columbia, MO 65211, USA

Dong Xu
Christopher S. Bond Life Sciences Center, University of Missouri, Columbia, MO 65211, USA
Informatics Institute, University of Missouri, Columbia, MO 65211, USA
Department of Computer Science, University of Missouri, Columbia, MO 65211, USA

Mikhail Dozmorov
Department of Biostatistics, Virginia Commonwealth University, Richmond, VA 23225, USA

Jonathan D. Wren
Arthritis and Clinical Immunology Program, Oklahoma Medical Research Foundation, Oklahoma City, OK 73104, USA

Jing Qiu
Department of Applied Economics and Statistics, University of Delaware, Newark, DE 19716, USA

Huidong Shi
GRU Cancer Center, Georgia Regents University, Augusta, GA 30912, USA
Department of Biochemistry and Molecular Biology, Georgia Regents University, Augusta, GA 30912, USA

U. Plöckinger, A. Ziagaki and N. Tiling
Kompetenzzentrum Seltene Stoffwechselkrankheiten, Interdisziplinäres Stoffwechsel-Centrum: Endokrinologie, Diabetes und Stoffwechsel, Charité Universitätsmedizin Berlin, Augustenburger Platz 1, Campus Virchow-Klinikum, 13352 Berlin, Germany

V. Prasad
Department of Nuclear Medicine, Charité Universitätsmedizin Berlin, Berlin, Germany
Department of Nuclear Medicine Universitätsklinik Ulm, Ulm, Germany

A. Poellinger
Department of Diagnostic, Interventional and Pediatric Radiology, Inselspital Bern University Hospital, University of Bern, Bern, Switzerland

Itsuki Taniguchi, Chihiro Iwaya and Hiroki Shibata
Division of Genomics, Medical Institute of Bioregulation, Kyushu University, 3-1-1 Maidashi, Higashi-ku, Fukuoka 812-8582, Japan

Keizo Ohnaka
Department of Geriatric Medicine, Graduate School of Medical Sciences, Kyushu University, 3-1-1 Maidashi, Higashi-ku, Fukuoka 812-8582, Japan

Ken Yamamoto
Department of Medical Biochemistry, Kurume University School of Medicine, 67 Asahi-machi, Kurume, Fukuoka 830-0011, Japan

Jamie K. Teer, Yonghong Zhang, Eric A. Welsh, Steven A. Eschrich and Anders E. Berglund
Department of Biostatistics and Bioinformatics, H. Lee Moffitt Cancer Center and Research Institute, Tampa, FL 33612, USA

Lu Chen and W. Douglas Cress
Department of Molecular Oncology, H. Lee Moffitt Cancer Center and Research Institute, Tampa, FL 33612, USA

Alexander M. Vaiserman and Alexander K. Koliada
Laboratory of Epigenetics, Institute of Gerontology, Vyshgorodskaya st. 67, Kiev 04114, Ukraine

Elisa Napolitano Ferreira, Bruna Durães Figueiredo Barros, Renan Valieris Almeida, Giovana Tardin Torrezan, Sheila Garcia, Emmanuel Dias-Neto and Dirce Maria Carraro
1International Research Center/CIPE, A.C. Camargo Cancer Center, São Paulo, SP, Brazil

Jorge Estefano de Souza
Instituto Metrópole Digital, Federal University of Rio Grande do Norte, Natal, RN, Brazil

Ana Cristina Victorino Krepischi
Institute of Biosciences, University of São Paulo, São Paulo, SP, Brazil

Celso Abdon Lopes de Mello and Ademar Lopes
Departament of Abdominal Surgery, A.C. Camargo Cancer Center, São Paulo, SP, Brazil

Isabela Werneck da Cunha, Clóvis Antonio Lopes Pinto and Fernando Augusto Soares
Department of Anatomic Pathology, A.C. Camargo Cancer Center, São Paulo, SP, Brazil

Sandro José de Souza
Federal University of Rio Grande do Norte, Natal, RN, Brazil

N. Nazaripanah, F. Adelirad, A. Delbari, R. Sahaf and M. Ohadi
Iranian Research Center on Aging, University of Social Welfare and Rehabilitation Sciences, Tehran, Iran

T. Abbasi-Asl
Department of Biostatistics, University of Social Welfare and Rehabilitation Sciences, Tehran, Iran

Jyothi Thrivikraman
POLARIS, Genome Institute of Singapore, Agency for Science, Technology and Research, Singapore, Singapore

Yasmin Bylstra
POLARIS, Genome Institute of Singapore, Agency for Science, Technology and Research, Singapore, Singapore
SingHealth Duke-NUS Institute of Precision Medicine, Singapore, Singapore
Inherited Cardiac Clinic, National University Hospital, Singapore, Singapore

Patrick Tan
SingHealth Duke-NUS Institute of Precision Medicine, Singapore, Singapore
Cancer and Stem Biology, Duke-NUS Medical School, Singapore, Singapore
Biomedical Research Council, Agency for Science, Technology and Research, Singapore, Singapore

Tamra Lysaght and Sangeetha Watson
Centre for Biomedical Ethics, Yong Loo Lin School of Medicine, National University of Singapore, Singapore, Singapore

Magnus Ingelman-Sundberg, Souren Mkrtchian, Yitian Zhou and Volker M. Lauschke
Department of Physiology and Pharmacology, Section of Pharmacogenetics, Karolinska Institutet, SE-171 77 Stockholm, Sweden

Simranjeet Kaur
CPH-DIRECT, Department of Pediatrics, Herlev University Hospital, Herlev Ringvej 75, DK-2730 Herlev, Denmark

Aashiq H. Mirza and Flemming Pociot
CPH-DIRECT, Department of Pediatrics, Herlev University Hospital, Herlev Ringvej 75, DK-2730 Herlev, Denmark
Faculty of Health and Medical Sciences, University of Copenhagen, Copenhagen, Denmark

Center for non-coding RNA in Technology and Health, University of Copenhagen, Copenhagen, Denmark

Xiaoya Chen, Jinjun Li and Lili Lu
Medical College, Wuhan University of Science and Technology, Wuhan 430065, China

Youping Deng
Medical College, Wuhan University of Science and Technology, Wuhan 430065, China
Department of Internal Medicine and Rush University Cancer Center, Rush University Medical Center, Chicago, IL 60612, USA

Ling Hu
Department of Anesthesiology, Tianyou Hospital, Wuhan University of Science and Technology, Wuhan 430064, China

William Yang
Texas Advanced Computing Center, University of Texas at Austin, 10100 Burnet Road, Austin, TX 78758, USA

Hongyan Jin and Zexiong Wei
Puren Hospital, Wuhan University of Science and Technology, Wuhan 430081, China

Jack Y. Yang and Mary Qu Yang
MidSouth Bioinformatics Center, Department of Information Science, George Washington Donaghey College of Engineering and Information Technology and Joint Bioinformatics Graduate Program, University of Arkansas at Little Rock and University of Arkansas for Medical Sciences, 2801 S. University Avenue, Little Rock, AR 72204, USA

Jun S. Liu
Department of Statistics and Harvard School of Public Health, Harvard University, One Oxford St., Cambridge 02138 Massachusetts, USA

Hamid R. Arabnia
Department of Computer Science, University of Georgia, Athens, GA 30602, USA

Taobo Hu, Yogesh Kumar, Iram Shazia, Wai-Kin Mat, Zhenggang Wu, Xi Long, Cheuk-Hin Chan, Si Chen, Peggy Lee, Siu-Kin Ng, Timothy Y. C. Ho, Jianfeng Yang, Xiaofan Ding, Shui-Ying Tsang and Xuqing Zhou
Division of Life Science, Applied Genomics Centre and Centre for Statistical Science, Hong Kong University of Science and Technology, Clear Water Bay, Kowloon, Hong Kong, China

Hong Xue
Division of Life Science, Applied Genomics Centre and Centre for Statistical Science, Hong Kong University of Science and Technology, Clear Water Bay, Kowloon, Hong Kong, China
School of Basic Medicine and Clinical Pharmacy, China Pharmaceutical University, Nanjing, China

Shen-Jia Duan, Dan-Hua Zhang and En-Xiang Zhou
Department of General Surgery, The Second Xiangya Hospital, Central South University, Changsha, Hunan, China

Yi Li and Wai-Sang Poon
Department of Surgery, The Chinese University of Hong Kong, Shatin, Hong Kong, China

Lei Chen and Hong-Yang Wang
Eastern Hepatobiliary Surgery Institute, Second Military Medical University, Shanghai, China

Jin-Fei Chen
Department of Oncology, Nanjing First Hospital, Nanjing Medical University, Nanjing, China

Rong Yin and Lin Xu
Jiangsu Key Laboratory of Cancer Molecular Biology and Translational Medicine, Jiangsu Cancer Hospital, Nanjing, China

Ava Kwong and Gilberto Ka-Kit Leung
Division of Neurosurgery, Department of Surgery, Li Ka Shing Faculty of Medicine, Queen Mary Hospital, The University of Hong Kong, 102 Pokfulam Road, Pokfulam, Hong Kong, China

Carmela Rinaldi and Rosalia D'Angelo
Department of Biomedical and Dental Sciences and Morphofunctional Imaging, Division of Molecular Genetics and Preventive Medicine, University of Messina, via C. Valeria 1, I-98125 Messina, Italy

Concetta Scimone, Luigi Donato and Antonina Sidoti
Department of Biomedical and Dental Sciences and Morphofunctional Imaging, Division of Molecular Genetics and Preventive Medicine, University of Messina, via C. Valeria 1, I-98125 Messina, Italy
Department of Cutting-Edge Medicine and Therapies, Biomolecular Strategies and Neuroscience, Section of Neuroscience-applied Molecular Genetics and Predictive Medicine, I. E. ME. S. T, via Michele Miraglia 20, I-90139 Palermo, Italy

Teresa Esposito
Department of Experimental Medicine, Division of Human Physiology and Integrate Biological Functions "F. Bottazzi", University of Campania Luigi Vanvitelli, ex II University of Naples, via Santa Maria di Costantinipoli 16, I-80138 Naples, Italy

Elina A. M. Hirvonen, Esa Pitkänen and Outi Kilpivaara
Genome-Scale Biology Research Program, Research Programs Unit and Department of Medical and Clinical Genetics, Medicum, University of Helsinki, Helsinki, Finland

Lauri A. Aaltonen
Genome-Scale Biology Research Program, Research Programs Unit and Department of Medical and Clinical Genetics, Medicum, University of Helsinki, Helsinki, Finland
Department of Biosciences and Nutrition, Karolinska Institutet, SE-17177 Stockholm, Sweden

Kari Hemminki
Division of Molecular Genetic Epidemiology, German Cancer Research Center (DKFZ), Heidelberg, Germany

I-Chun Tsai
Center for Human Disease Modeling, Duke University, 300 North Duke Street, Durham, NC 27701, USA

Georgios Kellaris
Center for Human Disease Modeling, Duke University, 300 North Duke Street, Durham, NC 27701, USA
Department of Medical Genetics, University of Athens Medical School, Aghia Sophia Children's Hospital, 11527 Athens, Greece

Kamal Khan
Center for Human Disease Modeling, Duke University, 300 North Duke Street, Durham, NC 27701, USA
Human Molecular Genetics Laboratory, Health Biotechnology Division, National Institute for Biotechnology and Genetic Engineering (NIBGE), Faisalabad 38000, Pakistan

Nicholas Katsanis
Center for Human Disease Modeling, Duke University, 300 North Duke Street, Durham, NC 27701, USA
Imaging Institute, Cleveland Clinic, 9500 Euclid Avenue, Cleveland, OH 44195, USA

Shahid M. Baig
Human Molecular Genetics Laboratory, Health Biotechnology Division, National Institute for Biotechnology and Genetic Engineering (NIBGE), Faisalabad 38000, Pakistan

Paul Ruggieri
Imaging Institute, Cleveland Clinic, 9500 Euclid Avenue, Cleveland, OH 44195, USA

Marvin R. Natowicz
Pathology and Laboratory Medicine and Genomic Medicine Institutes, Cleveland Clinic, Cleveland, OH 44195, USA

Francisca Millan Zamora
GeneDx, 207 Perry Parkway, Gaithersburg, MD 20877, USA

Khalid Mahmood, Chol-hee Jung, Gayle Philip, Peter Georgeson, Jessica Chung, Bernard J. Pope and Daniel J. Park
Melbourne Bioinformatics, The University of Melbourne, Melbourne, Australia

Bianmei Han, Xuewen Liu and Kun Zhao
State Key Laboratory of Cardiovascular Disease, Fuwai Hospital, National Center for Cardiovascular Diseases, Peking Union Medical College, Chinese Academy of Medical Sciences, Beijing, China

Wen Chen, Yi Ma and Zhou Zhou
State Key Laboratory of Cardiovascular Disease, Fuwai Hospital, National Center for Cardiovascular Diseases, Peking Union Medical College, Chinese Academy of Medical Sciences, Beijing, China
State Key Laboratory of Cardiovascular Disease, Beijing Key Laboratory for Molecular Diagnostics of Cardiovascular Diseases, Diagnostic Laboratory Service, Fuwai Hospital, National Center for Cardiovascular Diseases, Peking Union Medical College, Chinese Academy of Medical Sciences, Beijing, China

Wenke Li, Yujing Zhang and Yuanyuan Fu
State Key Laboratory of Cardiovascular Disease, Beijing Key Laboratory for Molecular Diagnostics of Cardiovascular Diseases, Diagnostic Laboratory Service, Fuwai Hospital, National Center for Cardiovascular Diseases, Peking Union Medical College, Chinese Academy of Medical Sciences, Beijing, China

Meixian Zhang and Jie Mi
Department of Epidemiology, Capital Institute of Paediatrics, Beijing, China

Jonas Langerud, Sarah Louise Ariansen and Nina Iversen
Department of Medical Genetics, Oslo University Hospital, Oslo, Norway

Elisabeth Jarhelle and Marijke Van Ghelue
Department of Medical Genetics, Division of Child and Adolescent Health, University Hospital of North Norway, Tromsø, Norway

Sanghoon Moon and Juyoung Lee
Division of Genome Research, Center for Genome Science, Korea National Institute of Health, Cheongju, Chungcheongbuk-do 28159, South Korea

Young Lee
Division of Genome Research, Center for Genome Science, Korea National Institute of Health, Cheongju, Chungcheongbuk-do 28159, South Korea
Veterans Medical Research Institute, Veterans Health Service Medical Center, Seoul 05368, South Korea

Sungho Won
Department of Public Health Science, Seoul National University, Seoul 08826, South Korea

Masoud Arabfard
Department of Bioinformatics, Kish International Campus University of Tehran, Kish, Iran
Laboratory of Complex Biological Systems and Bioinformatics (CBB), Department of Bioinformatics, Institute of Biochemistry and Biophysics (IBB), University of Tehran, Tehran, Iran

Kaveh Kavousi
Laboratory of Complex Biological Systems and Bioinformatics (CBB), Department of Bioinformatics, Institute of Biochemistry and Biophysics (IBB), University of Tehran, Tehran, Iran

Ahmad Delbari and Mina Ohadi
Iranian Research Center on Aging, University of Social Welfare and Rehabilitation Sciences, Tehran, Iran

Lejla Mahmutovic, Camil Durakovic, Aida Maric, Muhamed Adilovic, Nour Hamad and Sabina Semiz
Faculty of Engineering and Natural Sciences, International University of Sarajevo, Hrasnicka cesta 15, 71210 Ilidza, Sarajevo, Bosnia and Herzegovina

Betul Akcesme
Faculty of Engineering and Natural Sciences, International University of Sarajevo, Hrasnicka cesta 15, 71210 Ilidza, Sarajevo, Bosnia and Herzegovina
Department of Medical Biology, Faculty of Medicine, University of Health Sciences, Istanbul, Turkey

Faruk Berat Akcesme
Faculty of Engineering and Natural Sciences, International University of Sarajevo, Hrasnicka cesta 15, 71210 Ilidza, Sarajevo, Bosnia and Herzegovina
Department of Biostatistics and Medical Informatics, Faculty of Medicine, University of Health Sciences, Istanbul, Turkey

Matthias Wjst
Helmholtz Zentrum Muenchen, German Research Center for Environmental Health (GmbH), Ingolstaedter Landstraße 1, D-85764 Munich, Neuherberg, Germany

Oliver Feeney
Centre of Bioethical Research and Analysis, National University of Ireland (Galway), Galway, Republic of Ireland

Hang Yang, Yanyun Ma, Kun Zhao, Yinhui Zhang, Guoyan Zhu and Zhou Zhou
State Key Laboratory of Cardiovascular Disease, Beijing Key Laboratory for Molecular Diagnostics of Cardiovascular Diseases, Diagnostic Laboratory Service, Fuwai Hospital, National Center for Cardiovascular Diseases, Chinese Academy of Medical Sciences and Peking Union Medical College, Beijing 100037, China

Mingyao Luo, Xiaogang Sun and Chang Shu
State Key Laboratory of Cardiovascular Disease, Center of Vascular Surgery, Fuwai Hospital, National Center for Cardiovascular Diseases, Chinese Academy of Medical Sciences and Peking Union Medical College, Beijing 100037, China

Fanyan Luo and Lin Wang
Department of Cardiovascular Surgery, Xiangya Hospital Central South University, Changsha 410008, Hunan, China

Index

www.ingramcontent.com/pod-product-compliance
Lightning Source LLC
Chambersburg PA
CBHW080509200326
41458CB00012B/4144